William S. Green

Textbook of oral surgery

Textbook of
ORAL SURGERY

Edited by

Gustav O. Kruger

B.S., A.M., D.D.S., F.A.C.D., F.I.C.D.

Professor of Oral Surgery and Associate Dean for Graduate Studies, Georgetown University School of Dentistry, Washington, D. C.; Chief of Dental Staff, Georgetown University Hospital, Washington, D. C.; Consultant and Member of Executive Committee, District of Columbia General Hospital, Washington, D. C.; Consultant to Veterans Administration Hospitals in Martinsburg, W. Va., and Washington, D. C., United States Naval Dental School, Bethesda, Md., and Walter Reed Army Hospital, Washington, D. C.; Member, U. S. Public Health Service Clinical Cancer Training Committee (Dental), National Cancer Institute; Member, Review Commission on Advanced Education in Oral Surgery, Council on Dental Education; Past President, Middle Atlantic Society of Oral Surgeons; Diplomate and Past President, American Board of Oral Surgery

Third edition

With 434 illustrations and 3 color plates

Including drawings by Biagio J. Melloni

The C. V. Mosby Company

Saint Louis 1968

Third edition

Copyright © 1968 by The C. V. Mosby Company

Third printing

All rights reserved. No part of this book may be reproduced in any manner without written permission of the publisher.

Previous editions copyrighted 1959, 1964

Printed in the United States of America

Standard Book Number 8016-2790-7

Library of Congress Catalog Card Number 68-23779

Distributed in Great Britain by Henry Kimpton, London

CONTRIBUTORS

S. Elmer Bear, D.D.S., F.A.C.D.

Professor and Chairman, Department of Oral Surgery, Medical College of Virginia School of Dentistry; Chairman, Division of Oral Surgery, Medical College of Virginia Hospitals, Richmond, Va.; Consultant, United States Naval Hospital, Portsmouth, Va., National Institutes of Health, Clinical Center, Bethesda, Md., and McGuire Veterans Hospital, Richmond, Va.; Diplomate, American Board of Oral Surgery

Philip J. Boyne, D.M.D., M.S., F.A.C.D.

Captain, United States Navy Dental Corps; Director, Dental Research Department, Naval Medical Research Institute, National Naval Medical Center, Bethesda, Md.; Consultant-Instructor in Oral Surgery, United States Naval Dental School, Bethesda, Md.; Member, Committee on Research, American Society of Oral Surgeons; Diplomate, American Board of Oral Surgery

Jack B. Caldwell, D.D.S., M.Sc., F.A.C.D., F.I.C.D.

Colonel, United States Army Dental Corps, Retired; Chief, Oral Surgery, Denver General Hospital, Denver, Colo.; Consultant in Oral Surgery, Fitzsimons General Hospital, and Veterans Administration Hospital, Denver, Colo.; formerly Chief of Dental Service, Second General Hospital, and Oral Surgery Consultant to the Chief Surgeon, United States Army, Europe; formerly Visiting Professor, College of Physicians and Surgeons, School of Dentistry, San Francisco, Calif.; formerly Staff Member, Army Medical Service Graduate School, Walter Reed Army Medical Center, Washington, D. C.; formerly Chief of Oral Surgery, Walter Reed General Hospital, Washington, D. C., Fitzsimons General Hospital, Denver, Colo., and Letterman General Hospital, San Francisco, Calif.; Diplomate, and Member, Board of Directors, American Board of Oral Surgery; now at Denver, Colo.

James R. Cameron, D.D.S., Sc.D., LL.D., F.A.C.D., F.I.C.D.

Emeritus Professor of Oral Surgery, Temple University School of Dentistry, Philadelphia, Pa.; Emeritus Professor of Oral Surgery and former Chairman of the Course in Oral Surgery, Graduate School of Medicine, University of Pennsylvania, Philadelphia, Pa.; Founder and Chief of Oral Surgery Service, Pennsylvania Hospital, Philadelphia, Pa., from 1916 to 1950; Consultant in Oral Surgery, Pennsylvania Hospital and United States Naval Hospital, Philadelphia, Pa., and Valley Forge Army Hospital, Phoenixville, Pa.; Past President, American Board of Oral Surgery and American Society of Oral Surgeons; Diplomate, American Board of Oral Surgery

Donald E. Cooksey, D.D.S., M.S., F.A.C.D.

Captain, United States Navy Dental Corps (Retired), Beverly Hills, Calif.; formerly Commanding Officer, United States Naval Dental Clinic, Yokosuka, Japan; Chief of Clinical Services, Head of Oral Surgery Division, and Consultant-Instructor in Oral Surgery, United States Naval Dental School, National Naval Medical Center, Bethesda, Md.; Guest Lecturer, University of Pennsylvania, Philadelphia, Pa., and Georgetown University, Washington, D. C.; Diplomate and Past President, American Board of Oral Surgery

Leslie M. Fitzgerald, D.D.S., D.Sc., F.A.C.D., F.I.C.D.

Formerly Chief of Oral Surgery Staff, St. Joseph's, Finley, and Xavier Hospitals, Dubuque, Iowa; formerly Consultant in Oral Surgery to the Surgeon General of the United States Navy and to the Central Office of the Veterans Administration; formerly Chairman, Council on Dental Education, American Dental Association; Past President, American Society of Oral Surgeons and American Dental

v

Association; Diplomate and Executive Secretary, American Board of Oral Surgery

Athol L. Frew, Jr., B.A., D.D.S., M.D.

Associate Professor of Oral Surgery, University of Oklahoma Medical School, Oklahoma City, Okla.; Director, Section of Oral Surgery, Saint Anthony Hospital, Oklahoma City, Okla.; Diplomate and Past President, American Board of Oral Surgery

J. Orton Goodsell, D.D.S., D.D.Sc., F.A.C.D.

Director, Cleft Lip and Cleft Palate Rehabilitation Center, Saginaw General Hospital, Saginaw, Mich.; formerly Lecturer in Oral Surgery, University of Michigan School of Dentistry, Ann Arbor, Mich.; Diplomate and Past President, American Board of Oral Surgery

Merle L. Hale, B.A., D.D.S., M.S., F.A.C.D.

Professor of Oral Surgery, University of Iowa, College of Dentistry; Chief, Oral Surgery and Dental Department, Iowa University Hospitals, Iowa City, Iowa; Clinical Professor, Oral Surgery, College of Medicine; Consultant in Oral Surgery, Veterans Administration Hospital, Iowa City, Iowa; Editor, Oral Surgery Section of Year Book of Dentistry; Diplomate, American Board of Oral Surgery

James R. Hayward, D.D.S., M.S., F.A.C.D.

Professor of Oral Surgery, University of Michigan School of Dentistry and Medical School, Ann Arbor, Mich.; Director, Service of Dentistry and Oral Surgery, University of Michigan Hospital, Ann Arbor, Mich.; Diplomate and Past President, American Board of Oral Surgery

Fred A. Henny, D.D.S., F.D.S.R.C.S.(Eng.), F.A.C.D.

Chief of Division of Dentistry and Oral Surgery, Henry Ford Hospital, Detroit, Mich.; President, International Association of Oral Surgeons; Member, U. S. Public Health Service National Advisory Dental Research Council; Past Editor, Journal of Oral Surgery; Past President, American Society of Oral Surgeons; Consultant in Oral Surgery, Veterans Administration Hospital, Dearborn, Mich.; Diplomate, American Board of Oral Surgery

Edward C. Hinds, B.A., D.D.S., M.D., F.A.C.S., F.A.C.D.

Professor of Surgery, The University of Texas Dental Branch, Houston, Texas; Chief, Dental Service, Ben Taub General Hospital, The Methodist Hospital, and M. D. Anderson Hospital and Tumor Institute, Houston, Texas; National Consultant to the Surgeon General, United States Air Force; Consultant, Veterans Administration Hospital, Houston, Texas, William Beaumont Army Hospital, El Paso, Texas, and Wilford Hall Air Force Hospital, San Antonio, Texas; Consultant in Oral Surgery to the Central Office, Veterans Administration; Diplomate, American Board of Oral Surgery; Diplomate, American Board of Surgery

Don M. Ishmael, A.B., D.D.S.

Consultant in Dental Pathology, Bone and Joint Hospital, Oklahoma City, Okla.; Chief of Dental Staff, Saint Anthony Hospital, Oklahoma City, Okla.

Donald R. King, D.D.S., M.S.

Assistant Professor of Oral Surgery, Georgetown University School of Dentistry, Washington, D. C.; Consultant, District of Columbia General Hospital, Washington, D. C.

Gustav O. Kruger, B.S., A.M., D.D.S., F.A.C.D., F.I.C.D.

Professor of Oral Surgery and Associate Dean for Graduate Studies, Georgetown University School of Dentistry, Washington, D. C.; Chief of Dental Staff, Georgetown University Hospital, Washington, D. C.; Consultant and Member of Executive Committee, District of Columbia General Hospital, Washington, D. C.; Consultant to Veterans Administration Hospitals in Martinsburg, W. Va., and Washington, D. C., United States Naval Dental School, Bethesda, Md., and Walter Reed Army Hospital, Washington, D. C.; Member, U. S. Public Health Service Clinical Cancer Training Committee (Dental), National Cancer Institute; Member, Review Commission on Advanced Education in Oral Surgery, Council on Dental Education; Past President, Middle Atlantic Society of Oral Surgeons; Diplomate and Past President, American Board of Oral Surgery

Claude S. LaDow, D.D.S., M.Sc.(Dent.)

Chairman and Associate Professor, Department of Oral Surgery, University of Pennsylvania School of Dentistry, Philadelphia, Pa.; Associate Professor of Oral Surgery, Graduate School of Medicine, University of Pennsylvania, Philadelphia, Pa.; Chief of

Oral Surgery, Presbyterian General Hospital, Visiting Chief of Oral Surgery, Philadelphia General Hospital, and Associate in Oral Surgery, Episcopal Hospital, Philadelphia, Pa.; Consultant, Valley Forge Army Hospital, Phoenixville, Pa., and Fort Dix, N. J.; Chief of Oral Surgery and Dentistry, Lankenau Hospital, Philadelphia, Pa.; Diplomate and Past President, American Board of Oral Surgery

Theodore A. Lesney, D.D.S., F.A.C.D.

Captain, Dental Corps, United States Navy; Staff Dental Officer, 12th Naval District Headquarters and Western Sea Frontier; formerly Chief of the Dental Service, Head of Oral Surgery, and Consultant-Instructor to Dental Intern and Residency Training Programs at the following naval hospitals: Portsmouth, Va., San Diego, Calif., and the Naval Dental School, National Naval Medical Center, Bethesda, Md.; Diplomate, American Board of Oral Surgery

Sanford M. Moose, D.D.S., F.A.C.D.

Clinical Professor of Oral Surgery, School of Dentistry, University of the Pacific, San Francisco, Calif.; Special Civilian Consultant in Maxillofacial Surgery to the Surgeon General, United States Army; Consultant to the Central Office, Veterans Administration; Consultant in Oral Surgery and Faculty Member, Graduate Training Programs, Letterman General Hospital, San Francisco, Calif.; Consultant in Oral Surgery, Veterans Hospital, Palo Alto, Calif., Veterans Hospital, Livermore, Calif., and United States Public Health Service Hospital, San Francisco, Calif.; Associate Chief, Dental Staff (Oral Surgery), Mt. Zion Hospital, San Francisco, Calif.; Diplomate, American Board of Oral Surgery

George E. Morin, D.D.S.

Late Associate Professor of Oral Surgery, Georgetown University School of Dentistry, Washington, D. C.; Assistant Chief, Dental Staff, Georgetown University Hospital, Washington, D. C.; Consultant, District of Columbia General Hospital, Washington, D. C.; Consultant, Clinical Center, National Institutes of Health, Bethesda, Md.; Diplomate, American Board of Oral Surgery

James A. O'Brien, B.S., D.D.S., F.A.C.D.

Diplomate, and Member, Advisory Committee, American Board of Oral Surgery

Leroy W. Peterson, D.D.S., F.A.C.D.

Professor of Oral Surgery, Washington University School of Dentistry, St. Louis, Mo.; Consultant in Oral Surgery, Veterans Administration Hospital, St. Louis, Mo.; Consultant to the Council on Dental Education, American Dental Association; Editorial Board, Journal of Oral Surgery; Founder and Fellow, International Association of Oral Surgeons; Past President, American Society of Oral Surgeons; Diplomate, American Board of Oral Surgery

Donald C. Reynolds, D.D.S., M.S.

Associate Professor of Oral Surgery, Georgetown University School of Dentistry, Washington, D. C.; Consultant, District of Columbia General Hospital, Washington, D. C., and Veterans Administration Hospitals, Martinsburg, W. Va., and Washington, D. C.; Diplomate, American Board of Oral Surgery

R. Quentin Royer, D.D.S., M.S.(Dent. Surg.), F.A.C.D.

Formerly Consultant, Section of Dentistry and Oral Surgery, Mayo Clinic, Rochester, Minn.; formerly Assistant Professor in Dentistry, Mayo Foundation, Graduate School, University of Minnesota, Rochester, Minn.; Diplomate, American Board of Oral Surgery

Robert B. Shira, D.D.S., F.A.C.D.

Major General, United States Army; Assistant Surgeon General and Chief, Army Dental Corps; Visiting Professor of Oral Surgery, College of Physicians and Surgeons, School of Dentistry, University of the Pacific, San Francisco, Calif.; Lecturer in Oral Surgery, University of Pennsylvania School of Dentistry, Philadelphia, Pa.; Past President, American Society of Oral Surgeons; Chairman, Council on Dental Therapeutics, American Dental Association; Diplomate, American Board of Oral Surgery; Associate Editor, Journal of Oral Surgery, Anesthesia and Hospital Dental Service; Assistant Editor, Oral Surgery, Oral Medicine, and Oral Pathology

Phillip Earle Williams, B.S., D.D.S., M.S., F.A.C.D.

Faculty Member, Baylor Dental College and Southwestern Medical School of the University of Texas, Dallas, Texas; formerly First Vice President, American Dental Association; Director, American Society of Oral Surgeons; Regent, American College of Dentists; Diplomate and Past President, American Board of Oral Surgery

Dedicated to

Simon P. Hullihen

1810-1857

The first oral surgeon in the United States

PREFACE TO THIRD EDITION

For the third edition a new chapter on tissue transplantation has been prepared by a man who is familiar with this fascinating field in which so much experimentation is taking place.

This edition has been reset entirely and several new illustrations, including three in color, have been added. Anatomical terminology has been changed to conform with *Nomina Anatomica 1955* as adopted by the sixth International Anatomical Congress. The metric system is used throughout the book. The text has been reviewed carefully, and some of the chapters have been changed considerably to reflect recent changes in technique and philosophy. The collaborators and Mr. Melloni again have cooperated willingly and effectively in this task.

It is the hope of all the collaborators that this book may continue to serve a useful purpose in depicting the essentials of oral surgery in a graphic manner.

Gustav O. Kruger

PREFACE TO FIRST EDITION

This text was written with two purposes in mind: (1) to give a concise description of procedures and current thinking in each area and (2) to present the subject of oral surgery in the sequence in which it is given to the senior dental students in the lecture courses.

Pronounced changes have taken place in the approach to oral surgical problems with the advent of antibiotics, improved techniques, and a backlog of recorded experience that dates back to Hullihen. Basic principles of surgery, of course, have changed little. These basic principles are presented in the light of the newer ideas.

The lecture sequence in oral surgery was originally suggested by the American Association of Dental Schools in 1935 and modified by a Committee on the Teaching of Oral Surgery of the same organization in 1952. A deviation from this outline has been made in the presentation of the material in this book in that the sections on exodontia have not been included. In most schools exodontia is taught as a separate course in the third year, and there are several textbooks on this subject.

This book is designed to fit the needs of the undergraduate senior student, but general practitioners, interns, residents, and oral surgeons will also find it useful. Emphasis has been placed on the basic fundamentals of judgment and technique. Even if the senior student does not perform all the surgery described, he should have a clear idea of what is done and how it is done. He should understand what can be accomplished by surgical procedures in the mouth.

The contributors have been selected because of their competence in the field. Each has devoted his efforts to one chapter. It is to them that any credit for this work is due. Without exception, they have been most generous with their time and efforts.

I should like to thank Mr. Biagio J. Melloni, Director of the Department of Medical and Dental Illustration, Georgetown University Medical Center, for his superb art work and generous assistance.

Gustav O. Kruger
Washington, D. C.

CONTENTS

Chapter 1 PRINCIPLES OF SURGERY (James R. Cameron), 1

    Case history, 1
    Laboratory work, 2
    Asepsis, 4
    Atraumatic surgery, 4
    Infection, 5
    Suture material, 5
    Ligatures, 10
    Needles, 10
    Dressings, 10
    Blood loss, 13
    Operating room, 13
    Linen, 13

Chapter 2 PRINCIPLES OF SURGICAL TECHNIQUE (Theodore A. Lesney), 14

    Introduction, 14
        Infection, 15
        Patent airway, 15
        Hemorrhage control, 16
    Sterilization of armamentarium, 18
        Principles of sterilization, 18
        Sterilization of supplies on industry-wide level, 20
        General observations, 21
        Comment, 22
    Preoperative preparation for oral surgery problems, 22
        Preoperative routine for patients requiring oral surgery, 23
        Comment, 23
    Operating room decorum, 24
        Scrub technique, 24
        Isolation of patient from operating team, 27
        Modifications of aseptic routine for office practice of oral surgery, 27
        Disposable (single use) materials and equipment, 28
        Some fundamental precautions with gaseous mixtures in operating rooms, 30
        Oxygen cylinders, 30
    Basic oral surgery, 31
        Incision, 31
        Suture materials, 34
        Wire mesh, 34
        Dressings, 34
    Operative technique, 35
        General, 35

Contents

           Submandibular approach to the ascending ramus and body of the mandible, 35
           Soft tissue closure, 38
           Surgical approach to the temporomandibular joint, 39
      Postoperative care, 42
           Water, electrolyte, and nutritional balance, 43
      Armamentarium, 45

Chapter 3   INTRODUCTION TO EXODONTIA (Gustav O. Kruger), 46

      General principles, 46
           Psychology, 46
           Anesthesia, 49
           Examination of the patient, 49
      Indications and contraindications for extraction, 50
           Indications, 50
           Contraindications, 50
      The office; equipment; armamentarium, 52
      Armamentarium, 52
           Sterilization and care of instruments, 56

Chapter 4   FORCEPS EXTRACTION (Gustav O. Kruger), 58

      Anesthesia, 58
      Position of patient, 58
      Preparation and draping, 58
      Position of left hand, 59
      Forceps extraction, 59
      Postextraction procedure, 59
      Number of teeth to be extracted, 70
      Order of extraction, 70

Chapter 5   COMPLICATED EXODONTIA (Gustav O. Kruger), 72

      Alveoloplasty, 72
      Surgical flap, 76
      Root removal, 78
      Elevator principles, 82

Chapter 6   IMPACTED TEETH (Gustav O. Kruger), 85

      Preliminary considerations, 85
      Mandibular mesioangular impaction, 89
      Mandibular horizontal impaction, 91
      Mandibular vertical impaction, 92
      Mandibular distoangular impaction, 93
      Maxillary mesioangular impaction, 95
      Maxillary vertical impaction, 95
      Maxillary distoangular impaction, 96
      Maxillary canine impaction, 97
      Supernumerary tooth impaction, 99

Chapter 7   ABNORMALITIES OF THE MOUTH (J. Orton Goodsell and Donald R. King), 101

      Sharp ridges, 101
      Tori, 103
      Enlarged tuberosities, 107

Soft tissue deformities, 108
    Tissue supports, 109
        Folds and redundancies in sulci, 110
        Scar bands, frenums, and high muscle attachments, 111
    Deepening of buccolabial sulcus: ridge extensions, 111
        Secondary epithelization technique using a labial flap (Kazanjian's technique), 115
        Secondary epithelization technique using an alveolar flap, 116
        Procedures employing an immediate epithelial covering, 117
        Submucous vestibuloplasty, 117
    Deepening of lingual sulcus, 118
        Supraperiosteal method, 118
        Subperiosteal method, 119
    Other procedures, 119

Chapter 8 SPECIAL CONSIDERATIONS IN EXODONTIA (Donald C. Reynolds), 120

    Removal of teeth for children, 120
    Selection of anesthesia for exodontia, 122
    Removal of teeth under general anesthesia, 124
    Removal of teeth in the hospital, 125
    Management of acutely infected teeth, 126
    Complications of exodontia, 126
    Postexodontia complications, 127
    Emergencies in the dental office, 129

Chapter 9 SURGICAL BACTERIOLOGY (S. Elmer Bear), 132

    Infection, 132
        Local factors, 133
        Systemic condition of the patient, 133
        The physiology of infection, 133
        Systemic effects of oral infection, 137
        Focus of infection, 137
    Antibiotics, 139
        Historical background, 139
        General considerations, 139
        Nature of the lesion, 140
        Sensitivity of microorganisms, 141
        Dosage and route of administration, 142
        Indiscriminate use of antibiotics, 144
        Specific antibiotics, 145
    Sulfonamides, 154
    Adjunctive therapy, 155
        Vitamins, 155
        Antihistamines, 155
        Penicillinase, 156
    Sequelae, 156

Chapter 10 SPECIAL INFECTIONS AND THEIR SURGICAL RELATIONSHIP (George E. Morin), 158

    Tetanus, 158
    Gas gangrene, 159
    Syphilis, 159
    Oral tuberculosis, 160

Moniliasis (thrush), 160
Actinomycosis, 161
Blastomycosis (North American blastomycosis), 162
Histoplasmosis, 162
Oral herpes, 162
    Herpetic ulcers, 162
    Herpetic (aphthous) stomatitis, 163
Erythema multiforme, 163
    Stevens-Johnson syndrome, 164
    Behçet's syndrome, 164
Herpangina, 164
Pemphigus, 164

Chapter 11 ACUTE INFECTIONS OF THE ORAL CAVITY (Sanford M. Moose), 166

Acute infection of the jaws, 167
    Periapical abscess, 167
    Pericoronal infections, 169
    Periodontal abscess, 173
Acute cellulitis, 174
Treatment, 174
    Fascial planes, 176
    Ludwig's angina, 185
    Cavernous sinus thrombosis, 186
General management of patient with acute infection, 187
Osteomyelitis, 187

Chapter 12 CHRONIC PERIAPICAL INFECTIONS (Leslie M. Fitzgerald and James A. O'Brien), 191

Types of chronic periapical infection, 191
    Chronic alveolar abscess, 191
    Granuloma, 191
    Periapical cyst, 193
Treatment, 193
    Technique of apicoectomy, 194
    Technique of removal of periapical cysts, 195
    Chronic periodontal infection, 197
    Removal of broken needles, 197

Chapter 13 HEMORRHAGE AND SHOCK (R. Quentin Royer), 199

Preoperative examination and preparation, 199
Oral hemorrhage, 200
Shock, 206
Fluid and electrolyte balance in oral surgery, 207
Postoperative care, 210

Chapter 14 CYSTS OF BONE AND SOFT TISSUES OF THE ORAL CAVITY AND CONTIGUOUS STRUCTURES (Leroy W. Peterson), 212

Classification, 212
    Congenital cysts, 213
    Developmental cysts, 215
General consideration of cystic lesions, 223

Diagnosis, 223
Surgical technique, 225
Postoperative complications, 234

Chapter 15 DISEASES OF THE MAXILLARY SINUS OF DENTAL ORIGIN (Phillip Earle Williams), 237

Description, 237
Diseases, 239
Pathology, 242
Treatment, 244
    Accidental openings, 244
    Preoperative considerations, 246
    Closure of the oroantral fistula, 247
    Caldwell-Luc operation, 249
Summary, 250

Chapter 16 TISSUE TRANSPLANTATION (Philip J. Boyne), 252

Criteria used in bone graft evaluation, 253
Immunological concepts applied to oral surgical transplantation procedures, 253
    The immune response, 253
Storage and preservation of homogenous bone for grafting, 254
Forms of homogenous banked bone available, 255
Preparation of heterogenous bone for grafting, 257
Autogenous bone grafts, 259
Current experimental studies on bone graft procedures, 259
Tooth transplantation, 261
    Homogenous tooth transplantation, 261
    Autogenous tooth transplantation, 261
    Reimplantation, 263
Summary, 263

Chapter 17 WOUNDS AND INJURIES OF THE SOFT TISSUES OF THE FACIAL AREA (Robert B. Shira), 266

General considerations, 266
Classification of wounds, 267
    Contusion, 267
    Abrasion, 268
    Laceration, 268
    Penetrating wound, 268
    Gunshot, missile, and war wounds, 268
    Burns, 268
Treatment of wounds, 268
    General considerations, 268
    Treatment of contusions, 269
    Treatment of abrasions, 269
    Treatment of lacerations, 270
    Treatment of puncture type of penetrating wounds, 276
    Treatment of gunshot, missile, and war wounds, 277
    Foreign bodies, 280
Treatment of burns, 281
    Therapy, 282
    Burns in mass casualty care, 283
Miscellaneous wounds, 284
    Intraoral wounds, 284
    Severed parotid ducts, 287

Chapter 18 TRAUMATIC INJURIES OF THE TEETH AND ALVEOLAR PROCESS (Merle L. Hale), 289

> Traumatic injuries, 289
> > Clinical evaluation of the injury, 289
> > Radiographic evaluation of the injury, 292
> > Completing the diagnosis and treatment plan, 292
> > Splinting procedures, 293
> > Anesthesia, 294
> > Postoperative considerations and care, 294

Chapter 19 FRACTURES OF THE JAWS (Gustav O. Kruger), 296

> General discussion, 296
> > Etiology, 296
> > Classification, 297
> > Examination, 298
> > First aid, 303
> > Treatment, 304
> Healing of bone, 307
> Fractures of the mandible, 309
> > Causes, 309
> > Location, 311
> > Displacement, 311
> > Signs and symptoms, 317
> > Treatment methods, 318
> > Treatment of fractures of the mandible, 333
> > Feeding problems, 352
> > Time for repair, 354
> > Complications, 354
> Fractures of the maxilla, 356
> > Causes, 356
> > Classification; signs and symptoms, 356
> > Treatment, 359
> > Complications, 364
> Zygoma fractures, 364
> > Diagnosis, 365
> > Treatment, 365
> > Complications, 367

Chapter 20 THE TEMPOROMANDIBULAR JOINT (Fred A. Henny), 369

> Anatomy, 369
> The painful temporomandibular joint, 370
> > Etiology, 370
> > Symptoms, 371
> > Clinical findings, 371
> > Roentgenographic findings, 373
> > Treatment, 374
> Dislocation, 381
> > Treatment, 382
> Ankylosis, 383

Chapter 21 CLEFT LIP AND CLEFT PALATE (James R. Hayward), 386

> Embryology, 386
> Etiology, 389

Surgical correction, 392
    Cheilorrhaphy, 392
    Palatorrhaphy, 394
Incomplete cleft palate, 397
Submucosal cleft palate, 399
Other habilitation measures, 401
    Presurgical orthopedics, 401
    Secondary surgical procedures, 401
    Prosthetic speech aid appliances, 402
    Dental care, 402
    Repair of residual deformities, 404
    Speech therapy, 404
    Cleft palate team approach, 405

Chapter 22 ACQUIRED DEFECTS OF THE HARD AND SOFT TISSUES OF THE FACE (Edward C. Hinds), 407

Soft tissue repair, 407
    Free grafts, 408
    Local flaps, 409
    Distant flaps, 415
Contour replacement, 416
    Soft tissue, 416
    Cartilage, 416
    Bone, 418
    Artificial implants, 419
    Repositioning procedures, 422
Reconstruction of the mandible, 423
    Alloplasts, 423
    Bone, 427
    Alveolar ridge, 433
Immediate repair of compound defects resulting from cancer surgery, 434

Chapter 23 DEVELOPMENTAL DEFORMITIES OF THE JAWS (Jack B. Caldwell), 438

Growth and orthodontics, 440
Selection of an operative procedure and preoperative planning, 440
Preparation of the patient for surgery, 444
    Anesthesia, 444
    Skin preparation and draping the patient, 445
Technique of soft tissue surgery, 447
Prognathism (mandibular), 447
    Supportive and postoperative care, 478
    Relationship of musculature to surgical correction of jaw deformities, 478
    Fixation appliances and immobilization, 480
    Discussion, 482
Micrognathia and retrognathia, 484
    Preparation for surgery, 485
Microgenia and genioplasty, 500
Apertognathia (open bite deformity) and other occlusion and jaw abnormalities, 501
Conclusion, 513

Chapter 24 SURGICAL ASPECTS OF ORAL TUMORS (Claude S. LaDow), 517

    Tumors of the hard tissues of the oral cavity, 517
        Odontogenic tumors, 517
        Osteogenic tumors, 520
    Tumors of the soft tissues of the oral cavity, 525
    Carcinoma of the oral cavity, 531
        Treatment, 533
    Comment, 537

Chapter 25 SALIVARY GLANDS AND DUCTS (Donald E. Cooksey), 539

    Structure of the salivary glands, 539
        Gross anatomy, 539
        Microscopic anatomy, 541
        Anatomical weaknesses, 542
    Diseases of the salivary glands, 542
        Inflammatory diseases, 542
        Diseases due to obstruction, 544
        Tumors of the salivary glands, 545
    Differential diagnosis of salivary gland lesions, 549
        History, 549
        Physical examination, 550
        Radiographic evaluation, 552
        Laboratory procedures, 554
    Surgical procedures, 560
        Transoral sialolithotomy of submandibular duct, 561
        Transoral sialolithotomy of parotid duct, 563
        Removal of submandibular gland, 564
    Conclusion, 566

Chapter 26 NEUROLOGICAL ASPECTS OF DENTAL PAIN (Athol L. Frew, Jr., and Don M. Ishmael), 568

    Clinical examination for localization of dental focus, 568
        Motor nerves, 569
        Sensory nerves, 571

Color plates

Plate 1	Photomicrograph taken with ultraviolet illumination of ground, unstained cross sections of dog alveolar ridges	260
Plate 2	Photomicrograph taken with ultraviolet illumination following intravital labeling with tetracycline demonstrating homogenously transplanted incisor teeth in a dog	260
Plate 3	Transplanted, fully formed homogenous teeth in dogs after intravital labeling with tetracycline at 6 and 12 weeks postoperatively	260

Textbook of oral surgery

Chapter 1

PRINCIPLES OF SURGERY

James R. Cameron

The principles of surgery applicable to the general surgeon are equally applicable in the practice of the oral surgeon. Oral surgery as a specialty of dentistry was introduced as a major subject in the curriculum of the Philadelphia Dental College, now the School of Dentistry, Temple University, in the year 1864. As dental education advanced, the practice of oral surgery became increasingly important, necessitating advanced training over and above that received at the undergraduate level. Oral surgery as defined by the American Board of Oral Surgery and accepted by the Board of Trustees and the House of Delegates of the American Dental Association and by the Board of Trustees of the American Medical Association is as follows:

> Oral surgery is that part of dental practice which deals with the diagnosis, the surgical and adjunctive treatment of the diseases, injuries and defects of the human jaws and associated structures.

A careful study of this definition will impress the dental practitioner with the need for special training in surgical principles and the development of sound surgical judgment. Courses in the basic sciences on the graduate level offered by various universities and followed by approved residencies in oral surgery are developing an oral surgeon who is capable of practicing this specialty intelligently in its broadest concept.

A successful surgeon is one whose digital skill and dexterity are based upon a fundamental knowledge of anatomy, physiology, and pathological conditions commonly met in daily practice. A correct diagnosis is essential in all fields of surgery. There is only one diagnosis—the correct one—although different methods of treatment may be employed, each giving a satisfactory result. To arrive at a diagnosis, the clinician calls upon his entire knowledge and experience and by a process of elimination reaches certain conclusions. He should view the patient as a whole, but concentrate on the area of complaint as though it were of glass, enabling him to visualize the normal anatomy and think in terms of the structural changes that may occur in that particular part of the body. He should train his fingers to detect structural abnormalities and interpret these changes into pathological conditions or injuries. An adequate history will often lead to a correct conclusion.

CASE HISTORY

The fundamental principles of an adequate case history are as follows.

Chief complaint (C. C.). The symptoms presented by the patient as well as the duration of the symptoms are listed in brief form.

Present illness (P. I.). The patient describes his illness in his own way, and this often gives important clues to the relative significance of the symptoms. Rarely does an ill person narrate his illness as we would prefer, that is, clearly, concisely, and chronologically with mode of onset and course. Nor will the patient adequately describe symptoms as to their location, type of distress, areas of radiation, duration, relation to other functions, response to domestic or professional remedies, and the present status.

Past history (P. H.). This should give valuable information regarding the physical insults the patient has previously sustained by earlier disease and injury. Be specific in detail, including time of onset, duration, complications, sequelae, management, place of treatment, and name of attending physician. Important examples are rheumatic disease, tuberculosis, pneumonia, venereal disease, and bleeding tendencies.

Social and occupational history. In some cases, because of the nature of the present illness, a detailed knowledge of the patient's emotional and economic status may be relevant as well as the occupation in which he is engaged (kind and number of jobs, type of present work, exposure to toxic agents, and hazards, for example, ventilation, temperature, and illumination).

Family history (F. H.). This should give an opportunity to evaluate the patient's inherited tendencies or the possibilities of exposure to disease within his own family. Examples include cancer (kind and origin), diabetes, arthritis, vascular diseases (hypertension, heart attacks, kidney disease), hematological diseases (hemophilia, pernicious anemia), allergic conditions (hay fever, asthma), and infections (tuberculosis, rheumatic fever).

Habits. This should summarize any disorder in the patient's sleep, diet, or liquid intake. Be scrupulous regarding the drugs he is taking or has taken, for example, analgesics, stimulants, vitamins, tranquilizers, sedatives, narcotics, prescribed medications (digitalis, cortisone), and particularly the reaction to antibiotics, sulfonamides, sedatives, and other drugs.

The family physician should be consulted for evaluation of the patient's physical condition in all cases in which there is a questionable finding upon physical examination or case history regarding systemic abnormality or disease.

Certain laboratory aids may be useful in establishing a diagnosis.

LABORATORY WORK

Laboratory aids are available to the oral surgeon to help him at times to arrive at the correct diagnosis. Roentgenography sometimes supplies information in situations in which an adequate diagnosis cannot be made by inspection, palpation, or auscultation. The standard periapical films can be supplemented by occlusal, topographical, lateral jaw, or posteroanterior head films.

Routine blood and urine analyses may sometimes reveal a hidden condition that can complicate a proposed oral surgical procedure. For example, glycosuria would warrant medical consultation and treatment before surgery is performed. Blood and urine analyses should be standard operational procedures for all patients entering the hospital. Included in the blood test should be a report of the patient's hematocrit (HCT) test and white blood cell count (WBC). This is commonly ordered as a CBC (complete blood count). A normal white blood cell count (WBC) is in the range of 4,000 to 6,000 cells per cubic millimeter of blood. It is important to note, however, not only the number of white blood cells as to relative increase or decrease, but also the ratio in which they are present. Normally these cells are in the ratio of 60% to 70% polymorphonuclear leukocytes, 20% to 30% lymphocytes, 4% to 5% monocytes, 1% eosinophils, and 0.5% basophils. If abnormalities in these ratios are suspected, consultation with the physician is indicated. The polymorphonuclear leukocytes are normally increased in acute inflammatory processes and following traumatic injuries. In cases of osteomyelitis of the jaws the monocytes would show an increased ratio.

The hematocrit (Fig. 1-1) serves as an excellent index of the patient's red blood cell volume. It is a laboratory test in which the volume of packed red cells is expressed in percentage after whole blood is centrifuged; if there were 2 ml. of packed red cells in the tube containing 4 ml. of blood originally, the hematocrit value would be 50. The normal value for men is 45 ± 5; for women 40 ± 5. A patient with a low hematocrit value should receive immediate medical attention since a blood transfusion may be necessary. Again, a high hematocrit value may be reflecting an underlying polycythemia. The hematocrit test is superior to hemoglobin estimation for screening suspect oral surgical patients in that the latter test is subject to errors not encountered with the hematocrit test.

Other laboratory tests may be necessary, depending on the needs of the patient to be studied. Thus a patient whose complaint is prolonged bleeding following tooth extraction may warrant such tests as bleeding, coagulation, and prothrombin time. Bleeding and coagulation time tests may be performed by the practitioner himself with little difficulty and expenditure of time. Bleeding time by Duke's method is accomplished by making a small cut in the lobe of the ear with a needle or the point of a scalpel. At intervals of 30 seconds the blood is all blotted off with a piece of absorbent paper. The usual bleeding time is 1 to 3 minutes before the hemorrhage finally ceases. Several drops of blood are collected on a clean glass slide for the determination of coagulation time. At 1-minute intervals a needle is drawn through one or another drop. Coagulation has occurred when fibrin shreds cling to the needle and can be dragged along with it. The normal time is 7 minutes or less.

Normal prothrombin time (Quick method) may vary from 9 to 30 seconds, depending on the activity of one of the solutions (thromboplastin) that the laboratory utilizes. A normal standard is established for each new thromboplastin solution and at intervals of 48 hours during the use of a given solution by a given laboratory. Prothrombin time values from two different laboratories may vary a great deal numerically and yet be within the normal values established for each laboratory.

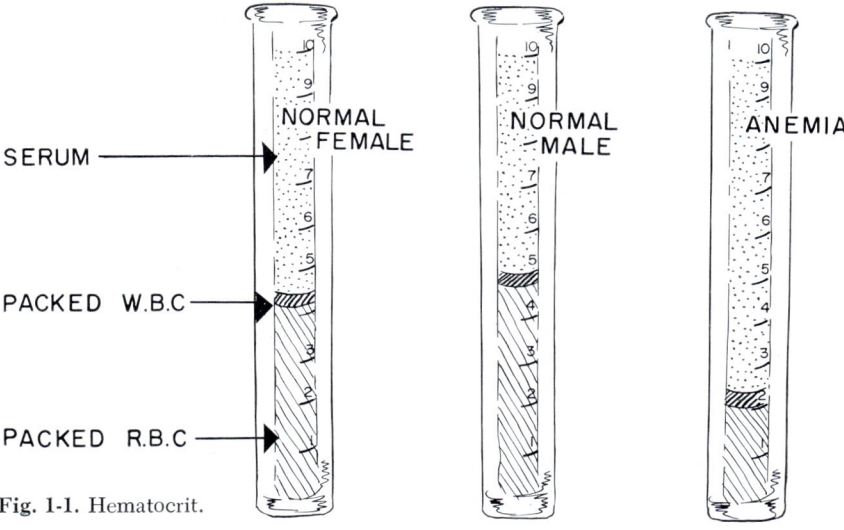

Fig. 1-1. Hematocrit.

ASEPSIS

Although the principles of asepsis are as well recognized in oral surgery practice as in any field of surgery, the advent of antibiotics and improved methods of anesthesia, both local and general, have revolutionized the practice of surgery to some extent. Many oral surgical procedures once considered problematical can now be successfully accomplished with the aid of safe anesthesia, antibiotic therapy, and an understanding of fluid balance. Valuable as they are, the use of antibiotics should not lessen the need for meticulous care in asepsis; infection introduced into a surgical wound may bring about complete failure of the operation or at least prolong the healing process.

The oral cavity is never a surgically clean area of the body. It is, however, readily available for cleansing of gross contamination prior to a surgical operation. Prior to any intraoral surgery, even an uncomplicated tooth extraction, the mouth should be cleansed by a rigid oral hygiene procedure or by swabbing the entire oral cavity and tongue with a solution of Mercresin. All instruments to be used should be adequately sterilized and placed on a tray covered by a sterile towel. Only sterile gauze or sponges should be introduced into the operative area. Careful attention to cleanliness of the operator's hands is necessary. The hands and arms up to the elbow should be carefully scrubbed with soap and water, with particular attention given to the cleanliness of the fingernails. It is customary in major surgery to scrub the hands and arms above the elbow for a 10-minute period, with frequent rinsing in running water, after which the hands and arms are immersed in alcohol prior to putting on a sterile gown, which a circulating nurse will secure at the back. In major operations in and about the mouth or jaws, all drapes used should be sterile and the operator and his assistants should wear sterile masks, caps, gowns, and rubber gloves.

The surgeon differentiates between everyday cleanliness of his person (social cleanliness) and surgical cleanliness by preparing himself to be surgically clean prior to operating. The most frequent failure of a surgical operation is one of infection. Though the surgeon is not responsible for infection found in a part, he is responsible for infection that he may introduce into a wound. Heat, chemicals, and drugs possessing antiseptic, germicidal, or bactericidal properties are aids used by the surgeon and his assistants to render the operative field and instruments free of infection. Aseptic surgery is understood to be free of all infection or contamination by instruments or materials used in an operation.

Hypodermic needles that have been sterilized in an autoclave are safer than those sterilized by cold solutions. Sterile disposable needles are now available. Extraoral operations require careful cleansing of the skin beyond the operative field. Male patients should be shaved prior to the skin preparation. A standard method of skin preparation is to first cleanse the entire part to be exposed, using an ether sponge on a forceps. This is followed by cleansing the area with a sponge soaked in alcohol, and finally the entire part beyond the operative field is painted with tincture of Mercresin. Sterile towels and drapes are now applied, leaving only the operative site exposed. A good light is essential and should be focused upon the operative field. Once attired in cap, mask, gown, and gloves, the operator and his assistants should not touch anything outside the sterile operative field.

ATRAUMATIC SURGERY

One of the first principles of good surgery is that the handling of living tissue be done with a minimum of trauma. Gentle handling of tissue made up of many cells will aid in the ultimate repair and healing of the structures that have been invaded by the instruments of the surgeon. Torn and lacerated tissue tends to lose its vitality

and becomes necrotic. This invites infection and retards functional healing. All surgical operations should be well planned in advance to minimize undue trauma. In the field of oral surgery the use of flaps of various designs in different areas of the mouth is common practice. There are three fundamental principles that must be strictly adhered to in the utilization of flaps.
1. The flap should be so designed that the blood supply will be maintained.
2. The design of the flap should permit its reflection away from the operative field.
3. The design should also permit the flap to completely cover the operative site and be retained by nontension sutures when returned to its original position.

INFECTION

Infection is determined by (1) virulence of the organisms present, (2) the number of organisms, and (3) the vital resistance of the host.

When operating in an infected wound where pus is found, it is usually advisable to insert a drain at the time of closing the wound. It may be made of various kinds of material, such as the following:
1. A Penrose drain, which is one of plain gauze enclosed in a thin rubber tube, made in various sizes
2. Rubber tissue (rubber dam), cut to an appropriate width and length
3. Rubber tubing, beveled at the inserted tip and perforated on alternate sides
4. Iodoform gauze, 5%, in various widths

The drain is inserted into the depth of the wound or abscess cavity to facilitate the passing of infected material from the depth of the wound to the external surface. A sufficient length should be allowed to extend beyond the external surface to prevent its being lost in the wound and to facilitate its removal. Rubber tissue and rubber tube drains should have a safety pin attached at the external surface to prevent entrance of the drain into the depth of the wound.

Drains should be changed daily according to the amount of contaminated fluid present. If no excess fluid is found on removal of the first drain inserted, a new drain need not be inserted and the wound may be allowed to close. Intraoral drains should be changed or discontinued in 1 to 3 days. An exception to this may be necessary in large, open wounds where a dressing of gauze is used more as a pack than as a drain, such as in large intraoral cystic cavities, osteomyelitis, or a wide open maxillary sinus. However, a drain should not be confused with a pack. A drain facilitates the passing of unwanted fluid from the depth of a wound to the surface, whereas a pack is a dressing placed in a wound under pressure. A pack may be used to control hemorrhage or keep a wound cavity open until new healthy tissue lessens its size. Iodoform gauze, 5%, of various widths is the most commonly used material for a pack.

SUTURE MATERIAL

Various suture materials are available for use by the oral surgeon (Figs. 1-2 to 1-4). The most frequently used suture material for closure of intraoral incisions is braided black silk of appropriate size, which is moisture- and serum-proof. Sterile black silk fulfills most requirements for intraoral suturing. It is nonirritating to the tongue and its color is readily recognized for removal. The material is inexpensive.

Closure of intraoral wounds or incisions by interrupted sutures is preferable to a continuous suture since alternate sutures may be removed when necessary without disturbing the entire suture line.

Closure of external incisions on the face is best done with fine material, usually nylon monofilament No. 3-0 threaded on an eyeless needle. Closure of such skin incisions can be made with through-and-through interrupted sutures or mattress sutures. Subcutaneous suturing has some cosmetic advantages but is a disadvantage when opening of the incision is necessary to permit escape of serous exudate.

Text continued on p. 10.

6 *Textbook of oral surgery*

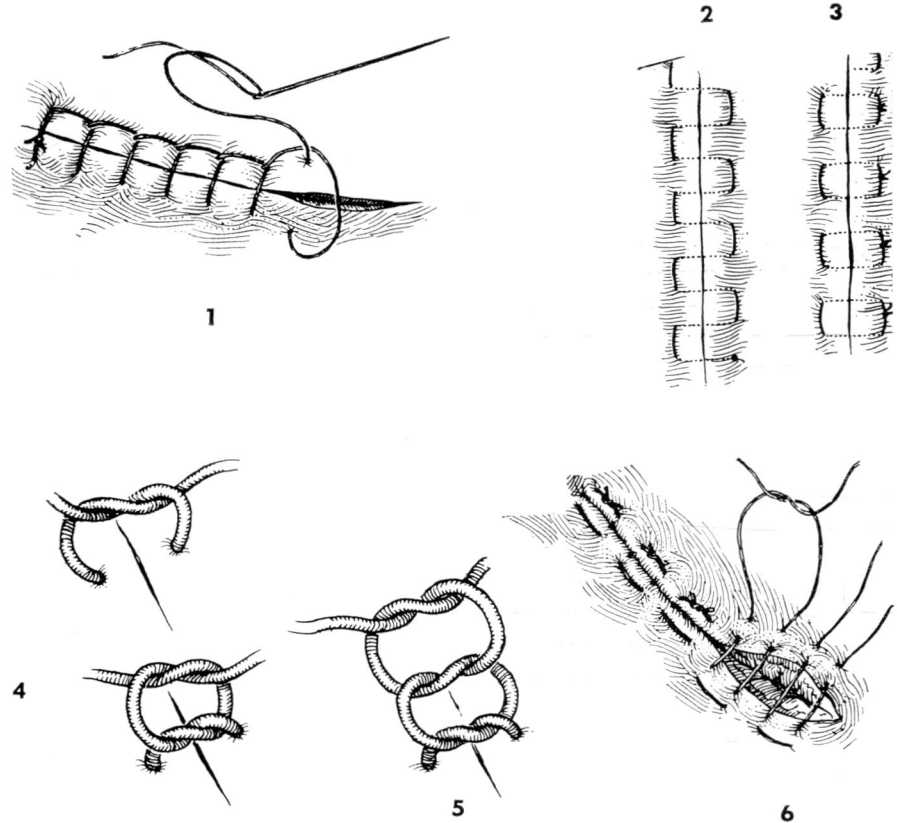

Fig. 1-2. Suture techniques. *1,* The blanket or continuous locked suture. *2,* Continuous suture. *3,* Interrupted mattress suture. *4,* Method of placing first and second half hitches in the square or true knot. *5,* The square knot reinforced by third half hitch. *6,* The Halsted interrupted mattress suture. (Courtesy Ethicon, Inc., Somerville, N. J.)

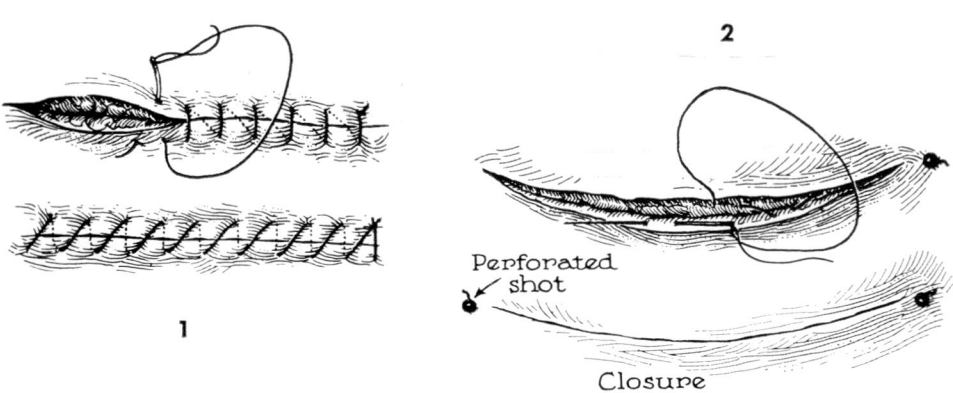

Fig. 1-3. Suture techniques. *1,* Two methods of continuous over-and-over closing suture. *2,* Subcuticular suture for closure of skin incision. Perforated buckshot used to anchor suture. (Courtesy Ethicon, Inc., Somerville, N. J.)

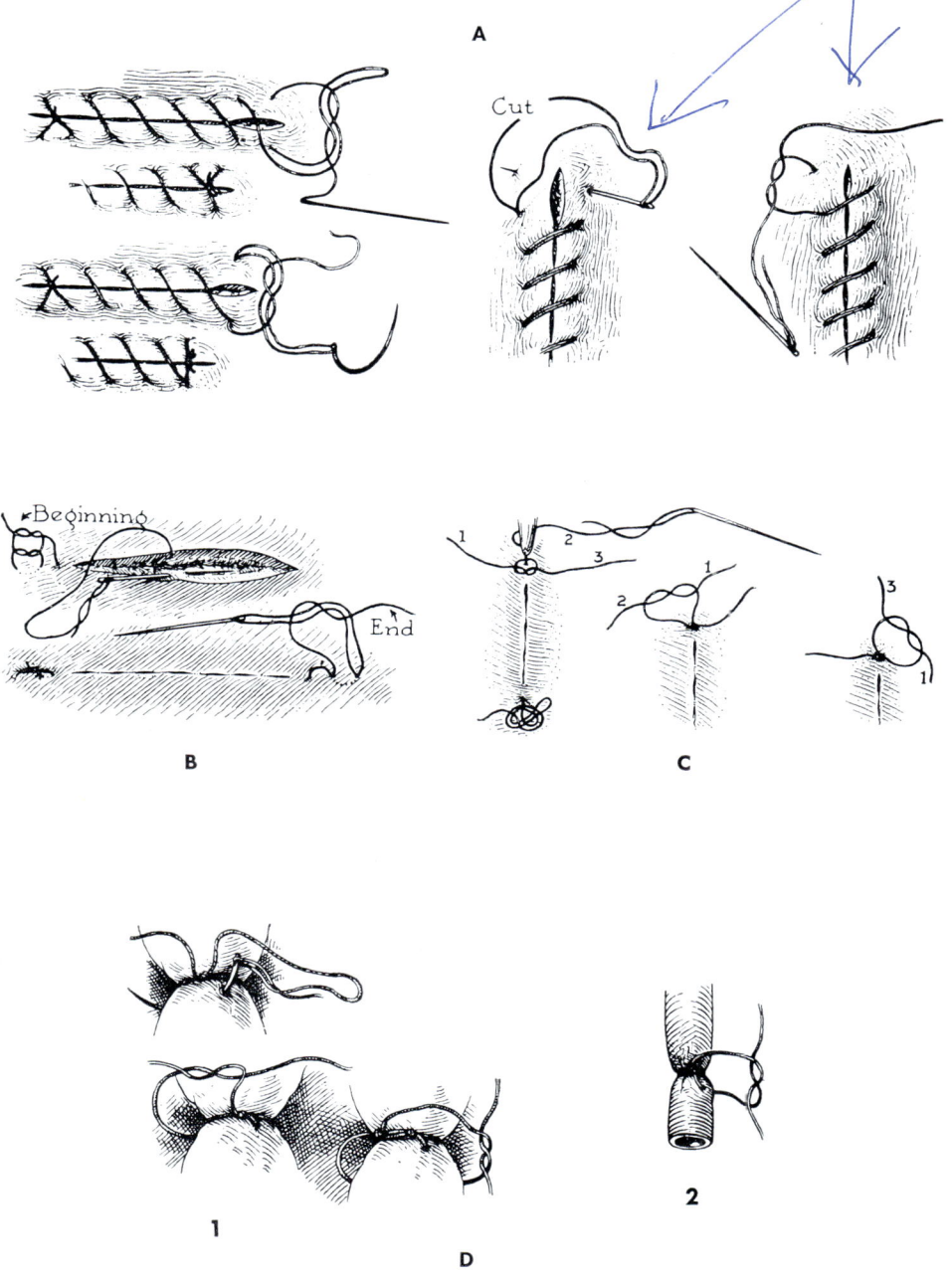

Fig. 1-4. Suture techniques. **A,** Variety of methods for securing the ends of completed continuous sutures. Technique for securing ends of both double and single sutures is demonstrated. Note method of dividing suture to avoid double thickness of knot. **B,** Method of beginning subcuticular suture by placing square knot lateral to incision and method of ending suture at opposite end of incision. **C,** Alternate method for the completion of subcuticular continuous suture by placing a holding knot around end of subcuticular suture. **D,** Methods of placing transfixing ligatures to prevent slipping: **1,** transfixing ligature of pedicle; **2,** method of placing transfixing ligature in vessel. (Courtesy Ethicon, Inc., Somerville, N. J.)

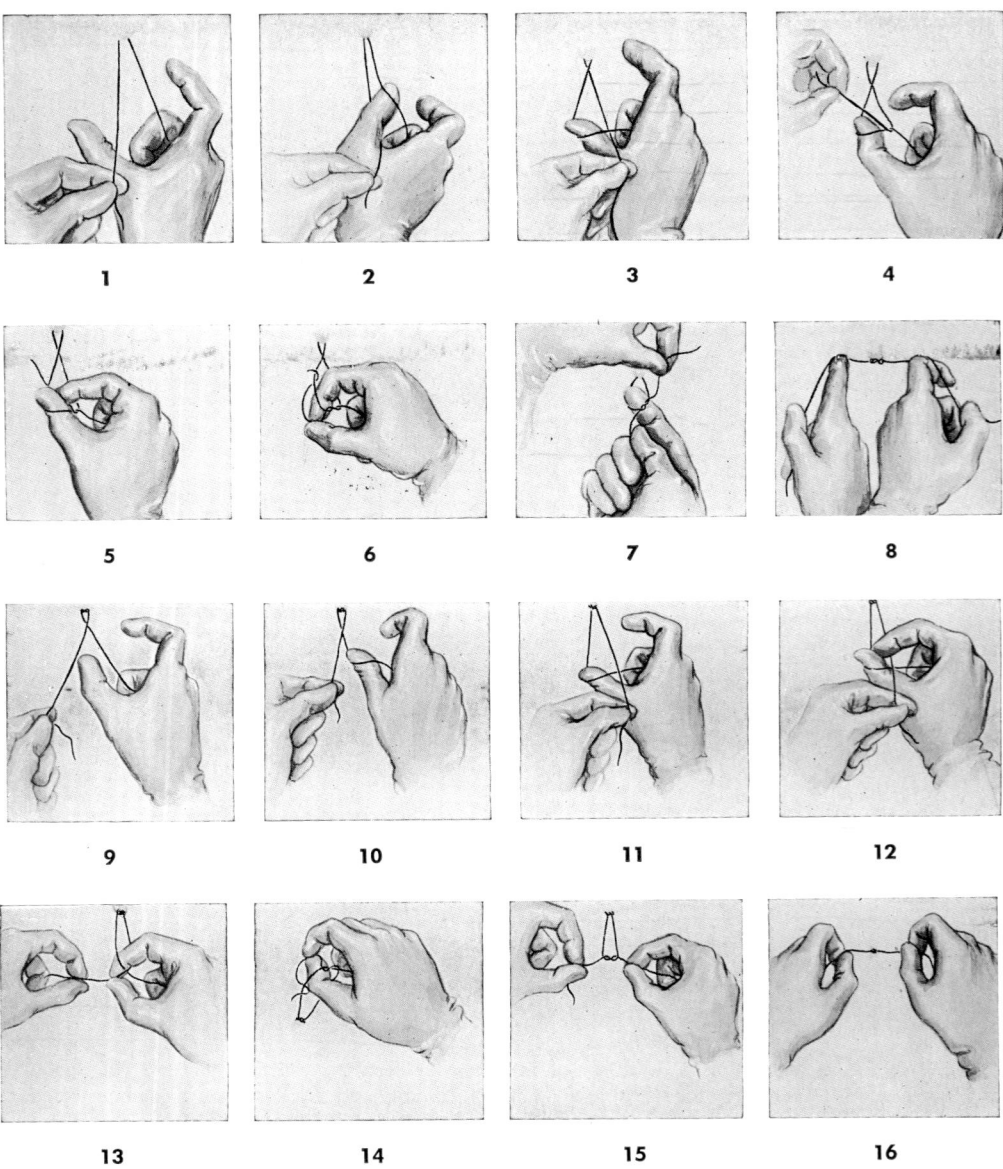

Fig. 1-5. Two-hand knot tie. (After Partipilo.) Note: The two-hand square knot illustrated may be begun with either the right or left hand. (Courtesy Ethicon, Inc., Somerville, N. J.)

Principles of surgery 9

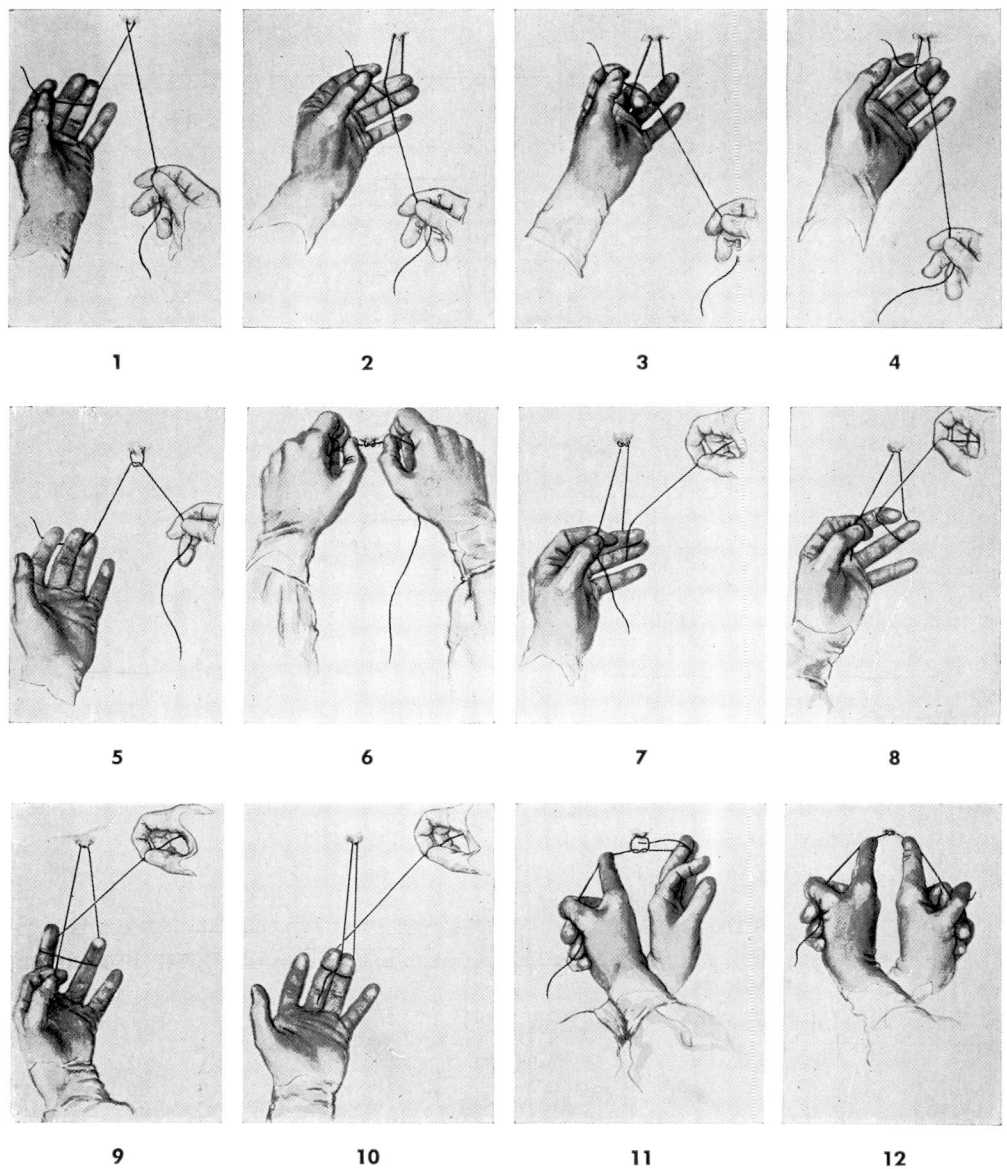

Fig. 1-6. One-hand tie. Note: Shown here is the left hand beginning the knot with the short end of the ligature. However, either hand may be used in this initial step. (Courtesy Ethicon, Inc., Somerville, N. J.)

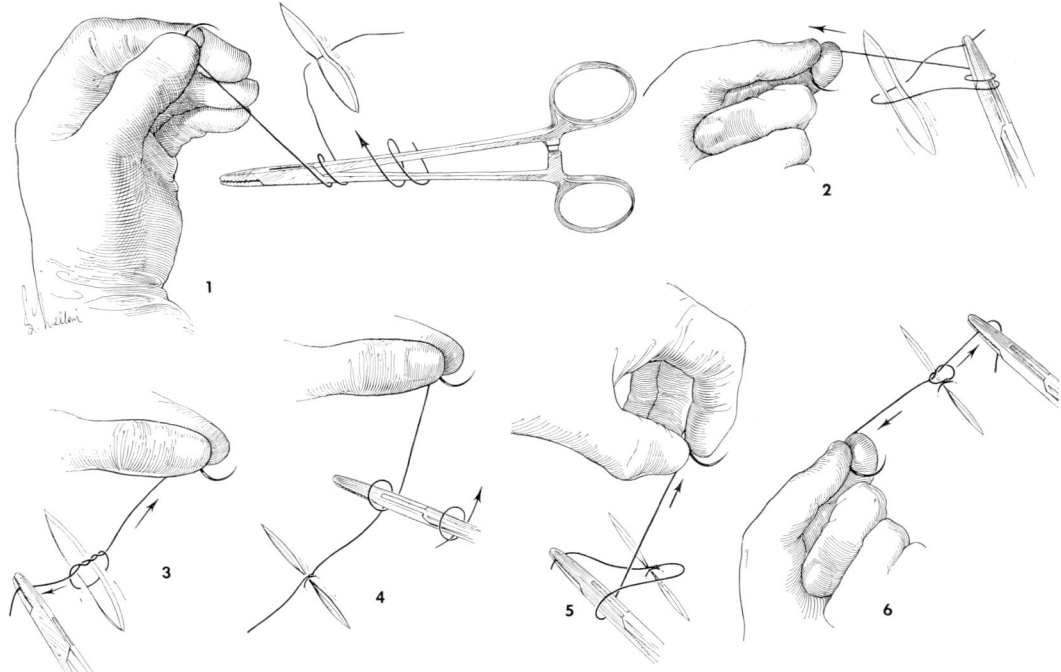

Fig. 1-7. Technique of instrument tie. **1,** The needle on the long end of the suture is held in the left hand while the needle holder makes two clockwise turns around it to form a loop. **2,** The needle holder has crossed over to grasp the short end of the suture. **3,** The hand and the needle holder have reversed positions to tighten the knot. The knot should lie to one side of the wound. **4,** The needle holder makes one counterclockwise turn around the long end of the suture to form a square knot. **5,** The instrument grasps the short end of the suture on the other side of the wound. **6,** The knot is tightened on the same side of the wound.

LIGATURES

Ligation of sectioned blood vessels is usually done with plain catgut, the size of the catgut depending on the size of the blood vessel to be tied (Figs. 1-5 to 1-8). Most small blood vessels requiring ligation can be secured with plain catgut No. 2-0. Larger blood vessels such as the external facial artery are best ligated with chromic gut. The use of plain catgut No. 3-0 is satisfactory for approximation of sectioned muscle about the face. Sectioned muscle can be approximated and secured by interrupted sutures or continuous sutures, depending on the location of the muscle to be approximated.

NEEDLES

A curved, cutting-edge needle that will fit around a five-cent piece or a dime is the size of choice for intraoral suturing. Different manufacturers have different numbers for their needles. A cutting-edge needle is usually preferable to a smooth round needle.

DRESSINGS

Sponges and dressings of gauze are preferable to cotton. They are of various sizes, depending on the locale of the operative field. They can be sterilized and kept in sterile muslin packages. Sponges and cotton rolls of different sizes can be cut

Principles of surgery 11

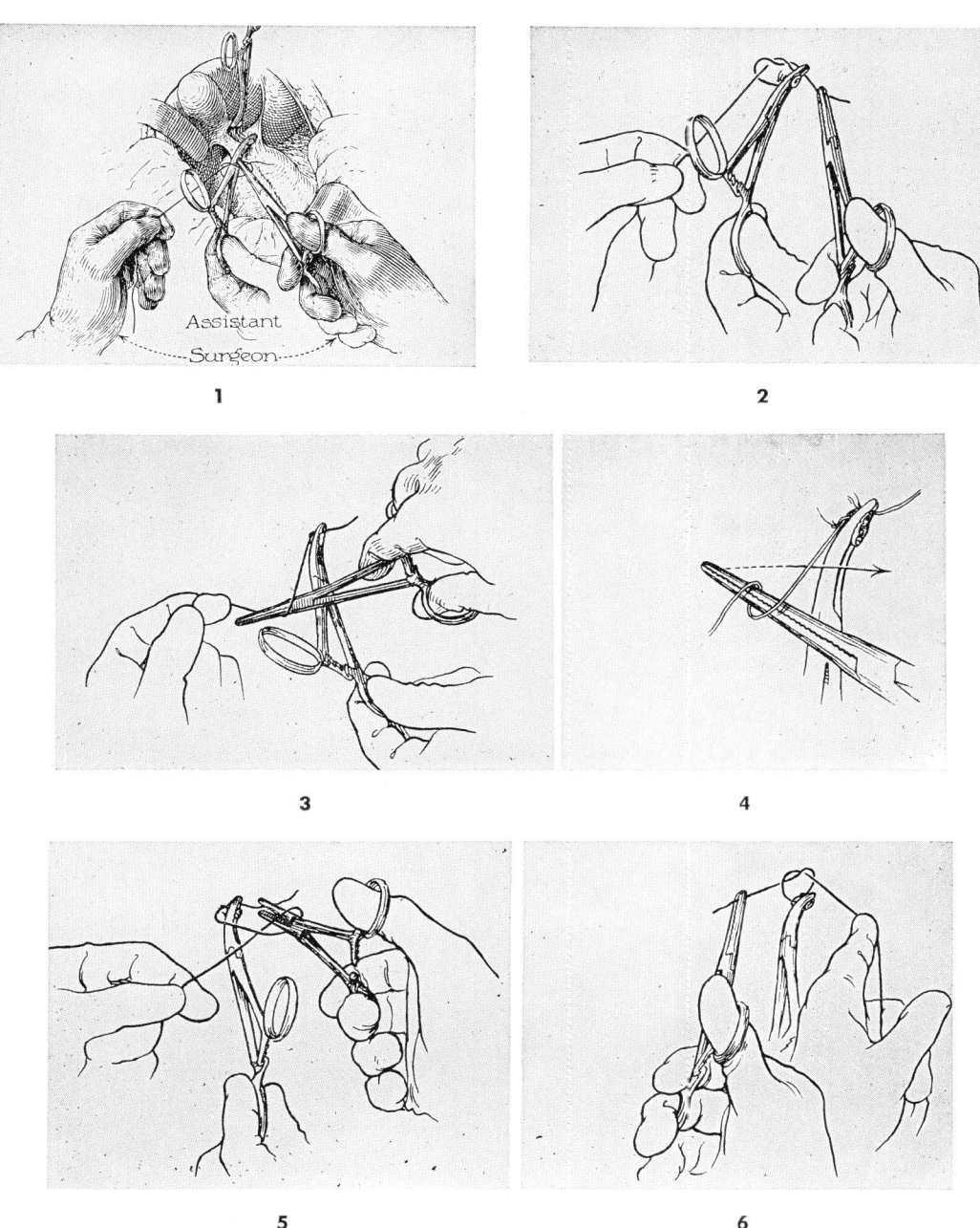

Fig. 1-8. Technique of placing deep ligatures (Printy, Grant). **1,** First half hitch is taken loosely and slipped down over the tip of holding forceps. **2,** Short end of ligature is grasped by forceps and the ligature tightened around pedicle. **3,** A second half hitch is begun by looping long end around forceps in the right hand. **4,** Method of beginning second half hitch by looping around forceps. Holding forceps left in place. **5,** After loop is thrown around forceps, short end is grasped by opening forceps and is pulled through. **6,** Second half hitch completed by crossing hands. This method is helpful in regions difficult of access. (Courtesy Ethicon, Inc., Somerville, N. J.)

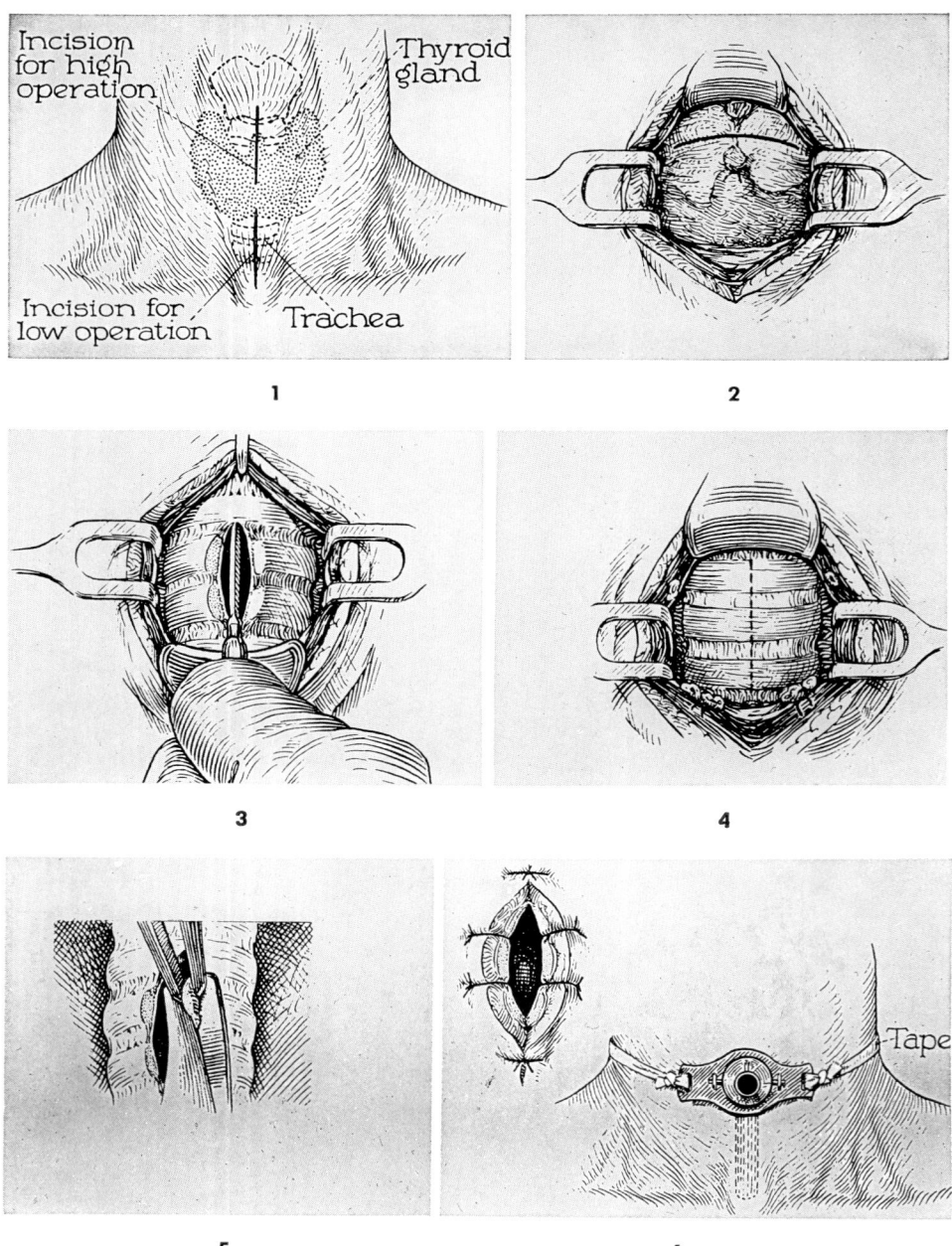

Fig. 1-9. Tracheotomy. 1, Surface anatomy showing relationship of high and low incisions to underlying structures. 2, Technique of high tracheotomy. The pretracheal fascia is incised at the level of the cricoid cartilage. 3, Cricoid cartilage retracted to steady trachea. First, second, and third cartilaginous rings incised. 4, Technique of low tracheotomy. Dotted line indicates incision. Low site is inadvisable in children. 5, Method of trimming edges of tracheal incision to establish an oval-shaped opening (Digby). 6, Method of fixing trachea by through-and-through sutures and method for holding tracheal tube by tape. (Courtesy Ethicon, Inc., Somerville, N. J.)

obliquely for exodontia. They should be sterilized in an autoclave and kept in a sterile container ready for use.

A clean surgical wound on the face requires attention only to prevent contamination. A sterile gauze dressing covering the wound is all that is necessary. Small, dry external wounds may be left uncovered after the second day, provided clothing will not contaminate the area.

BLOOD LOSS

When a large amount of blood has been lost, secondary to an accident or during surgery, replacement by whole blood is necessary. Toxic patients with marked elevation of temperature not only require antibiotic therapy and possibly surgery, but also adequate fluid intake. Intravenous replacement should be done for patients who are unable to take fluids by mouth. Usually glucose in 500 to 1,000 ml. of sterile distilled water will be found beneficial. The rate of administration should not exceed 250 ml. per hour. Patients who are markedly dehydrated and toxic, especially in hot weather, will respond well to intravenous saline solution. Toxic patients also respond well to a cleansing enema of soapsuds. If intravenous fluid intake is found difficult, 500 ml. of ordinary tap water at room temperature given by proctoclysis is advantageous.

OPERATING ROOM

The room where operations are to be performed should be devoid of elaborate furnishings. Above all, it should be clean and so arranged that it can be kept clean. Pictures on the wall, draperies, and carpets or rugs on the floor have no place in a modern operating room since they are collectors of dust. A room with a tiled floor, and preferably tiled walls, lends itself to easy cleaning. A good artificial light is essential for oral surgery procedures. A well-arranged oral surgeon's operating room will be minus an instrument cabinet since all instruments to be used will be placed on a table covered by a sterile towel. If a stainless steel tray is used, it can be sterilized before instruments are placed upon it.

The traditional cuspidor of a dental office can be dispensed with since small hand emesis basins are all that are necessary. Likewise, the conventional unit of a dental office is not necessary in an operating room. With the elimination of a cuspidor and unit, the operating chair or table stands free of equipment that otherwise hampers free movement of assistants. All well-equipped operating rooms should have a suction apparatus with various-sized aspirator attachments. A sphygmomanometer is a necessity in a modern operating room. A portable oxygen apparatus should be available in an office even though general anesthesia is not administered. Oxygen should be considered a necessary part of the local anesthesia equipment as it is with any apparatus used in general anesthesia.

LINEN

Routine, uncomplicated exodontia procedures may be carried out with a plastic apron covering the patient's clothing (which should be loosened at the neck and waist). A sterile chest towel can cover the apron. Wiping the lips and surrounding skin with an alcohol sponge will remove surface contamination. The patient's head and chest should be covered with a sterile sheet for more complicated surgical procedures done in the dental office.

REFERENCES

1. Davis, L., editor: Christopher's textbook of surgery, ed. 8, Philadelphia, 1965, W. B. Saunders Co.
2. Moyer, C. A., Rhoads, J. E., Allen, J. G., and Harkins, H. N.: Surgery principles and practice, ed. 3, Philadelphia, 1965, J. B. Lippincott Co.

Chapter 2

PRINCIPLES OF SURGICAL TECHNIQUE

Theodore A. Lesney

INTRODUCTION

Contrary to uninformed opinion, surgery is intended to salvage human tissues, in whole or in part. To salvage life or to salvage the gross anatomy, it often becomes necessary to sacrifice human tissue in part. It took many years for this concept to gain universal acceptance, and only after that was surgery elevated to its rightful place among equally important branches of the healing arts. In the preanesthetic era surgery was a matter of speed and deftness and somewhat a sleight-of-hand procedure. With anesthesia came the more meticulous, more deliberate approach to a surgical problem with knife in hand.

In the pre-Lister era of the nineteenth century practically every wound became infected. As a matter of fact, the formation of pus in surgical wounds became known as "laudable pus" and was actually considered as a necessary stage in wound healing. When Lister contributed his doctrines of asepsis in 1867, he was ridiculed by the surgical rank-and-file doctor of that day. He was called that "so-and-so advocate of Listerism." And this because of his insistence that the surgeon wash his hands thoroughly after the cadaver dissection and before starting viable surgery in the operating room. Surgeons were remarkably slow in accepting the fact that a suppurating wound was actually an unfavorable complication.

In this country William S. Halsted, the first professor of surgery at Johns Hopkins Medical School in the early days of American medicine, is now considered to be the first surgeon to use rubber gloves as one means of avoiding cross infection. Shortly thereafter this innovation was further developed to include the use of operating room apparel and isolation of the patient through the use of sterile sheets. In those days there was opposition from both patients and doctors over so much "fussing" for minor surgical procedures. But infected wounds do not differentiate between minor and major surgery. In dentistry today there is still an occasional cry of opposition to the "fussing" in preparing for surgery within the mouth. Furthermore, Halsted preached the doctrine of the use of sharp scalpels to minimize tissue damage. He designed fine-pointed hemostatic forceps so that only the bleeding vessel might be grasped without trauma to adjacent tissues. His suture technique, introduced in 1883 and involving the use of thin, black silk, is in common practice today with only minor modifications. He considered that interrupted sutures were superior to the continuous suture in regard to strength and in limiting the spread of infection along the suture material. He advocated that the silk used in suturing should be no stronger than the tissue itself and that a greater number of fine stitches was better than a few coarse ones. He warned against bringing the tissues together under tension since this endangered blood supply, delayed healing, and encouraged necrosis of injured tissues.

The basic principles of surgical technique remain rather constant after having withstood the rigors of time and surgical practice. Only evolutionary modifications, developed after current knowledge has been proved, will affect these fundamentals.

Technically, the fundamental goal of the good surgeon is the development of an atraumatic technique, the careful control of hemorrhage, the gentle and considerate handling of tissue, and a wholesome respect for surgical asepsis.

Infection

Infection is the greatest deterrent to normal wound healing. It is furthermore the most serious complication to modern surgery. Today the surgeon knows sufficient anatomy to avoid severing major vessels unwittingly. He knows basic physiology to the point of administering blood and plasma and maintaining fluid and electrolyte balance to abort shock and comparable disaster. He is always alert to control hemorrhage and maintain an adequate airway and to provide necessary oxygenation. His efforts, however, at controlling secondary infection may not be so complete.

Despite the care with which mouth surgery may be provided, patients still develop osteomyelitis of the jaw bones after uneventful tooth extraction. They develop actinomycosis and other deep mycotic infections in mouths that were preoperatively asymptomatic. Other, sometimes less dramatic, infection involving streptococcal, staphylococcal, spirochetal, and viral contamination is not an unusual sequel to mouth surgery as commonly practiced.

There is no doubt that the general physical condition of the patient is a predisposing factor to infection. Every surgeon has operated upon a patient who "should certainly have come down with postoperative infection" but did not. Conversely, that patient who "should *not* have been sick with secondary infection" has developed complications. Shock, exhaustion, malnutrition, dehydration, and systemic disease will lower the patient's resistance to infection.

Wound healing is influenced to a considerable degree by the nutritional state of the patient, whether it be due to the lack of food or the lack of its assimilation. The anemic patient is a prime example of a "slow healer." He may be unable to absorb sufficient protein and vitamins to maintain balance. Another typical "slow healer" is the patient with metabolic disease. The uncontrolled diabetic responds poorly to trauma and is a constant problem in postoperative secondary infection. Diseases of the liver and kidney, with their resultant influence on normal hematology and serology, will certainly affect wound healing.

It is quite evident that while modern bacteriostatic and bacteriolytic antibiotics and chemotherapy are of great support to the surgeon in his constant battle with wound infection, they are nevertheless not a substitute for good surgical principles concerned with aseptic technique and atraumatic surgery. Localized suppuration must still be drained; it is not good practice to attempt to "dry it up" with antibiotics. Infected wounds are not sutured until the infection has been controlled.

Patent airway

Since man lives only a minute-to-minute existence, depending upon his ability to acquire and assimilate oxygen, it becomes a fundamental principle in surgery that an unobstructed airway be maintained in all patients at all times.

The glottis is commonly obstructed by the following:
1. Inability of the patient to adequately evacuate the mouth and pharynx of oral fluids, blood, or foreign bodies
2. Edema following trauma or infection
3. The patient seemingly having "swallowed" the tongue
4. Mechanical obstruction, such as displaced dental prostheses
5. Drug poisoning, as with (a) respiratory depressants or (b) muscle relaxants (such as the curare-like drugs)

In any event the conscious patient will struggle desperately to clear the airway. This will not be true of the unconscious patient. The immediate sign of anoxemia may be cyanosis, quickly followed by rapid depression of all vital functions.

Emergency treatment will concern primarily the following:
1. Pulling the patient's tongue out of the mouth as far as possible, which helps in elevating the epiglottis
2. Digital palpation of the oropharynx in seeking obstructing foreign bodies
3. Attempt to pass endotracheal tube past the vocal cords, and subsequent administration of oxygen therapy
4. Respiratory assistance through artificial respiration
5. Tracheotomy or cricothyroidotomy when other measures fail

Hemorrhage control

Galen, the great Roman anatomist, warned the surgeon to be aware of a basic knowledge of the anatomy that he is about to invade. He is quoted: "If under such circumstances one does not know the position of an important nerve or muscle, or a large artery or vein, it can happen that one helps the patient to death, or sometimes mutilates him, instead of saving him." Some of the difficulties concerned with secondary infection and normal wound healing may be traced to inadequate management of operative hemorrhage. The loss of a patient's blood is a constant complication to every surgeon's procedure. The blood in the artery is bright red, relatively thin, and expelled by pulsations, whereas venous hemorrhage is a darker red, with a constant flow that can often be controlled by the application of pressure tampons. Modern methods of hemostasis have improved remarkably since the era of Hippocrates, when wounds were seared with hot irons to stop bleeding. Even as late as the sixteenth century, boiling oil was used to coagulate a bleeding wound.

The best means for controlling hemorrhage is that concerned with "clamping and tying" a visibly bleeding vessel. All severed arteries require ligation since blood loss under such pressure is rapid. Not all venous hemorrhage can be controlled by measures short of "clamping and tying," and many of the larger veins, like all of the arteries, must be ligated to control bleeding. The small, fine-pointed, hemostatic forceps perfected by Halsted is the instrument of choice for clamping *only* the severed end of the bleeding vessel. When surrounding tissue is also clamped with the vessel, the tissue so traumatized may necrose.

The fine-pointed tip of the hemostatic forceps grasping a bleeder is slightly raised to permit introduction of ligature material around the clamped tip of the forceps, and the first stage of a surgical knot is tied. The hemostat is then disengaged and the bleeding point reevaluated to assure that hemostasis is complete before applying the second stage of the surgical tie. In ligating bleeders, gauze pads are more effective in sponging than is a mechanical aspirator since they permit a periodic application of pressure over the bleeding point and a momentary hemostasis. When the pressing gauze is removed, a sudden flow of blood helps to quickly locate the severed vessel.

In the oral surgery field there is small choice as regards the material best indicated for ligating vessels. Classically, subcutaneous tissues are closed and vessels are ligated with absorbable materials such as surgical gut. Tanned surgical gut (chromicized) is more slowly resorbed than is plain surgical gut and for that reason is preferred by many operators for ligating larger vessels and suturing fascia, tendons, and ligaments. Skin and mucous membrane are classically closed by suture with nonabsorbable materials such as silk, cotton, nylon, and wire. However, these classical concepts are currently in varied stages of alteration, and many outstanding surgeons are using nonabsorbable materials where only surgical gut was previously permitted. Some prefer to use cotton subcutaneously and silk on the surface. One teaching institution may not permit the burying of nonabsorbable materials because these are foreign bodies; another school may consider that surgical gut is a poor choice in that it is a culture media for the gross multiplication of bacteria in postoperative infection.

Cautery of bleeding vessels is effectively practiced in many of the surgical specialties. Electrocoagulation employs the principle of searing the cut ends of blood vessels to seal off hemorrhage. It is best used in managing hemorrhage from smaller vessels. In the larger vessels, especially those under arterial pressure, such coagulated eschar may separate more easily than might the surgical knot in good ligation. Postoperative hemorrhage in a ward or in the living room is infinitely more difficult to manage than it would be in an operating room. Electrocoagulation is best indicated where ligation cannot be effectively employed, as, for instance, in friable glandular tissues or in a venous plexus. Neurosurgeons use electrocoagulation to a wide extent and to great advantage. At present the Bovie unit providing faradic current in noncoagulative, coagulative, and surgical intensity is in common use at many hospitals.

Pressure packs and tampons have remained through the years as one of the more satisfactory and convenient means for controlling capillary hemorrhage. In stubborn cases a pressure pack soaked in hot water hastens clotting. Hematomas should be evacuated by adequate incision and drainage. Such accumulations of blood from injury or from inadequate hemorrhage control during and after surgery may exist as extravasations of blood within the tissue planes or as pools in hematomas.

A hematoma has no circulation until it becomes organized. It may harbor bacteria and provide optimum conditions for multiplication of such infectious colonies. It is quite difficult to manage an infected hematoma with antibacterial medication since there is no appreciable circulation to the hematoma. Hematomas are slowly digested and sometimes remain as residual, fibrous-walled cavitations.

Extravasation of blood in the tissue planes will produce edema and, if superficial enough, will be seen as ecchymosis. In the face such edematous and ecchymotic areas may drop by the sheer force of gravity into the tissue planes to become dispersed in the cervical areas and sometimes down on the anterior chest wall. This sequence is occasionally seen as a complication to tooth extraction when postoperative hemorrhage is inadequately controlled. Over a period of several days the edematous, ecchymotic discoloration (first black and blue, then fading to yellow) is observed to drop from the site of operation in the face into the neck and then subsequently to the area of clavicles from which the fascia originate.

Summarizing the management of hemorrhage. Visible bleeding from an isolated vessel is controlled by clamping and ligation. Capillary hemorrhage in bony cavitations responds to pressure tampons. It may be necessary to first pack the bony cavitation with a hemostatic agent (such as oxidized cellulose, or gelatin sponge saturated in Adrenalin or thrombin) before a pressure tampon is applied. Sterile bone wax, made of beeswax, has proved effective in controlling capillary hemorrhage from bone. This bone wax is absorbable.

Concealed bleeding is subcutaneous and is usually the result of ligature failure of a large vessel. This will require the reopening of the wound and religation of the bleeding vessel. Prolonged hemorrhage with appreciable loss of blood volume requires antishock procedures.

In acute blood loss the early replacement of blood volume is indicated. Transfusion with fresh, matched whole blood is preferred.

Preoperative preparation to control postoperative hemorrhage in patients being maintained on anticoagulant medication for purposes of therapeutic hypoprothrombinemia is a subject deserving of special mention elsewhere in this text. At this point it is only pertinent to generally recognize such anticoagulant antagonists as are in wider usage today. The phytonadiones (vitamin K–like preparations) are considered to be chiefly effective in the prevention and treatment of hypoprothrombinemia incident to anticoagulant therapy when induced by the coumarin series of drugs. However, the use of phytonadiones for coumarin antagonism must not be substituted for whole blood transfusion when this latter demand exists. Currently, the antagonist for heparin is protamine.

It is fittingly proper to recognize the fact that despite the great progress being made in the fields of biological chemistry and hematology, the total understanding of the clotting mechanism of the blood has not yet been fully attained.

Snake venoms and escharotics such as tannic acid are sometimes used locally with occasional benefit. However, in one large hospital no snake venom was used for any hemorrhage problem whatsoever over the past 25 years. And escharotics may be only a short step beyond hot irons and boiling oil.

STERILIZATION OF ARMAMENTARIUM
Principles of sterilization

Autoclaving. Autoclaving is the preferred method of sterilization and the most reasonably certain for destroying resistant sporeformers and fungus. It provides moist heat in the form of saturated steam under pressure. This combination of moisture and heat provides the bacteria-destroying power currently most effective against all forms of microorganisms. Instruments and materials for sterilizing in the autoclave are usually enclosed in muslin wrappers as surgical packs. Muslin for this purpose is purchased most economically in bolt lots and cut to desired size. It is used in double thickness, and each surgical pack is marked as to contents and date of sterilization. Paper is now apparently supplanting muslin for wrapping surgical packs.

Several manufacturers are producing various types of paper wrappers. These papers have clothlike handling properties and present several advantages over muslin. They are less porous than muslin and thereby less likely to be penetrated by dust and microorganisms. However, they are sufficiently porous to permit required steam penetration under pressure. The crepe papers are currently in favor; they have some degree of elasticity and can be reused several times. Sterility under adequate paper wrapping appears to be effective for periods of 2 to 4 weeks' shelf life. This compares favorably with muslin-wrapped surgical packs.

Autoclaving time will vary directly with the size of the surgical pack. The smaller packs used for oral surgery usually require 30 minutes at 250° F. under 20 pounds' pressure. Various sterilization indicators can be inserted into a pack to provide evidence that adequate steam penetration has been effected. Rubber gloves are more fragile than linens and most instruments. They are sterilized effectively after 15 minutes under 15 pounds of pressure at 250° F.

Boiling-water sterilization. Ordinarily,

boiling-water sterilizers do not reach a temperature level above 212° F. Some of the heat-resistant bacterial spores may survive this temperature for prolonged periods of time. On the other hand, steam under 15 to 20 pounds' pressure will attain a temperature of 250° F., and most authorities concur that no living thing can survive 10 to 15 minutes' direct exposure to such saturated steam at that temperature. If boiling-water sterilization must be used, it is recommended that chemical means be employed to elevate the boiling point of water and thereby increase its bactericidal efficiency. A 2% solution of sodium carbonate will serve this purpose. Sixty milliliters of sodium carbonate per gallon of distilled water will make a 2% solution. This alkalinized distilled water reduces the required sterilization time and the oxygen content of the water as well, thereby reducing the corrosive action on the instruments.

Dry-heat sterilization. Sterilization in dry-heat ovens at elevated temperatures over long periods of time is widely used in dentistry and oral surgery. This technique provides a means for sterilizing instruments, powders, oils (petrolatums), bone wax, and other items that do not lend themselves to sterilization through the use of boiling water or steam under pressure. Dry heat will not attack glass and will not cause rusting. Furthermore, the ovens have additional uses in dentistry such as baking out and curing plastic pontics and other applications. The general design of the ovens permits a heating range of from 100° to 200° C. Overnight sterilization in excess of 6 hours at 121° C. is widely employed. Adequate sterilization of small loads is attained at 170° C. for 1 hour. The manufacturers of the dry-heat sterilizers provide detailed instructions for their effective use. The major disadvantage of dry-heat sterilization obviously is the long periods of time required to ensure bactericidal results.

Cold sterilization. None of the chemicals used for cold sterilization satisfactorily meets all of the requirements. Alcohol is expensive; it evaporates readily and also rusts instruments. The widely used benzalkonium chloride, 1:1,000 solution, requires an antirust additive (sodium nitrate) and long periods of immersion (18 hours). The more recently introduced cold-sterilizing chemicals employ hexachlorophene compounds as the active base. These chemicals claim adequate sterilization of heat-sensitive instruments in 3 hours. Fundamentally, most of the cold sterilizing media that may be safely used probably kill vegetative bacteria, but there is doubt of their effectiveness against spores and fungus.

Gas sterilization. The limitations of chemical solution sterilization techniques have made it necessary to exploit other methods for sterilizing the heat-sensitive or water-sensitive armamentarium. One of these other methods employs a gas, ethylene oxide, which is proved to be bactericidal when used in accordance with controlled environmental conditions of temperature and humidity as well as an adequate concentration of the gas for a prescribed period of sterilizing exposure. Ethylene oxide sterilizers are currently manufactured in varied sizes from the small (chamber measuring about 7.5 cm. in diameter), portable table model, to the large, built-in, stationary apparatus found in many of our hospitals. The smaller chambers use the gas as provided from convenient metal cartridges. The large, built-in sterilizers are hooked up to multiliter tanks.

The relatively high cost of using ethylene oxide sterilizers frequently results in their being used only "once or twice per day", more often for overnight sterilization of a capacity load. A hermetically sealed apparatus is necessary to economically ensure the retention of the expensive gas at its most effective concentration over a prolonged period of time ranging from 2 to 12 hours. Since ethylene oxide is highly diffusable, it requires a containing apparatus of precise manufacturing detail.

Under arid conditions desiccated microorganisms are known to resist the bactericidal effectiveness of ethylene oxide. Therefore the relative humidity within the sterilizing chamber should be controlled at an optimum of 40% to 50%. Also the efficiency of the gas sterilizer is reduced directly by temperature drops below 22° C.

In general, gas sterilization as currently employed in ethylene oxide techniques does indeed fill a necessary void in our presently available sterilization practices, but its shortcomings dictate the urgent need for better and less expensive methods.

Sterilization of supplies on industry-wide level

Our expanding population and the successful practice of geriatrics have greatly increased the demands for more medical services. Although the construction of hospitals to meet this demand has been slow and the training of medical personnel has been even slower, it is encouraging to observe the notable achievements of the pharmaceutical and hospital industry in the mass production of medical supplies. One of these major achievements concerns the development and profession-wide acceptance of sterile, disposable (single use) items. There are now so many disposable products in daily use that space precludes their individual discussion. Another achievement involves automation in manufacture, processing, sterilization, and packaging on an industrial scale. It is with the *sterilization* of disposables and other mass-produced medical supplies that our interest shall be concerned.

Modern manufacturing methods for medical supplies and their marketability have pointed out the shortcomings of former sterilization practices as applied to this industry. Whereas formerly heat, steam, gas, and bactericidal solutions were the only widely accepted means for sterilization, these methods could not be adapted to current mass production and marketing techniques. Many of the supplies, containers, illustrations, and enclosed printed matter could not withstand the sterilization procedures. The hermetic sealing of products and packages was impossible since asepsis was dependent upon permeation by heat, steam, gas, or bactericidal solutions. Heat-sensitive and water-sensitive equipment and supplies required special handling that was inadaptable to mass-production practices.

Today a radical change has been instituted in sterilization procedures for manufactured and packaged medical supplies. The change has been expensive but effective. Its success in industry has focused the attention of the professions on some of our rather archaic sterilization techniques. Briefly, the improved sterilization techniques employ ionizing radiation. The pharmaceutical and hospital industries are credited with developing, at considerable expense, a successful radiation sterilization technology. The military establishment of the federal government has also played a major role in its studies of irradiation sterilization of foodstuffs for preservation purposes. Both have contributed knowledge and standardization of irradiation techniques to the degree that now permits the safe and efficient use of gamma rays and accelerated beta rays on the wide scale used in food and drug technology. Today the manufacturer is able to package his product in a variety of containers that he could not use under previous sterilization methods. He can include directions, legends, illustrations, and heat-sensitive and water-sensitive materials and yet meet the profession's requirements of sterilization. As a matter of fact, in much of the industry all of the contents are packaged for final shipment before they are run through an irradiation building on a conveyor-belt system for the efficient sterilization of the entire shipping container and its contents.

Radiation sources. Ionizing radiation for sterilization as currently practiced is available through two sources: (1) machines of low energy but high output (electron accelerators) and (2) radioisotopes. The machines convert the electron output in a manner somewhat comparable to the output of an x-ray machine, but with a higher potential of several kilowatts of x-ray output. Of the isotopes, cobalt-60 and cesium-137 emit the highly penetrating gamma rays. At the present time the isotopes are more widely used. However, the electron accelerators (machines) have a number of advantages, and it is expected that they will ultimately supplant the radioisotopes for these purposes.

Insight into our current sterilization practices strongly suggests the need for improving the methods presently employed in the hospital and in the clinic. As previously indicated, the pharmaceutical industry is spending much time and money in furthering the use of radiation sources for sterilization of a wide array of products. Certainly irradiation is currently an expensive process. The capital investment and operating costs are beyond the scope of small institutions and private practice. But the overwhelming advantages of radiation sterilization dictate the continued exploitation of this field until it can be made available on a wide scale to the professions as well as to industry.

The presentation of this subject matter has been oversimplified. For this reason the discussions of Artandi[1] and Olander[2] are recommended for a more detailed and authoritative review of the technological aspects of radiation for sterilization.

General observations

1. Oils and grease are the major enemies of sterilization. Instruments exposed to oils should be wiped with a solvent and then vigorously scrubbed in soap and water before being put through a sterilizing procedure.

2. When instruments are completely immersed in boiling water, they will not rust. This is due to the fact that dissolved oxygen is driven out of the solution by the heat and is no longer available for corrosion. On the contrary, if wet instruments are exposed to air for any considerable period of time, rusting will occur. After boiling-water sterilization, instruments should be dried with a sterile towel while they are still hot.

3. Instruments with movable joints will require much less oiling if sterilized by autoclave rather than by boiling. This is especially true if tap water is used in the sterilizer since such water has a high concentration of lime salts, which are deposited on the instruments in boiling.

4. Particular precautions must be exerted in the adequate sterilization of hypodermic needles and syringes. Injections with contaminated equipment may produce latent symptomatology. With slow-incubating infections such as hepatitis, the infected patient may become jaundiced months after the injection. It is particularly recommended that hypodermic syringes and needles be sterilized, preferably by autoclaving, or by boiling water. Effectiveness of cold sterilization is alway doubtful.

5. Instruments are best stored in autoclaved muslin or paper packs. If unused, these packs should be reautoclaved every 30 days, unless there is a good reason for resterilization prior to that time.

6. Instrument packs should be organized in case pans so that the necessary instruments are included for routine procedures. The instruments can be removed from the pack and arranged on a tray (such as a Mayo tray or a dental bracket table). To this arrangement can be added additional instruments as required to meet the needs of a special situation. An unscrubbed assistant should handle sterile instruments only with a sterile pick-up forceps, which is kept constantly in a container of cold-sterilizing solution.

Comment

At this writing notable achievements are being made in the better aseptic control of the entire hospital environment—from the operating rooms, through the clinics, and into the supporting services. For instance, successful efforts are being made to control the direction of flow, the temperature, and the purity of the air circulated through the surgical operatories. Filterable microorganisms are removed, and the temperature of the air is adjusted before it is permitted to flow at a measured rate in a predetermined direction.

Postoperative infection receives the constant vigilance of staff medical and nursing care. Dressings are changed with strict adherence to aseptic principles. Resistant infections are identified and subjected to vigorous treatment when such is indicated, sometimes employing isolation of the patient and/or total bed rest. Infection committees composed of cognizant staff personnel are organized to ensure the proper care and disposition of unusual, acute, or persistent infections.

The central supply service must keep fully informed of the latest and best developments in the area of sterilization techniques so that there may be no doubt whatsoever about the sterility of such materials and equipment that are provided upon request. Dietetics, food services, the many laboratories, and even the general, overall housekeeping of the hospital environment require a thoughtful discipline and a constant surveillance in the maintenance of aseptic control.

PREOPERATIVE PREPARATION FOR ORAL SURGERY PROBLEMS

Frequently, many, but not all, oral surgical procedures are elective surgery.

It is of course unwise to provide any type of elective surgery for a patient who may not survive the anesthetic or the operative procedure. However, even the seriously sick must be rendered reasonable freedom from pain and infection, and fractured bones must be splinted. Even in poor-risk cases these procedures must be undertaken; it is best that such patients receive adequate preoperative evaluation in order that preparation may be made for anticipated complications in such calculated risks.

In the hospital a careful case history is obtained from all patients upon admission; a thorough physical examination and routine laboratory studies are done and there is consultation when required. For many reasons this procedure cannot be conveniently employed in the office practice of oral surgery. Furthermore, while many elective surgical procedures continue to be efficiently performed in the dental outpatient clinic or "dental office" practice, there remains no doubt that emergency oral surgery, like any major surgical procedure, is best performed in the hospital properly prepared to lend all physical, material, and personnel support to the oral surgeon. Today the general hospital already has an oral surgery service or is planning to make available this necessary care in the staff organization.

In the outpatient dental clinic a history is obtained from each patient so that unnecessary risks are avoided unless carefully calculated. This history may divulge information of great interest to a doctor contemplating surgery. Has this patient required medical care presently, or recently, and for what diagnosis? Was hospitalization required and what treatment was provided? Data concerning bleeding tendencies and drug sensitivities may require further exploration before surgery is instituted. An anesthetic history is imperative. How has this patient tolerated or responded to previous anesthetic agents? The psychological status of the patient relative to forthcoming surgery may very well establish the need for adequate preoperative sedation. It may well be unwise to administer a general anesthetic to patients who are emotionally disturbed to the extent that they are certain they cannot survive such procedure.

In a general sense such a brief history is

taken so that, if gross or remarkable findings are discovered, the patient may be referred to competent authority for further evaluation and preparation for the required oral surgery.

The preoperative sedation of an apprehensive patient is necessary; it serves to relieve great emotional tensions. Episodes of syncope, convulsion, and such other complications that extreme apprehension may produce can be aborted.

Hypnotics, analgesics, opiates, and antisialogogues are readily available to every doctor practicing dentistry, and there is little excuse for their not being used on a much wider, more intelligent basis. A tried-and-proved combination of barbiturates and an antisialogogue, using sodium pentobarbital and atropine sulfate, has been employed effectively for many years as a good preoperative medication. The usual plan is to administer 100 mg. of barbiturate to the patient upon retiring on the preoperative night. The following day, 1 hour before surgery, another dose of 100 mg. of barbiturate and 0.4 mg. of atropine are given. Of course the dosage is varied with the age, size, and general physical condition of the patient. Children and elderly patients require less drug. In difficult sedation problems, opiates may be substituted for barbiturates. Morphine, 15 mg., or meperidine, 75 to 100 mg., gives a more effective sedation than the somnifacience produced by barbiturates. Again, this dosage must be reduced for greater-risk cases.

Certainly a heavily sedated patient must be escorted to and from the dental clinic. The fact remains that many more complex oral operations can be performed under local anesthesia if such patients are prepared better preoperatively.

If the surgery is to be performed under local anesthesia, a light breakfast, or a light meal, about 2 hours prior to surgery is permissible. However, if a general anesthetic is to be used, the patient should fast for at least 6 hours prior to surgery. An enema is prescribed before the patient is taken to the operating room for general anesthesia.

Preoperative care and postoperative care of the patient are as much a part of good surgical technique as is the actual technical phase of the operative procedure.

Preoperative routine for patients requiring oral surgery

1. The patient is made fully aware of the need for, and the extent of, the operation that has been recommended.
2. The patient is informed of the type of anesthetic to be used.
3. The extent of anticipated postoperative disability is discussed with the patient.
4. If the patient is reluctant to submit to the recommended procedures, the treatment plan is delayed until such a time as the patient has become convinced of its necessity.
5. All male patients shall be cleanly shaved on the morning of surgery. Female patients shall not use facial cosmetics.
6. Valuables such as watches, money, jewelry, etc. shall be checked and placed in safekeeping.
7. Patients to be given general anesthesia shall be deprived of at least one meal prior to surgery. Children shall fast for 6 hours.
8. Premedication is according to plan. If somnifacience is adequate, barbiturates are employed. Otherwise, opiates are substituted. Antisialogogues such as atropine or scopolamine are given in general anesthesia cases and are used electively for local anesthesia problems.
9. Sedated patients are escorted to and from the clinic by an acquaintance, preferably a member of the family.
10. Surgery is not provided to minors without the consent of parents or guardian.

Comment

The usual hospital preoperative routine requires that the surgeon visit the patient on the evening prior to surgery. At this time preoperative and postoperative orders may be written and arrangements made for posting the case on the operating room schedule.

On the morning of surgery the doctor arrives in the hospital early enough to review the patient's current history and to bring the ward chart up to date. He arranges to have the necessary records and the roentgenograms accompany the patient to the operating room. He confers with assistants regarding the need for any special equipment and instruments not routinely set up for the particular surgical problem at hand. The plan for anesthesia is discussed with the responsible team, and the location of the anesthetic armamentarium, relative to the patient's head, where oral surgery will be done, is predetermined.

OPERATING ROOM DECORUM

The work of Lister has proved conclusively the role played by bacteria in wound infection. It is now mandatory in all surgery, within the mouth as well as elsewhere, that all intelligent, precautionary measures be taken to avoid the contamination of wounds.

While the means for providing strictly aseptic mouth surgery are still unavailable, this is no reason for completely abandoning an aseptic routine. At the very least an aseptic routine for mouth surgery markedly eliminates some of the dangers of cross infection; that is, the infection of the doctor from the patient, the infection of the patient from the doctor, or the infection of the patient from another patient through the doctor or through the contaminated armamentarium employed by the doctor. It has long been established that surgical wounds are contaminated chiefly from microorganisms harbored in the skin or mucous membranes that have been incised. Furthermore, the oral cavity is a normal breeding ground for a wide assortment of microorganisms. The noses, throats, and hands of the *operating team* are the next most frequent source of wound infection. Unsterile instruments and supplies follow in order of importance. For the latter there is no excuse.

Complete asepsis in surgery may very well be an ideal that is never fully attained. There may always be some doubt regarding the sterility of the skin or the mucous membranes to be incised. The air contamination of wounds is an omnipresent problem. But if wound infection in surgery is to be minimized, all logical precautions and preparations must be instituted.

This should include the proper preparation of the operating team as well as the patient. Wherever surgery is done, in the hospital operating room or in the clinic, the surgeon wears a face mask of four-ply, fine-meshed gauze and a surgical helmet of linen or cloth such as the stockinette used under plaster casts. However, here as elsewhere throughout the hospital, paper is gaining favor over cloth for disposable face masks and headgear. The surgeon's hands are adequately scrubbed. Presently, highly detergent soaps containing hexachlorophene are commonly used in prescribed scrub techniques. Sterile gloves are used for all surgery, and these, like sterile sheets, wraps, towels, etc., serve bacteriologically to isolate the doctor from the patient.

Scrub technique

1. Street clothes are replaced with a scrub suit (Fig. 2-1). This consists of clean linen trousers and a short-sleeved blouse. In the operating room where static electricity may be a complicating problem, the surgical personnel will wear appropriate conductive footwear. Each shoe will have a sole and heel of conductive rubber, conductive leather, or equivalent material. Such shoes have metal electrodes fabricated into the inner soles so that conductive contact is maintained with the stockinged foot.

2. A surgical helmet and a face mask are donned. It is an unwritten rule that

Principles of surgical technique 25

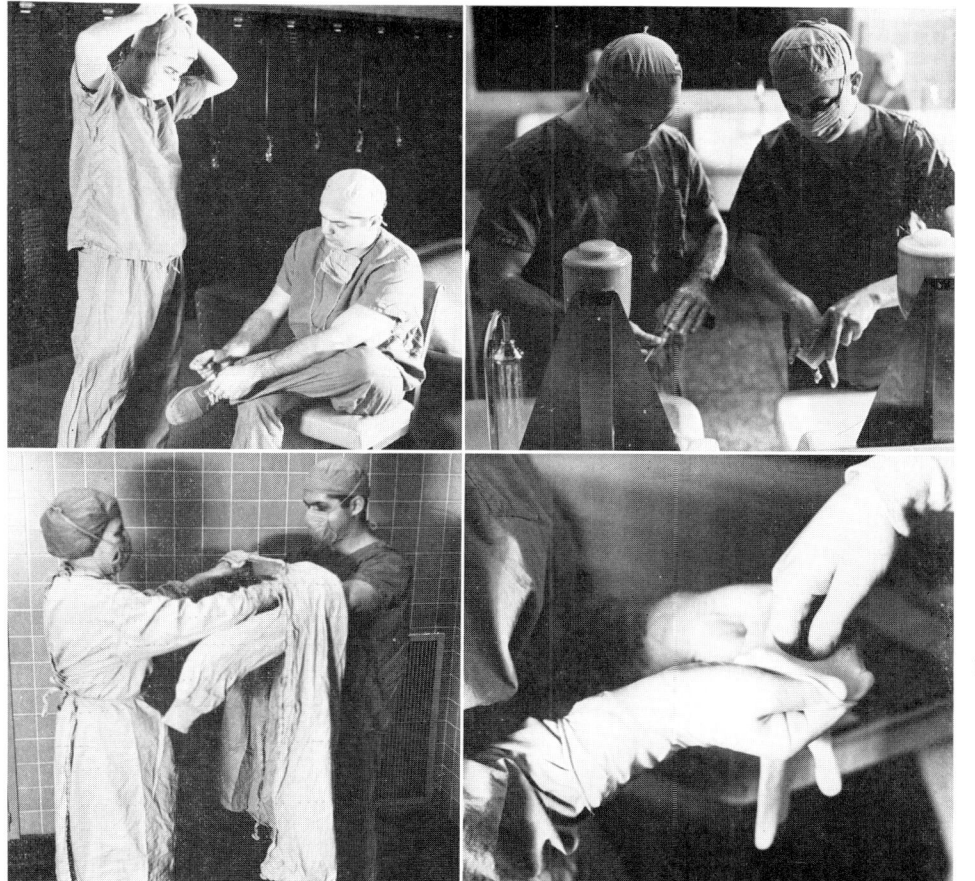

Fig. 2-1. Typical scrub suit attire. (Official U. S. Navy Photograph.)
Fig. 2-2. Scrub technique is in accordance with instructions usually posted over the scrub sink. (Official U. S. Navy Photograph.)
Fig. 2-3. The doctor is helped into his sterile gown by a scrubbed assistant. (Official U. S. Navy Photograph.)
Fig. 2-4. The doctor is helped into the gloves so that only the interior of the gloves is touched by his hand. (Official U. S. Navy Photograph.)

sneezing and coughing are not permitted in the operating room.

3. The surgical scrubbing is carried out in the manner prescribed for major surgery. The hands and forearms are scrubbed to the elbows with brush and soap (or hexachlorophene detergents) and water according to prescribed plan. At many hospitals the recommended scrub technique is posted directly over the scrub sinks (Fig. 2-2). Two-minute scrubs in between operations may be acceptable. However, it should be mentioned that numerous hospitals frown on any scrub technique requiring less than 10 minutes. During the scrub the fingernails must be adequately cleansed. Sterile orangewood sticks are conveniently provided for this purpose. If nondetergent soap

is used for the scrub, a longer scrub period is required and a postscrub rinse with a low surface tension antiseptic such as alcohol or Septisol is recommended.

4. The hands are dried in the operating room with a sterile hand towel. At this stage the hands are considered surgically clean but *not sterile*.

5. The surgeon is helped into his sterile gown by a properly gowned and gloved surgical assistant (Fig. 2-3). A circulating assistant secures the gown ties at the sur-

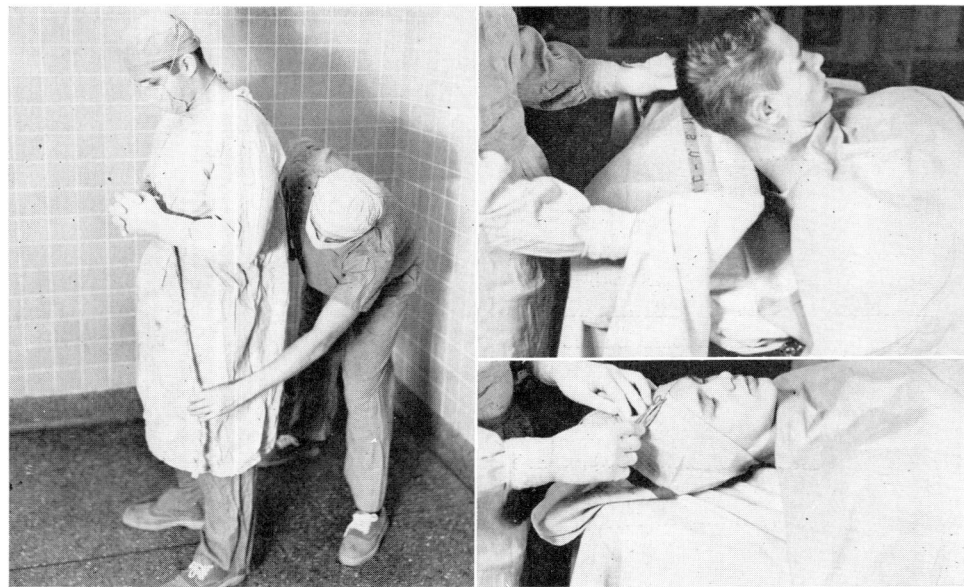

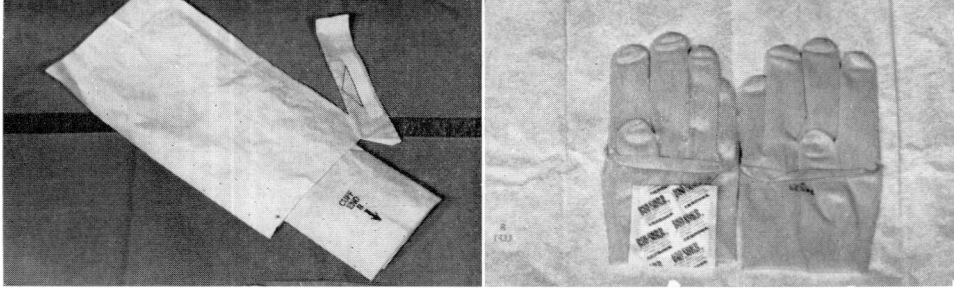

Fig. 2-5. The entire back of the surgeon's gown and also that portion of the front of the gown below the level of the surgical table will be considered as unsterile. (Official U. S. Navy Photograph.)

Fig. 2-6. A drape and a hand towel are combined for wrapping the patients. Double hand towels may be similarly used. (Official U. S. Navy Photograph.)

Fig. 2-7. Towels and drapes are secured by clipping. (Official U. S. Navy Photograph.)

Fig. 2-8. **A**, Sterile, disposable, latex surgeon's gloves are packaged in exterior and interior paper wrappings to permit usage under aseptic conditions. **B**, A packet of dusting powder or cream is included with the cuff-turned gloves enclosed in the sterile interior wrapping. Sterilization is by irradiation.

geon's back. The surgeon's back as well as the gown below the level of the waist are considered *unsterile* (Fig. 2-5).

6. The surgeon is helped into his gloves in such a manner that *only the interior* of the gloves is touched by his hands (Fig. 2-4). The exterior and not the interior of the rubber glove is considered sterile.

Only a minimal amount of dusting agent is permitted in preparing the hands for the wearing of rubber gloves. Modified starch powder has replaced talcum as the dusting agent of choice. However, sterile creams are being used for this purpose more than dusting agents. In the surgery of open wounds consideration must be given to the irritating, granuloma-producing propensity of foreign materials such as talcum, starch, and creams when used in excessive amounts and when inadvertently introduced into the wound.

Sterile isolation is provided only through the wearing of gloves. Sterile gloves are employed for the protection of the patient and the doctor. The dangers of cross infection make it imperative for the professional worker to wear gloves whenever the blood, tissue fluids, or saliva is contacted. Tuberculosis thrives in oral fluids. Serum hepatitis may be present in the blood of asymptomatic patients.

Isolation of patient from operating team

1. The site of incision is prepared. The operative field is cleansed by scrubbing with detergent soap, rinsing, and then painting with a suitable antiseptic.

2. The patient is further isolated from the doctor through the use of sterile drapings of cloth or clothlike materials. The initial drape may be a single-thickness draw sheet measuring approximately 115 by 180 cm. A second drape, called a front sheet, measures about 115 by 175 cm., completing the major isolation (Fig. 2-6).

3. The patient's head is wrapped in a double-sheet technique, using a drape as the lower sheet and a hand towel as the upper sheet (Fig. 2-6).

4. Sterile drapings are secured with towel clips (Fig. 2-7). In some oral surgical problems requiring the manipulation of the patient's head from side to side, it is good practice to suture to the skin those sterile drapings outlining the periphery of the incision.

5. The anesthetist and his equipment are isolated from the operating team by a drape-covered screen.

6. Only that field above the level of the surgical table is considered sterile. Hands, equipment, and supplies lowered below the level of the surgical table are considered as having been contaminated.

7. Organization is such that once the surgeon has completed the scrub, put on sterile gloves, and draped the patient, it will be unnecessary to break scrub to obtain needed items.

8. It is important at this point to establish the fact that a gown, drape, or covering is considered as *contaminated when wet*—unless the gown, drape, or covering is made of waterproof material or otherwise backed by a waterproof lining or sheathing.

Modifications of aseptic routine for office practice of oral surgery

One school of thought will insist that there can be no compromise with the aseptic measures employed in surgery. Another group may insist that a rigid aseptic technique is not practical in a busy office practice dealing with minor oral surgery in a large volume of patients. The fact remains that infection does not differentiate minor from major surgery, large numbers from small numbers of patients, or short operations from long operations.

It is generally believed that the reason for the relatively low incidence of oral infection following surgical procedures within the mouth can be traced directly to "man's acquired tolerance for his own microorganisms." No doubt these same organisms transmitted to another individual in cross infection may quite likely result in virulent infection. In other words, man can tolerate his own organisms better than he can somebody else's. This fundamentally proper concept justifies the need for aseptic technique in surgical areas that defy complete bacterial sterilization, areas such as the mouth, the nasal and antral cavities, the digestive and urinary tracts, etc.

Despite the care that the operator may exert in preparing himself, his instruments, his supplies, and his patient for oral surgery, the dangers of cross infection are omnipresent. All reasonably intelligent efforts at limiting this danger of infection are the least that the patient should expect from his doctor.

Much of the operating room decorum employed for major surgery is within practical limits for oral surgical procedures. In the hospital operating room the level of the surgical table is the line of demarcation for asepsis. In the dental clinic the level of the armrests of the dental chair might be considered as a similar line of demarcation. Everything above the armrests should be subject to aseptic requirements.

The perioral facial skin should be as carefully prepared as the mucosa directly involved in surgery. This can be conveniently done by asking the patient to wash the face with detergent hexachlorophene provided in the washroom. Thereafter, a colorless, nonirritating antiseptic is applied to the perioral skin as well as to the mucosa. The patient's mouth is lavaged with a pleasant-tasting, antiseptic solution, and the immediate area of the needle puncture or incision is painted with an antiseptic having staining qualities so that the area for surgery is clearly visualized as having been antiseptically prepared.

The patient's hair may be enclosed in a sterile wrapping such as that employing double hand towels.

Most patients are highly pleased with any extra effort that the doctor may choose to employ in assuring a safer operation (Figs. 2-9 and 2-10). Many patients prefer that the doctor's hands be gloved before they invade the mouth. In short-duration, large-volume surgery, rubber gloves need not be changed for each patient. Instead, the gloved hands may be scrubbed between patients, using a 2-minute scrub technique with detergent, hexachlorophene soaps (Fig. 2-11). The difficulty with this method is that the rubber gloves, when washed and dried in this manner, become "tacky" and thereby somewhat difficult to use unless used wet.

Surgical caps and masks need not be changed for each operation. The surgeon's gown can be isolated from the sterile sheets used over the patient by clamping a sterile hand towel over that portion of the surgeon's gown which contacts the patient's sterile coverings (Fig. 2-12). There will be opposition, of course, from uninformed patients and from some doctors to such recommendations concerning the need for sterile approach to so-called minor surgery in the mouth. But less than a hundred years ago there was similar opposition to the doctor who "fussed so much" washing his hands preparatory to surgery—and then proceeded to turn up the contaminated sleeves of his frock coat before reaching for the scalpel. In those days "laudable pus" was erroneously accepted as a necessary sequel to surgery. There can be no justification whatsoever for permitting the "laudable pus" concept in oral surgery today.

Disposable (single use) materials and equipment

Modern manufacturing, sterilizing, and packaging techniques are currently providing an ever-wider array of supplies conveniently packaged for single use and disposal thereafter. The increasing cost of labor in the multiple handling of reusable hospital supplies has resulted, in many instances, in making the use of disposables a more economical practice.

Paper and similar man-made fibers are replacing woven cloth for sheeting, drapes, toweling, etc. Lap sheets, stand covers, and

Principles of surgical technique 29

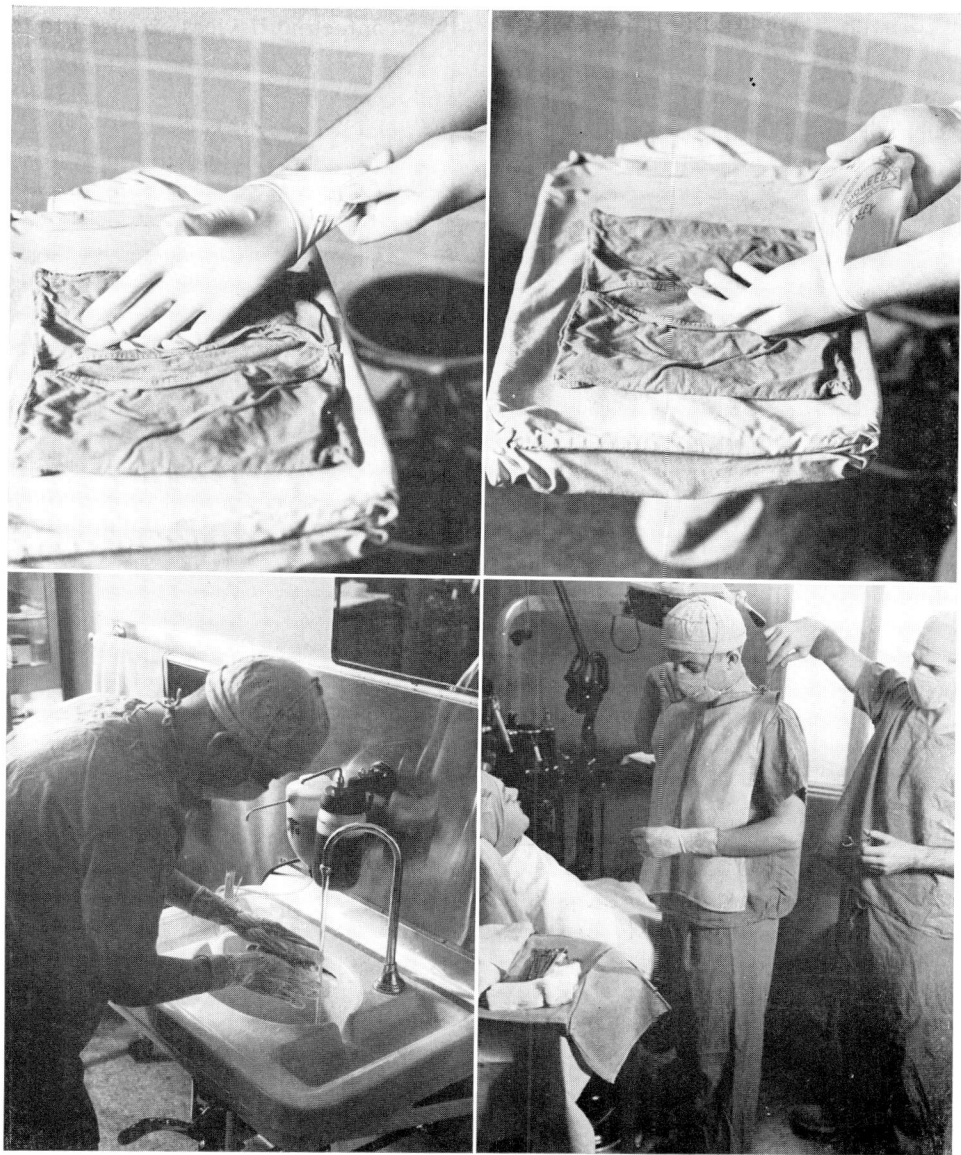

Fig. 2-9. Only the interior of the glove is touched by the bare hands. (Official U. S. Navy Photograph.)

Fig. 2-10. The sterile gloves may touch each other on their exterior surfaces. (Official U. S. Navy Photograph.)

Fig. 2-11. In large-volume, short-duration mouth surgery, it may be permissible to employ 2-minute scrub of the gloved hands between patients. This is in lieu of changing gloves for each patient. (Official U. S. Navy Photograph.)

Fig. 2-12. In office practice, a sterile hand towel is often used for isolating the surgeon's attire from the patient's draping. (Official U. S. Navy Photograph.)

surgical wrappings are now available in sterile, ready-to-use packages conveniently and economically disposable after single usage. Seamless, disposable latex gloves that can be placed on surgically scrubbed hands without the need of dusting powders or creams are now being used in many hospitals and clinics.

Hypodermic needles, syringes, and plastic collection tubes and containers for biological specimens are currently packaged as disposables. Intravenous techniques concerned with the collection and infusion of blood, administration of drug and fluid therapy, etc. are largely accomplished through the use of disposable plastic supplies and equipment. Almost every department of the hospital or clinic concerned with dispensing professional care seems to be using more and more of the increasingly available disposables. The potential for single-use supplies seems limitless.

Of course the more disposables used within an activity the more an increased, adequate storage area is required for supplies with such a rapid turnover.

Some fundamental precautions with gaseous mixtures in operating rooms

The following anesthetic agents are considered combustible, and precautionary procedures must be employed in their administration: (1) cyclopropane, (2) divinyl ether (Vinethene), (3) ethyl ether, (4) ethyl chloride, and (5) ethylene. An explosion in an operating room is indeed a dramatic hazard, and unfortunately, like the automobile or airplane accident, it is classified as "something that happens to somebody else." As a regular operating room routine, the following precautionary measures are employed:

1. Modern operating rooms are built with conductive flooring. Operating room personnel and visitors must wear conductive footwear. Such shoes are usually made with conductive rubber or conductive leather soles and heels. They contain stainless steel conductors built into the inner sole so that frictional static electricity may be grounded and sparking avoided. Other floor-contacting devices are used to ground equipment used in the vicinity of explosive, gaseous mixtures.

2. Wool, silk, and synthetic textures are known to produce electrical charge when subjected to friction. For this reason no woolen blankets and silk or nylon garments are permitted in the operating rooms.

3. Electrical equipment and anesthetic and other apparatus commonly used in the presence of combustible gases must be periodically examined to assure freedom from any defect that might emit spark in the presence of explosive mixtures.

4. Electrocautery, electrocoagulation, and other equipment employing open spark are of course not permitted in the vicinity of combustible gases.

Oxygen cylinders

Ordinarily, oxygen is not considered an explosive agent, but it does support combustion and perhaps, thereby, it may be considered as secondarily contributory to explosion. Some basic precautions must be taken with the care of oxygen cylinders[3]:

1. Fundamentally, oils, greases, and lubricants may be highly combustible with oxygen. Therefore, their proximity to oxygen must be avoided. Regulators, gauges, and other fittings on oxygen cylinders must not be lubricated when the cylinder contains the gas under pressure.

2. Oxygen cylinders must not be handled with oily hands and greasy gloves or rags.

3. Before applying fittings to the cylinder, clear the duct opening by allowing a momentary escape of gas.

4. Open the high-pressure valve on the cylinder *before* bringing the oxygen apparatus to the patient. Open this valve slowly and take common precautionary measures concerned with unexpected explosion.

Principles of surgical technique 31

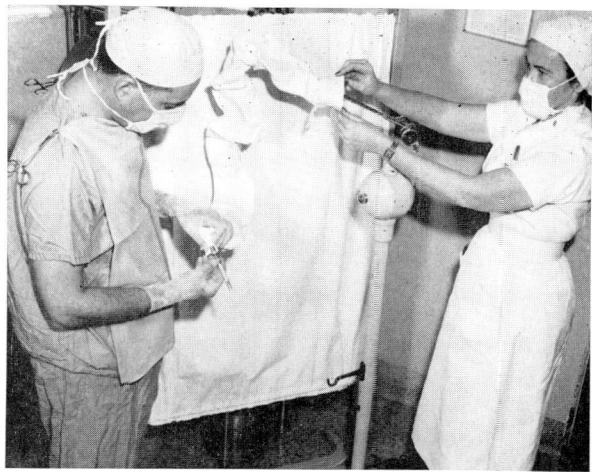

Fig. 2-13. The cable and extensions from the portable dental engine are covered with a sterile sleeve for operating room procedures. (Official U. S. Navy Photograph.)

5. Avoid covering the oxygen cylinder with gowns, linens, etc., which may serve to contain leaking gas.

6. Never use oxygen from a cylinder that does not have a pressure-reducing regulator.

7. Do not attempt to repair any of the attachments on a cylinder containing oxygen under pressure.

BASIC ORAL SURGERY
Incision

The efficient employment of a scalpel requires a basic knowledge of convenient fulcrum points already taught the dental surgeon during his instruction in the use of motor-driven instruments within the mouth. The scalpel is gripped firmly but lightly in any one of several grasps. It should not be grasped too rigidly in such a manner as to produce digital tremors and otherwise influence the unrestricted movement that is required in producing a clean, atraumatic incision.

Two of the scalpel grasps most commonly used in oral surgery are illustrated. The "pen grasp" (in which the handle of the blade is engaged between the thumb and first two fingers) is favored for the delicate, short strokes frequently required for intraoral surgery (Fig. 2-14).

Skin is more difficult to incise than mucosal tissue, and the steady pressure required for such cutting may be better obtained by grasping the scalpel in the illustrated "table-knife" manner (Fig. 2-15).

The choice of using one scalpel grasp over another becomes a matter of individual preference. It is more important that an atraumatic technique for incision and excision procedures be developed so that a sharp scalpel may be safely and efficiently employed. It is much safer to use a fulcrum point during surgical incision so that the scalpel may be braced through fingers resting on bone or tooth structure conveniently adjacent to the line of incision. A clear visualization of the area about to be incised is imperative.

Intraoral incisions involving the reflection of the mucoperiosteum for exposure of bone or dental structures are direct, straight-line, or curvilinear incisions taking the shortest distance through the tissues. However, where underlying bone may be remote from the site of the incision, such

32 *Textbook of oral surgery*

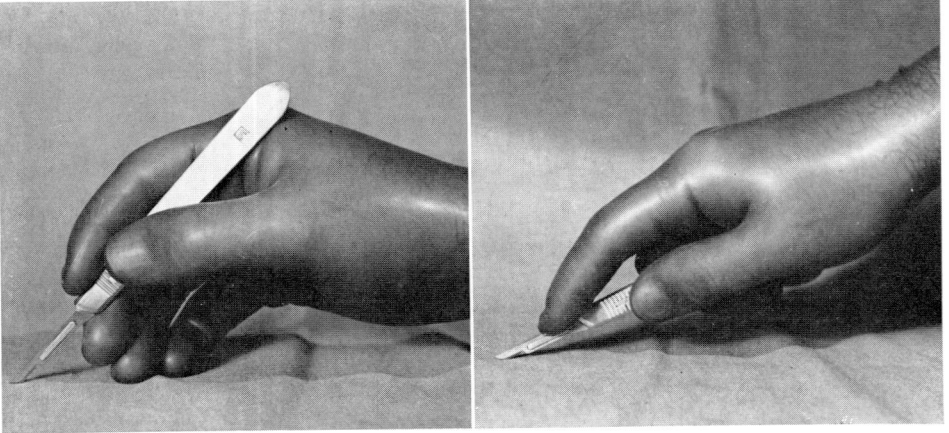

Fig. 2-14. The "pen grasp," commonly used in oral surgery, permits the grasping of the scalpel handle between the thumb and first two fingers. The third and fourth fingers provide a rest position (fulcrum) on a firm base from which short, deft, incising strokes may be safely instituted.

Fig. 2-15. The "table-knife" grasp permits the thumb and second finger to engage the scalpel handle, which is further supported in its upper end by the palm of the hand. The index finger rests on the dull edge of the blade and provides the necessary pressure for more vigorous incising.

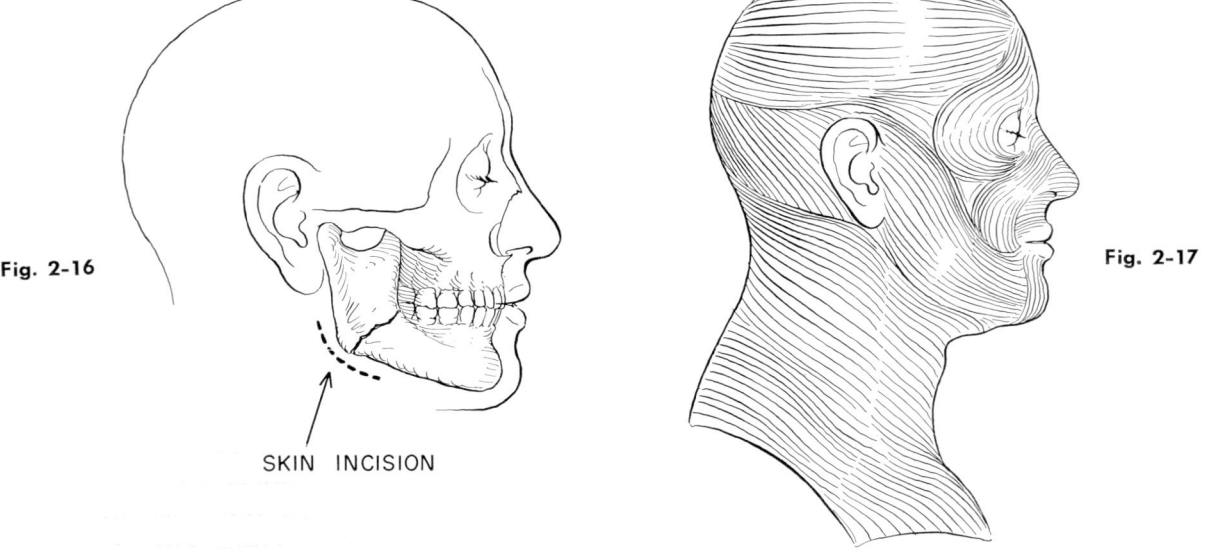

Fig. 2-16. Submandibular incision in natural shadow line of mandible. This approach is often employed for open surgical procedures on the body of the mandible.

Fig. 2-17. Langer's lines of skin tension throughout the face.

as when operating upon the soft palate, tongue, cheeks, lips, and floor of the mouth, the incision is not necessarily direct. In these cases the incision is made only through the mucosa. Thereafter, blunt dissection is combined with further sectioning, or scissors section, so that important anatomical structures are not needlessly sacrificed. Such dissection may be carried out with blunt instruments; the tissue layers are separated by actual tearing. Hemostatic forceps, rounded scissors, the handle end of a scalpel, or the gloved finger of the surgeon is commonly used for blunt dissection.

Cleavage dissection, in which the tissue layers are exposed by accurate snipping of the tissues with a sharp scissors or scalpel, produces less blind trauma than does blunt dissection. This, however, requires more detailed anatomical knowledge. The actual cutting is necessary only to expose a line of cleavage between tissue layers, permitting easy separation of the layers until another line of cleavage is exposed. The next tissue layer is then cut and dissected until another cleavage is encountered. Thus an orderly and atraumatic approach is made to the pathological area.

Skin surgery on the face carries the cosmetic requirement that the postoperative scar be minimal in size and so uncomplicated as to be esthetically acceptable. Whenever possible, these incisions are concealed in natural wrinkles, in the hairline, along the mucocutaneous junctions, or in shaded areas such as the nasolabial fold and the immediately submandibular-cervical zones (Fig. 2-16). Furthermore it is desirable that skin incisions be made along, and not across, the "grain" of the skin (sometimes referred to as the "lines of tension" or Langer's skin lines) (Fig. 2-17). Incisions made *in* Langer's lines will permit wide exposure of the operative field since these are really cleavage lines of the superficial tissue planes. If incisions are made across these lines of tensions, the sutures will be placed under maximum stress and the possibility of unfavorable cicatricial formation will be enhanced.

Hair clipping, of course, is necessary when hairy areas are invaded. However, eyebrows are not shaved and eyelashes are not clipped.

Particular attention must be given to the prevention of wound infection since septic wounds may heal with irregular and extensive scarring. Depression contraction and hypertrophy along the line of incision produces unsatisfactory cosmetic results and oftentimes requires corrective surgery that might have been avoided if adequate early care had been thoughtfully administered. Incisions must be made with a sharp scalpel, perpendicular to the skin surface, and preferably in the natural skin creases (Langer's lines of tension). The capable surgeon is especially adept at the gentle handling of soft tissue. "Heavy-handed" retracting may very well result in the necrotizing of such injured tissue with subsequent healing by second intention and considerably more scarring than was necessary. In suturing a skin incision about the face, a slight eversion of the skin edges is preferred. This will compensate for anticipated swelling and permit the levelling out of the eversion without loss of the edge contact of the skin incision. It is simply a means for aborting a spreading of the line of incision.

Skin edges must not be sutured too tightly, and the sutures should be removed on the third or fourth day to avoid suture scars. Halsted's basic teachings can well be repeated—the suture material should be no stronger than the tissue itself; a greater number of fine stitches is better than a few coarse ones; fine silk or cotton, Nos. 3-0, 4-0, and 5-0, is used to best advantage for skin incisions on the face. When it is necessary to support such fine skin suturing, this may be done by the following methods:

1. The use of deep, dermal tension sutures

2. Antitension elastic and adhesive bandaging across the suture line
3. The use of pressure bandaging
4. Subcuticular (intradermic) suturing with fine-gauge, stainless steel wire

Any history of keloid scar formation should be recorded in the patient's history, and both doctor and patient should be fully aware of the calculated risks assumed in this regard. The Negroid race is thought to be most predisposed to keloid formation, but this problem is not limited by racial boundaries.

Suture materials

Currently in oral surgery there appears to be a preference for the use of nonabsorbable suture materials for cutaneous, mucosal, and deeper layer approximations. However, there is still wide usage of absorbable suture materials in subsurface closures. Of the absorbable sutures, catgut is commonly used. Actually, catgut is a misnomer since the material is made from the serosa layer of sheep intestine. It is provided by manufacturers as plain and tanned (chromic) in a suitably wide range of sizes.

Of the nonabsorbable suture materials, black silk is widely used. It has an adequate tensile strength, produces minimal tissue reaction, and can be readily seen for convenient removal. No. 4-0 is quite popular in oral surgery. If purchased in spool lots, it is inexpensive. Ordinary cotton sewing thread No. 40, quilting, has many of the advantages of silk and is even less expensive.

Atraumatic-type sutures of both absorbable and nonabsorbable materials are put up by various manufacturers in sealed ampules containing a cold sterilizing medium. The atraumatic feature comprises a fine, ½-circle or ⅜-circle needle which is swaged-on one end of the suture material.

Wire mesh

In oral surgery wire mesh is sometimes used to fill in bony defects and to develop lost bony contours. Tantalum mesh is most satisfactory because it is best tolerated when buried in the tissues. However, it is expensive. Stainless steel mesh has been gaining popularity as a satisfactory, less expensive substitute for tantalum. Wire mesh is made of very thin wires about 0.008 cm. in diameter. The mesh is woven with about twenty-two wires to the centimeter. This allows sufficient spacing to permit tissue to grow through the wire meshing. The mesh must be sutured with wire of the same material or with nonabsorbable silk or cotton to eliminate the possibility of galvanic current activity.

Dressings

The primary intent of dressings is to keep the surgical field free of infection. Second, dressings support the incision, protect it from trauma, and absorb drainage. Intraorally, dressings are not used for these purposes. Within the mouth they are used as drains or as vehicles for carrying medicaments, obtundants, etc. to the operative site. Sterile strip gauze, 1 or 2 cm. wide, is preferred. This gauze may be plain or iodoform. The iodoform gauze has antiseptic qualities, but it also has a strong, persistent, medicinal odor. When used as a drain, strip gauze may be saturated in petrolatum to facilitate removal after its purpose has been served.

For extraoral wounds, gauze pads in 5 by 5 cm. and 10 by 10 cm. squares are practical. Such gauze pads are maintained in position by adhesive or elastic bandage. Elastoplast bandage is a cotton elastic with adhesive on one side. Because it is elastic it does not constrict; yet it provides the desirable gentle, even pressure required in firmly supporting a dressing and avoiding incisional hernia. Pressure bandaging is frequently employed for dressing facial incisions. The chief purpose for using pressure dressings is the need for splinting the soft tissues and minimizing edema that might tear through sutures and reopen the incision. They also serve to eliminate dead space, control secondary, capillary oozing, and abort hematoma. Pressure dressings consist essentially of bulky materials such as fluffed gauze, mechanic's waste, sea sponges, and foam rubber. The bulky material is placed directly over the sterile gauze pads covering a wound and is retained in position by an elastic bandage.

A few objections to compression bandaging should be pointed out so that they may be recognized and eliminated if possible. These dressings are constrictive by design, and when used over a progressively swelling area, they are painful. They may be responsible for lymphatic and venous blockage and thereby increase, rather than decrease, the swelling for which they were used. Pressure bandages should be heavily padded to be effective. They should be carefully observed for stasis and swelling beyond the edges of the bandage. If this occurs, the bandage should be either eliminated or the compression released for short periods of time to relieve the stasis.

Compression bandaging, when intelligently employed, will promote good wound healing with excellent cosmetic results at the line of incision. When poorly employed, such dressings will not only retard healing but may also stimulate fibrosis through lymphatic and venous obstruction in areas somewhat remote from the site of actual wound healing.

OPERATIVE TECHNIQUE
General

It is not the purpose of this chapter to deal with the detailed anatomy in the oral surgery field. This information is readily and authoritatively available through many well-known sources. Fundamentally, the major facial vessels concerned in oral surgical exposures run a course that is (1) deep to the superficial muscles of expression (including the platysma but excluding the caninus and buccinator muscles) and (2) superficial to the muscles of mastication and, of course, the deeper facial bones. In a similarly general sense, the facial vein drains the areas supplied by the facial artery, and the posterior facial vein drains those deeper facial areas supplied by the terminal branches of the external carotid artery. The major sensory nerve to the face is the fifth cranial nerve. The major motor nerve to the face (other than to the muscles of mastication, which are supplied by the fifth) is the seventh cranial nerve. Surgical injury to the fifth cranial nerve may be considered of minor significance since sequel to such injury most likely would be sensory paresthesia with good chance for regeneration. However, surgical injury to the seventh cranial nerve and subsequent loss of function of the muscles of expression presents extreme cosmetic problems without much hope for spontaneous and functional regeneration.

A thorough knowledge of the anatomical relations of the tissues that the surgeon is about to invade is of course a mandatory responsibility. It is common practice among young surgeons of limited experience to perform the proposed surgery in cadaver dissection prior to the actual operation. Such procedure is good technique and is not to be misinterpreted as indicating deficiency.

Submandibular approach to the ascending ramus and body of the mandible

Most extraoral surgery requiring exposure of the mandible is done through a submandibular approach. The area about the angle of the mandible is considered more complex than are the more anterior zones, and this area will be discussed surgically.

The location of the incision must be given careful consideration to be sure that deeper anatomical structures are exposed to view in normal relationship. Positioning of the patient or rotating or extending his head may considerably alter the location of the incision as compared to its location

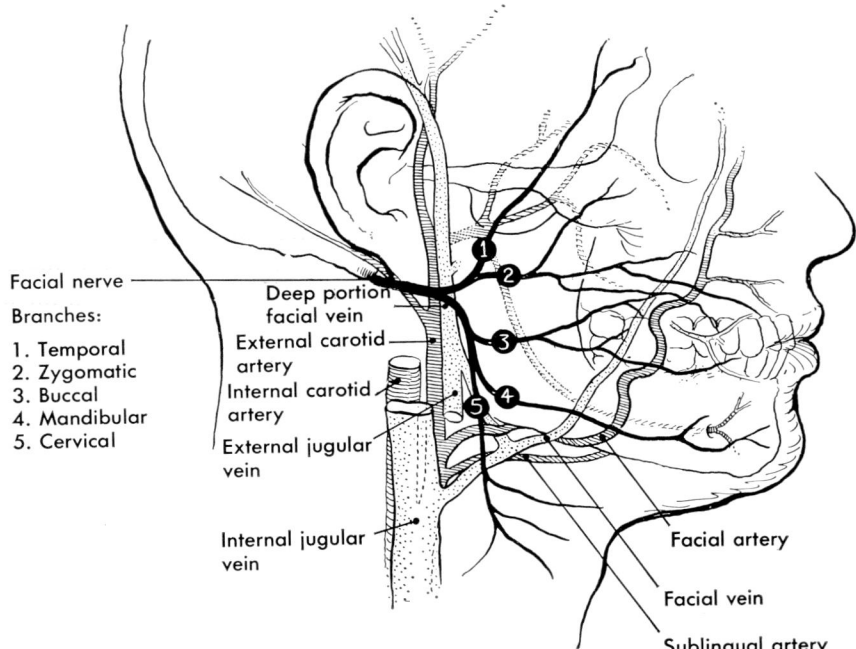

Fig. 2-18. General distribution of facial nerve, arterial blood supply to face, and venous return from face.

when the patient is seated at rest. The incision in the submandibular approach should be made in one of the lines of skin tension, and it should be predetermined and marked either by superficial scratching with the back edge of a scalpel or by marking with an analine dye. The gonial angle of the mandible and the notch in the inferior border of the mandible (produced by the pulsating facial artery) should be marked as points of reference, the former indicating the posterior terminus of the operative field and the latter suggesting the location of the facial artery and the facial vein (Fig. 2-18). The incision is placed in the shadow line of the mandible about 2 cm. below the inferior border of the mandible and curved in best cosmetic conformity with that bone. This distance below the mandible will avoid cutting the mandibular branch of the facial nerve. The total length of the incision may vary between 6 and 8 cm.

"Crosshatching" the line of incision. With the line of incision predetermined and marked, the patient's head is extended and turned as far as possible to one side. This is for the convenience and comfort of the operating team. A final, brief consultation is held with the anesthesiologist relative to the patient's readiness for immediate surgery. The line of incision, clearly marked, is then "crosshatched" by scratching vertical lines with the back edge of a scalpel, perpendicular to the prospective line of incision. These vertical scratch lines should be about 1.5 cm. apart and extend, so spaced, throughout the length of the incision. Such "crosshatching" serves only to ensure that subsequent skin closure is perfectly approximated with the least possible scar.

The incision. The skin is stretched superiorly so that the marked line of incision rests on solid bone and thereby provides a firm base for a clean incision in one deft incising move. The depth of the incision should be vertical and completely through the skin. Cutting on the bias may result in widening of the ultimate scar. A Bard-Parker blade No. 10 or No. 15 is well suited to skin incisions in this area, but the choice of scalpel best rests with the operator's individual preference. Some bleeding points may be anticipated at this subcutaneous level. If the bleeding is arterial, the vessel is clamped with a Halsted mosquito hemostatic forceps and ligated with either fine cotton (No. 3-0 or 4-0) or plain surgical gut (No. 3-0). A square knot is recommended for vessel ligation, and the free ends are cut short on the knot.

Deeper soft tissue dissection. With the skin and subcutaneous areolar tissue incised, they may be widely undermined by blunt dissection, using a 14 cm., curved Mayo scissors, a hemostatic forceps, or the butt end of a knife handle. This will permit the insertion of retractors (such as a Kny-Scheerer trachea rake retractor) on each side of the incision to permit wide exposure and visualization of the underlying platysma muscle. A few points of interest relative to retraction technique might be developed now:

1. Good retraction includes gentle elevation as well as tractile force.

2. Good retraction should be reasonably firm and steady. Tissue is unnecessarily damaged and the operation time prolonged by the assistant who is persistently changing the position of the retractors.

3. When the operative technique so permits, the tractile force on the retractors should be periodically released without removing the retractors; thus circulation may be restored to the soft tissue flaps during that brief period.

4. Retraction must be continual and adequate during unexpected arterial hemorrhage until that immediate problem is solved.

With adequate exposure of the platysma muscle and its overlying, rather poorly defined superficial fascia, this muscle is now made ready for sectioning. It should be remembered that this muscle will later require suturing in closure-by-layers. At this time it should be carefully dissected, elevated, and cleanly sectioned so that it can be conveniently found for later suturing. Immediately under the platysma muscle and along the border of the mandible, exploration should be provided for identification of the mandibular branch (ramus marginalis mandibulae) of the facial nerve. It is small and sometimes difficult to locate, especially if there has been surgical shredding of fascial tissue in the immediate field. It is often best found in the potential fascial space just deep to the platysma and superficial to the anterior border of the masseter, or over the depressor anguli oris. Suspected segments of this nerve can be identified when stimulated with faradic current or by gentle clamping with a hemostatic forceps. The effect of such stimulation will be seen in noticeable contracture of the musculature at the corner of the mouth. The Bovie unit employing low current (noncoagulative) is frequently used in operating rooms in providing faradic current for such stimulation. Many surgeons consider that the most constant point of reference for convenient identification of the mandibular branch of the seventh cranial nerve is its relationship to the large, pulsating facial artery. The nerve is found lying directly over the facial artery as that vessel passes over the mandible. If the artery and vein are reflected superiorly from their location at the inferior border of the mandible, such retraction is certain to include, and thereby salvage, the more superficial mandibular branch of the seventh cranial nerve (ramus marginalis mandibulae). At any rate this important nerve has considerable cosmetic and some functional significance, and it should not be inadvertently sacrificed.

The next step in orderly surgical approach concerns the identification and retraction of the facial artery and vein as they pass over the notching in the inferior border of the mandible just anterior to the angle. The parotideomasseteric fascia and other sheaths from the ascending deep cervical fasciae are first brought into surgical view. After adequate orientation by palpating the inferomandibular notch, this fascia is separated by blunt dissection, permitting the large, pulsating facial artery to bulge into the created opening. The larger facial vein will be found slightly superficial and posterior to the artery, but in close approximation. Both vessels are sacrificed if necessary. This is best done by first clamping each vessel, and then ligating proximally and distally before sectioning. White cotton sutures, No. 2-0, are well chosen for this ligation. For smaller vessels, finer cotton sutures, Nos. 3-0 and 4-0, are used. Of course other subcutaneous suture materials such as chromicized surgical gut and similar absorbable ligating sutures are equally acceptable for this purpose.

Glandular tissue will be observed in the dissection at this point. This is the submandibular gland (glandula mandibularis). Some difficulty may be encountered in separating the lower pole of the parotid gland from the submaxillary gland. The stylomandibular ligament is often surgically viewed as a heavy fascial plane that serves to separate these glands. The glandular tissues should be separated by blunt dissection and carefully retracted. If incised, they may produce persistent hemorrhage that may be difficult to control. With the glandular tissue retracted, the facial vessels subsequently ligated and sectioned, and the seventh cranial nerve salvaged and protected in careful retraction, the remainder of the surgical exposure can proceed with greater speed and impunity. Other smaller vessels will be encountered, but these will be of no surgical significance except as requires ligation to preserve blood volume and maintain a dry surgical field. Surgery on the body of the mandible anterior to the facial artery and veins is seldom complicated by excessive bleeding. Minor and smaller bleeders will often coagulate under pressure tampons. Sometimes the clamping of such a minor bleeder with a hemostatic forceps for a few minutes will serve to enhance coagulation so that ligation is not required. However, when the hemostatic forceps is removed, the bleeding site must be carefully evaluated to establish that hemostasis is complete. If in doubt, ligate the bleeding point.

Variations of the soft tissue surgery described will be required in a minor manner to meet the demands of surgery in the more anterior aspects of the lower face. If the body of the mandible is to be approached, the location of the incision is placed more anteriorly. The amount of exposure required determines the length of the incision. Usually 6 to 7 cm. will be found adequate, but accessibility should not be sacrificed only to produce a slightly smaller scar. To do so may result in unnecessary trauma to adjacent soft tissue, postoperative swelling, poor healing, and ragged scarring. It is good technique to identify and retract or identify, ligate, and retract blood vessels overlying the operative field. It is *necessary technique* to identify and salvage nerve supply—especially *motor nerve* supply.

Soft tissue closure

As in all surgery, closure of the soft tissues in submandibular approach to oral surgery is carried out in an orderly manner. The field is first scrutinized to assure that hemorrhage is controlled and ligated vessels are adequately secured. It is better that the time be taken to ensure these necessary precautions at this stage of surgery rather than facing the problem of postoperative hemorrhage on the ward in the middle of the night.

Closure of the soft tissues is then done in layers with anatomical repositioning in proper relation. Periosteal tissues are very difficult to suture. Fine surgical gut, No. 3-0 or 4-0, on a ⅜-circle, side-cutting needle is best used for this procedure. Whether the surgical gut is tanned (chromic) or plain is of small consequence. The chromic gut will resorb more slowly than will the plain, and this may be desirable in ligating large vessels and in suturing fascia. The cervical fascia is likewise closed. In operations on the ramus of the mandible in which the masseter muscle is detached and elevated, it is especially important that this muscle be well sutured at its origin in the vicinity of the angle of the mandible. This can be accomplished by suturing the lower end of the masseter muscle to the lower end of the medial pterygoid muscle (on the medial aspect of the mandible) at the angle of the mandible. The position of these muscles may be slightly altered by this procedure, but no appreciable residual will be evident in their function.

It is important in closing by layers that approximation be reasonably accurate so that all dead space may be eliminated. Dead space is a harbor for a hematoma.

As the platysma is recognized and closed, it is well to have assistants hold Dural-Adson skin hooks tautly at each end of the incision. By so doing, the longitudinal relation of this muscle is reestablished and smoother skin closure can be effected. Muscle closure at this superficial level can be established with No. 4-0 plain surgical gut (although silk or cotton may be acceptable) on a small ⅜-circle, round needle. To approximate skin with minimal scarring, it is wise to use first a subcuticular suture of plain surgical gut or stainless steel wire. If the wire is employed, it can be conveniently removed after the tenth day. The subcuticular approximation serves to relieve suture tension on the skin incision.

If subcuticular suture has not been employed, the skin wound may be closed with vertical mattress sutures. Interrupted sutures are preferable to continuous sutures since approximation may be maintained even if one of the sutures should slip. The skin sutures should be of nonabsorbable material of very fine gauge (No. 4-0 or 5-0) on a ⅜-circle, cutting needle and spaced about 3 mm. apart. A fine atraumatic needle swaged-on very fine Dermalon is equally useful for skin closure. The skin closure is initiated at each of the preoperatively marked "crosshatchings" to facilitate the exact repositioning of the skin.

It is considered good technique to slightly evert the line of skin incision in suture closure. Sutures must be removed on the fourth postoperative day to avoid suture scarring, and at that time there may be a tendency for some separation in the suture line. Everting the skin edges permits some subdermal contracture without separation in the line of incision. Irrespective of the care devoted to skin closure, unless there has been careful attention paid to the closure by anatomical layers of all of the tissues, the cosmetic result may be unsatisfactory.

The skin incision line is first covered with a single-layer pad of sterile, lubricated gauze. The lubricant may be sterile petrolatum jelly. Over this is placed a 4 by 4 inch sterile gauze pad and this is covered with a pressure dressing to limit postoperative edema. The dressing is part of the surgical procedure and is the responsibility of the surgeon. It is most important that all dressings, primary and reapplied, be sterile. The greatest complication to all wound healing is infection.

Surgical approach to the temporomandibular joint

Many of the so-called classical approaches to surgery of the temporomandibular joint mechanism have been complicated by the danger of surgical damage to the cosmetically significant seventh cranial nerve.

Blair[4] used an incision resembling a reverse question mark or an inverted L, commencing in the temporal hairline and curving downward in close proximity to the an-

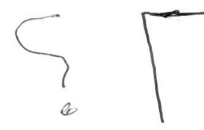

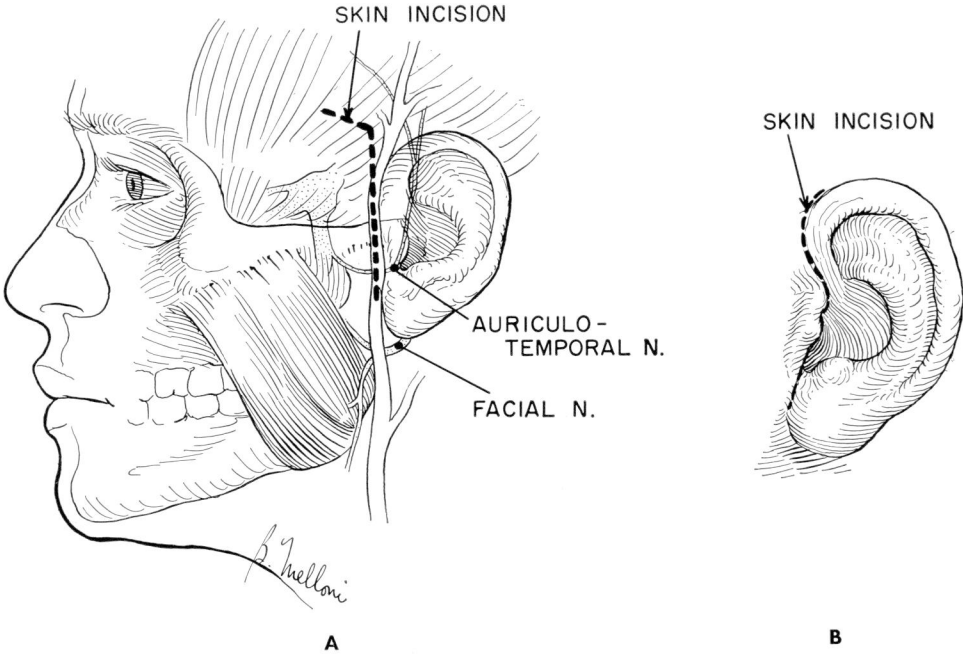

Fig. 2-19. **A,** Basic incision employed by Blair, Ivy, and others in surgical approach to the temporomandibular joint. **B,** Dingman's approach to the temporomandibular joint.

terior auricle (Fig. 2-19, A). Wakely[5] used a modification resembling a **T** incision with the horizontal bar of the **T** placed over the zygomatic arch. Lempert's[6] endaural approach to the middle ear suggested to numerous observers that, with some modifications, this could be basically employed as perhaps the safest surgical route to the glenoid fossae.

In 1951 Dingman and Moorman[7] reported such a new approach, which appeared to be initiated somewhat similarly to Lempert's second endaural incision. The major objective of this approach concerned sectioning the minor fibrous attachment of the lamina of tragus at its superior aspect and reflecting this cartilage anteriorly and down over itself (Fig. 2-19, B). Rongetti[8] in 1954 reported another modification of the second stage of Lempert's endaural approach to the middle ear, which promised safe and direct invasion of the temporomandibular joint. However, for practical purposes Rongetti's approach is similar to Dingman's, differing chiefly in that he invades the external auditory meatus to a greater depth and does not extend his incision as far superiorly and inferiorly as does Dingman. Both are endaural approaches, and both are designed to avoid injury to the facial nerve and to leave behind the least noticeable scar.

The endaural incision for exposing the glenoid fossae has been used successfully for meniscectomy and condyloidectomy, but it is not necessarily limited to that surgery.

The hair in the temporal fossae is shaved and the head is prepared and draped for sterile surgery. The incision is started in the skin crease immediately adjacent to the anterior helix. It is carried downward to the level of the tragus, at which point it passes in a gap to the deeper aspects of the ex-

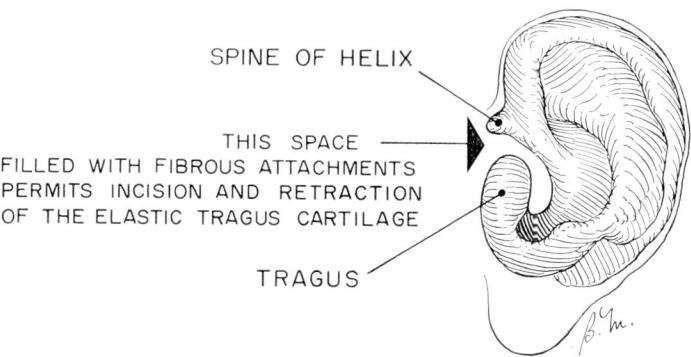

Fig. 2-20. Cartilaginous laminae of ear. The normally present space between the cartilaginous supports of the helix and the tragus allows for the convenient retraction of the tragus, anteriorly and inferiorly, for subsequent direct exposure into the temporomandibular joint.

ternal auditory meatus where it is cosmetically concealed. The gap is filled with a fibrous attachment for the lamina of tragus and no damage is done in this sectioning (Fig. 2-20). While in the auditory meatus, the incision remains in contact with the bony tympanic plate. As the incision leaves the external auditory meatus, it becomes just visible at the lower aspect of the tragus. It is not necessary to section the cartilage at this point since it has sufficient elasticity to permit adequate retraction without hazarding the risk of incision at this close proximity to the stylomastoid foramen (exit point for the facial nerve). In the upper aspects of this incision, the superficial temporal vessels and the auriculotemporal nerve may be encountered. These vessels are either retracted or the artery and vein may be ligated and sectioned. The next landmark will be the temporalis fascia and then the exposed cartilage of the tragus. The fascia is sectioned with a scalpel, or scissors, and the temporalis muscle is undermined with a periosteal elevator and raised from the root of the zygomatic arch. Some small portion of the upper pole of the parotid gland may be identified in this field. It is better to dissect and retract the glandular tissue since incising may produce troublesome bleeding. Mandibular ex-

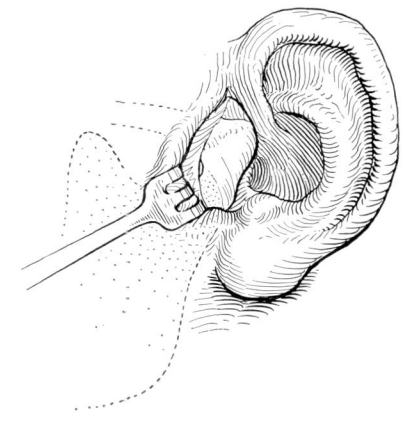

Fig. 2-21. This endaural incision permits the tragus to be incised at the fibrous bundle attachment at its superoanterior border so that it may be reflected anteroinferiorly, thereby exposing the articular ligamentous covering of the temporomandibular joint.

cursions at this point will clearly demonstrate the condyle enclosed in a rather loose articular capsule. Further exposure may be effected by blunt dissection. Any further incising at this stage is best made directly over the condylar head or along the inferior margin of the zygomatic arch. (See Fig. 2-21.)

No surgical danger is anticipated deep

to the temporalis fascia and lateral to the condyle. There may be some retraction paralysis of some of the branches of the facial nerve since the area of exposure is small although adequate. This will be a temporary paresthesia.

If further surgery deep to the neck of the condyle is required, this must be done with diligent respect for the maxillary artery, the middle meningeal artery, and the auriculotemporal nerve. Invasion of the pterygoid plexus of veins will result in persistent hemorrhagic seepage, but this is controlled by pressure tampons or Gelfoam strips saturated with a hemostatic. All gauze sponges used in this area should be tied on one end with long, black suture silk to facilitate convenient removal.

The endaural approach to the temporomandibular joint, as for menisectomy or condyloidectomy, is thought by many to be the most direct and perhaps the safest approach to a difficult area. The chief objections to it may be a limited range of exposure of the joint mechanism and the possibility of secondary infection of aural cartilage. However, these are small objections. Any surgical approach to this area that promises to eliminate the danger of damage to the facial nerve and provides a cosmetically acceptable postoperative scar is to be desired.

The Lempert operation for otosclerosis forms the basis for this modified approach to the temporomandibular joint via the external auditory meatus.

POSTOPERATIVE CARE

The patient who has had local anesthesia will require little else besides routine symptomatic care concerned with good oral hygiene measures and relief of postoperative pain. After mouth surgery a patient may require some dietary management such as

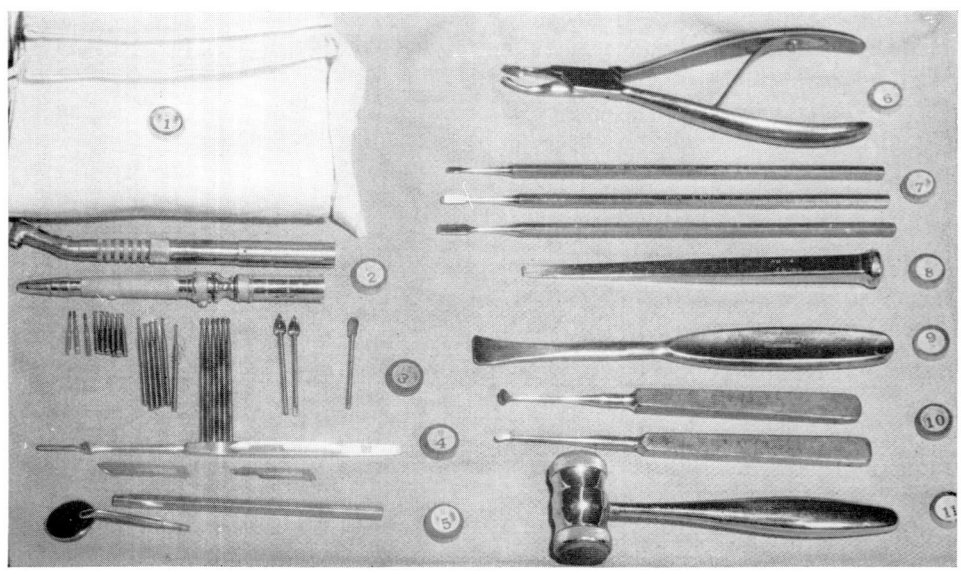

Fig. 2-22. 1, Sterile sleeves for draping engine arms, cables, and extensions from portable dental engine. 2, Straight and angle dental handpieces. 3, Assorted burs; carbide preferred. 4, Scalpel handle and blades Nos. 10 and 15. 5, Mouth mirror and handle, plain. 6, Bone rongeur No. 4. 7, Osteotomes, Stout, assorted. 8, Osteotome, single-bevel. 9, Periosteotome, blunt, Lane, 7¾ inches. 10, Curets, Molt, straight, Nos. 2 and 4. 11, Mallet, metal. (Official U. S. Navy Photograph.)

Principles of surgical technique 43

high protein, high caloric, liquid or soft diets until he can manage masticatory effort. If a liquid diet is necessary over a prolonged period of time (as in jaw fracture problems), this diet should be supported with protein hydrolysates; multiple supplementary feedings should be made available to avoid dehydration and marked loss of body weight.

The patient who has had general anesthesia will require routine recovery room procedures primarily concerned with maintaining an adequate airway and evacuating excess oral fluids and hemorrhage until he recovers. All unconscious or semiconscious patients must be carefully attended to avoid their falling out of bed or conveyances.

Water, electrolyte, and nutritional balance

The normal individual living in a favorable environment ingests, assimilates, and excretes required amounts of water, salts, and foods to meet body demands.

The diseased patient may be unable to take, absorb, utilize, and excrete the necessary nutrients in normal quantity. This patient poses particular problems in postsurgical response to tissue injury and repair. He also is abnormally susceptible to infection, to wound hemorrhage, and to marked delay in wound healing.

Excessive perspiration, diarrhea, vomiting, wound seepage, or blood loss will probably require correction of depleted water and electrolyte. If these deficiencies

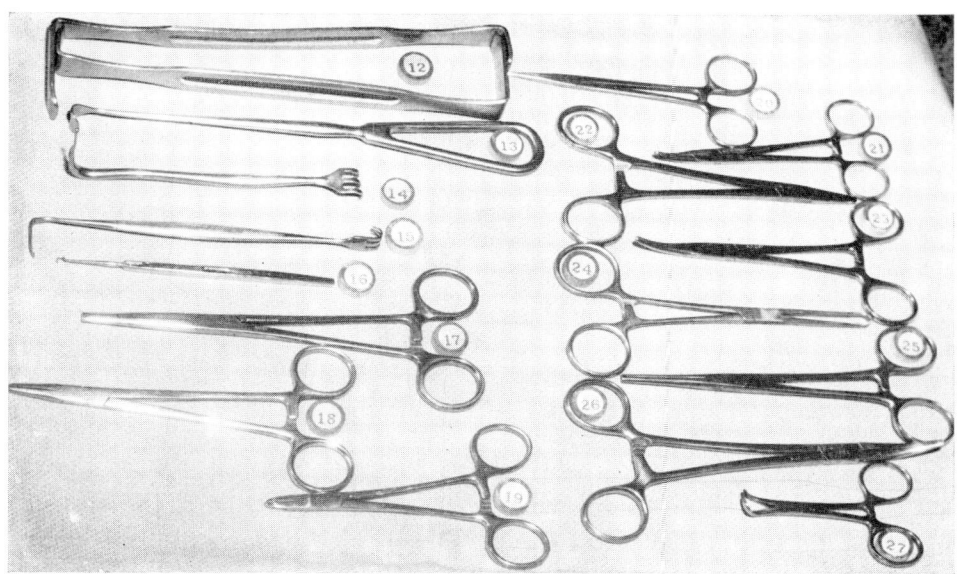

Fig. 2-23. 12, Retractor, set, general operating (Army-Navy). 13, Retractor, vein, Cushing. 14, Retractor, trachea, Hupp, 3-prong, blunt, 6½ inches. 15, Retractor, trachea, Kny-Scheering, 3-prong, blunt, 6½ inches. 16, Hook, skin, Dural-Adson. 17, Forceps, straight, hemostatic, Rochester-Ochsner, 7½ inches. 18, Holder, needle, Mayo-Hegar, 7 inches. 19, Holder, needle, Sterz-Brown, 5½ inches. 20, Forceps, hemostatic, straight, Halsted (mosquito), 5 inches. 21, Forceps, hemostatic, curved, Halsted (mosquito), 5 inches. 22, Holder, needle, Mayo-Hegar, 6 inches. 23, Forceps, hemostatic, Kelly, curved, 5½ inches. 24, Forceps, tissue, straight, Allis, 6 inches. 25, Forceps, hemostatic, straight, Rochester-Ochsner, 5½ inches. 26, Forceps, hemostatic, curved, Rochester-Pean, 6¼ inches. 27, Forceps, towel, Backhaus, 3¼ inches. (Official U. S. Navy Photograph.)

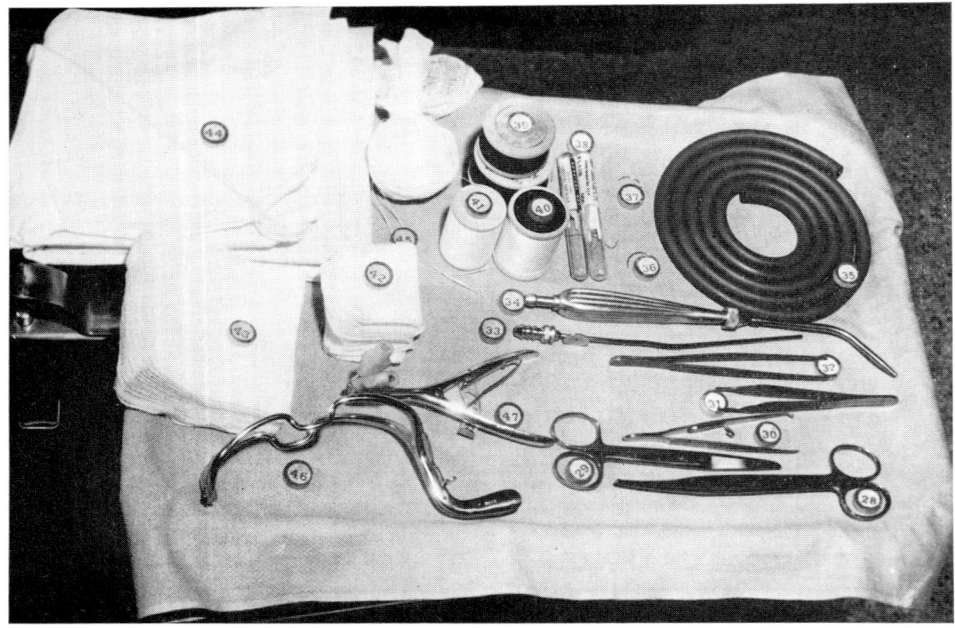

Fig. 2-24. 28, Scissors, general surgical, curved, Aufricht, 5½ inches. 29, Scissors, general surgical, straight, one point sharp, 5½ inches. 30, Forceps, fixation, straight, Graefe, 4½ inches. 31, Forceps, tissue, Brown-Adson, 4½ inches. 32, Forceps, dressing, straight, 5¼ inches. 33, Suction tip, antrum. 34, Suction tip, laryngeal. 35, Rubber suction tubing. 36, Needle, suture, ½-circle, taper, No. 12. 37, Needle, suture, ⅜-circle, cutting No. 20. 38, Suture, surgical gut (plain and chromic), No. 3-0. 39, Suture, silk, black, spools, Nos. 3-0, 4-0, and 5-0. 40, Suture, cotton, white, No. 2-0. 41, Suture, cotton, white, No. 3-0. 42, Sponges, 2 by 2 inches. 43, Sponges, 4 by 4 inches. 44, Sterile drape, front sheet, 45 by 70 inches. 45, Throat pack, with string attached. 46, Mouth prop, Jennings. 47, Mouth prop, Denhardt. (Official U. S. Navy Photograph.)

cannot be corrected through mouth feedings, the intravenous route will be necessary.

If water is required by vein, it may be given as distilled water with 5% glucose. If there is need for electrolytes, 500 ml. of normal saline solution may be added to the intravenous glucose-water per day. Electrolytes (such as sodium lactate and sodium chloride), proteins, and nitrogens (amino acids) are best taken by mouth. If oral feedings are impossible, the alternate route is via stomach tube.

Dehydration is no more or no less serious than malnutrition. One or the other may very well set off a "chain reaction" that encompasses a wide range of disturbed metabolic activity.

Except in rather obvious cases, it may be difficult indeed to establish that a patient is not in balance in regard to his requirements of water, plasma salts, plasma proteins, vitamins, nitrogen, etc. Complicated laboratory procedures and expert interpretation of these results are required to make deficiency determinations. These determinations are often inconclusive.

However, gross findings of such imbalance should be considered and looked for in preoperative and postoperative evaluation. A brief dietary history and comparison of the patient's weight against his height may reveal suggestions of nutritional imbalance.

The quantitative examination of fluid intake and urinary output is carefully recorded in surveillance against dehydration. A daily excretion of 1,500 ml. of fluid having a normal (1.020) specific gravity can be considered as satisfactory hydration. Febrile patients and those with debilitating diseases commonly require forced-fluids therapy to provide replacement and additional volume to carry away waste products of infection. In kidney disease in which urinary concentration is deficient, it may be necessary to force fluids to provide additional volume.

ARMAMENTARIUM

Some of the more frequently used instruments and supplies for oral surgery are illustrated and identified (Figs. 2-22 to 2-24). These are normally set up in sterile packs, or case pans, for routine use in oral surgical problems. To these routine setups the surgeon will add the special armamentarium required for a particular surgical problem.

REFERENCES

1. Artandi, Charles Production experiences with radiation sterilization, Bull. Parenteral Drug Ass. **18**:2, 1964.
2. Olander, J. W.: New facilities and equipment for radiation sterilization, Bull. Parenteral Drug Ass. **17**:14, 1963.
3. Safe practice for hospital operating rooms, Booklet No. NFPA-56, July, 1956, National Fire Protective Association, 60 Batterymarch St., Boston 10, Mass.
4. Blair, V. P.: Consideration of contour as well as function in operations for organic ankylosis of lower jaw, Surg. Gynec. Obstet. **46**:167, 1928.
5. Wakeley, C. P. G.: Surgery of temporomandibular joint, Surgery **5**:697, 1939.
6. Lempert, J.: Improvement of hearing in cases of otosclerosis; new, one stage surgical technic, Arch. Otolaryng. **28**:42, 1938.
7. Dingman, R. C., and Moorman, W. C.: Meniscectomy in treatment of lesions of temporomandibular joint, J. Oral Surg. **9**:214, 1951.
8. Rongetti, J. R.: Meniscectomy; new approach to temporomandibular joint, Arch. Otolaryng. **60**:566, 1954.

Chapter 3

INTRODUCTION TO EXODONTIA

Gustav O. Kruger

GENERAL PRINCIPLES

A careful technique based upon knowledge and skill is the most important factor in successful exodontia. Living tissue must be treated with gentleness. Rough handling, ragged or incomplete incision, excessive retraction of flaps, or uneven suturing, even though not painful to the anesthetized patient, will result in tissue damage or necrosis, which in turn provides an excellent medium for bacterial growth. Healing that could have taken place by primary intention must granulate from the bottom of the wound after necrotic tissue is phagocytized. This causes pain, excessive swelling, and possibly deformity. Gentle handling and instrumentation with a sharp, well-cared-for armamentarium are rewarded with a better tissue response.

Psychology

Science of behavior. The reaction with which different people respond to the same stimulus varies considerably. Individuals react to pain according to their basic makeup, which may range from stoicism to extreme sensitivity. An occasional patient who does not want anesthesia may sit through an extraction with few outward signs of pain. Another patient with profound local anesthesia may jump when a forceps is placed upon the tooth. The stoic patient is able to disregard a certain amount of the pain he feels. A story is told of one Christian Science patient who refused anesthesia of any kind. She telephoned her practitioner and left the telephone off the hook, even though it was across the room and therefore the reading was unintelligible to the patient in the chair. The patient did not move or make outward sign of discomfort during the extraction, although tears streamed down her cheeks.

The psychological effect of the placebo has been studied many times. A double blind study to compare the sedative effects of a therapeutic agent with those of a bland pill of similar size and color was so conducted that neither the operator nor the patient knew which pill contained the active agent. The patients were told that a sedative or analgesic agent would be administered; they did not know that there was an equal possibility that a sugar pill might be administered. At the end of the experiment, after the reactions of all patients had been recorded, the code was opened and the completed record cards were marked with the ingredients. In numerous such studies involving many ills and various drugs, no less than 35% of patients experienced relief using the placebo. The point was made that real pain was relieved in these patients, not merely imagined pain, indicating that physiological and psychological processes can be modified by psychological attitudes. In another double blind experiment an injection of either a normal saline or a local anesthetic solution was given in the oral tissues of dental students. A significant number of men injected with saline had complete objective and subjective signs of anesthesia.

Circumstances have much to do with pain perception. Soldiers in the stress of warfare have been subjected to major injuries that were unfelt and unknown to them until the immediate objective was won. Children sometimes will react with fear to the white coat worn by the practitioner, and consequently some pedodontists wear street clothes in the office.[1]

The pain threshold varies significantly in individuals. What is major pain to one person at one time may be minor pain to another person. The introduction of a hypodermic needle into the vein of the arm may be barely felt by one individual although it may be felt as excruciating pain by another.

Emotional control in the presence of pain varies considerably. Patients with the same threshold of pain can range from the individual who overreacts, such as the child who has no inhibitions, to the patient who will give no outward sign of pain.[2]

The anxious patient. Fear can be related to any one of several factors:

1. Fear of fear itself. Past experiences from a painful childhood incident that have been relegated to the subconscious mind, or even tales of painful experiences told by someone else, can condition the patient to fear the fear he associates with the procedure. This is mainly an introverted reaction, although extraneous factors such as long-remembered odors, colors, and situations may stir latent memories.[3]

2. The operation. Any normal individual has some degree of concern over an impending operation. General surgeons say that the patient who approaches major surgery with no concern at all does not have the same chance of survival as the patient who has stimulated his adrenal cortices to some extent. Everyone has stresses in life, but the size of the factor required to stress him and the response of the individual to that stress vary. It is the concern of the dentist and his entire staff to reduce this normal fear to its absolute minimum. Every successful practitioner induces in his patients confidence in him that ameliorates natural fear. The patient should be prepared psychologically before any operation is performed, and in many cases the preparation is done by thoughtful considerations by the staff and practitioner even without words. Most dentists will not extract teeth for the patient who grips the arms of the chair until white knuckles show, preferring to prepare him psychologically and by premedication for a more relaxed, subsequent appointment.

3. Esthetics. The menopausal matron whose children are married, whose husband at the peak of his career is busy and inattentive, and who has lost her girlhood beauty thinks beyond the full maxillary extractions for which she is sitting. This last insult to her beauty has been likened to a subconscious castration. She is fearful she is losing her power in society that beauty once gave her, and this is the last straw in that process. This fear can be aggravated by mental instability associated with the menopause. The wise dentist proceeds slowly in recommending such extractions, showing all the pathological reasons for removal of the teeth and allowing the patient herself to first express the conclusion that all teeth should be removed. Her first statement to this effect seems to prepare her better from a psychological standpoint. Of course, the practitioner in doing this occasionally encounters the matter-of-fact matron who says, "Come, come, young man, what are you saying? What is your diagnosis?"

It must be remembered that the pain the anxious patient experiences is really felt by that patient, even though in some psychosomatic illnesses no objective organic basis for the pain can be found.

Evaluation and preparation. The general psychological makeup of the patient should be evaluated before treatment is undertaken. His self-confidence, self-reliance, general attitude, and demeanor give clues to his later reactions. The neurotic patient has a nervous instability that must be taken into consideration when premedication and management are planned. The big policeman who swaggers in, saying that he is afraid of nothing, often is the first to go into syncope when the forceps appear. The banker's wife whose position has made her immune to physical and mental insult may react vocally upon extraction even in the presence of adequate anesthesia; firmness by the operator at the moment, followed after the operation by kind words of commendation on her excellent behavior, with no mention of the unpleasantness, will make a firm friend. Age, race, health, physical considerations, and even vocation present variables that must be considered in evaluating the patient.

In verbal presentation of the exodontia problem, the patient should be told what to expect. Possible complications and postoperative problems can be identified without describing every catastrophic detail. The patient may have occasion to verify these experiences later and thereupon will have more confidence in the dentist who anticipated them. Terminology is important. For instance, when considerable alveoloplasty is anticipated, the patient is told that the parts will be smoothed in order to create a better base for the denture in anticipation of natural resorption. The gory details are best left unsaid. During the operative procedure the patient is forewarned of noise made by instruments such as the chisel or rongeur.

Psychological office management. The office and its personnel should be geared to the instillation of confidence in the patient from the moment he arrives. Nothing defeats this objective as much as ignoring the patient in a bustling, impersonal office. As one of its primary functions the office should show concern for the patient. Another irritation in the office is extraneous noise. One practitioner had a quiet office in which the entire wall facing the chair was replaced by two pieces of plate glass, extending from floor to ceiling, which formed a tropical fish tank. This was most restful to the patient.

Instruments should never be exposed to view. Odors suggestive of medication should be eliminated as much as possible. Adequate premedication is given if necessary. A towel head wrap can be placed over the patient's eyes if considerable instrumentation will be done.

The operator should exhibit sympathetic actions: gentleness and tranquility. He should be calm and self-reliant in order to inspire confidence. The terminology should be arranged so that if he wishes a new needle he will call for a "point." The entire office should be devoted to eliminating psychological problems in patients and to ensuring them only minimum mental discomfort while in the office.

Psychiatric aspects. Neurotic patients need dental extractions, just as much as normal patients do, but there are several differences to be observed in their management. First, the neurotic patient often has tensions that make management difficult. Second, the neurotic or slightly neurotic patient can exhibit bizarre postoperative reactions such as prolonged symptoms of local anesthesia, unnatural or prolonged wound pain, and other hysteria-like phenomena. The patient may return for months and then start legal action. Third, the neurotic patient will insist on prescribing operations on himself that will, in his mind, cure him miraculously of his troubles. He may complain of a vague pain in the maxilla for which no organic basis can be found and insist that the second molar be extracted. Complete examination will show a healthy tooth. After visiting several dentists he will find one who will extract the tooth. Immediately the pain will disappear, vindicating the patient's diagnosis and making this dentist the best one he has ever known. Unfortunately, within months the patient will return, complaining of the same pain and demanding that the second premolar be removed or, if all teeth on that side have been removed, that the maxilla be opened surgically to remove "bad bone." Once the initial nonpathological tooth is removed, it is almost impossible to convince the patient that this type of treatment will do no good and that psychiatric evaluation and treatment are necessary. If the dentist feels that the patient may take umbrage at such recommendation, he can always refer him to a neurologist for evaluation of the neurological pathways.

Anesthesia

Whether the operation is performed under local or under general anesthesia depends upon many factors, primary among which are the custom, training, and equipment of the dentist, the wishes and physical status of the patient, the presence of an acute pericementitis or pulpitis that may make local anesthesia difficult, the presence of infection in the surrounding tissues, and the extent of the procedure.

Some operators use local anesthesia for every type of procedure, using major block anesthesia and premedication to manage the difficult cases. Others use general anesthesia for everything.

Premedication with local anesthesia for extraction is helpful, especially if the operation is expected to involve complicated procedures.[4] Premedication must be tailored for each individual. It can vary from a barbiturate or ataraxic drug taken by mouth at home or in the waiting room to an intramuscular injection of a synthetic narcotic or antihistaminic or an intravenous injection of a barbiturate given when the patient is in the chair.

Examination of the patient

The more experience a man has in exodontia the more aware he is of the complications that might befall him and the more thorough is his examination. He becomes adept at sizing up the patient and the area of the mouth involved. Legal considerations require that the examination be recorded. For the beginner the examination should be stylized and recorded in some detail. Examination is divided into several portions.

History is divided basically into the chief complaint, present illness, past history, and family history (see Chapters 1 and 2). To intelligently assess the problem an adequate knowledge must be obtained of both the background of the patient and of the present complaint. No problem is so simple that it cannot cause serious injury or death under the wrong circumstances. However, under apparently normal circumstances in which no diagnostic problem needs to be fathomed, a few leading questions are used rather than an attempt to write a complete, hospital-type history. The patient is asked if he has had major operations or illnesses, when he last was examined by his physician, if there were positive findings, and what drugs he is taking now. He is asked whether he has allergies or a history of rheumatic fever, how many pillows he sleeps on, and if he has difficulty climbing steps.

Clinical examination consists of visual evaluation (color, swelling, condition of tooth and surrounding structures), palpation and percussion, instrumentation, and vitality tests. The tooth in question is examined closely. In addition, adjacent teeth and surrounding structures are examined carefully for problems that may be pertinent. The overhanging margin of the filling on the next tooth, which will fracture upon extraction, osteoradionecrosis in the underlying jaw, or a fractured jaw under the loose tooth in a patient who has come from a barroom fight should not be overlooked. A clinical survey of the general health status of the fully clothed patient in the dental chair likewise is a necessary art in the successful dental practice.

Radiographic examination is necessary, both preoperatively and postoperatively. Many conditions that could not be diagnosed otherwise are thus revealed—the curved root, the large cyst, a new abscess or carious exposure of the pulp on an adjacent tooth that was not present on radiographs made several years earlier. The man whose jaw was fractured in the fight will sue when he becomes sober, claiming the jaw was fractured during the extraction, unless a preoperative radiographic record exists. A postoperative radiograph is equally important for clinical evaluation as well as for record purposes. It might be necessary to prove that a fracture received by the patient convalescing in a nightclub was not sustained during the extraction. With better radiographic procedures and protection there is negligible radiation associated with these radiographs. However, children and pregnant women often are not given postoperative radiographs following uncomplicated procedures.

Laboratory tests are necessary adjuncts to diagnosis and management. Some tests (e.g., urinalysis) can be done in a well-equipped office, but most tests are done in a laboratory. Tests for bleeding are not done accurately in the office. If such tests are indicated, they should be done in a laboratory, in the hospital, or in the physician's office. Although such tests are expensive and time-consuming, there should be no hesitancy in ordering them if they are indicated.

INDICATIONS AND CONTRAINDICATIONS FOR EXTRACTION
Indications

Any tooth that is not useful in the total dental mechanism is considered for removal.

1. Pulp pathology, either acute or chronic, in a tooth that is not amenable to endodontic therapy condemns the tooth. A tooth that is not restorable by dental procedures can be considered in this category even if pulp pathology is not demonstrable.

2. Periodontal disease, acute or chronic, that is not amenable to treatment may be cause for extraction.

3. Trauma effects on the tooth or alveolus sometimes are beyond repair. Many teeth in the line of jaw fracture are removed in order to treat the fractured bone.

4. Impacted or supernumerary teeth often do not take their place in the line of occlusion.

5. Orthodontic considerations may require the removal of fully erupted teeth, erupting teeth, and overretained deciduous teeth. Malposed teeth and third molar teeth that have lost their antagonists can be included.

6. Nonvital teeth are possible foci of infection. Devitalized teeth, radiographically negative, are removed occasionally as a last resort upon the request of the physician.

7. Prosthetic considerations may require the removal of one or many teeth for design or stability of the prosthesis.

8. Esthetic considerations at times transcend purely functional factors.

9. There may be pathology in surrounding bone that involves the tooth, or treatment of which requires removal of the tooth. Examples are cysts, osteomyelitis, tumors, and bone necrosis.

10. Teeth "in line of fire" of planned therapeutic radiation to a nearby area are removed so that a supervening osteoradionecrosis of the bone will not be complicated by radiation caries or by necrosing pulps and their sequelae.

Contraindications

Few conditions are absolute contraindications for extraction of teeth. Teeth have been removed in the presence of all types of complications because of necessity. In these situations much more preparation of the patient is necessary to prevent serious damage or death or to obtain healing of the local wound. For example, the injection of a local anesthetic, let alone the extraction of a tooth, can cause instant death in a patient in an addisonian crisis. Surgical intervention of any kind, including exodontia, may activate systemic or local disease. Therefore, a list of relative contraindications is given. In some instances these conditions become absolute contraindications.

Local contraindications. Local contraindications are associated mainly with infection and, to a lesser extent, with malignant disease.

1. Acute infection with an uncontrolled cellulitis must be controlled so that it does not spread further. The patient may exhibit a toxemia, which brings complicating systemic factors into consideration. The tooth that caused the infection is of secondary importance at the moment; to better control the infection, however, it is removed as soon as such removal does not endanger the life of the patient. Before antibiotics became available the tooth was never removed until the infection had become localized, the pus was drained, and the infection had subsided to a chronic state. This sequence of events took much longer than the present method of removing the tooth as soon as an adequate blood level of a specific antibiotic has brought systemic factors under control.

2. Acute pericoronitis is managed more conservatively than other local infections because of the mixed bacteriological flora found in the area, the fact that the third molar area has more direct access to the deep fascial planes of the neck, and the fact that removal of this tooth is a complicated procedure involving ossisection.

3. Acute infectious stomatitis is a labile, debilitating, and painful disease, which is complicated by intercurrent exodontia.

4. Malignant disease disturbed by the extraction of a tooth embedded in the growth will react with exacerbated growth and nonhealing of the local wound.

5. Irradiated jaws may develop an acute osteoradionecrosis after extraction because of a lack of blood supply. The condition is severely painful and may terminate fatally.

Systemic contraindications. Any systemic disease or malfunction can complicate, or be complicated by, an extraction. These conditions are too numerous to list. Some of the more frequently encountered relative contraindications are as follows:

1. Uncontrolled diabetes mellitus is characterized by infection of the wound and absence of normal healing.

2. Cardiac disease (e.g., coronary artery disease, hypertension, cardiac decompensation) can complicate exodontia. Management may require the help of a physician.

3. Blood dyscrasias include simple as well as more serious anemias, hemorrhagic diseases such as hemophilia, and the leukemias. Preparation for extraction varies considerably with the underlying factors.

4. Debilitating diseases of any kind make patients poor risks for further traumatic insults.

5. Addison's disease or any steroid deficiency is extremely dangerous. The patient who has been treated for any disease with steroid therapy, even though the disease is conquered and the patient has not taken steroids for a year, may not have sufficient adrenal cortex secretion to withstand the stress of an extraction without taking additional steroids.

6. Fever of unexplained origin is rarely cured and often is worsened by extraction. One possibility is an undiagnosed subacute bacterial endocarditis, a condition that would be complicated considerably by an extraction.

7. Nephritis requiring treatment can create a formidable problem in preparing the patient for exodontia.

8. Pregnancy without complications presents no great problem. Precautions should be taken to guard against low oxygen tension in general anesthesia or in extreme fright. Obstetricians hold varied opinions

regarding the timing of extractions, but they usually prefer that necessary extractions be done in the second trimester. Menstruation is not a contraindication, although elective exodontia is not done during the period because of less nervous stability and greater tendency toward hemorrhage of all tissues.

9. Senility is a relative contraindication that requires greater care in overcoming a poor physiological response to surgery and a prolonged negative nitrogen balance.

10. Psychoses and neuroses reflect a nervous instability that complicates exodontia.

THE OFFICE; EQUIPMENT; ARMAMENTARIUM

The chief difference between the office devoted solely to exodontia and the one designed for general practice is the lack of fixed equipment around the chair in the former. The space on the left of the chair, usually occupied by the dental unit and cuspidor, is left vacant so the assistant can stand there. The patient either expectorates into a sterilized stainless steel basin that is held in the lap or held by the nurse, or a suction machine is used. If suction is used, it is more powerful than that produced by the average dental unit, and often it is central suction (e.g., a large compressor located in another room or area). If bone burs are used, a high-speed movable engine is employed. A general anesthesia machine is brought near the chair after the patient is seated. Instead of a bracket table in front of the patient where its contents are in view, a Mayo stand is placed behind the chair (Fig. 3-1).

Little change is necessary to adapt the general office for exodontia, provided that several basic considerations are included in the design. The cuspidor on the unit can be pushed back so that the assistant can work on the side of the patient opposite from the operator. A good light on the unit will suffice for exodontia. If suction on the unit is inadequate and central suction is

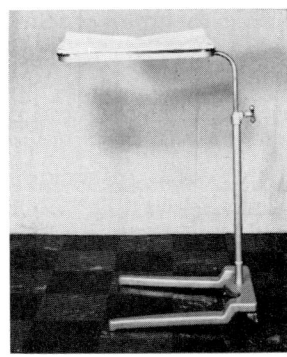

Fig. 3-1. Mayo stand holding covered instrument tray.

not available in the building, a mobile suction machine can be purchased. A Mayo stand should be available behind the chair so that the bracket table is not used. The sink need not be larger than the conventional size, but it should have knee controls. No sink in a dental office should have hand controls. Foot pedals are difficult to clean under, and elbow controls sometimes get in the way.

Adequate storage space should be available for the sterile armamentarium either out of sight in the room, or in a nearby area. A place should be provided for a sterile canister of sponges in the room.

A radiographic viewbox should be placed in a prominent position facing the operator. This can be placed on the wall opposite him, to the left of the assistant. The room should contain an x-ray machine so that the patient does not have to move for postoperative or intercurrent radiographs.

ARMAMENTARIUM

The more experience the exodontist acquires and the greater volume of work he sees, the simpler and more standardized his armamentarium becomes. Because he does not wish to lose time picking up several instruments, because it costs him more money to add another forceps to his complete sets, and because each additional instrument must be handled many times by the office personnel, he learns to do more with each instrument. Some men boast that they can work with only two forceps. Although this philosophy seems foolhardy since modern forceps are carefully designed to fit the anatomy of the various teeth, it nevertheless proves the ultimate in the "back pocket" philosophy.

Many practitioners have substituted universal forceps for paired (right and left) forceps. Another saving is the elimination of many, if not all, special forceps. Naturally, wide variation is found in individual likes and dislikes as well as various techniques that call for specialized instruments. The beginner is well advised to start out with a basic armamentarium and to become thoroughly familiar with its use for at least a year before considering new or additional instruments.

An armamentarium that has proved satisfactory and complete over the years is as follows:

Forceps (Fig. 3-2)

Standard forceps No. 1 for maxillary central and

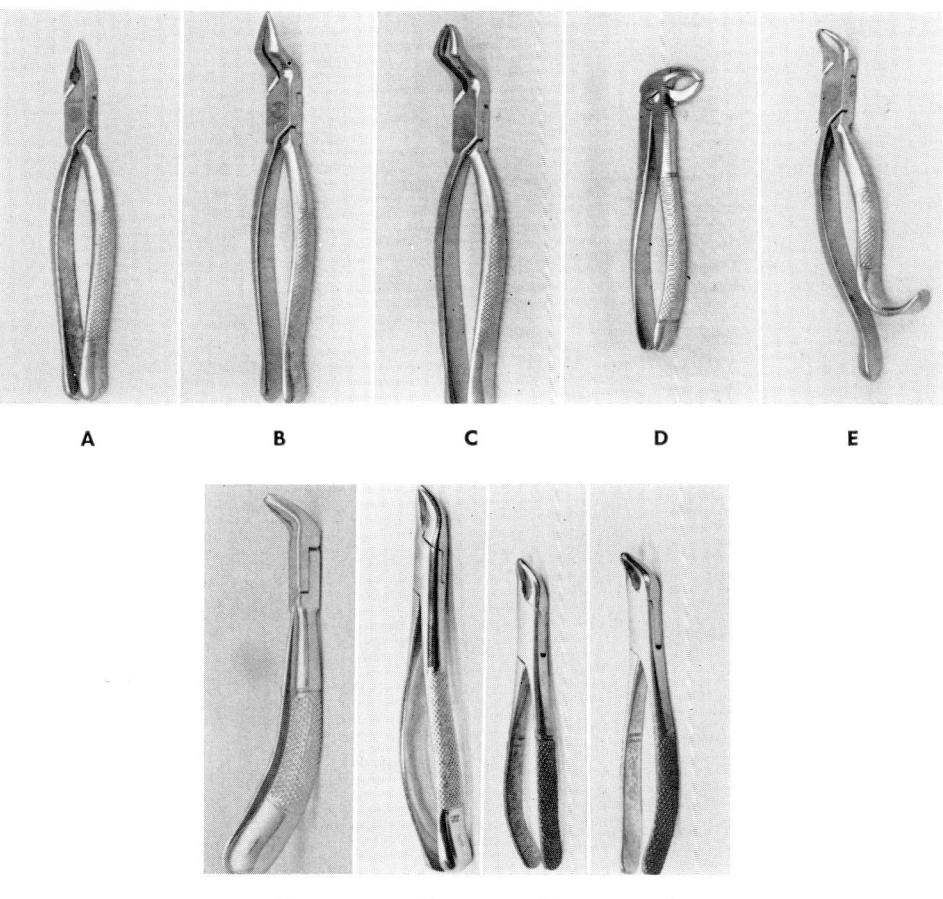

Fig. 3-2. Extraction forceps. **A,** No. 1. **B,** No. 65. **C,** No. 10S. **D,** Mead forceps. **E,** No. 16 cowhorn. **F,** No. 151. **G,** No. 150. **H,** Children's maxillary forceps. **I,** Children's mandibular forceps.

54 *Textbook of oral surgery*

lateral incisors, canines, and premolars in some instances
Standard forceps No. 65 for maxillary root tips
Standard forceps No. 10S for maxillary molars
Ash forceps, Mead No. 1, for mandibular teeth
Standard forceps No. 16, cowhorn, for mandibular molars
(To these basic five forceps can be added standard forceps No. 150 for maxillary premolars and standard forceps No. 151 for mandibular premolars if desired.)
(A maxillary and a mandibular child's forceps are desirable.)
Exolevers (Fig. 3-3)
Winter exolevers 14R and 14L, "long Winter exolever," designed primarily for removing deep-seated mandibular molar roots
Winter exolevers 11R and 11L, "short Winter exolevers," designed for elevation of tooth roots near the rim of the alveolus
Straight-shank No. 34, "shoehorn exolever," designed for elevating roots as well as entire teeth
Krogh exolever, Krogh 12B, designed for removal of third molar impactions
Root exolevers Nos. 1, 2, and 3, Hu-Friedy, for removal of fractured root apices

Many designs are made, which vary in delicateness. The beginner needs a fairly stout instrument to minimize breakage; but sharp, deli-

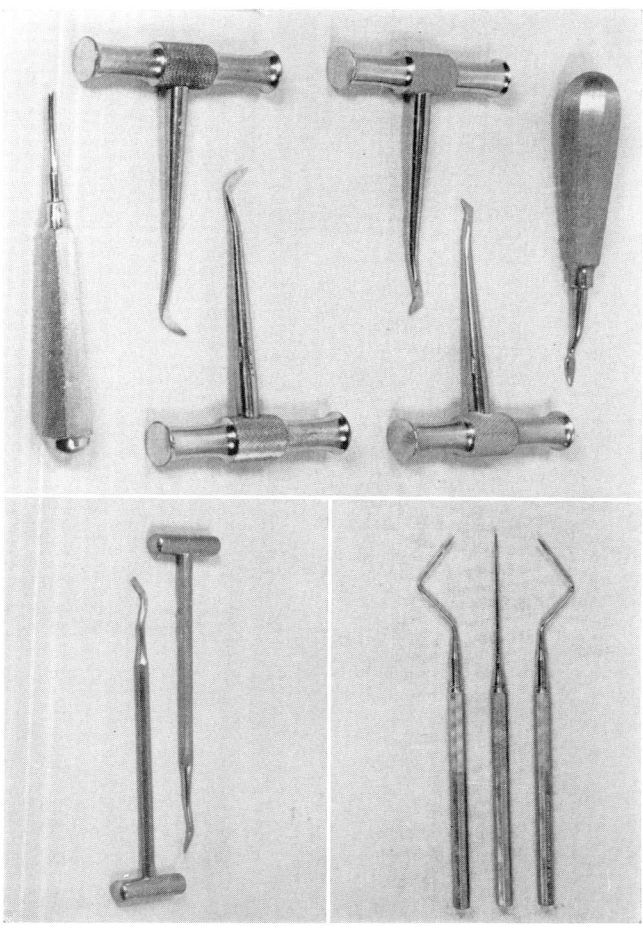

Fig. 3-3. Exolevers. Top row, left to right: straight-shank; long Winter (right and left); short Winter (right and left); Krogh spearpoint. Bottom row, left to right: Potts elevators (right and left); root exolevers.

cate instruments are better. They are made in sets of three: right, left, and straight (Potts exolevers R and L can be added for deciduous root tips.)

Surgical instruments (Fig. 3-4)
  Bard-Parker handle No. 3; No. 15 blade used most frequently
  Rongeur No. 4, universal, for cutting bone
  Bone file No. 10
  Chisel, Gardner No. 52
  Mallet, standard No. 1
  High-speed handpiece and burs if the bur technique is used
  Retractors, Austin
  Curets, Molt No. 2 for universal use, including breaking periodontal attachment before exodontia; Molt Nos. 5 and 6, same size, angled to right and to left; Molt No. 4 for periosteal elevator and for removal of large cysts
  Needle holder, Mayo-Hegar 6-inch (A needle holder should be 6 inches long; a delicate hemostat is not adequate.)
  Needles, ½-circle, cutting edge
  Suture material, silk No. 3-0
  Scissors, tissue
  Scissors, suture
  Hemostats, small curved
  Allis forceps for grasping tissue
  Single-tooth forceps, Adson 4½-inch, for delicate grasp of tissue
  College pliers
  "Russian forceps," V. Mueller Co., 6-inch, for grasping teeth

Several general observations can be made for purchasing equipment. Stainless steel equipment is more costly initially, but

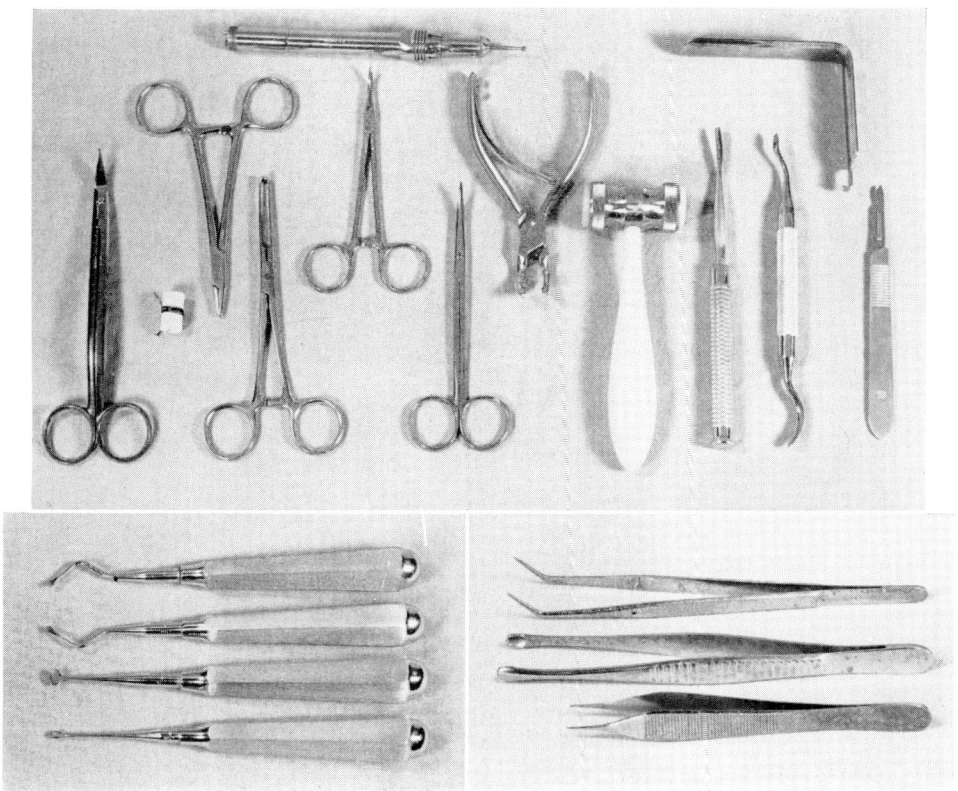

Fig. 3-4. Surgical instruments. Top row, left to right: suture scissors; suture and needle around cotton roll; needle holder; Allis forceps; hemostat; high-speed drill; tissue scissors; rongeurs; mallet; chisel; bone file; retractor; scalpel. Bottom row, left: Molt curets; right: Adson forceps (bottom), Russian forceps, college pliers.

it holds up better. It is mandatory that two complete sets of instruments be bought, although an office devoted to exodontia will have many sets. If an instrument is dropped or otherwise contaminated, time is too precious to await resterilization, even with highspeed autoclaving. If the bur technique for bone removal is employed, especial care must be given by the operator and by all office personnel to provide a sterile handpiece for each procedure. Perhaps the greatest argument in favor of the chisel technique is that a sterile chisel is always available, whereas the general practitioner in a hurry might be tempted to employ his usual handpiece for what he considers just a small bone or tooth cut in the wound. Some of the worst infections in patients admitted to the dental service of a general hospital in the South Pacific in World War II were the result of exodontia complicated by handpiece infection.

Sterilization and care of instruments

The best way to sterilize instruments is by autoclaving. Sharp instruments such as

Fig. 3-5. **A,** Forceps in sterile towel. Note forceps number written on towel before autoclaving. **B,** Pick-up forceps.

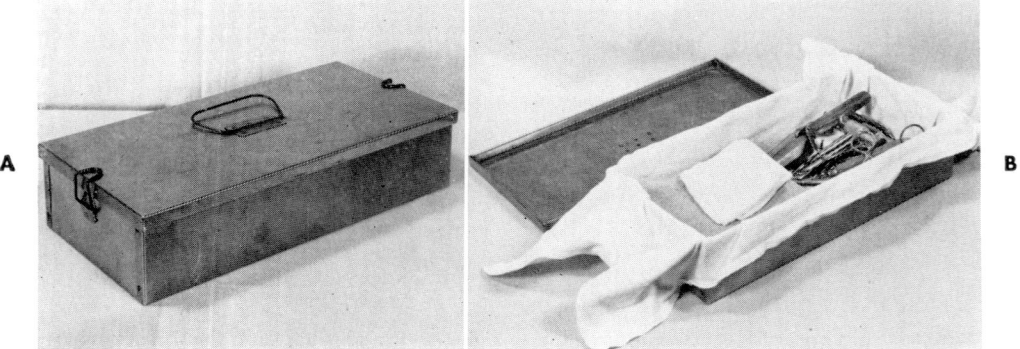

Fig. 3-6. **A,** Stainless steel box as removed from autoclave. **B,** Box opened, showing folded towels, gauze sponges, and accessory surgical instruments.

chisels and scalpels can be sterilized by the hot oil sterilizer. Cold solutions are used for storing sterilized instruments or for primary sterilization if many hours of undisturbed time can be given. The autoclave is used for sterilization of gauze sponges, cotton applicators, and linen.

Storage of the sterilized instruments is a problem. In the office devoted to exodontia a sterile table can be set up each day. This is not feasible in a general practice. Here each forceps should be wrapped in a linen towel large enough to fit the Mayo stand, and towel and forceps should be sterilized together. A pencil mark on the outside of the pack before sterilization will identify the instrument (Fig. 3-5, A). A complete tray of sterile accessory instruments covered with a towel should be available for more extensive surgery. The instruments can be sterilized on the tray if there is space to store the complete trays (which is the ideal way); or the instruments can be placed in a stainless steel box, which is more convenient to store and fits the smaller autoclave (Fig. 3-6). In the latter case a sterile pick-up forceps (Fig. 3-5, B) is used to arrange the instruments on the Mayo tray, which has been covered with a sterile towel. Sharp instruments are placed in the autoclaved box or on the tray after they have been sterilized by other methods.

Instruments should be scrubbed with a brush and soap in order to remove blood and debris that would harden during sterilization. Hospitals do this with ultrasonic equipment. The hinge of forceps should be free-swinging at all times. The patient lacks confidence in the operator who uses two hands to pull the handles of a frozen forceps apart just before an extraction. Rust has no place in the dental office.

The working points of all instruments should be sharp. Forceps with dull tips can be returned to the factory for refurbishing. A chisel that has been on a tray should be scrubbed and placed on the dentist's desk for inspection. If it has been used, it should be sharpened on a stone so that it will cut hair. Scalpel blades and needles should be changed frequently if disposable items are not used.

REFERENCES

1. Baldwin, D. C.: An investigation of psychological and behavioral responses to dental extraction in children, J. Dent. Res. 45:1637, 1966.
2. McKenzie, R. E., Szmyd, L., and Hartman, B. O.: A study of selected personality factors in oral surgery patients, J. Amer. Dent. Ass. 74:763, 1967.
3. Kruger, G. O., and Reynolds, D. C.: Maxillofacial pain. In McCarthy, F. M., editor: Emergencies in dental practice, Philadelphia, 1967, W. B. Saunders Co., p. 123.
4. Shannon, I. L., Isbell, G. M., and Hester, W. R.: Stress in dental patients. IV. Effect of local anesthetic administration on serum free 17-hydroxycorticosteroid patterns, J. Oral Surg. 21:50, 1963.

Chapter 4

FORCEPS EXTRACTION

Gustav O. Kruger

After the history, radiographs, and examination have been completed, the exodontia procedure is discussed with the patient, and the operator makes notes concerning the planning of the procedure, including premedication if indicated. The anxious patient who will be accompanied to the office can start premedication the night before the procedure or ½ hour before arriving at the office. Other patients can be premedicated in the office while waiting in the reception room. Medications by mouth or by intramuscular or intravenous routes vary in depth of effect and time of onset according to the agent and the amount used.

ANESTHESIA

The armamentarium should be in place, covered with a sterile towel, when the patient enters the operatory. The patient is seated and the chair is adjusted to the proper position for the administration of anesthesia. A paper napkin is placed on the patient and he is given ⅓ cup of mouthwash in a paper cup to rinse his mouth. Local anesthesia is administered. The operating light is turned off, and the patient is allowed to read or he is engaged in conversation for a minimum of 3 to 10 minutes, depending upon the tooth or teeth to be extracted. The operator should use at least a full minute of this time to study intently the radiograph of the tooth involved and its surrounding structures for anatomical and pathological variations from normal.

POSITION OF PATIENT

The chair usually has to be repositioned in order to be satisfactory for exodontia. For mandibular extractions it should be as low as possible. For maxillary extractions the upper jaw of the patient should be at the height of the operator's shoulder. These positions allow the upper arm to hang loosely from the shoulder girdle and obviate the fatigue associated with holding the shoulders in an unnaturally high position during the course of a day. The low positions allow the operator to bring his back and leg muscles into the operation to assist his arm. The chair can be tipped backward slightly for maxillary extractions.

PREPARATION AND DRAPING

The operating light is turned on, the operator and his assistant scrub, and a sterile towel is placed over the paper napkin while the dentist admonishes the patient not to touch it. Since the towel is sterile, gauze sponges or instruments can be placed on it. If complicated exodontia is planned, or if the patient manifests anxiety, another sterile towel is placed over the eyes from behind the head and fastened with a sterile pin or towel clamp over the forehead. The operator and his assistant may place sterile towels over their uniforms, fastening them with sterile towel clamps. The exposed portion of the patient's face is wiped with sponges dipped in benzalkonium chloride 1:10,000 solution.

A 3 by 3 inch gauze sponge is placed in the mouth so as to isolate the operative field. The sponge allows the field to be dried, it keeps the tongue out of the way, it absorbs saliva and blood, it prevents teeth and fragments from slipping into the posterior pharynx, and it keeps the patient from leaning over the bowl to spit, which wastes time. If a continuous suction technique is chosen, the gauze sponge may or may not be used.

POSITION OF LEFT HAND

The fingers of the left hand serve primarily to retract the soft tissues and to provide the operator with sensory stimuli for the detection of expansion of the alveolar plate and root movement under the plate. It is for these reasons that one finger is always placed on the labial or buccal alveolar plate overlying the tooth and another finger retracts the lip or tongue. A third finger or the thumb helps guide the forceps into place on the tooth and protects teeth in the opposite jaw from accidental contact with the back of the forceps if the tooth loosens suddenly. In mandibular extractions equal and opposite torquing force must be provided by the left hand to counteract the forces placed on the mandible by the extracting forceps in the right hand so that temporomandibular joint pain and injury do not occur. Each extraction and each type of forceps require different left-hand positions to accommodate the positions of the right hand, which holds the forceps.

FORCEPS EXTRACTION

A sharp No. 2 Molt curet is used to check the anesthesia. Then it is slid around the free gingival cuff to sever the gingival attachment of each tooth to be extracted in that quadrant. No force should be employed since this will alarm the patient.

The forceps are brought from the Mayo stand behind the patient, shielded from his view as much as possible, and guided into the mouth with the help of a finger or thumb of the left hand. The palatal or lingual beak is placed first, followed by the buccal or labial beak. The long axis of the forceps must be placed parallel with the long axis of the tooth. Failure to accomplish this is the most common cause in fracturing teeth. (Use of the wrong anatomical forceps, such as a molar forceps on a premolar, is another common cause for fracture.) Pressure is placed toward the apex of the tooth to "set" the forceps at the cementoenamel junction.

Enough pressure is placed on the handles to hold the forceps on the tooth without slipping, but uncommon force may shatter a weak tooth. The forceps should be held near the ends of the handles in order to obtain the maximum mechanical advantage. No greater delicacy of touch is obtained by holding them midway up the handles. In furniture factories, when an apprentice holds the hammer halfway up the handle, an old foreman takes it from him and cuts off the portion he was not using. This is a lesson he learns early, and he can hardly wait until evening to purchase a new, balanced handle.

Each tooth requires a separate series of movements for extraction, which are described in the accompanying photographs and diagrams (Figs. 4-1 to 4-8).

POSTEXTRACTION PROCEDURE

After the extraction all loose bone spicules and portions of tooth, restoration, or calculus are removed from the socket as well as from the buccal and lingual gutters and the tongue. If pathological tissue is present in the apical region, it is removed carefully with a small curet. The granula-

Text continued on p. 70.

60   Textbook of oral surgery

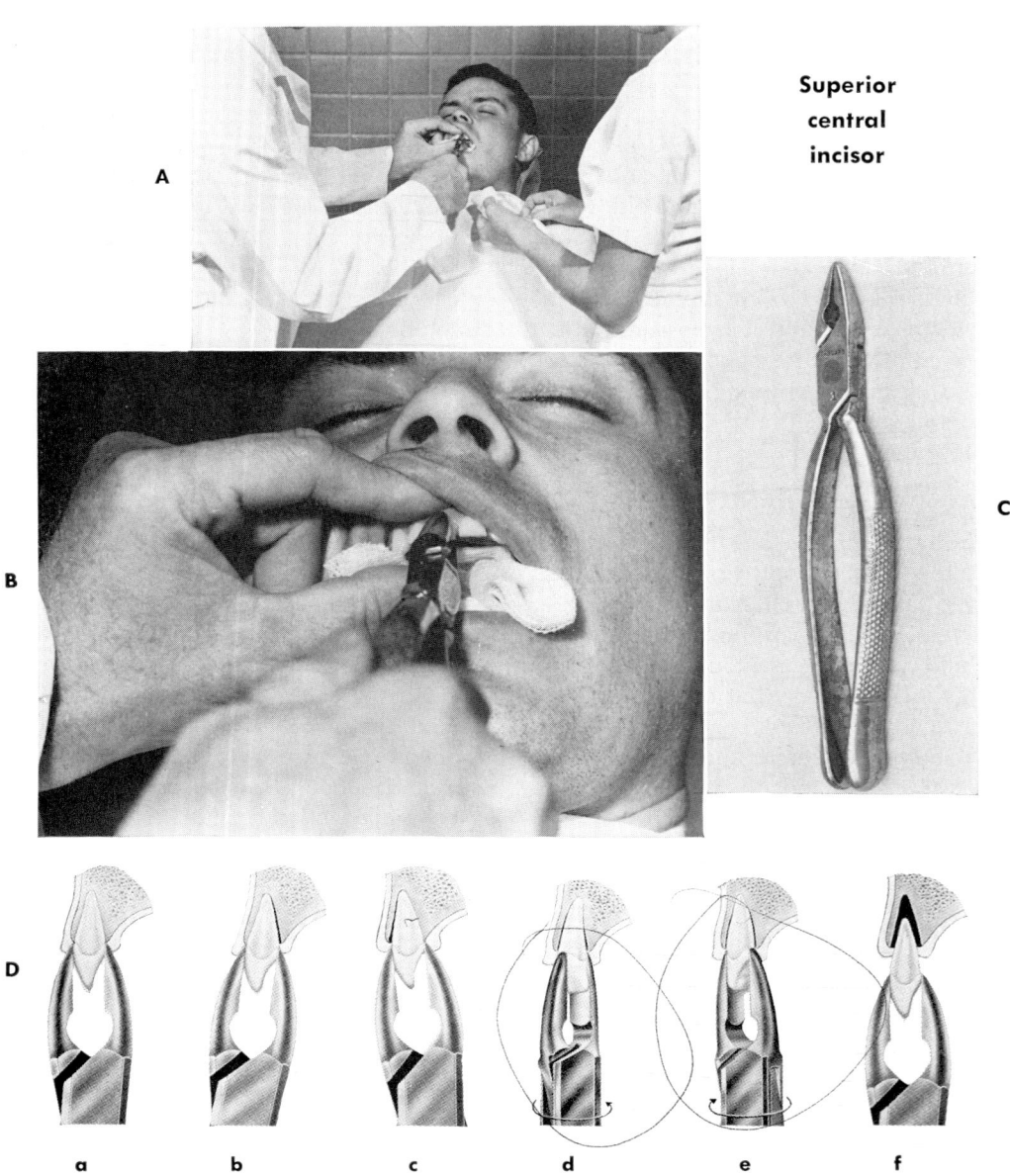

Fig. 4-1. **A,** Positions of patient, operator, and assistant. **B,** Fingers of left hand retracting tissues. **C,** Forceps No. 1. **D,** Extraction movements: **a,** forceps applied; **b,** first movement to labial side; **c,** movement to palatal side; **d,** rotatory movement from labial to distal side; **e,** reversed rotatory movement from labial to mesial side; **f,** downward movement in line with original position of tooth. (**D** from Winter, George B.: Exodontia, St. Louis, 1913, American Medical Book Co.)

Forceps extraction 61

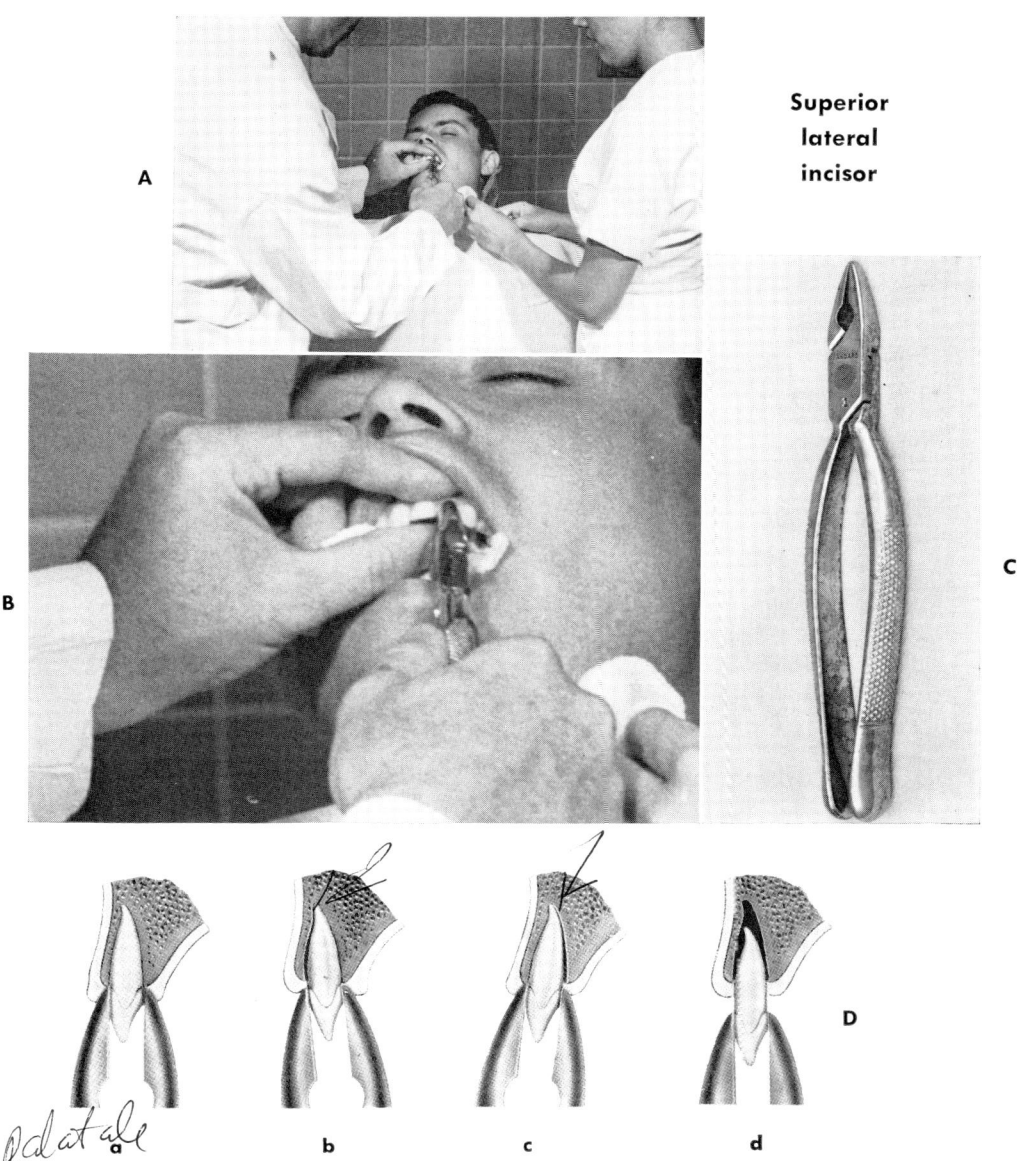

Fig. 4-2. **A,** Positions of patient, operator, and assistant. **B,** Fingers of left hand. **C,** Forceps No. 1. **D,** Extraction movements: **a,** forceps applied at anatomical neck; **b,** first movement to palatal side; **c,** movement to labial side; **d,** downward movement in line with original position of tooth. (**D** from Winter, George B.: Exodontia, St. Louis, 1913, American Medical Book Co.)

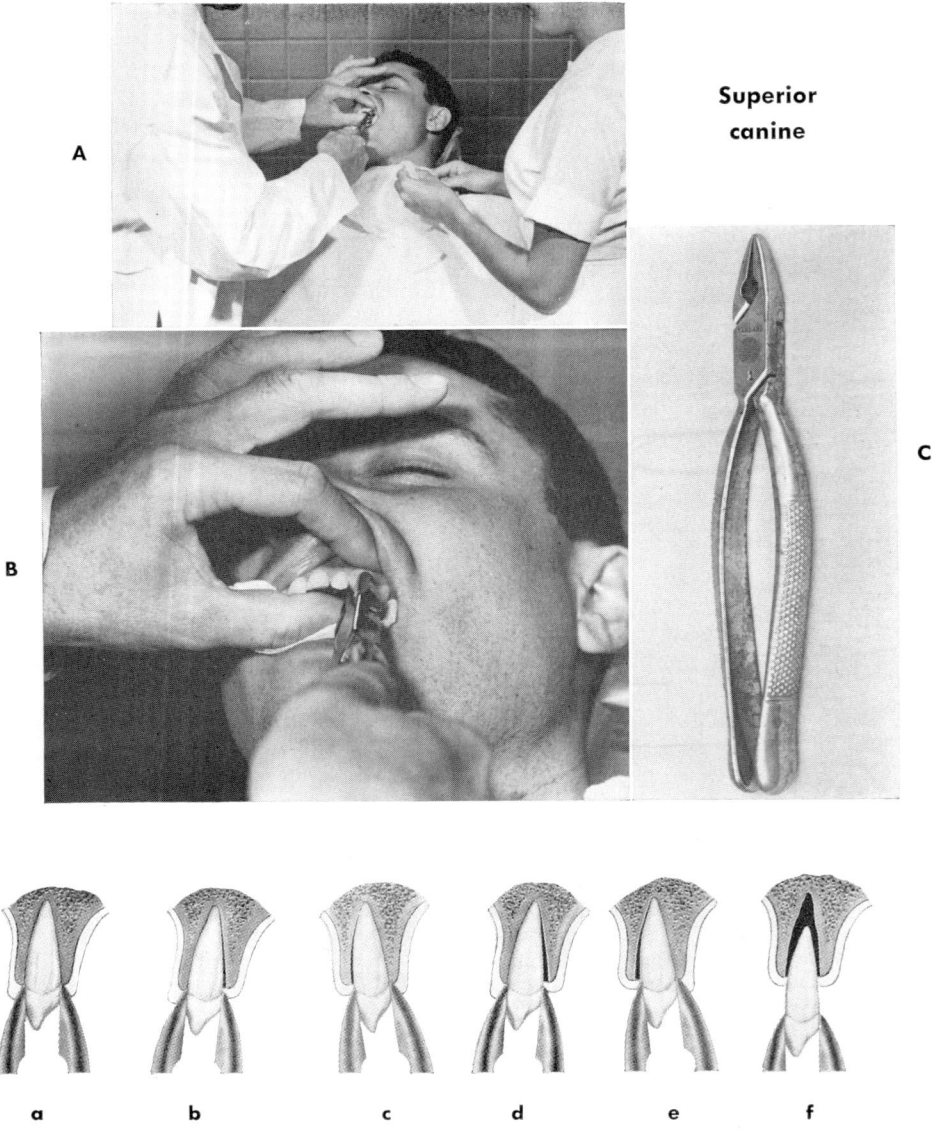

Fig. 4-3. **A**, Positions of patient, operator, and assistant. Note the straight line made by tooth, forceps, and lower arm while upper arm hangs from shoulder girdle. **B**, Positions of fingers of left hand. **C**, Forceps No. 1. **D**, Extraction movements: **a**, forceps applied at anatomical neck; **b**, first movement to labial side; **c**, movement to palatal side; **d** and **e**, labial and palatal movements more forcibly repeated; **f**, downward movement in line with original position of tooth. (**D** from Winter, George B.: Exodontia, St. Louis, 1913, American Medical Book Co.)

Forceps extraction 63

Superior premolars

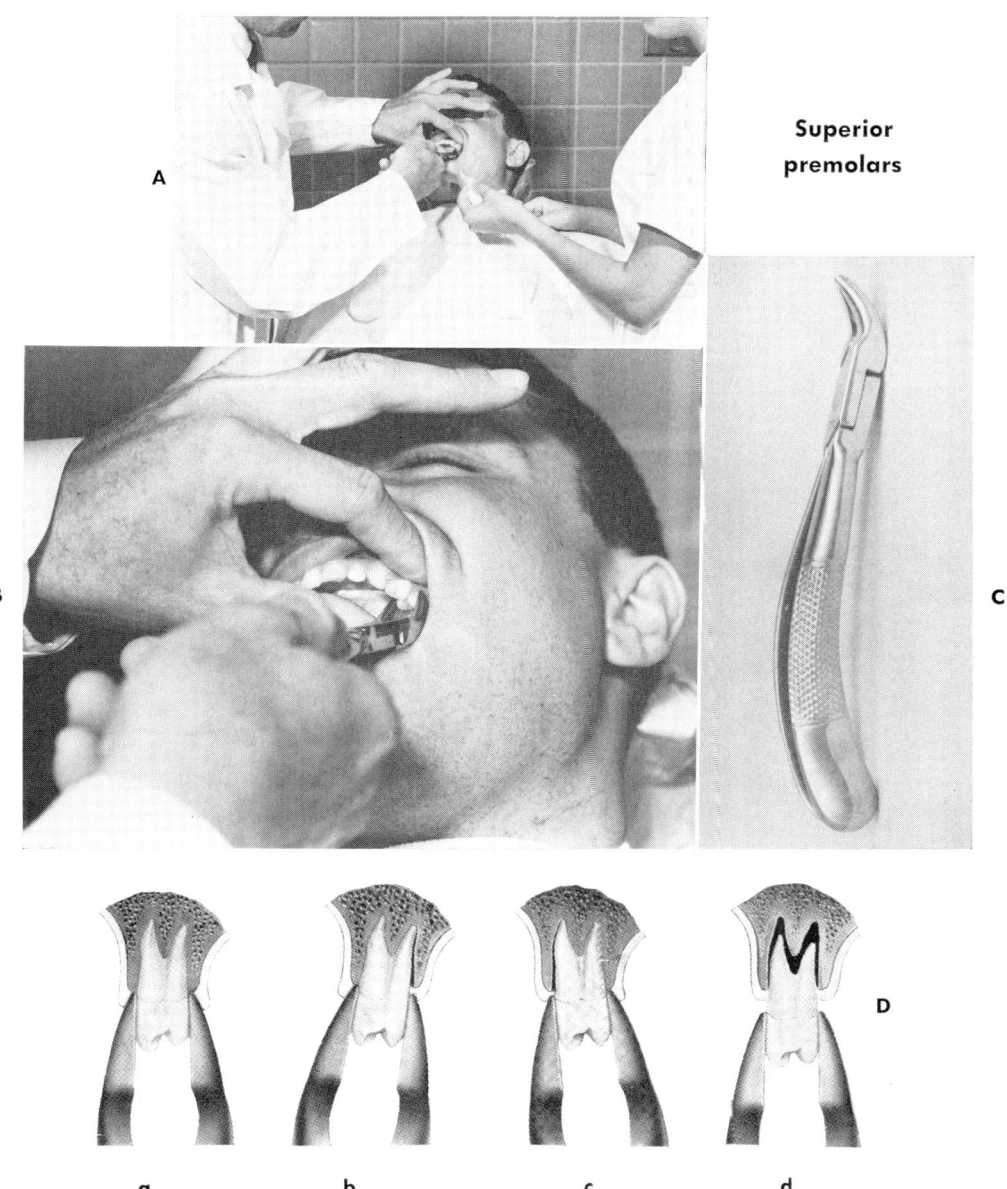

Fig. 4-4. A, Positions of patient, operator, and assistant. B, Positions of fingers of left hand. C, Forceps No. 150 (No. 1 can be substituted). D, Extraction movements: a, forceps applied to anatomical neck; b, first movement to buccal side; c, movement to palatal side; d, downward movement in line with original position of tooth. (D from Winter, George B.: Exodontia, St. Louis, 1913, American Medical Book Co.)

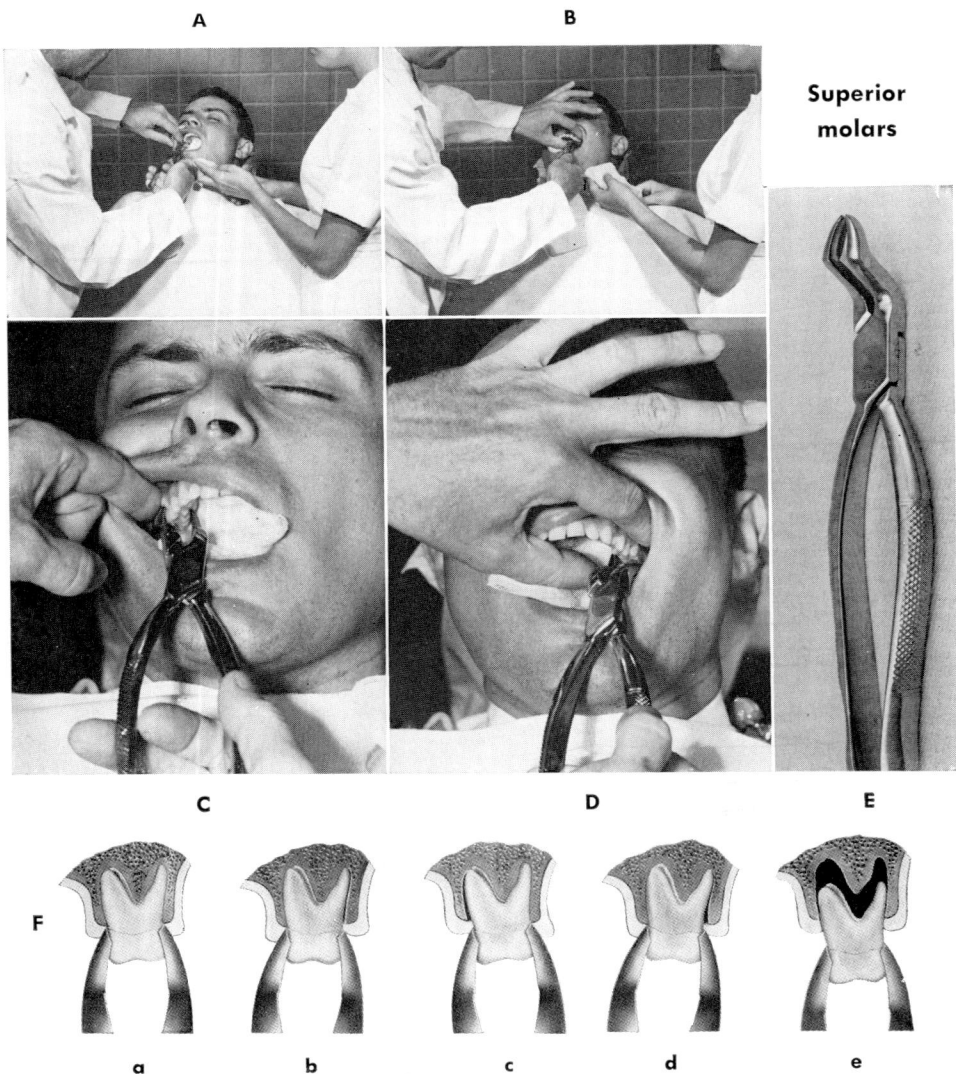

Fig. 4-5. **A**, Right side positions. **B**, Left side positions. **C**, Retraction of tissues and palpation of buccal plate with radial side of forefinger, right side. **D**, Retraction of tissues, left side. **E**, Forceps No. 10S. **F**, Extraction movements: **a**, forceps applied at anatomical neck; **b**, first movement to buccal side; **c**, movement downward and to palatal side (do not thread lingual root back into socket; the downward and palatal movement may be stopped when the tooth is in its original buccopalatal position, but lower, rather than in palatoversion); **d**, buccal movement repeated more forcibly; **e**, downward movement in line with original position of tooth. (**F** from Winter, George B.: Exodontia, St. Louis, 1913, American Medical Book Co.)

Forceps extraction 65

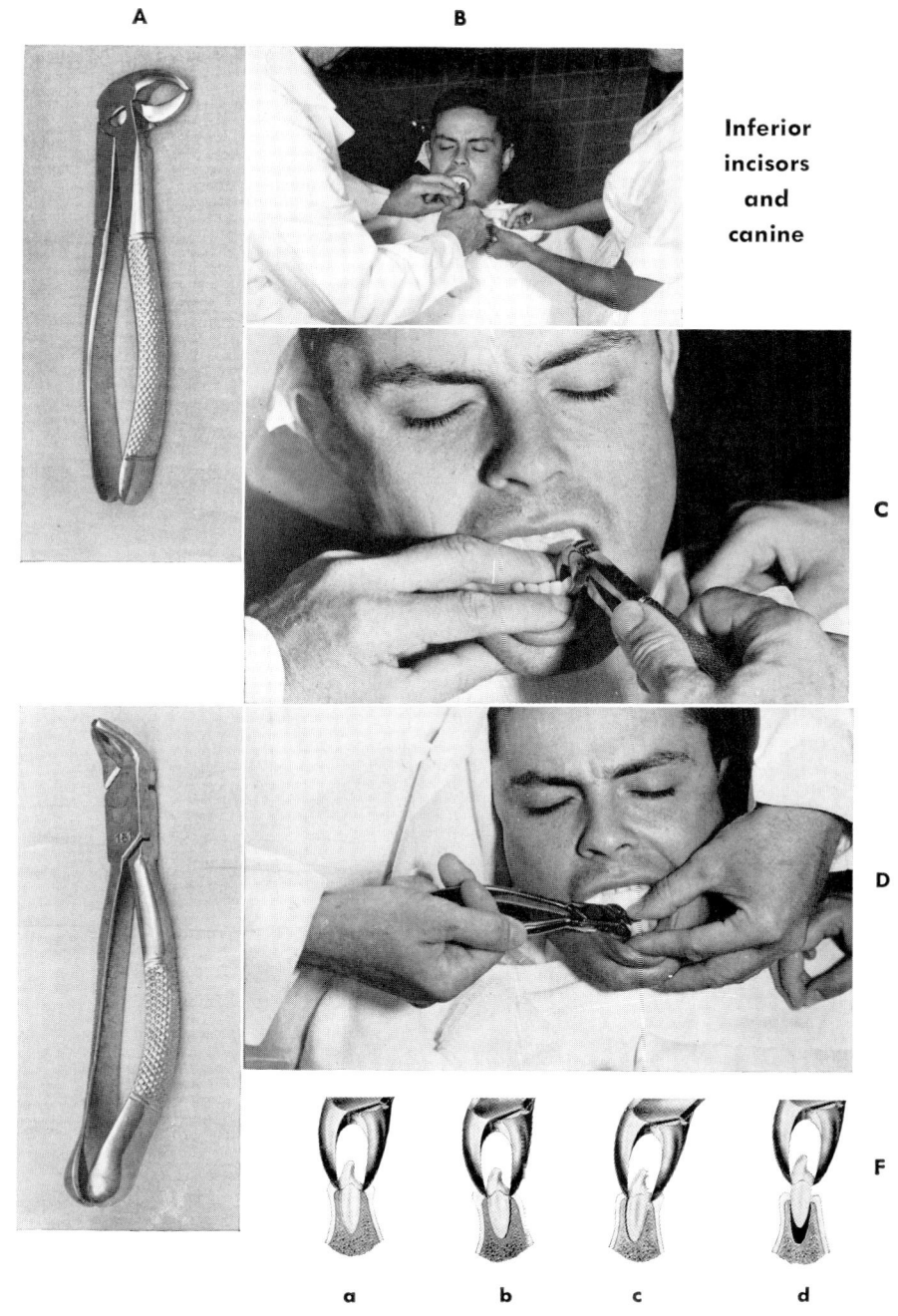

Inferior incisors and canine

Fig. 4-6. **A**, Mead forceps. **B**, Relative positions of patient, operator, and assistant. **C**, Fingers of left hand retract tongue and lip, while thumb supports jaw. **D**, Reverse position employed with forceps No. 151. **E**, Forceps No. 151. Either this forceps or Mead forceps may be used. **F**, Extraction movements: **a**, forceps placed at anatomical neck; **b**, first movement to labial side; **c**, movement to lingual side; **d**, upward movement in line with original position of tooth. (**F** from Winter, George B.: Exodontia, St. Louis, 1913, American Medical Book Co.)

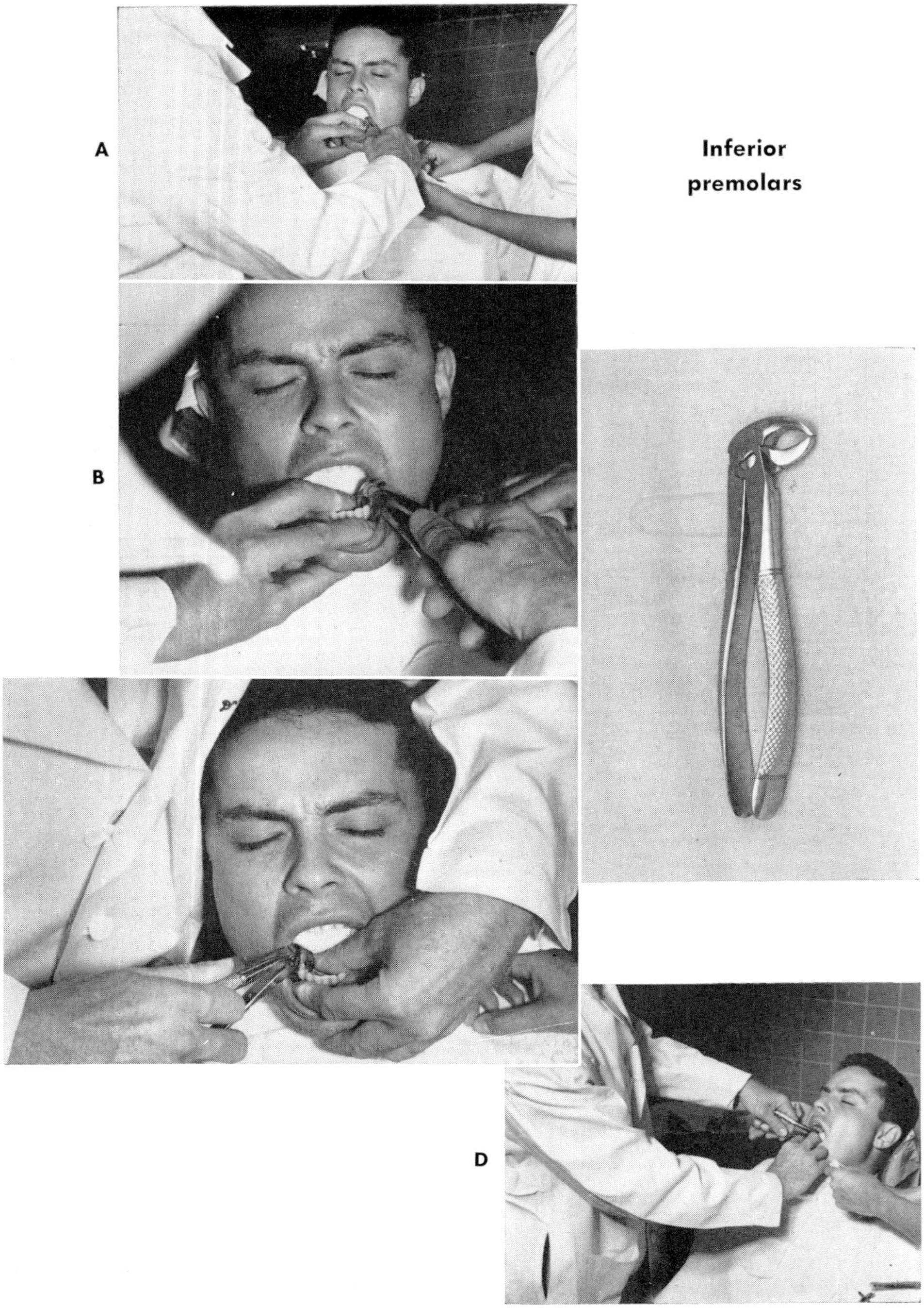

66   Textbook of oral surgery

Inferior premolars

Fig. 4-7. For legend see opposite page.

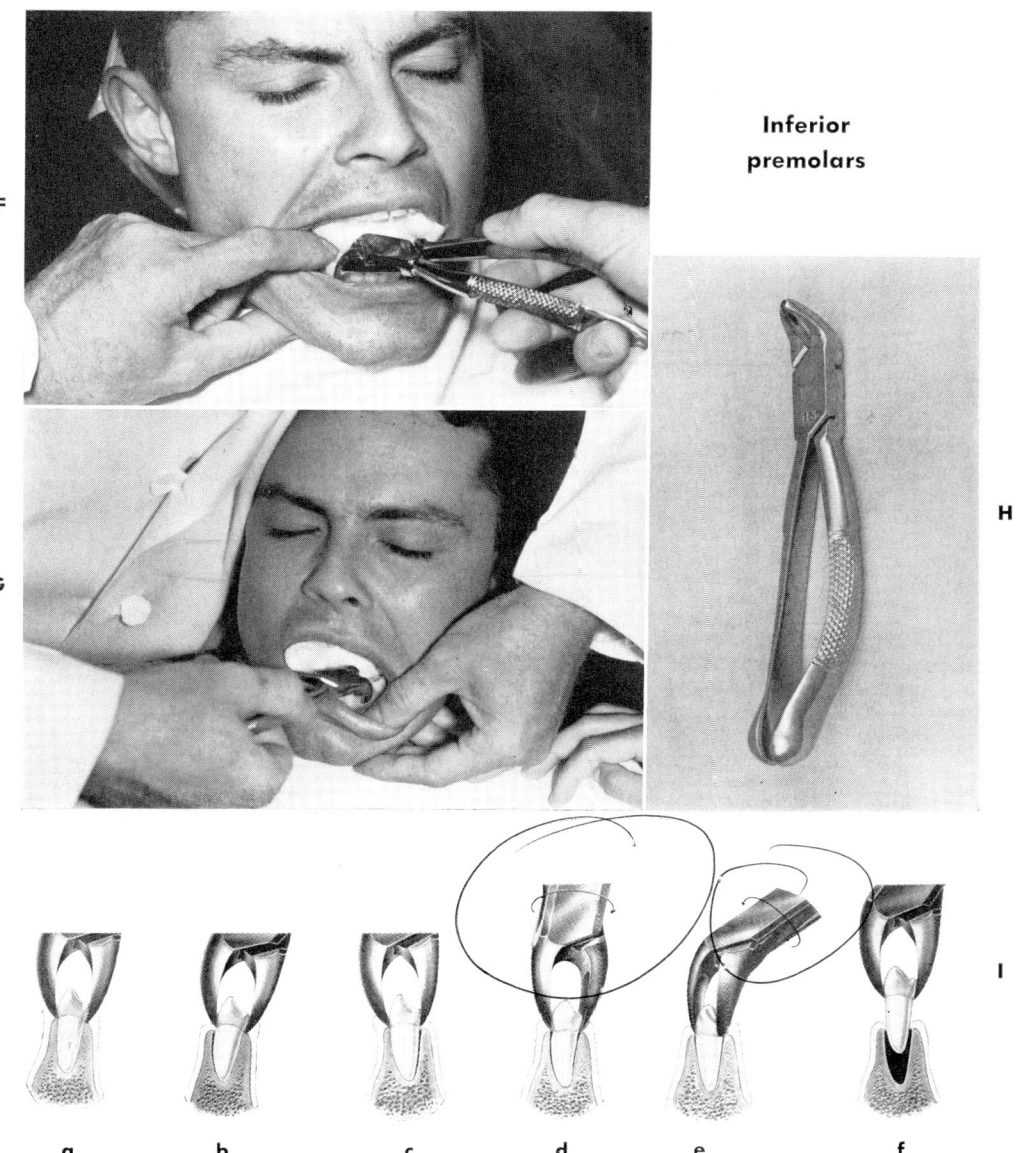

Fig. 4-7. A, Positions for left side extractions using Mead forceps. B, Fingers of left hand supporting jaw. C, Positions for right side extractions. D, Alternate position for right side extractions using Mead forceps in left hand. E, Mead forceps. F, Positions employed for right side extractions using forceps No. 151. G, Positions employed for left side extractions using forceps No. 151. H, Forceps No. 151. I, Extraction movements: a, forceps placed at anatomical neck; b, first movement to lingual side; c, movement to buccal side; d, rotatory movement from the mesial to the buccal side; e, reversed rotatory movement; f, upward movement in line with original position of tooth. (I from Winter, George B.: Exodontia, St. Louis, 1913, American Medical Book Co.)

68 Textbook of oral surgery

Inferior molars

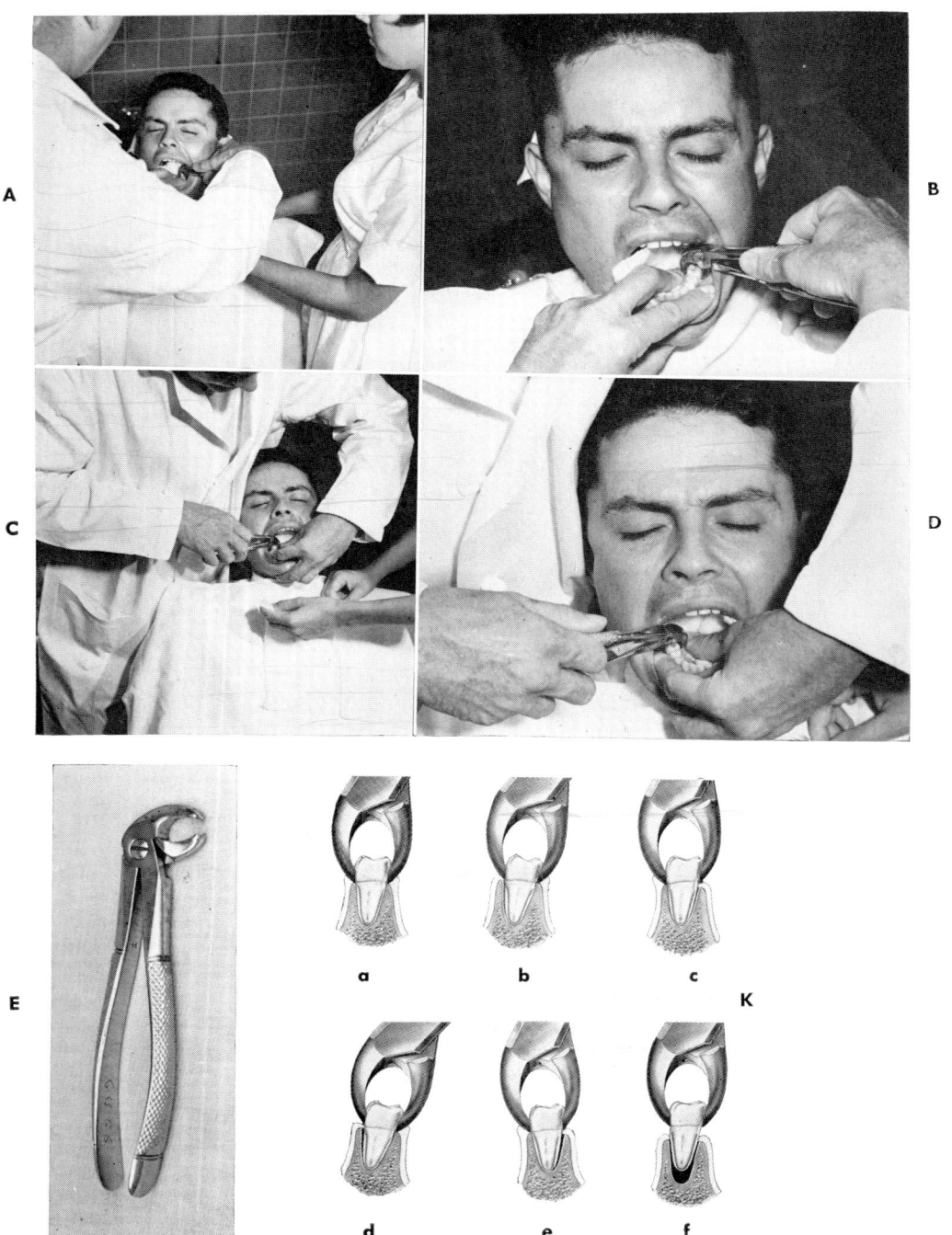

Fig. 4-8. For legend see opposite page.

Inferior molars

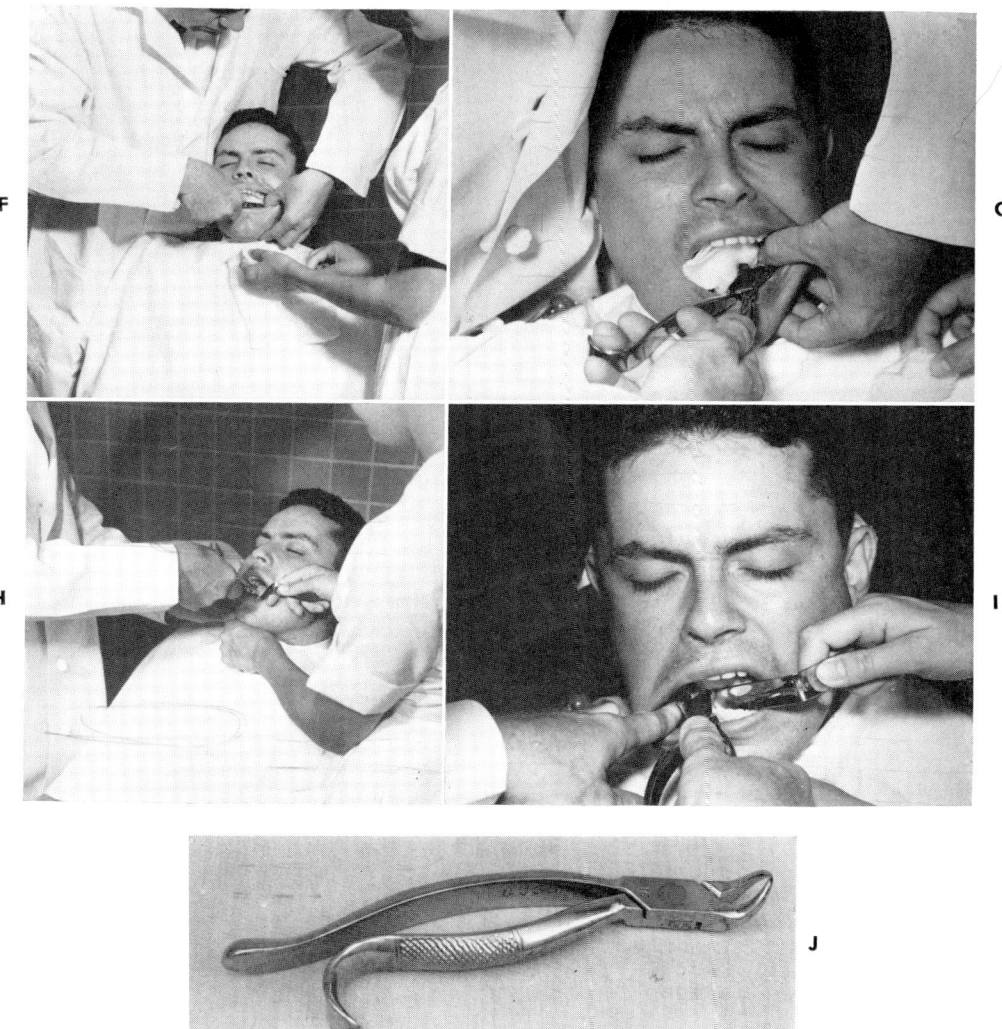

Fig. 4-8. **A**, Positions for extractions on left side using Mead forceps. **B**, Note positions of left hand. **C**, Positions for extractions on right side using Mead forceps. **D**, The thumb retracts the tongue, the forefinger retracts the lip, and the third finger supports the jaw. **E**, Mead forceps. **F**, Positions for extractions on left side using cowhorn forceps. **G**, Thumb is placed on occlusal surface of next posterior tooth or on ridge of mandible. **H**, Positions for extractions on right side using cowhorn forceps. **I**, Forefinger is placed on ridge of mandible. **J**, Forceps No. 16 (cowhorn). **K**, Extraction movements: a, forceps in position; b, first movement to lingual side; c, movement to buccal side; d and e, movements to lingual and buccal sides more forcibly repeated; f, upward movement in line with original position of tooth. With the cowhorn forceps the beaks are set into the bifurcation by squeezing the handles while moving them up and down. When the two beaks are in place, movements to the lingual and buccal sides are started. (**K** from Winter, George B.: Exodontia, St. Louis, 1913, American Medical Book Co.)

tion tissue "velvet" is removed or broken up, but the bone is not scraped. This is *not* done in the maxillary incisor area because the veins here have no valves; consequently, infected material and thrombi may ascend into the cranial cavity to form a cavernous sinus thrombosis. If a recent radiograph does not show apical radiolucency, it is wise not to put a curet into any socket since this will only inoculate the socket with organisms and debris from the free gingival margin if the original curet is used.

The socket must be compressed by the fingers to reestablish the normal width present before the plate was surgically expanded. In the case of multiple extractions, the sockets can be overcompressed by one third, which will eliminate the need for alveoloplasty in many borderline cases. Sutures usually are not necessary unless the papillae have been incised. When postoperative infection is anticipated, antibiotic or sulfonamide cones can be placed in mandibular molar, premolar, and canine sockets.

The socket is covered with a 3 by 3 inch gauze sponge that has been folded into quarters and moistened slightly at its center with cold water (to prevent hemorrhage from the socket from penetrating the gauze at that point, which would be torn away from the remainder of the clot when the gauze is removed, resulting in new bleeding). The side of the gauze placed over the wound is not touched by the operator for aseptic reasons. When the covering sponge is in place, the sponge originally placed over the tongue is removed. Saliva and debris are kept out of the socket by this method. The patient is asked to bite down on the sponge for 5 minutes.

After that time has elapsed a postoperative radiograph is made, for legal as well as professional reasons, and another moistened sterile sponge is placed, to be retained until the patient arrives home. Few cases of postoperative hemorrhage will occur if this procedure is followed. A printed instruction sheet is given to the patient, together with a prescription if pain is anticipated. Analgesic drugs should be started as soon as the patient returns home, well before the local anesthetic disappears. An appointment for postoperative examination is given.

NUMBER OF TEETH TO BE EXTRACTED

Many variables exist in the health and fitness of the patient in addition to the condition of his teeth and their surrounding structures. The planned procedure may involve complicated extractions and alveoloplasty, which may take a considerable length of time and result in a loss of blood of up to 500 ml. In the uncomplicated case the remaining posterior teeth in the maxilla and mandible on one side can be removed in one visit. If an immediate denture will not be made, occasionally the mandibular canine will be removed too, so that infiltration anesthesia can be given to remove the incisors later.

Further surgery is done no earlier than 1 week afterward, at which time swelling and discomfort have disappeared and the white cell count has returned to normal. The posterior teeth on the opposite side are removed 1 week later. The anterior teeth are removed after another week, or whenever the posterior wounds have healed well.

ORDER OF EXTRACTION

The order of extraction is important. Since anesthesia becomes effective in the maxilla earlier, the maxillary teeth are extracted first (with the exception of impacted teeth). Also, debris such as enamel or amalgam fragments cannot be lost in open mandibular sockets. The most posterior teeth are removed first, for better vision, since hemorrhage collects in the posterior region. In a mouth containing teeth that are difficult to extract, the first molar and canine teeth are extracted after their adjacent teeth are removed so that better purchase can be made on the tooth and so that advantage can be taken of earlier plate expansion resulting from adjacent extractions. These two teeth are encased in the so-called bony pillars of the face. Accordingly, the third molar, second molar, second premolar, first molar, first premolar, lateral incisor, and canine would be extracted in that order in difficult cases.

If a tooth or a root should break, it is best to stop and recover the root before proceeding to the next extraction. Consequently, the adjacent socket does not produce hemorrhage that obscures the field, and the location of the root is not lost. If there is a good possibility that adjacent teeth may break or if an alveoloplasty will be necessary, the operator may continue with the extractions, making careful note of the location of the root, and then design the surgical flap to accommodate the problem or problems that need attention.

REFERENCE

1. Rounds, F. W., and Rounds, C. E.: Principles and technique of exodontia, ed. 2, St. Louis, 1962, The C. V. Mosby Co.

Chapter 5

COMPLICATED EXODONTIA

Gustav O. Kruger

ALVEOLOPLASTY

Alveoloplasty or alveolectomy is the surgical removal of a portion of the alveolar process. When multiple extractions are performed, the contours of the alveolar ridge should be considered in the light of the needs of the future prosthesis. The ideal ridge is U shaped. Natural resorption will contour the ridges, occasionally unevenly, but a longer period of time is required and the patient may experience discomfort until the sharp bony edges underlying the sensitive periosteum round off. Judgment is required to determine whether alveoloplasty is necessary and how extensively it should be done.

Conservation of the maximum amount of bone consistent with a good ridge is the goal. Although the ridge that is extensively contoured by surgery is beautiful, with end-to-end mucosal closure over the sockets, the procedure is worthless if severe resorption of the remaining bone makes denture wearing impossible after a few years. On the other hand, laziness on the operator's part in smoothing obvious sharp edges, protuberances, and excessive undercuts that cause discomfort and an unsatisfactory denture base cannot be equated with conservatism.

Several years ago at a meeting of oral surgeons, discussion revealed that everyone had become more conservative in alveoloplasty procedures. The participants reported seeing greater numbers of elderly edentulous patients whose life span had increased and in whom no alveolar bone remained. Finally, an elderly oral surgeon in the back of the room said, "I am a diabetic. As you know, diabetics experience rapid and extensive bone resorption. When my son removed all my teeth he said, 'Dad, I am going to remove only the teeth and not one sharp ridge or piece of bone because we have to save every bit of bone we can.' Gentlemen, I suffered the agony of the damned until the sharp edges rounded off. On the basis of my personal experience, I make sure that the bone is smooth, even if I have to remove a little bone in a patient who is expected to undergo extensive resorption."

The most conservative procedure is compression of the alveolar walls by finger and thumb pressure. Extraction usually expands the labial or buccal cortex. Pressure will restore the walls to their former position. Overcompression by heavy pressure can reduce the width of the sockets by one third.

If there is a question in the operator's mind about the amount of natural resorption that will take place, he can make a better judgment 3 weeks after the extractions are accomplished. Most of the initial resorption will be completed in 3 weeks. At that time an extensive alveoloplasty may still be necessary, but more frequently he will find that only a few small areas require contouring.

Simple alveoloplasty. Following multiple extractions the buccal alveolar plates and interseptal bone are examined for protuberances and sharp edges. If alveoloplasty is necessary, incisions are made across the interseptal crests. The mucoperiosteum is raised carefully from the bone with a No. 4 Molt curet or a periosteal elevator. Difficulty is experienced in starting the flap at the edge of the bone because periosteum is

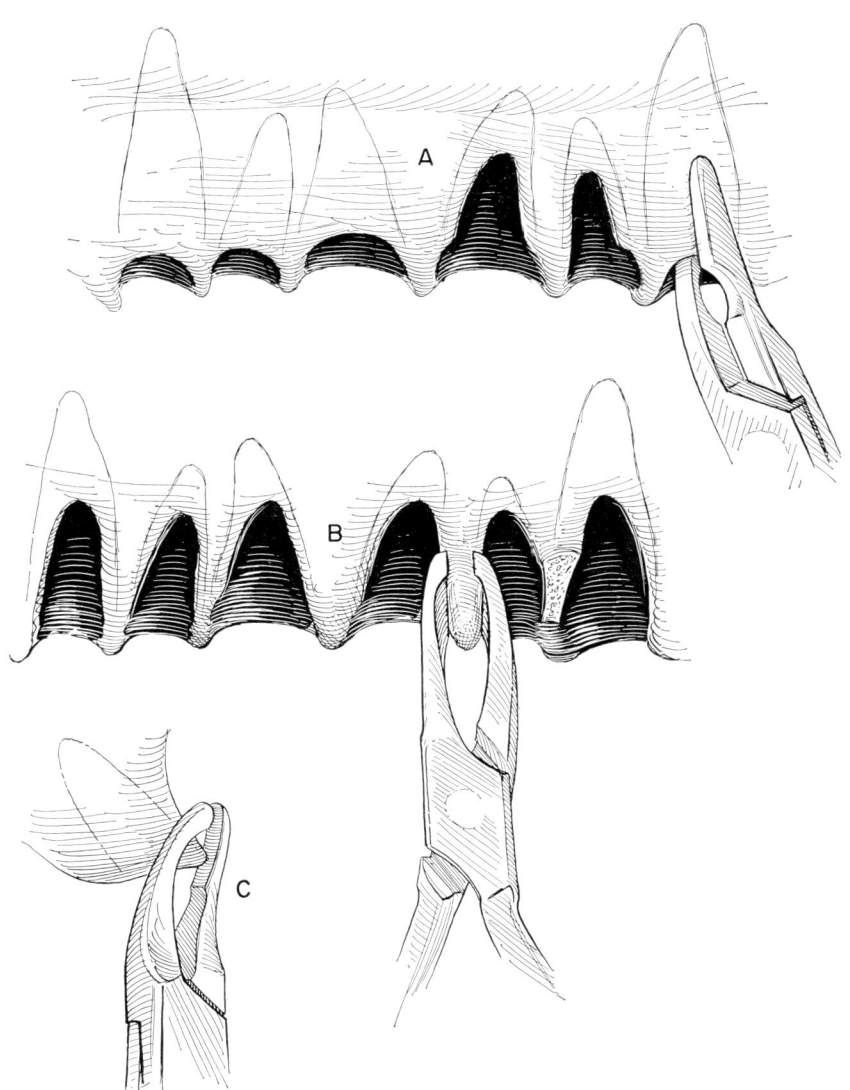

Fig. 5-1. Simple alveoloplasty. **A,** Rongeur removing labial plate. **B,** Removal of interseptal tip. **C,** Side view of interseptal tip removal.

attached at the ends of bones, but caution must be exercised in not raising the flap higher than two thirds of the way up the empty socket. To raise it further would strip the lightly attached mucobuccal fold, with the consequence of serious loss of space for denture flange height.

The flap is retracted gently and an edge of a gauze sponge placed between bone and flap. A universal rongeur is placed sideways halfway up the empty sockets, and the buccal or labial alveolar plate is resected to a uniform height in all sockets (Fig. 5-1, A). The rongeur now is placed at a 45-degree angle over the interseptal crest, one beak in each socket, and the labial or buccal interseptal tip is removed (Fig. 5-1, B and C). This procedure is accomplished on all interseptal crests. Bone bleeders are controlled by rotating a small curet in the bleeding point. A file lightly pulled in one direction over all cuts will smooth the bone. Loose particles are removed, the gauze is removed so that the flap resumes its place on the bone, and a finger is rubbed over the mucosal surface to examine the smoothness of the alveolus.

The buccal plate should be contoured to approximately the same height as the palatal plate to form a broad, flat ridge. Excessive undercuts in the upper posterior and lower anterior segments should be given particular attention. Excessive soft tissue and chronic granulation tissue are removed from the buccal and palatal flaps, which are then sutured over the interseptal areas, but not over the open sockets. Interrupted or continuous sutures are placed without tension.

Radical alveoloplasty. At times radical contouring of the alveolar ridge is indicated because of extremely prominent undercuts or, in some instances, a marked discrepancy in horizontal relation of maxillary and mandibular ridges due to marked overjet. Such patients may require complete removal of the labial plate to achieve satisfactory prosthetic replacement (Fig. 5-2).

In such cases a mucoperiosteal flap is raised prior to extraction. Extraction of the teeth can be facilitated by first removing the labial bone overlying the roots of the teeth (Fig. 5-3, A and B). This bone removal will also ensure preservation of interradicular bone. Following removal of the teeth the remaining bone is trimmed and contoured to the desired labial and occlusal height with the chisel or rongeur

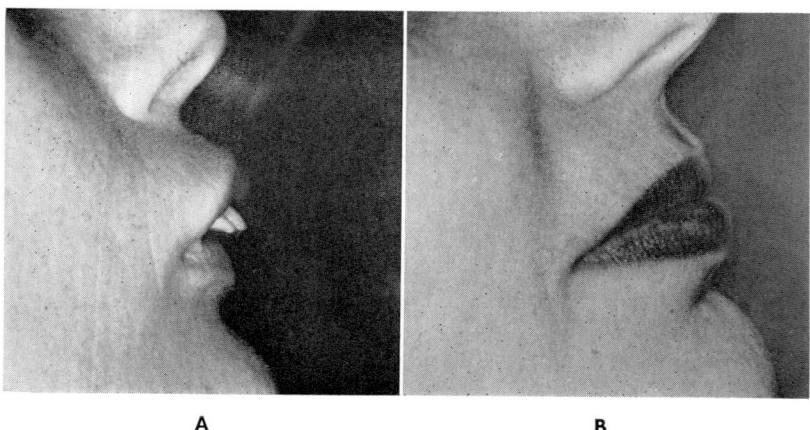

Fig. 5-2. Radical alveoloplasty. **A,** Preoperative overjet that was an esthetic and functional deformity. **B,** Postoperative result with denture in place.

and file (Fig. 5-3, C). Excessive tissue is trimmed from the labial and palatal flaps, which are approximated with interrupted or continuous sutures over the septa.

In closing such a flap it may be necessary to remove a wedge of tissue in the premolar areas to allow for the decreased outer circumference of the labial bone. Care must be taken with this larger flap to preserve as much attachment at the height of the mucobuccal fold as possible, or else an excessively long flap is encountered at closure. If the flap is not supported by an immediate denture and the excess tissue is resected, the height of the mucobuccal fold will be diminished drastically.

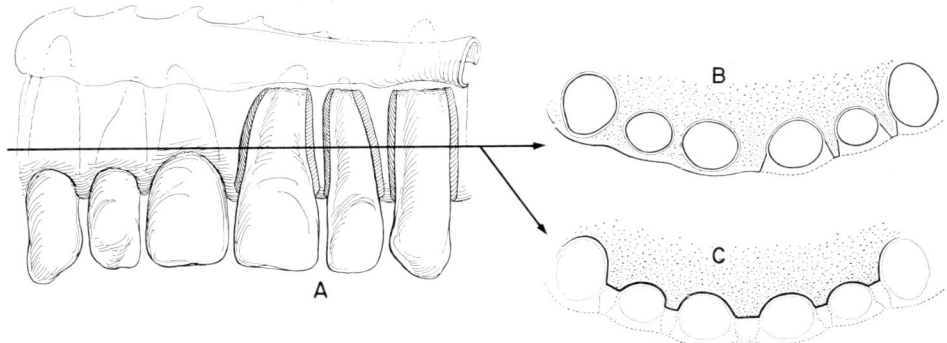

Fig. 5-3. Radical alveoloplasty. **A**, Mucoperiosteal flap raised and labial bone overlying teeth removed. **B**, Cross section showing removal of labial bone to encompass greatest width of tooth. **C**, Teeth removed and septa contoured back to palatal plate.

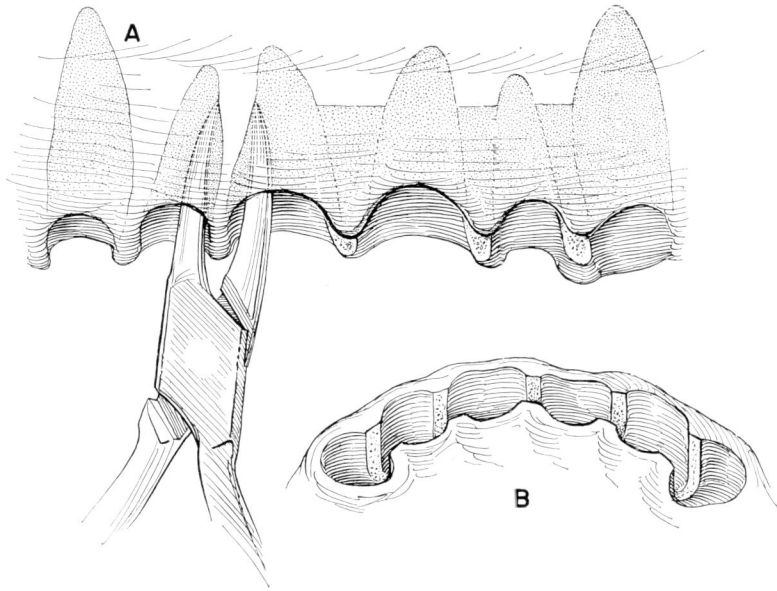

Fig. 5-4. Interradicular alveoloplasty. **A**, Narrow-beaked rongeur removes septa without raising a flap or destroying labial plate. **B**, The weakened labial plate is collapsed to the palatal plate by thumb pressure.

Interradicular alveoloplasty. In this procedure interradicular bone is sacrificed rather than labial plate. The teeth are extracted. No attempt is made to raise a mucoperiosteal flap over the bone to be collapsed. Interradicular bone is removed with a narrow-beaked rongeur (one beak in each socket) to a height halfway up the sockets (Fig. 5-4). A notch is cut by rongeur or chisel in the labial plate in each premolar area to allow for the greater circumference of the labial plate to fit into its new position. The bone is collapsed to the desired contour by thumb pressure.

Less resorption and less postoperative pain are associated with this procedure since periosteum is not stripped from bone and does not rest on roughened bone.

SURGICAL FLAP

A surgical flap is a soft tissue flap that is incised and retracted so that underlying bone can be removed to expose teeth, roots, and pathological tissue. Extractions and root removal procedures accomplished through the intact alveolus are called closed procedures. Operations requiring a surgical flap are called open procedures.

Basically, the indication for the surgical flap is inability to remove the structure or tissue without traumatizing the surrounding tissues. If a closed procedure fails, adequate visualization and access are obtained by means of an open procedure. A root remnant that cannot be recovered by ordinary means is removed by making a surgical flap. A large tooth that is encased in dense bone and will not move with forceps pressure is dissected out under a surgical flap, making forceps delivery possible. However, there are indications for making a surgical flap without first attempting a closed procedure. For instance, if there is a reasonable possibility that the crown of a tooth will fracture because it is weakened by extensive caries or large restorations, or if the crown is not present, a surgical flap should be considered. Some operators routinely prepare all devitalized teeth because the crown and root are friable after endodontic procedures. If the roots of a tooth are widely divergent, curved, or enlarged by hypercementosis, a flap may be prepared. If the overlying bone structure is enlarged or especially dense, or if the periodontal membrane is atrophic or absent (ankylosis), surgery is indicated. A large area of pathology that cannot be removed through the narrow socket may be removed through a surgical flap.

Principles. Healing should take place without complication if basic surgical principles are followed. The incision should be designed so that the blood supply of the flap is adequate. If the free end of the flap is wide and the base containing the blood supply is narrow, nutrition to the flap may be inadequate. The flap should contain all the structures overlying bone, including mucosa, submucosa, and periosteum, with especial care given to include the periosteum in the flap. The flap should be sufficiently large that adequate vision and space for removal of bone are present without damaging the soft tissue edges. The incision should always be made over bone that will not be removed, so that the sutured incisions are supported by bone. Incisions made in tissues that harbor uncontrolled infection may cause rapid spread of the infection.

Types. The two basic types of intraoral surgical flaps are the "envelope" flap and the flap that has a vertical component on the buccal or labial surface. The envelope flap is made by incising the tissues around the necks of several teeth anterior and posterior to the area and spreading the resultant labial or buccal flap away from the bone. This flap is used in removing impacted teeth more than in other extractions. The vertical flap employs a vertical incision extending from the mucobuccal fold to a horizontal gingival incision around the necks of the teeth. Less tissue is raised, and the free gingival fibers of adjacent teeth are not incised. Some operators prefer one type, some the other.

Surgical procedure. Incision with a No. 15 blade is made around the buccal or labial gingival cuff surrounding the tooth posterior to the one to be operated on, around the tooth itself, and then angled upward toward the mucobuccal fold away from the tooth to be removed (Fig. 5-5, A).

Elevation of the mucoperiosteal flap is started in the vertical component, where the periosteal attachment is not tight, and the periosteal elevator is worked toward the gingival cuff incisions as well as backward. The thin periosteum overlying the bone must be included in the flap. The flap is raised. The edge of the elevator is inserted 2 mm. under the attached anterior tissue midway between cuff and fold for later entrance of the suture needle.

The flap is held up from the incisal plane with the periosteal elevator, or a piece of gauze is placed under the flap to retract it away from the field of operation with a finger. Retraction should be gentle to prevent damage and edema. The flap should remain retracted without relaxation of the retracting force until the operation is completed.

Bone removal may be accomplished by chisel, bur, or rongeur, the last being used to start ossisection if an empty socket is present. In dissecting a tooth, cuts parallel to the long axis of the tooth are made in the labial or buccal plate on the mesial and distal sides of the root. Following removal of the buccal plate, further bone cuts are made on the two sides of the wound until the greatest width of the root is exposed. Care must be taken to avoid roots of the adjacent teeth (Fig. 5-5, B).

The tooth is removed with forceps or elevators. Pathological tissue at the apex is removed with curets. The edges of the bony incision are smoothed with a file or small curet. All debris and small spicules are removed. The flap is returned to position. A suture is placed through the edge of the free flap about halfway between cuff and fold and sutured to an opposite point in the fixed tissue anterior to the incision. It is tied without tension. A suture to the lingual tissues is not necessary. A folded, moist gauze sponge is placed over the socket to prevent bleeding.

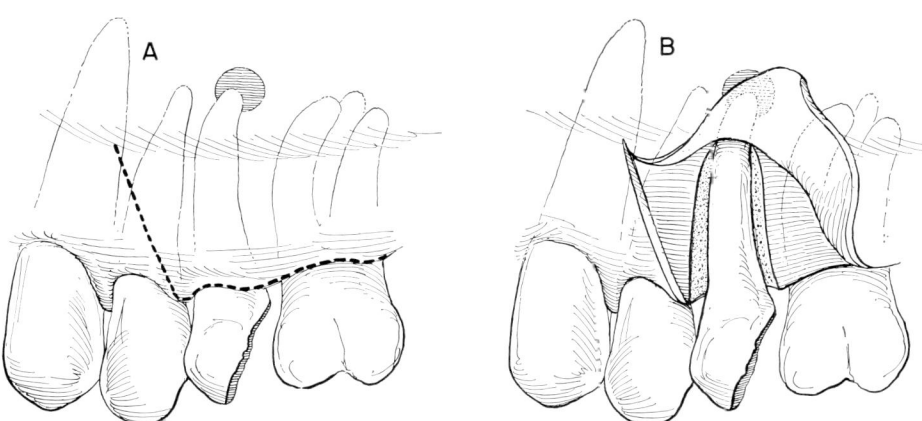

Fig. 5-5. Surgical flap. **A,** Incision. **B,** Retraction of flap and removal of labial bone to greatest width of tooth. Note that the edge of the flap, which will be sutured, will be supported by undissected bone.

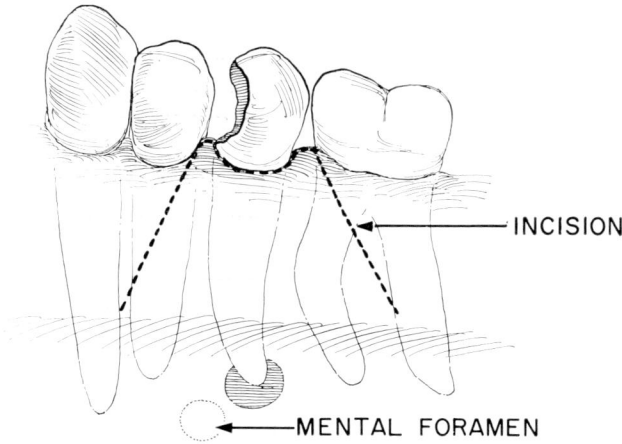

Fig. 5-6. Inverted incision for mandibular flap in the premolar-molar area.

Variations in basic flap design are necessary in special areas. In the mandibular premolar area a distal vertical incision is added so that the mental foramen structures can be protected (Fig. 5-6). The mandibular molar area benefits from a similar flap for better dissection of the distal root. The double flap is more difficult to suture.

ROOT REMOVAL

The removal of a freshly fractured root is attempted by the closed method (i.e., without a surgical flap) if there is likelihood of success. Many skilled operators boast that they can remove all such roots through the intact socket. However, it is best to prepare a surgical flap if the technique is not successful within 4 or 5 minutes. Otherwise, half an hour can be wasted, the soft and bony tissues are traumatized, and the flap has to be made anyway.

Closed procedures. A tooth fractured at its anatomical neck often can be grasped by an anatomical or a root forceps and delivered. An alveolar purchase may be obtained by loosening the buccal or labial gingival cuff with a small, sharp curet. The buccal beak of the forceps is then placed under the tissues on the buccal plate (Fig. 5-7). Pressure on a sharp forceps will bite down on the root, and the root with the cut alveolar plate attached is delivered. Occasionally pressure will fracture the plate enough to loosen the tooth, and the forceps is returned to its normal position at the anatomical neck for a normal extraction without removing alveolar plate. Alveolar purchase will not be successful if the buccal plate is excessively heavy or the palatal edge of the root cannot be grasped.

A straight-shank elevator is used to remove roots fractured just below the alveolar margin, especially in the maxilla. The instrument is held in a plane parallel to the long axis of the tooth and worked up along the palatal aspect of the root with purchase placed on the palatal rim if necessary (Fig. 5-8, *A*). Another method of using the straight-shank elevator is to place it in the interdental area at a right angle to the long axis of the tooth, using a buccal approach. The root is elevated by using the interdental septum as a fulcrum (Fig. 5-8, *B*).

If the root is fractured more than halfway up the socket, root exolevers are used. These are delicate instruments that can break easily (Fig. 3-3). Pressure on the root tip itself may force the fragment into the antrum, the mandibular canal, or the soft

Complicated exodontia 79

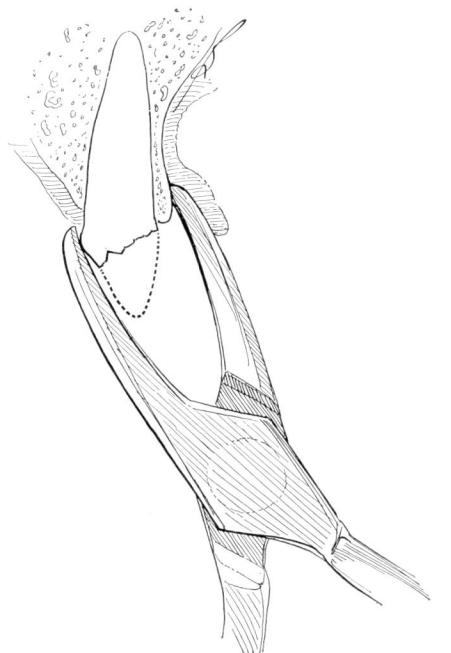

Fig. 5-7. Alveolar purchase. The labial tissues have been released, and the forceps beak is positioned on the labial alveolar plate.

tissues. A careful technique is necessary, the most important aspect of which is adequate vision. If bleeding obscures the field, pressure for several minutes on a piece of gauze held by an instrument in the socket, with or without 1:1,000 epinephrine, will allow the fragment to be seen. The light, positions of the patient and operator, retraction of tongue and cheek, and dryness must all be coordinated. Once the fragment is seen it often takes only a moment to remove it.

The object of the procedure is to place the instrument between the socket wall and the highest side of the fragment (i.e., closest to the rim of the socket) and tip the fragment in the opposite direction. It can then be teased out. A clue to the inclination of the surface of the root can be obtained by observing the fracture in the tooth that has been removed. It is better to excavate slightly into the socket wall to obtain a good purchase than to risk placing apical pressure on the fragment.

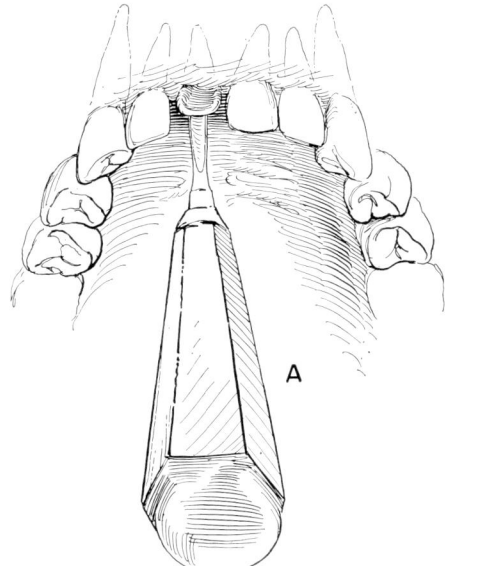 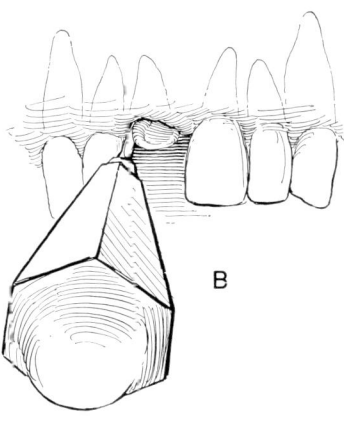

Fig. 5-8. Elevation of necrotic root remnant with straight-shank elevator. A, Palatal approach parallel with long axis of root. B, Labial-buccal approach at right angles to long axis of root.

Maxillary molar fragments, particularly those in the third molar area, are best visualized and approached indirectly using a mirror. The operator stands behind the patient. Buccal roots may be curved, necessitating considerable teasing. Palatal roots of molars are large and are surrounded by unyielding socket walls. Because of their proximity to the antrum no direct pressure is placed on the root. Space is gained between the socket wall and the root at the expense of the socket wall, and several sides are attacked before a curved root can be delivered.

Maxillary first premolar roots are small and thin. The buccal root can easily be pushed through the thin buccal wall so that it lies between periosteum and alveolar plate. A finger is placed over the buccal plate to prevent this occurrence or to feel the root if it does penetrate the plate. The palatal root is removed at the expense of the intervening septum between the roots.

Mandibular roots fractured at high level require separation of the roots if the crown is fractured below the alveolar rim and the two roots are still joined. Separation can be accomplished by chisel, bur, or elevator. The first root is removed with a short Winter elevator (No. 11); purchase is obtained between the two separated roots with the fulcrum on the second root (Fig. 5-9, A). An alternative method obtains purchase in the interdental area (Fig. 5-9, B). After the first removal the second root is removed with the same elevator by means of a high purchase in the interdental area, or, better, the long Winter elevator (No. 14) is placed in the depth of the empty socket (Fig. 5-10). With care that the heel of the elevator does not damage the adjacent tooth, the point of the elevator engages the septum and removes it with a turn. The elevator again is placed in the socket, engages the root, and delivers it. The latter method is used to remove all roots in the mandibular molar area.

Mandibular roots in the anterior and premolar areas are removed with root exolevers.

Open procedures. When unyielding socket walls, curved root tips, inaccessibility, or inadequate visibility precludes removal of roots by closed procedures, a surgical flap should be made before much time is wasted. The standard flap procedure is employed for buccal roots. Labial or buccal bone can be removed with a rongeur, although a chisel or bur is equally rapid. The root tip will come into view soon after the alveolar plate is removed.

An apicoectomy-type semilunar incision

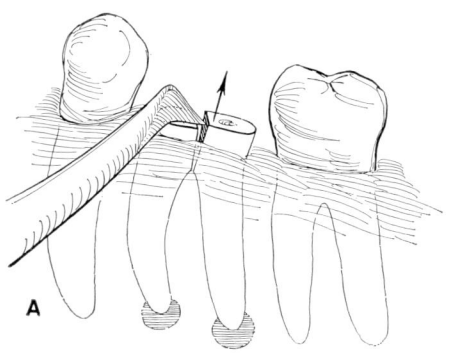 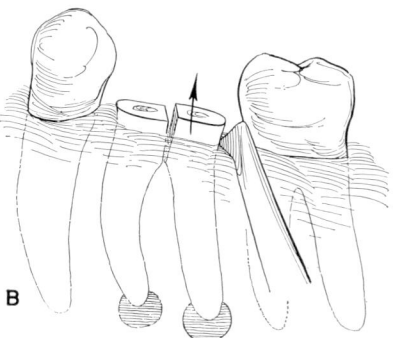

Fig. 5-9. Elevation of mandibular root with short Winter elevator. **A,** Fulcrum placed on shorter root by heel of elevator. **B,** Alternate procedure: fulcrum placed in interdental area.

Chapter 6

IMPACTED TEETH*

Gustav O. Kruger

Anthropologists state that the constantly increasing cerebration of man enlarges his brain case at the expense of his jaws. The prepituitary line that sloped forward from receded forehead to protruded jaw in prehuman forms has become almost vertical in modern man as the number of teeth has decreased. A softer and more refined diet that requires less chewing enhances this trend, making a powerful masticatory apparatus unnecessary. Greater numbers of people have impacted teeth for this as well as other reasons. Eventually all third molars will be lost to man, followed eons later by the impaction and subsequent loss of the lateral incisors.

All teeth that do not assume their proper position and function in the arch should be considered for removal. There are exceptions to this general statement, but they are rare. For instance, the youth who must lose all of his teeth for full dentures should not lose the unerupted maxillary third molars since the eruption of these teeth will help to form the tuberosity. The denture can be made over the unerupted teeth if the patient is made cognizant of the situation so that the teeth can be removed later when they appear beneath the mucosa.

In the older individual discretion may be the better part of valor. A tooth that has not erupted for 50 years is sometimes ankylosed, often presents an atrophied periodontal membrane separating tooth and bone, and is always encased in inelastic, heavily mineralized bone. Unerupted teeth can and should be removed to ensure success for the denture, but in the occasional instance removal may not be feasible.

PRELIMINARY CONSIDERATIONS

Presence of infection. Infection in the form of a pericoronitis should be treated before surgery. An acute pericoronitis around a mandibular third molar usually responds to the extraction of the maxillary third molar if the latter is impinging on the infected mandibular tissues. Probing with a sterile silver probe under the flap on the buccal side for the release of pus, subsequent irrigation, and antibiotic therapy may aid in treatment. Occasionally a tissue or high level impaction can be removed as soon as a satisfactory antibiotic level has been established. If surgical complications arise, the fractured roots can be allowed to remain undisturbed for a few days before removal. The removal of the crown will allow the pericoronitis to subside.

---

*Extensive portions of this chapter are quoted directly form Kruger, G. O.: Management of impactions, Dent. Clin. N. Amer. pp. 707-722, Nov., 1959.

86 Textbook of oral surgery

When no infection exists, oral or parenteral antibiotic therapy is unnecessary.

Premedication and preparation of patient. Premedication is helpful when impacted teeth are removed under local anesthesia. By mouth an average dose for an outpatient is pentobarbital sodium 0.1 Gm. However, 1 to 2 ml. of pentobarbital sodium can be given intravenously. The patient remains ambulatory, but requires someone to accompany him home. There are many other drugs that can be given intravenously or intramuscularly.

Music, quiet surroundings, and interesting talk by the operator help to establish a favorable atmosphere. General anesthesia is preferred by many patients and operators.

Preparation of the patient starts with a mouthwash of any suitable antiseptic agent to reduce the intraoral bacterial count.

Draping. Drapes in the form of sterile towels will provide a sterile field as well as cover the eyes, thereby reducing psychological trauma. A sterile towel is placed under the patient's head, brought forward over the nose and eyes, and fastened by a sterile towel clip or safety pin (Fig. 6-1). The exposed portions of the face and chin are washed with an antiseptic solution. A sterile towel is placed over the patient's chest. Another sterile towel can be clipped over the chest of the operator. Sterile gloves may be worn. This draping, incidentally, does not represent too much attention to detail since the incidence of dry socket is reduced considerably.

Chair position. The chair position should be low enough that the operator's right elbow is opposite the patient's right shoulder.

Sponges. A curtain sponge is placed to isolate the field of operation. A 3 by 3 inch exodontia gauze sponge is placed with one corner near the mandibular incisors and

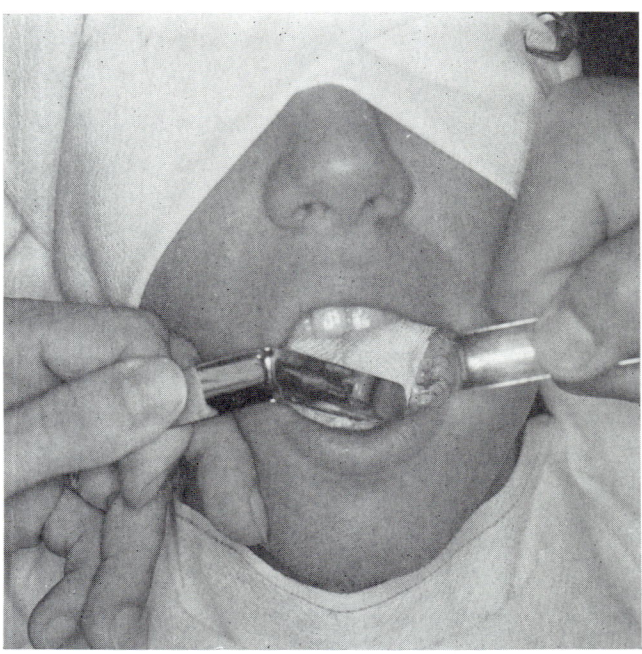

Fig. 6-1. Sterile drapes and retractors are in position. Note isolation of field with sterile gauze sponges. (From Kruger, G. O.: Dent. Clin. N. Amer., p. 707, Nov., 1959.)

another corner under the tongue on the side of the operation. The sponge keeps saliva from the field, keeps fragments and blood from the throat, and eliminates time loss associated with expectoration. The heavy, stringy, "sympathetic" type of saliva often encountered in surgery patients is difficult to remove from the mouth. By changing the sponge if it becomes wet, expectoration is eliminated and time is saved.

Retractors. The assistant should be trained to hold the retractor in the right hand. The edge of the gauze on the lingual side is held under the tip of the retractor, which in turn is held against the lingual plate when operating on the patient's right side. The tongue is not held toward the midline. When operating on the patient's left side, the tip of the retractor is held under the mucoperiosteal flap against bone. Heavy pulling on the flap by the assistant will cause excessive postoperative lymphedema. Sponging and malleting can be accomplished by the left hand. If suction is used, another assistant is helpful.

Armamentarium. The armamentarium is illustrated in Fig. 6-2. The chisels are resharpened after each use, and they are changed frequently during the course of an operation. Many operators prefer the use of burs.[1,2] Attention must be given to the sterility of the handpiece and burs if this technique is used.

Principle of removal of mandibular impacted teeth. The underlying principle in the removal of mandibular impacted teeth is a sectioning technique. Bone is removed to expose the crown. The tooth is split with a fresh, sharp chisel so that a good portion of the crown is separated from the tooth. When this portion is removed, space is obtained so that the remainder of the tooth can be elevated into the defect. Before this technique was developed, space for eleva-

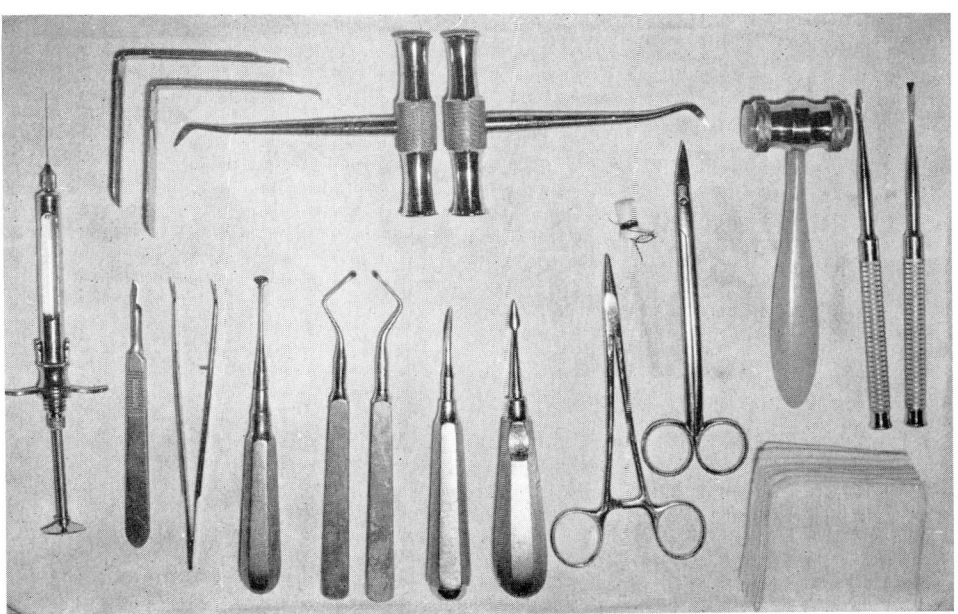

Fig. 6-2. Armamentarium: syringe, scalpel, thumb forceps, Molt curet No. 4, Molt curets No. 5 and No. 6, elevator No. 34, Krogh spearpoint elevator, needle holder, suture, scissors, mallet, Gardner No. 52 chisels, Winter elevators No. 14R and No. 14L, and Austin retractors. (From Kruger, G. O.: Dent. Clin. N. Amer., p. 707, Nov., 1959.)

tion was obtained by more extensive bone removal and consequently with more trauma.

Classification of mandibular impacted teeth. The classification of mandibular impacted teeth may be stated simply as (1) mesioangular, (2) horizontal, (3) vertical, and (4) distoangular. In addition, the tooth may be displaced to the buccal or to the lingual. Further, it may be located at a high occlusal level (near the ridge surface) or a low occlusal level. (See Fig. 6-3.)

A tooth in any basic class is more easily removed if it is displaced to a buccal position and more difficult if it is situated near the lingual plate or even directly behind the second molar. A tooth at a high occlusal level is easier to remove. A tooth may be prevented from erupting by bone (bone block), by the presence of an adjacent tooth (tooth block), or by both.

Preoperative evaluation. Careful preoperative evaluation will permit adequate planning for the subsequent surgery. The radiograph should be studied carefully to localize the impaction and to determine the shape, number, and inclination of the roots. Frequently a root will be directed toward or away from the observer rather than mesially or distally. Small roots often are superimposed and can be missed in the radiographic diagnosis. The relationship of the tooth to the mandibular canal should be noted so that the patient may be warned of a possible postoperative paresthesia. The presence of a large restoration, particularly an old amalgam filling, on the second molar should be cause for warning the patient that the operator is aware of the situation and will attempt to save the restoration from inadvertent damage during the surgery.

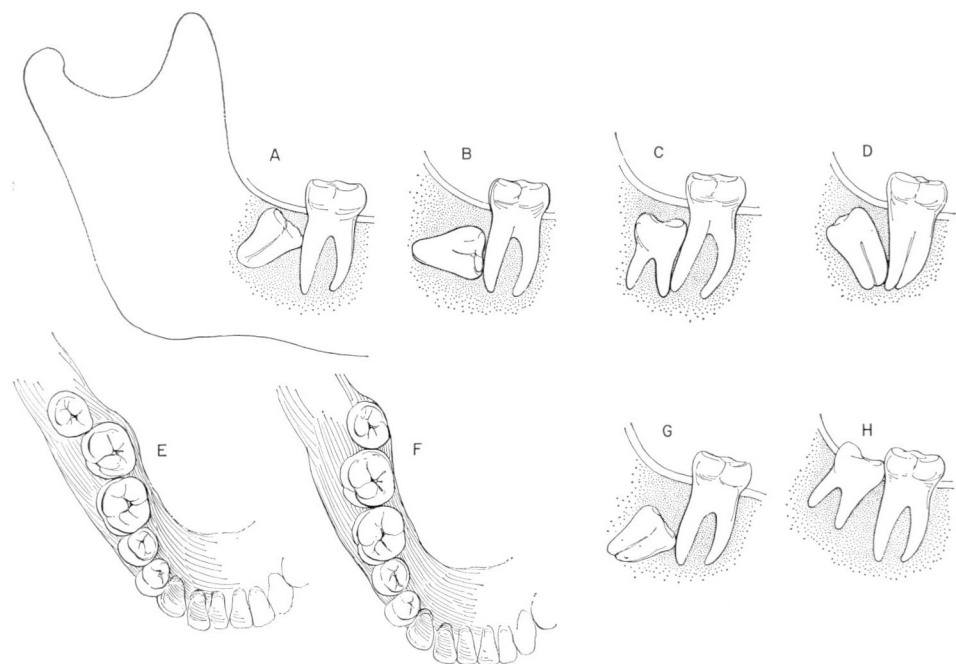

Fig. 6-3. Classification of mandibular impacted teeth. **A**, Mesioangular. **B**, Horizontal. **C**, Vertical. **D**, Distoangular. **E**, Buccoversion. **F**, Linguoversion. **G**, Low-level. **H**, High-level.

MANDIBULAR MESIOANGULAR IMPACTION

A typical mesioangular impaction, low level, with bone and tooth block is illustrated in Fig. 6-4. Prior to removal of the impaction the patient and the field of operation have been prepared adequately as described above, and a local anesthetic has been administered.

A curtaining sponge is placed in the mouth to isolate the operative site. Another sponge is used to dry the exposed oral mucous membranes. Pressure over the area with a small Molt curet (No. 5), combined with positive statement rather than negative questions, will ascertain the depth of anesthesia.

An incision is made into the tissues distal to the second molar with the scalpel. It is important to palpate the tissues before incision to keep the incision over bone. The vertical ramus of the mandible flares outward, and therefore a straight distal incision might extend into tissues medial to the mandible that contain important anatomical structures. A safe rule to follow is to place the incision back of the buccal cusp of the second molar, following the underlying bone, which may flare laterally (Fig. 6-4, A).

The second arm of the incision is made vertically from the first incision at its junction with the distobuccal cusp, extending downward and forward to the buccal tissues over the mesial root of the second molar.

Variations in flap design include the technique of detaching the buccal free gingival fibers around all the teeth forward to include the first molar and separating the large flap buccally. It is claimed that this flap is easier to suture, that it is less painful in the postoperative period, and that there is less distortion in healing. Another variation is the placing of the slanting vertical incision mesial to the second molar rather than mesial to the third molar.

The mucoperiosteal flap is raised carefully with a sharp No. 4 Molt curet, starting in the vertical incision where the periosteum is not attached to bone. The instrument is worked posteriorly and toward the alveolar ridge. When the operative site is widely exposed, a suitable retractor is placed under the flap and held against bone.

Ossisection is started in a vertical fashion parallel to and just back of the distal root of the second molar (Fig. 6-4, B). The bone incision should be one, two, or three chisel widths long, depending upon the depth necessary to get under the enamel crown of the impacted tooth as determined on the preoperative radiograph. The chisel then is turned to face posteriorly, placed in the bottom of the first cut, and directed slightly toward the alveolar crest. Most of the buccal plate will be removed in one piece, which is desirable.

Further horizontal cuts are made as necessary in order to expose the crown (Fig. 6-4, C). In a wide mandible with a heavy cortical plate the impacted tooth can be exposed further by angling one edge of the chisel toward the tooth in making a horizontal cut so that a "ditch" is created in the spongiosa between the tooth and the cortical plate (Fig. 6-4, D).

Two points are checked with the small curet. The bone over the distal or top surface of the impaction should be removed so that the crown can be removed after splitting. The bone at the junction of the vertical and horizontal cuts should be removed sufficiently to allow the curet to enter the spongiosa under the impacted crown. If either of these two check points is unsatisfactory, further bone is removed.

The tooth then is sectioned (Fig. 6-4, E). A new chisel is placed in the buccal groove, directed distally toward the distal anatomical neck of the tooth (not lingually, which may fracture the lingual cortical plate), and struck sharply. This blow should be a glancing blow, with no "follow-through." The tooth will often split on the first at-

90 Textbook of oral surgery

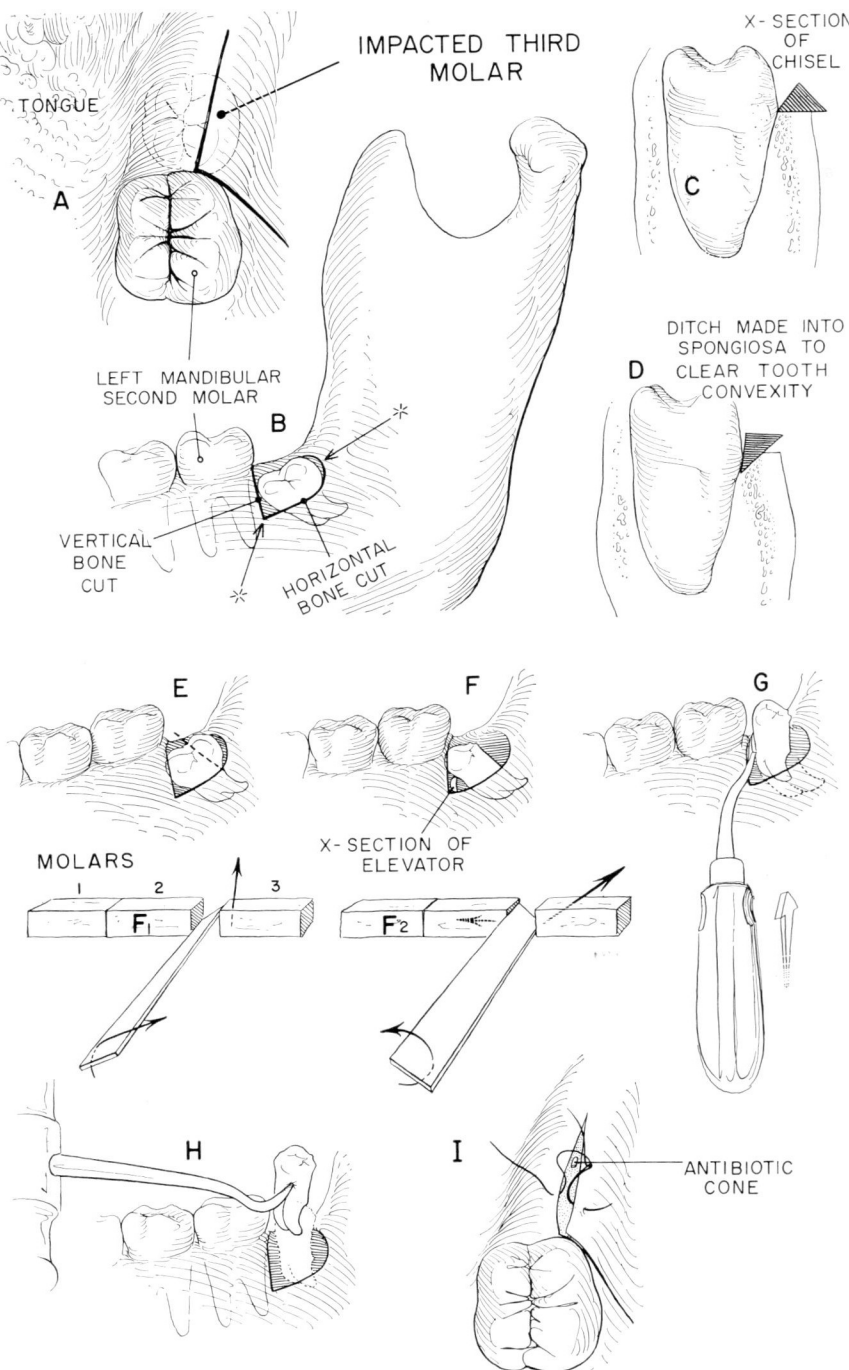

Fig. 6-4. For legend see opposite page.

tempt. The sectioned distal portion of the crown is lifted from the wound.

A binangled spearpoint elevator (such as the Krogh elevator) is placed under the crown and upward motion is made (Fig. 6-4, F). The upper edge of this elevator is the portion of the instrument that lifts the tooth. To obtain a better purchase on the tooth the leading (upper) edge is turned slightly distalward, toward the tooth. The handle of the instrument is moved in a straight vertical plane (Fig. 6-4, G). It is not rotated at this time.

When the tooth moves, it will be forced to move in an arc. When it has moved upward and distally to the point where the instrument can no longer maintain contact with it, the instrument is rotated so that the inferior edge completes the tooth removal. Earlier rotation sometimes will fracture the root and may endanger the second molar.

Often the tooth will move upward far enough to clear the second molar, but it will not rotate distally. It is now in a vertical position, separated from the second molar far enough to lose the mechanical advantage of the elevator placed between the teeth. A long Winter elevator (No. 14) placed in the root bifurcation and using the buccal cortical plate as a fulcrum will elevate this tooth out of the wound (Fig. 6-4, H).

Bone fragments are lifted from the wound with a small curet. Particular attention is given to chips that lodge under the flap buccal to the second molar. The soft tissue remnants in the socket (granulation tissue, eruption follicle) are removed carefully by means of sharp or blunt dissection. Heavy curettage is avoided in the depths of the wound where the inferior alveolar nerve and vessels lie. The edges of the bony wound are smoothed with the curet. One antibiotic cone is placed in the wound if preoperative questioning had indicated no sensitivity to the drug.

A suture is placed over the socket from lingual to buccal (Fig. 6-4, I). This violates a surgical rule to suture the free flap to the fixed flap, but it seems to be simpler here because the retractor is not removed from the wound until the needle is recovered in the depth of the wound. A ½-inch round cutting needle and No. 3-0 silk is used, although No. 3-0 catgut does not have to be removed. One suture is usually sufficient. The vertical cut is almost never closed. No drain is placed. A gauze sponge is placed over the area.

MANDIBULAR HORIZONTAL IMPACTION

The horizontal impaction situated at a low occlusal level requires a deep vertical bone cut, often extending almost to the level of the second molar apex (Fig. 6-5,

---

Fig. 6-4. Removal of impacted mandibular third molar, mesioangular position. **A**, Incision is made back of the buccal cusp of the second molar and then into the buccal tissues. **B**, Ossisection. The two check points that must permit entrance of the curet before ossisection is complete are marked with asterisks. **C**, Horizontal ossisection. **D**, "Ditching" to save height of buccal cortical plate. **E**, Sectioning of distal cusp. **F**, Position of elevator under cementoenamel junction on mesial surface. **F$_1$**, Diagram represents the action of the top edge of the instrument in elevating the posterior object. Note that the bottom edge of the instrument rests on the ground surface and not on the anterior object. This is the recommended technique. **F$_2$**, "Scooping" with the instrument forces the posterior object backward rather than upward. Note that the opposite edge of the instrument now rests on the anterior object and tends to force it forward. **G**, The tooth is moved upward and backward as far as the distal rim of bone will allow. **H**, Further straight upward movement is accomplished with the No. 14 elevator if the tooth cannot be removed in an arc with the spearpoint elevator. **I**, Suture placed. (From Kruger, G. O.: Dent. Clin. N. Amer., p. 707, Nov., 1959.)

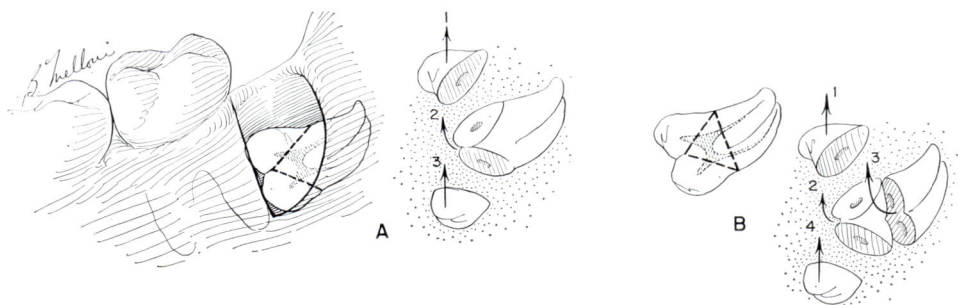

Fig. 6-5. A, Horizontal impaction. The superior (distal) cusp is sectioned, and the inferior (mesial) cusp is sectioned. The superior crown fragment is removed first, followed by the bulk of the tooth. The inferior crown fragment is removed last. **B,** Horizontal impaction (variation). If insufficient room is present for removal of the bulk of the tooth, a split is made near the anatomical neck of the tooth. (From Kruger, G. O.: Dent. Clin. N. Amer., p. 707, Nov., 1959.)

A). The horizontal cuts should be sufficient to expose the anatomical neck of the tooth. The classic description for the removal of this tooth includes a split at the anatomical neck to divide the crown from the root. This can be accomplished with a sharp chisel. However, the bur is especially efficient for this procedure, provided that a sterile bur and handpiece are available.

An alternate method involves placing the chisel in the buccal groove, directing it backward and upward and as little lingually as the access allows. The distal portion of the crown can be split off and removed. The chisel then is placed at the same site, directed backward and downward. This will split the mesial (lower) portion of the crown, which cannot be removed at this time. If the angles of the sections have been wide enough, there may be enough clearance to remove the impaction, provided that sufficient bone over the crest of the ridge has been removed. Attention is directed to this area now. If all the ossisection is accomplished before the sectioning is attempted, the tooth may be loosened slightly, and a tooth loose in its bed is difficult to split. The sectioning is accomplished as soon as access to the crown is obtained, even though the parts cannot be removed, and then further ossisection is accomplished.

A further split in a near vertical (downward) direction can be made at this time (Fig. 6-5, B). The exposed dentin surface can be split more easily than enamel, and if the pulpal chamber is exposed it is even easier to obtain a split.

The various superficial tooth fragments are removed. If the vertical bone cut has been made deep enough for elevator access and sufficient alveolar crest bone has been removed, the root portion can be removed with the No. 14 elevator with or without further root sectioning. Heavy pressure should not be used. Further tooth sectioning or ossisection should be carried out until the impaction can be removed with relative ease. The mesial portion of the crown is removed last. Primary closure is effected following careful debridement.

MANDIBULAR VERTICAL IMPACTION

The removal of the vertical impaction is one of the more difficult operations because of the difficulty in placing an instrument between the second molar and the closely

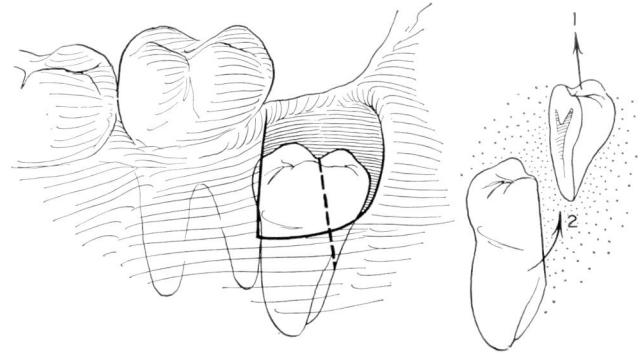

Fig. 6-6. Vertical impaction. A long split is obtained. The distal cusp is removed first, followed by elevation of the tooth. (From Kruger, G. O.: Dent. Clin. N. Amer., p. 707, Nov., 1959.)

adjacent impacted third molar. This space is too small for adequate bone removal.

The area is exposed to view under a large mucoperiosteal flap. A long vertical bone cut is made to expose at least the anatomical neck of the impaction. Bone is removed well behind (distal to) the impaction and over its occlusal surface as well. A long, almost vertical split is obtained from the buccal groove through the distal portion of the tooth below the anatomical neck (Fig. 6-6). This portion is removed. A thin spearpoint elevator is forced between the teeth if possible and the tooth is elevated. If access is not possible, a No. 14 elevator can engage the area of bifurcation on the buccal side and force straight upward can be exerted.

MANDIBULAR DISTOANGULAR IMPACTION

The distoangular impaction is difficult to remove because its bulk lies in the vertical ramus. The crown of the impaction is situated away from the second molar so that no mechanical advantage is afforded to the elevator.

A generous mucoperiosteal flap is raised, and the usual vertical and horizontal bone cuts are made. The tooth is sectioned in a vertical direction (Fig. 6-7, A). Depending upon the curvature of the roots, the mesial bulk of the tooth first is moved upward by the spearpoint elevator placed on the mesial side of the tooth or by the No. 14 elevator placed in the area of bifurcation. At times the distal sectioned crown portion may be dissected out of the bone first. The tooth then is rotated distally into the space created. It is often helpful to section the crown from the root in the distoangular impaction, remove the crown, split the root if feasible, and remove the separate root portions (Fig. 6-7, B).

Several points of caution in the operations for the removal of mandibular impactions should be noted. Force applied with elevators should always be controlled force, and it should be minimal. Greater than normal force is necessary in a few special situations, especially in forcing an elevator between two closely placed teeth. Some operators use more force than others. However, it is best to obtain multiple sections of the tooth and to clearly remove the bone blocks before attempting to elevate the tooth. A good many properly prepared impactions, even at low level, can be removed with a small curet rather than a heavy elevator.

94 *Textbook of oral surgery*

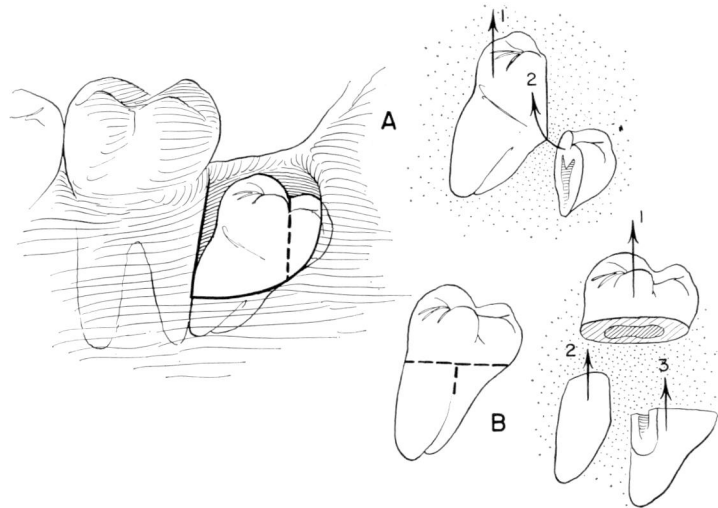

Fig. 6-7. A, Distoangular impaction. The distal cusp is split off. The tooth is elevated first, and then the sectioned distal cusp is removed. **B,** Distoangular impaction (variation). The tooth is sectioned at the anatomical neck. The crown is removed and the roots are divided and removed separately. (From Kruger, G. O.: Dent. Clin. N. Amer., p. 707, Nov., 1959.)

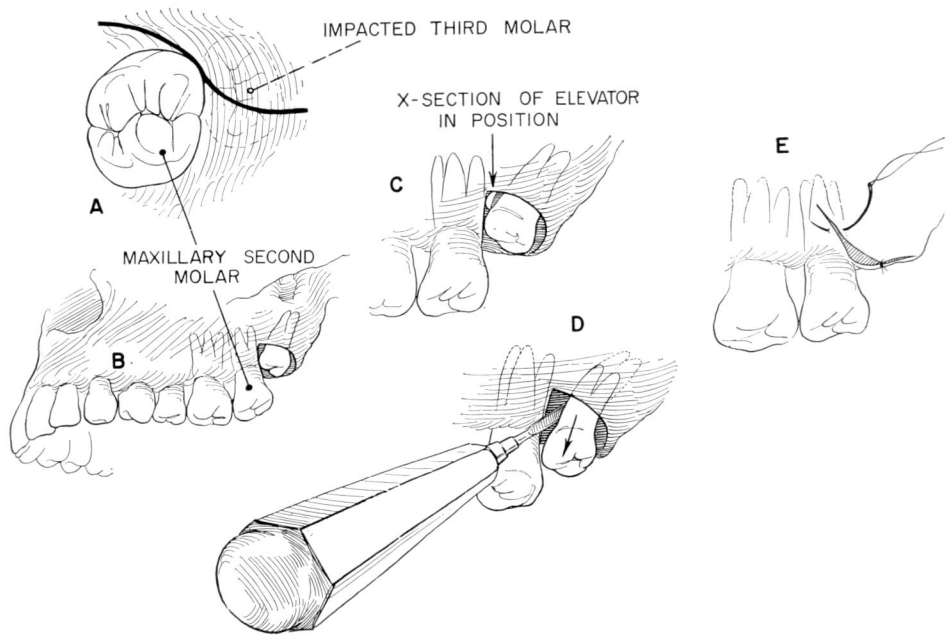

Fig. 6-8. Removal of impacted maxillary third molar, mesioangular position. **A,** Incision over alveolar crest extended to buccal tissues. **B,** Bone removal. Particular attention is given to access between the second and impacted third molars. **C,** Position of elevator at cementoenamel junction. **D,** The handle of the elevator is moved up and down. **E,** Suture closure. (Modified from Kruger, G. O.: Dent. Clin. N. Amer., p. 707, Nov., 1959.)

Bone that has become traumatized excessively should be removed with a sharp chisel or bur after the tooth has been removed.

MAXILLARY MESIOANGULAR IMPACTION

The maxillary impacted tooth on the same side usually is removed at the same sitting as the mandibular tooth on that side. Anesthesia is administered concomitantly with the mandibular anesthesia. The curtain sponge is replaced quickly with a dry gauze sponge. The buccal fold is dried, and the operator holds the buccal retractor himself.

Incision is made over the crest of the ridge extending from the tuberosity to the second molar, and a vertical component is slanted upward and forward to end over the mesiobuccal root of the second molar (Fig. 6-8, *A*). The mucoperiosteal flap is raised with a No. 4 Molt curet.

A new chisel is placed for a vertical cut parallel to the distal root of the second molar (Fig. 6-8, *B*). Light malleting will afford penetration into the soft spongiosa, and the enamel crown often is felt soon after entrance. The light cortical plate is raised slightly over the buccal aspect of the tooth, or in a heavy impaction it should be removed altogether. A small curet is used to ascertain if access exists between the second molar and the impacted third molar. In some cases it does not exist. Further bone removal between the two teeth is almost impossible, and considerable controlled elevator pressure is necessary to force the point of the instrument into the interdental space. Distal bone should be removed in such an instance.

The tooth is removed with a spearpoint elevator, a No. 34 elevator, or a No. 14 elevator (Fig. 6-8, *C*). The point of the elevator is forced between the teeth into the area of ossisection, and a straight downward and buccal force is applied (Fig. 6-8, *D*). The point and the inferior edge of the elevator make contact with the anatomical neck of the tooth and elevate it downward with these vantage points. Care is exercised in turning the elevator distally (backward) since to do so would increase the possibility of fracturing the tuberosity.

The area is debrided for extraneous soft and hard tissue material, and the bone edges are smoothed with the curet. A suture is placed across the crestal incision, and another is placed across the vertical incision (Fig. 6-8, *E*).

The curtain sponge is removed. Another sponge, slightly moistened in water, is placed over the wound (mostly to the buccal), and the patient is directed to bite down on it with pressure. A few minutes later postoperative radiographs are made and another sponge is placed between the jaws to remain until the patient has returned home. An ice bag to the face is ordered, on 10 minutes and off 10 minutes, for the remainder of the day. A therapeutic level of aspirin or other analgesic drug is established with the administration of the first dose upon arrival home, before the effect of the local anesthetic has disappeared.

MAXILLARY VERTICAL IMPACTION

The maxillary vertical impaction, particularly if the crown rests close to the anatomical neck of the second molar, permits no access between the teeth for ossisection or for purchase by an instrument.

A vertical bone cut is made parallel to the mesial edge of the impacted tooth. The thin bone overlying the buccal surface of the tooth is removed carefully or sometimes separated from the tooth and bent 1 to 2 mm. buccally. The chisel is introduced carefully back of the distal surface in order to create space for backward movement (Fig. 6-9, *A* and *B*).

A thin-bladed instrument of any kind described above is introduced between the teeth. Since the removal of bone has not been possible in this space, considerable force is necessary. As soon as the instru-

96   *Textbook of oral surgery*

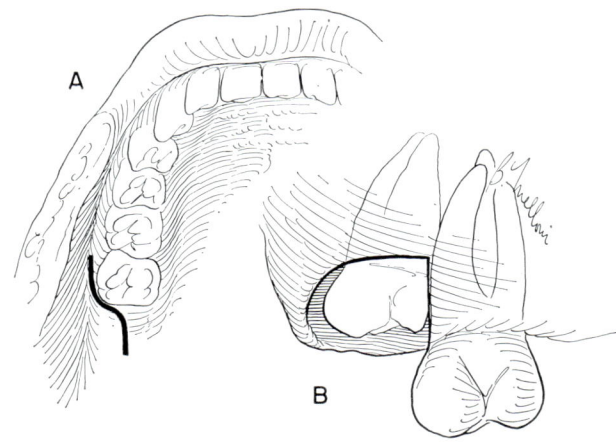

Fig. 6-9. A, Vertical impaction, incision. **B,** Bone removal. (Modified from Kruger, G. O.: Dent. Clin. N. Amer., p. 707, Nov., 1959.)

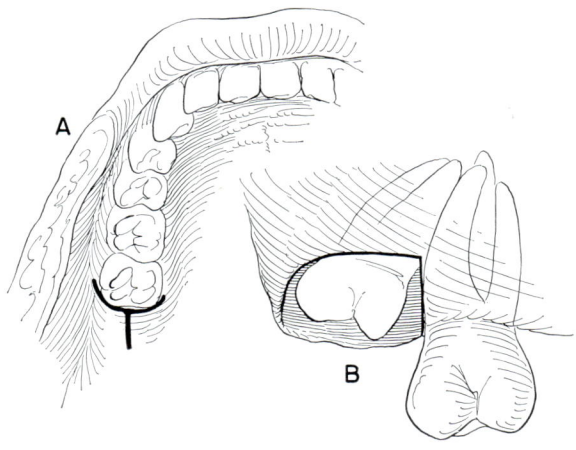

Fig. 6-10. A, Distoangular impaction, modified incision of soft tissues. **B,** Bone removal. (From Kruger, G. O.: Dent. Clin. N. Amer., p. 707, Nov., 1959.)

ment can be pushed into this space, the tooth can be removed easily. Occasionally it will move downward so rapidly that it may be swallowed or aspirated if a suitable gauze curtain does not cover the oropharynx.

If the instrument cannot be introduced into the space and considerable bone surrounding the tooth has been removed, a driving chisel can be placed on the buccal surface of the enamel in a vertical direction and gently tapped downward.

MAXILLARY DISTOANGULAR IMPACTION

A rare situation, the distoangular impaction requires a larger surgical flap and extensive removal of surrounding bone. A midcrest incision is made extending from the second molar to the tuberosity curvature, and vertical extensions to the buccal and lingual are made distal to the second molar. This flap exposes the entire bony tuberosity (Fig. 6-10, *A*).

A vertical bone incision is made distal to the second molar to the area of the apex. Buccal and alveolar crest bone is removed. The area distal to the impaction is carefully exposed with a chisel, mainly by hand pressure (Fig. 6-10, *B*).

The tooth is elevated from a purchase on the mesial side as near to the apex as access will allow. The tooth can be pushed into the antrum or into the tissues back of the tuberosity. A second instrument (No. 5 Molt curet) occasionally is placed simultaneously on the distal surface to guide the tooth downward. Several alternate methods can be used. If the tooth is in severe distoangular position a No. 14 elevator may be used on the distal (superior) crown surface to bring the tooth downward and forward. At times the tooth should be dissected extensively and removed with forceps. Gelfoam may be used to fill an extensive defect, and the wound should be closed tightly with multiple interrupted sutures.

MAXILLARY CANINE IMPACTION

Impactions of the maxillary canine are classified as labial, palatal, and intermediate. Localization is important since the surgical techniques for removal of the three types vary so much that they are almost unrelated operations. Intraoral radiographs can be read to determine the form of the tooth as well as its location (Clark's rule; buccal object rule). The true occlusal view made with an intraoral cassette and extraoral views often are necessary. Clinical palpation on the labial side is not reliable since the bulge felt may be either the impacted tooth or the labially displaced root of the incisor or premolar.

Palatal canine position. The palatal position is the most frequent situation. Incision is made in the palatal interdental spaces beginning with the space between the premolars on the one side and around the palatal free gingival fibers and interdental spaces to the premolar area on the other side (Fig. 6-11, *A*). The heavy mucoperiosteal flap is stripped from the bone with the No. 4 Molt curet. The contents of the incisive foramen are divided by scalpel where they enter the flap.

Bone is removed with the chisel, starting with a small rectangle back of the incisor that appears nearest to the impaction on the radiograph (unless an obvious protuberance locates the tooth). The rectangle is one chisel width in size initially, and it is enlarged as soon as the enamel crown is located. Care must be taken in dissecting anteriorly in the region of the incisors, and a 1 to 2 mm. margin of bone around their sockets should be maintained. When one half to two thirds of the tooth is exposed, a split is made at the anatomical neck. If the crown is near the incisors so that its tip lies in an undercut, a second split is immediately made 3 mm. toward the apex from the first cut (Fig. 6-11, *B*). The small piece is removed, the crown is backed into the space created and removed, and the root is teased out with a No. 34 elevator or a Molt curet (Fig. 6-11, *C*).

Bone chips and debris are removed, the edges of the bony wound are smoothed with a curet, an antibiotic tablet is placed in the defect, and the wound is closed by means of three or four sutures through the interdental spaces, tying on the labial (Fig. 6-11, *D*). Pressure on a large wad of gauze over the palate for 15 minutes helps to prevent formation of a gross hematoma. To support the palatal flap against bone a preformed clear acrylic palatal splint is useful. A stab incision and rubber drain through the palatal mucosa is used by some operators to prevent formation of a dependent hematoma.

Labial canine position. After the impaction has been localized a large semilunar incision is made extending from the labial frenum to the premolar area with the

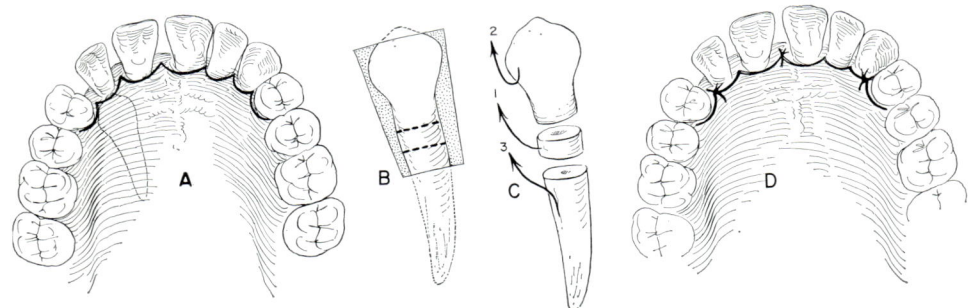

Fig. 6-11. **A,** Canine impaction, palatal position. Soft tissue flap design. **B,** Sectioning of tooth. **C,** Note that the middle section is removed first. **D,** Closure of flap. (Modified from Kruger, G. O.: Dent. Clin. N. Amer., p. 707, Nov., 1959.)

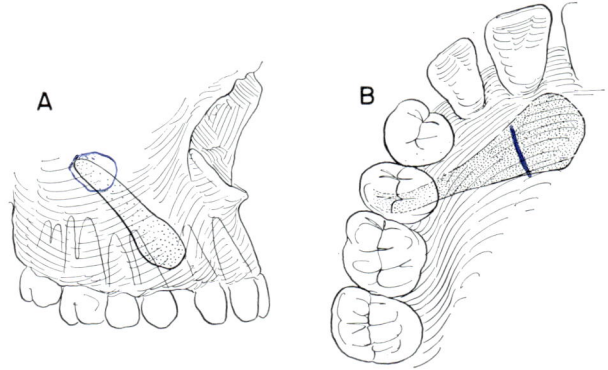

Fig. 6-12. **A,** Canine impaction, labial position. **B,** Canine impaction, intermediate position. (Modified from Kruger, G. O.: Dent. Clin. N. Amer., p. 707, Nov., 1959.)

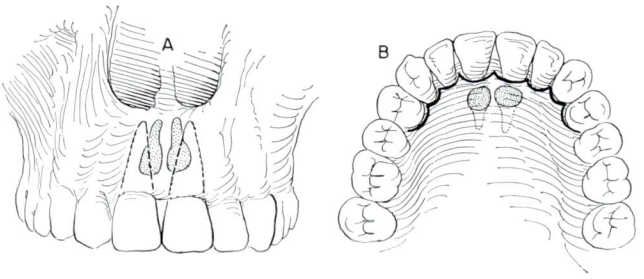

Fig. 6-13. Supernumerary teeth. **A,** Location anterior or posterior to central incisors can be difficult to determine. **B,** Incision around necks of teeth for palatally located mesiodentes. (Modified from Kruger, G. O.: Dent. Clin. N. Amer., p. 707, Nov., 1959.)

curvature pointing toward the gingival margin (Fig. 6-12, A). Labial bone is removed in the usual fashion until the tooth is located; it may be high on the facial surface of the maxilla. Sufficient dissection is accomplished until the tooth can be elevated with suitable instruments.

Intermediate canine position. The usual position for an intermediate impaction is the crown on the palate and the root lying over the apices of the premolar teeth near the buccal cortex (Fig. 6-12, B). Even if the condition is not diagnosed preoperatively, it should be suspected when difficulty arises in the removal of the root portion of any palatally placed canine.

The palatal exposure is made in the usual manner and the crown is removed. A separate buccal flap is made in the region suggested by the radiographic and clinical findings, usually above and between the premolars on the same side. Careful bone removal will uncover the root end of the impaction, which can be pushed from the buccal opening into the palatal wound. The two operative sites are closed.

SUPERNUMERARY TOOTH IMPACTION

Although supernumerary teeth may be found impacted in any area of the alveolar ridges, the most common ones occur in the maxillary anterior region. They may occur singly between the central incisors (mesiodens), or they may be double (mesiodentes).

Under ordinary circumstances removal of mesiodentes is not scheduled until the apices of the permanent incisors have closed since then there is less danger of damaging the growing mesenchymal portion of the permanent teeth. Sometimes the permanent incisors will not erupt because of interference by the supernumerary teeth. The operation is complicated by the difficulty in locating, identifying, and removing the supernumerary tooth without damaging the permanent tooth (Fig. 6-13, A).

Supernumerary anterior maxillary teeth usually are removed by a palatal approach. When the radiographs are inconclusive in establishing the location of the supernumerary teeth anterior or posterior to the normal teeth, a palatal approach is made since few are located in an anterior position.

The technique for removal is similar to that used for removal of the palatally placed impacted canine. An incision is made around the necks of the teeth on the palate from first premolar to first premolar, and a palatal flap is raised (Fig. 6-13, B). If no identifying protuberances are found on the bone surface, ossisection is started behind the central incisor, back of the incisive foramen. A collar of bone is left around the central incisor. Dissection is carried upward and backward until enamel is encountered. If the permanent central incisors have not erupted, the tooth encountered must be differentiated from the unerupted permanent central incisor by its anatomy. Sufficient bone is removed to deliver the tooth. When bilateral impactions occur, the second tooth often will be less difficult to find because of the experience gained in locating the first one. The wound is treated and closed in the usual manner.

If a labial approach is indicated (usually for a single mesiodens), a large semilunar incision is made between the lateral incisors, and the flap is raised upward. Bone is removed as indicated by the radiograph, starting as high on the labial cortical plate as necessary. Careful dissection is mandatory so that the permanent roots are not damaged. Closure is by the usual method.

Impacted supernumerary premolars are difficult to remove because of the presence of compact bone and vital structures such as the contents of the mental foramen on the buccal side and salivary gland and neurovascular structures on the lingual side. Occlusal radiographs will locate the tooth as being on the buccal or on the lingual side or midway between the plates (the last is most frequent).

A double flap is made on the buccal side, consisting of two vertical components some distance apart joined by an incision around the necks of the teeth. Unless the tooth has erupted through the lingual plate it is difficult and hazardous to make a lingual approach. Buccal bone over the tooth to be removed is removed through a square window until it is dissected out. If the supernumerary tooth is not fully formed, it is easier to remove (with a curet) than if it is completely formed. After removal an antibiotic cone is placed in the wound, and all borders of the incision are approximated with sutures.

Molar supernumerary teeth are managed much like an impacted third molar since the supernumerary tooth occurs at the end of the molar series.

REFERENCES

1. Szmyd, L., Shannon, I. L., Schuessler, C. F., and McCall, C. M.: Air turbine in impacted third molar surgery, J. Oral Surg. **21**:36, 1963.
2. Szmyd, L., and Hester, W. R.: Crevicular depth of the second molar in impacted third molar surgery, J. Oral Surg. **21**:185, 1963.

Chapter 7

ABNORMALITIES OF THE MOUTH*

J. Orton Goodsell and Donald R. King

Prosthetic art aims to supply functional or esthetic portions of human anatomy that have been lost or are congenitally absent. The success of any device that is to be worn in an orbit, on a leg, or in the mouth depends on the foundation upon which the device rests. A denture can be no better than its base. Many mouths, at first glance, seem to present insurmountable difficulties to the satisfactory insertion of dentures. Great numbers can be improved, however, if the prosthodontist is fully aware of the surgical aids that are available and if he utilizes them. Many dentures that are worn with discomfort or annoyance can be made comfortable or nondistracting if surgical alterations are performed. Many impossible situations can be made partially tolerable or esthetically acceptable.

The normal or ideal mouth must (1) provide adequate bony support for the dentures; (2) have bone covered by normal soft tissues; (3) present no undercuts or overhanging protuberances; (4) have no sharp ridges; (5) have adequate buccal and lingual sulci; (6) have no scar bands to prevent normal seating of a denture at its periphery; (7) have no muscle fibers or frenums to mobilize the prosthesis; (8) possess satisfactory relationships of maxillary and mandibular alveolar ridges; (9) contain no soft tissue folds, redundancies, or hypertrophies on the ridges or in the sulci; and (10) possess no neoplasms.

If the partially or completely edentulous mouth is normal or ideal in its contours, no surgery is required. But if surgery is required, it is unwise to fail to employ it.

It is the purpose of this chapter to illustrate some of the causes of prosthetic failure and to suggest and describe a few surgical methods for correction.

The general principles of surgery apply here as in other surgical fields. The judicious choice of anesthesia, relative asepsis, supportive treatment, sedation, antibiotic use when indicated, nutrition and fluid balance, and consideration of the physical status of the patient are important. The principles of plastic surgery also must be adhered to in the use of intraoral plastic procedures. Hemostasis, preservation of blood supply, lack of excessive suture tension, and prevention of hematoma formation by pressure dressings and appliances merit detailed attention.

SHARP RIDGES

Extremely sharp edentulous alveolar ridges may be revealed by heavy palpation

---

*Extensive portions of this chapter are quoted directly from Goodsell, J. O.: Surgical aids to intraoral prosthesis, J. Oral Surg. 13:8, 1955.

or by the patient attempting to wear dentures. Razorlike or sawlike ridges are among the most frequent and serious causes of denture discomfort. The process of mastication apparently compresses the mucoperiosteum against the sharp ridges of bone and the act of occlusion therefore is painful. Patients frequently go from one dentist to another in an effort to obtain dentures that can be worn comfortably. The prosthodontist may construct new dentures in the hope of satisfying the patient, usually with no more success than previously until it is decided that sharp ridges are at fault. When this conclusion is reached, the remedy becomes simple. Surgical correction of the sharp alveolar ridge followed by construction of new dentures usually is productive of comfort.

Many times the clinical observer may be deceived into believing that the bony ridge is satisfactory because the soft tissue covering is well rounded, obscuring the fact that a very sharp ridge is present beneath the mucoperiosteum (Fig. 7-1). Firm finger pressure may be required to elicit the typical discomfort experienced with sharp ridges, but usually the patient can point to the offending areas himself. It is of prime importance to employ surgery where it is needed and not to evade the issue by building new equipment that cannot be worn with comfort.

A sharp incision is made through the mucoperiosteum over the area to be exposed, slightly toward the labial or buccal side of the crest (Fig. 7-2). The periosteum is reflected only enough to bring the bone into adequate view. This is extremely important if the already shallow buccal or labial sulcus is to be preserved. It is safer to reflect the lingual or palatal periosteum than that on the labial or buccal side, but the less that it is undermined on either side, the better.

Rongeur forceps or bone files are then employed to remove the irregularities and to level off the sawlike protuberances. Just enough bone should be removed to provide a smooth alveolar process and no more. In some cases, when the soft tissue is approximated, it is necessary to excise 1 or 2 mm. of soft tissue along the wound edges if an excess is present. The mucosa from the lingual side provides a good ridge covering if it can be so positioned. Closure of the wound is best accomplished by utilizing nonabsorbable No. 4-0 or 5-0 suture material on atraumatic needles to suture the mucosal surfaces together accurately. Additional tissue support can be obtained by immediate insertion of the patient's old dentures, which should be lined with surgical cement or one of the soft, quick-cure acrylics.

Sharp mylohyoid ridges are infrequent offenders, but they can be bothersome to the wearer of lower dentures, and at times contouring reduction may be needed (Fig. 7-3). The same principle of retaining the buccal sulcus depth as mentioned previously should be kept in mind if surgical intervention is attempted. The originating incision is made along the crest of the ridge, extending from the retromolar region forward as far as necessary. The mucoperiosteum on the lateral side should not be reflected. It remains to serve as a fixed anchor

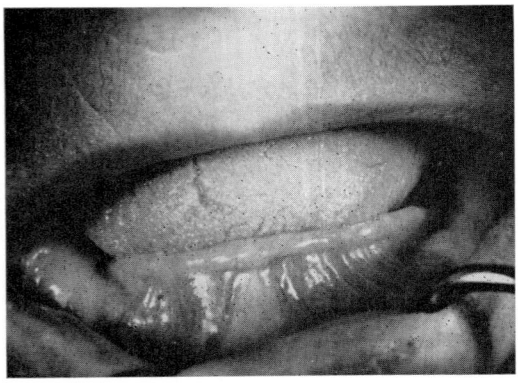

Fig. 7-1. Sharp ridge with redundant fold of soft tissue simulating well-rounded ridge. (From Goodsell, J. O.: J. Oral Surg. 13:8, 1955.)

to which the lingually raised periosteum can be sutured. The fibers of the mylohyoid muscle that are attached to the sharp bony crest are then dissected away, but only enough to obtain access to the bone, which is smoothed with burs, chisels, or rongeur forceps. Approximation of the lingual flap by suturing it to the fixed buccal side will draw up the soft tissues so that the flap is in tight contact with the medial surface of the mandible. One or 2 mm. of mucosal edge may need to be trimmed before suturing if the lingual side is loose. Close contact of the mucoperiosteum to the bone is essential if hematoma formation is to be prevented.

TORI

Maxillary or mandibular tori have no pathological significance and ordinarily

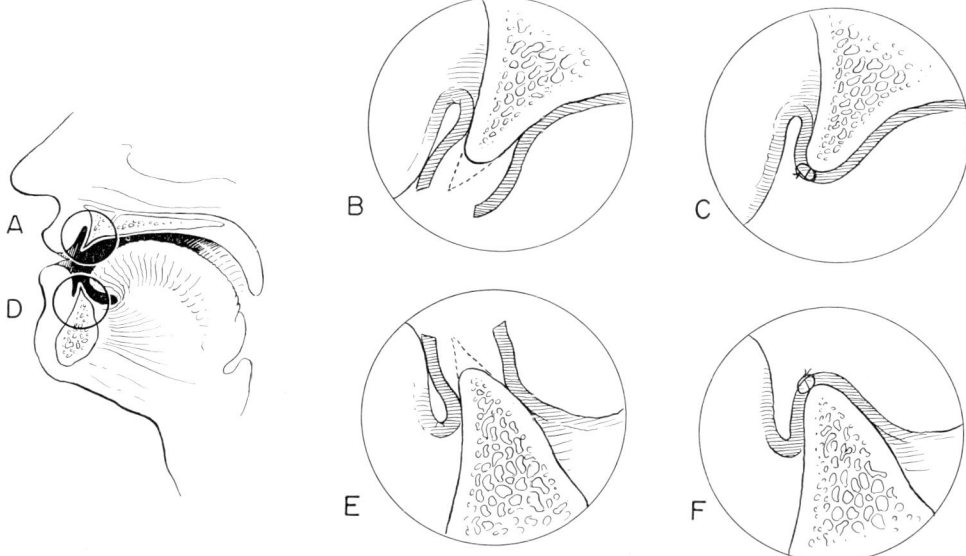

Fig. 7-2. **A** and **D**, Sharp edentulous ridges. **B** and **E**, Extent of bone trimming and amount of periosteal reflection. **C** and **F**, Utilization of palatal or lingual flaps to cover bony ridges.

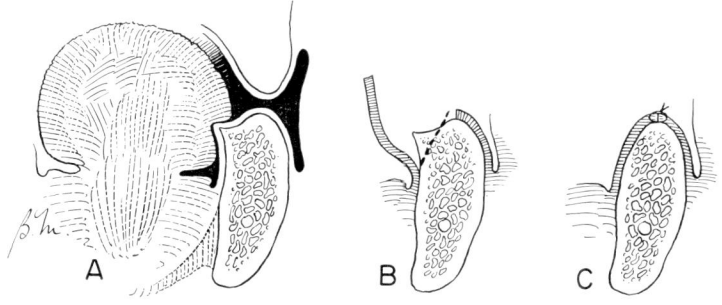

Fig. 7-3. **A**, Sharp mylohyoid ridge. **B**, Reflection of lingual flap and extent of bone removed. **C**, Lingual flap repositioned and sutured.

need no surgical attention. Removal is indicated if they become traumatized and the membrane surfaces become hyperkeratotic or if inflammatory processes occur as a result of debris retention under their folds and projections. Their excision is essential in many instances when dentures or portions of dentures will be made in that area.

Palatal tori vary in size and shape. Many are small and some are large. Some are multilobular with wide overextensions on narrow bases, whereas others are more or less sessile. Usually the mucoperiosteum is very thin over the rounded projections, whereas it is thicker as it overlies the periphery of the base. The main problems involved in the removal of palatal tori are those presented by the lobulations and the thin mucosa. Caution must be observed when the bony portion is removed.

The torus should not be excised en masse because occasionally the nasal floor dips downward in the area; a perforation into the nose may be produced if too large an area of bone is lost. A difficult soft tissue closure would then be required needlessly. Division of the torus into segments can be accomplished by burs and then the smaller pieces eliminated with chisels and rongeur forceps. Large surgical burs and files serve very well as instruments in the final preparation of the surface. Smooth burnishing of the bone should be avoided. (See Fig. 7-4.)

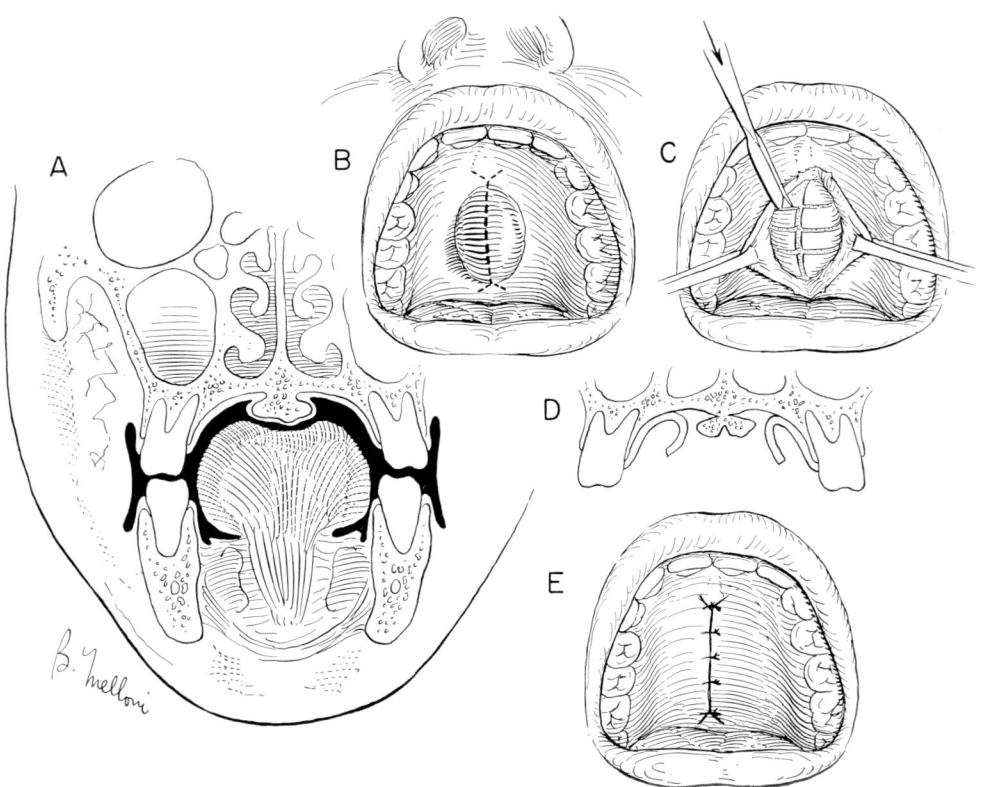

Fig. 7-4. **A**, Cross section of head with prominent torus palatinus. **B**, Dotted incision line. **C**, Denuded segments of torus being removed with chisel. **D**, Lateral grooving of mass at its base (optional). **E**, Suturing completed.

After the torus is reduced an excess of soft tissue must be trimmed from the approximating medial edges. After this is done the wound is sutured, preferably by a continuous "over and under" type suture, using fine, nonabsorbable sutures on an atraumatic needle. The thin membrane does not endure the passage of heavy needles.

To preserve the life of the flap and prevent hematoma formation it is essential that it be supported against the palatal vault. The freshened bony base furnishes serous exudate as nourishment for the thin membrane. Actually the treatment is not unlike that for the application of a free graft. Compression of the tissue reduces the incidence of venous stasis and future necrosis.

A clear acrylic vault support is useful, particularly when teeth are present in the anterior portion of the mouth and not in the molar areas (Fig. 7-5). The appliance is prepared preoperatively, and after suturing is completed the appliance is inserted into the mouth and petroleum jelly–type gauze packed between it and the palate in sufficient thickness to ensure adequate pres-

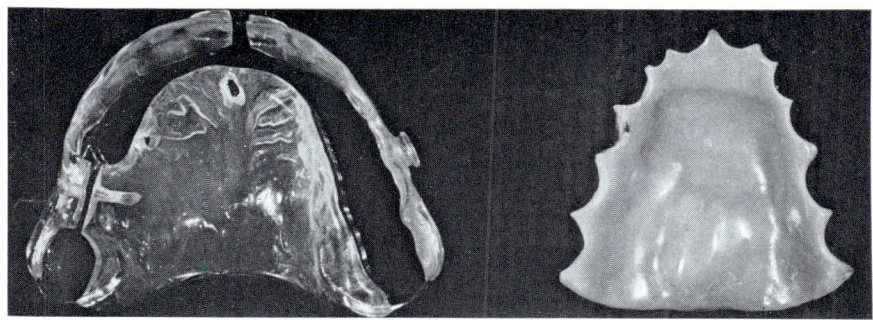

Fig. 7-5. Acrylic vault supports for palatal flaps.

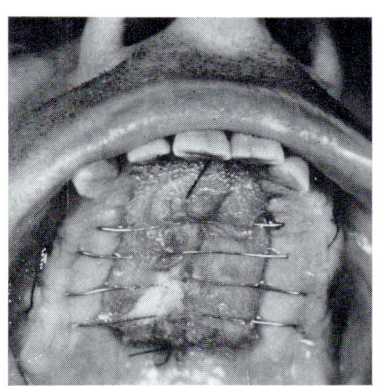

Fig. 7-6

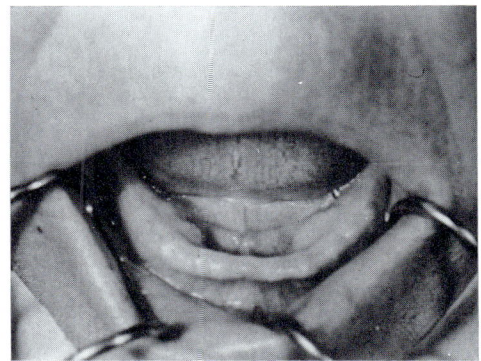

Fig. 7-7

Fig. 7-6. Crisscross stainless steel wire support with gauze pack inserted. (From Goodsell, J. O.: J. Oral Surg. 13:8, 1955.)
Fig. 7-7. Lingual mandibular tori that should be removed prior to preparation of lower denture. (From Goodsell, J. O.: J. Oral Surg. 13:8, 1955).

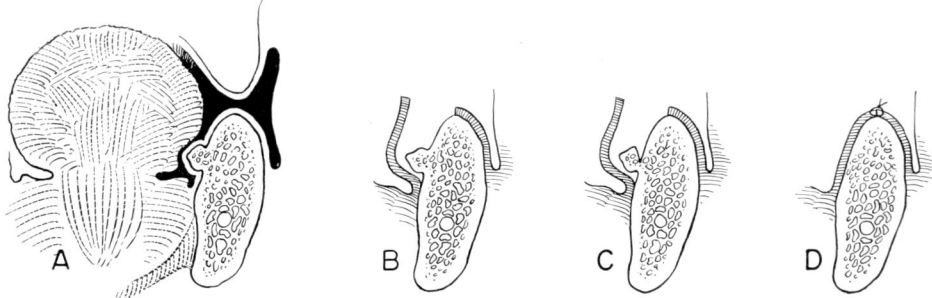

Fig. 7-8. **A,** Cross section of mandibular torus. **B,** Lingual periosteum reflected, exposing torus but leaving lateral periosteum attached. **C,** Superior grooving on torus. **D,** Incision sutured.

sure against the roof of the mouth. The appliance should be left in place for 1 week if possible, without removal or interference.

If teeth are present in the molar regions, the flaps can be supported by gauze placed under a cradle, which is constructed by crisscrossing the palate with wire that has been passed through and around the posterior teeth. If teeth are not present in the molar areas, the cradle may be inserted by passing the wire through the ridge mucoperiosteum (Fig. 7-6). The gauze can be tied to the front teeth or sutured to the anterior soft tissue. Excess gauze may be trimmed off posteriorly. The wire should be stiff enough to retain pressure against the pack as it is pressed upward by the surgeon's fingers. This type of retainer also should be left in place for about a week before removal. More discomfort is experienced by the patient, however, if the wire must be placed through the mucoperiosteum because of the absence of molar anchorage. Therefore it is advisable, if the patient's molars and bicuspids are to be removed, to dispose of the torus before the teeth are extracted.

Mandibular tori, when present, occur primarily in the zone lingual to the bicuspids. Removal is essential to future denture comfort if the area is to bear a prosthesis (Fig. 7-7). Although these tori may be lower than the inner flange of a newly constructed denture, the appliance encroaches on them as alveolar atrophy occurs. Any attempt to circumvent the tori is almost certain to result in denture failure.

The removal of mandibular tori is not complicated, but a few suggestions may be worthwhile. The incision over the ridge crest should be sharp and extend through to the bone (Fig. 7-8). If teeth are present, the incision should be at the necks of the teeth, reflecting the entire lingual mucosa. If the lateral periosteum is not reflected, the buccal sulcus will not be lost, and a fixed anchor can be maintained to which the lingual mucoperiosteum can be attached later. There is greater danger of the development of a postoperative hematoma here than in operating on a sharp mylohyoid ridge since in the bicuspid area the mylohyoid muscle is relatively low in the floor of the mouth, and a defect that will accept blood can develop easily if the lingual flap is loose and is not forced against and held closely to the lingual aspect of the mandible.

After the mass is exposed, troughs can be cut by burs in the superior and medial and distal aspects of the bony protuberance. A sharp blow on a chisel from above will fracture off the torus. Files and larger burs may be utilized to smooth the bony wound.

Irrigation and suction will dispose of the bone dust and debris from the depths of the cavity. An excess of lingual flap will need to be trimmed away at its edge prior to approximation and fixation by sutures to the immobile lateral mucoperiosteum. The employment of a denture-type tissue support is of no particular aid in such circumstances since the location of a potential hematoma is too far below the rim of an appliance to allow the retainer to be effective. The secret of success is to keep the periosteum in close contact with the lingual aspect of the mandible by suture methods.

ENLARGED TUBEROSITIES

Fibrous hyperplasia or bony enlargement of the maxillary tuberosities may interfere with denture construction because of excessive undercut or bulging into the intermaxillary space to such a degree that insufficient space remains for dentures (Fig. 7-9).

For the reduction of these tuberosities (Fig. 7-10) two curved incisions are made

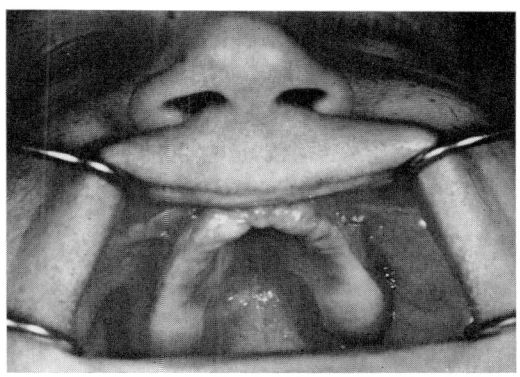

Fig. 7-9. Fibrous hyperplasia of tuberosity, molar region. (From Goodsell, J. O.: J. Oral Surg. 13:8, 1955.)

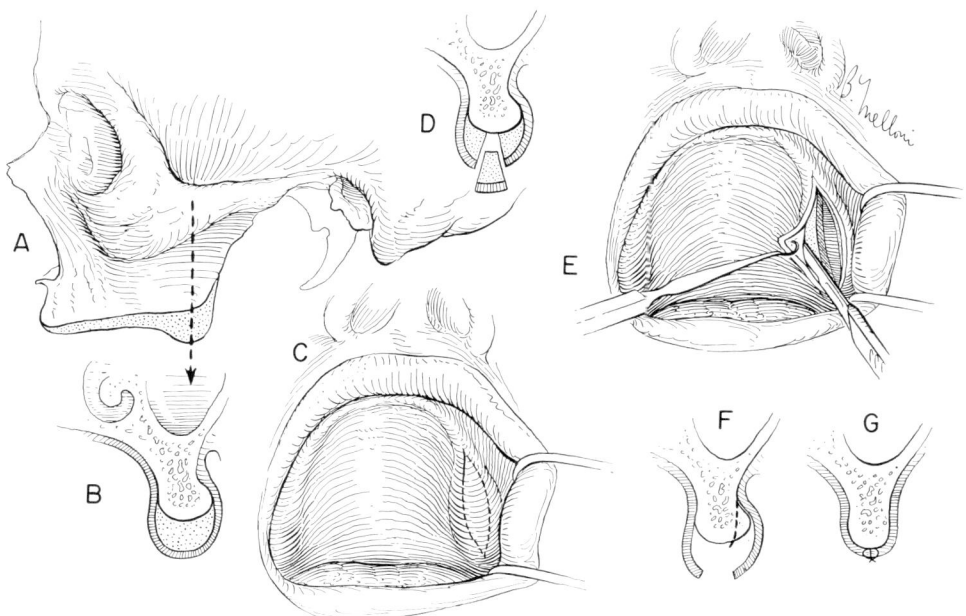

Fig. 7-10. Removal of bulbous tuberosities. **A** and **B**, Lateral and cross-sectional views of enlarged tuberosities. **C**, Elliptical incisions from tuberosity to bicuspid area. **D**, Cross section with area between elliptical incisions removed. Dotted area represents fibrous tissue to be removed. **E**, Removal of fibrous tissue by undermining buccal and palatal flaps. **F**, Removal of bony undercut. **G**, Closure.

down to bone from a point at the extreme distal end of the tuberosity, running anteriorly to a point where they join in the bicuspid area. The mucosa and fibrous tissue between the incisions are then removed by means of a periosteal elevator, leaving a wedge-shaped defect. The fibrous tissue underlying the buccal and lingual flaps is then removed by sharp dissection. Care must be taken when removing fibrous tissue from the palatal side not to interfere with blood supply to the mucous membrane. Excess bone is then removed from the crest of the ridge and from the buccal plate if excessive undercut exists. This may be accomplished with chisels, rongeurs, and files. After the desired contour is established any excess tissue is removed from the buccal and lingual flaps, and the flaps may then be approximated with interrupted sutures. The flaps should be properly trimmed to permit close adaptation to bone.

Occasionally such tuberosity reduction is made impossible by the presence of a large maxillary antrum. In such cases additional intermaxillary space for the molar areas of dentures can be obtained by reducing the height of the alveolar ridges. Soft tissue excesses are removed first, followed by contouring the bone as much as anatomical structures will permit (Fig. 7-11).

SOFT TISSUE DEFORMITIES

Intraoral soft tissue deformities frequently interfere with the proper seating of dentures. Flabby (or wobbly) ridge coverings, whether they are densely fibromatous or the softer, more redundant type, provide an unstable base for dentures. Excessive atrophy in the ridges of either arch causes partial obliteration of the bony foundation with resultant loss of labial or buccal sulci. Fibrous bands, muscle attachments, or scars mobilize dentures and prevent stability. In many instances soft tissue alterations that produce interference are traumatic in origin. Dentures that have been worn too long without adjustment are the chief offenders. The removal of teeth sometimes produces cicatrices that may obliterate the sulci.

Massive ulcerative stomatitis can produce scars about the cheeks and jaws, and electrical burns, automobile accidents, and gunshot wounds may produce the same result. Deformities may be anatomical or congenital in origin as well as acquired. The varied physical characteristics of bone play an important part in the behavior of a base in response to occlusal denture pressures. Patients who possess large, dense bones have less trouble with alveolar ridge atrophy than do patients with smaller bony structure.

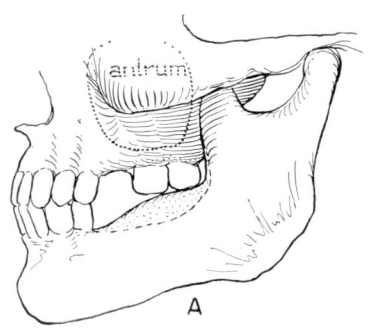 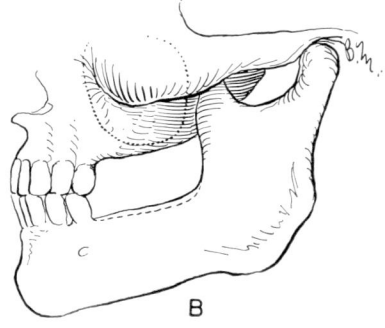

Fig. 7-11. **A,** Position of antrum and outline of the portion of the mandibular area that is designated for removal. **B,** Space that is gained by removal of soft tissue and bone from the maxillary and mandibular ridge areas.

Regardless of the cause of soft tissue intraoral abnormalities, it is certain they present obstacles to the prosthodontist that should be overcome if at all possible. Mucous membrane irritations arising from ill-fitting dentures cannot be ignored as contributing factors in the formation of many oral malignancies.

Surgery is not the cure-all for every denture problem, but many mouths can be improved greatly by some type of intraoral corrective surgery.

Perhaps only a slight adjustment employing but one technique will suffice in a given case, but many times multiple procedures (with revision) are necessary to accomplish the desired results. Plastic surgery, whether in the mouth or elsewhere, requires accurate planning, precision, and meticulous attention to details.

Tissue supports

To immobilize flaps and grafts after an operation and for the period of readjustment of tissue during the healing process, intraoral soft tissues almost invariably require mechanical supports in addition to sutures. It is essential that close adaptation of mucous membrane to freshened submucous tissue be maintained for several days if hematoma formation and shifting of the flaps are to be prevented. Failure to appreciate this factor may cause the loss of a hard-won buccal or labial sulcus. A few retaining devices that have proved helpful will be described.

Equal parts of zinc oxide and finely triturated resin can be spatulated on a hot slab with eugenol liquid to form a surgical cement that has many uses. Long shreds of absorbent cotton can be incorporated into the soft, thick mass to give it body and stability. This type of splint can be used to form a support for surgerized tissue that must be held tightly against a base to which it has been sutured. However, the cement can be used in any case if a device is available to which it can be attached. After the material is placed in the desired location, on an old denture for instance, it is inserted into the mouth and allowed to remain there until the cement is set. The whole splint is then removed, smoothed, and reinserted, to be left in place for at least 4 days. Frequently this revised appliance can be used as a denture until healing is sufficient to allow construction of a new one (Fig. 7-12).

Modeling compound also can be utilized on occasion as a good support in much the same manner as surgical cement. Intermaxillary wire or rubber-band fixation of the teeth will keep them in occlusion and aid the retention of the support. The compound can also be used as a stent around which split-thickness skin grafts can be wrapped.

Acrylics that retain their qualities of elasticity and flow after polymerization can be used in selected cases to line splints. These materials are kind to the tissue and are particularly useful in surgery of the hard palate. Their use should be avoided where good results depend upon rigidity of material.

When it is impossible to deepen or form a labial or buccal sulcus from neighboring

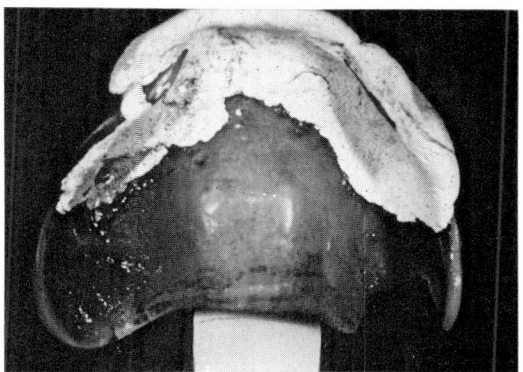

Fig. 7-12. Patient's old denture with surgical cement flange added for the purpose of immobilizing labial sulcus flaps after removal of redundancies. (From Goodsell, J. O.: J. Oral Surg. 13:8, 1955.)

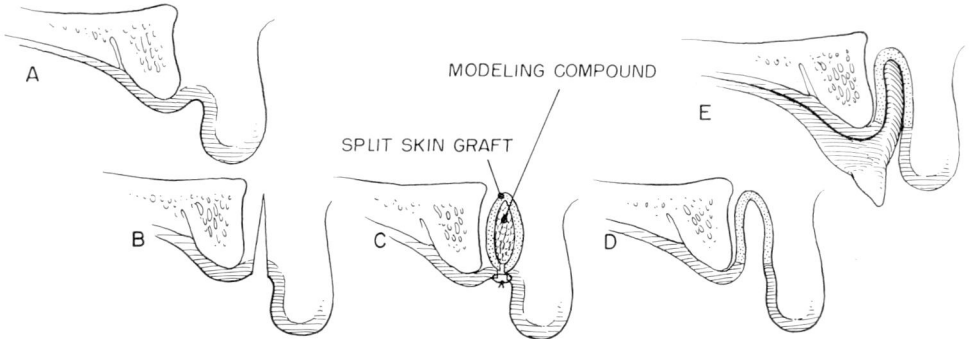

Fig. 7-13. **A,** Shallow labial sulcus. **B,** Sharp incision creating cavity of desired depth, leaving periosteum intact. **C,** Modeling compound stent impression with split-thickness skin graft over it, sutured into cavity. **D,** Support removed and margins trimmed. **E,** New denture for permanent sulcus depth retention.

mucosa, a split-thickness skin graft may be required (Fig. 7-13). This must be supported and kept in contact with the prepared base by one means or another, depending on the location and the situation encountered. An incision is made through the region to be freed, care being taken to stay above the periosteum. A modeling compound impression is made of the newly created defect. The graft is then wrapped around the impression, with the raw surfaces on the outside, and is inserted into the cavity and maintained in position for at least 10 days without undue motion of the surrounding tissues. After the graft has taken, the edges of the wound should be surgically refined and a prosthesis inserted immediately. If a prosthesis is not inserted, considerable shrinkage of the graft will occur.

Pressure dressings (applied externally) frequently are valuable since they assist in stabilization of the tissues, thereby preventing undue motion and reducing the incidence of hematoma formation. External pressure bandages after intraoral surgery are not required frequently, but should be utilized when indicated. Gauze or mechanic's waste under the plastic-type adhesive bandage seems to furnish the best and most positive form of pressure, although elastic bandages may be adequate.

Folds and redundancies in sulci

The prolonged wearing of ill-fitting dentures creates complications that are dangerous to the wearer. Folds and redundancies about the gingiva, cheeks, and sulci may develop, which must be corrected if the individual is to enjoy the wearing of a dental prosthesis to any degree (Fig. 7-14). On some occasions the irregularities, atrophies, or hypertrophies are so complex that surgical correction is almost impossible. Nevertheless, most patients who, through neglect or lack of advice, develop intraoral deformities of this type usually can have them corrected. The removal of folds and redundancies should be undertaken while keeping in mind the various principles mentioned previously.

Sharp dissection and tissue support should be utilized. Electrosurgery may be employed at times, but its application is rare since it may produce excessive scar tissue formation. Clean, precise surgery with fine suture approximation produces a minimum of cicatrization. The creation of good buccal sulci is the goal, and anything that will be an aid should be utilized. The

Abnormalities of the mouth

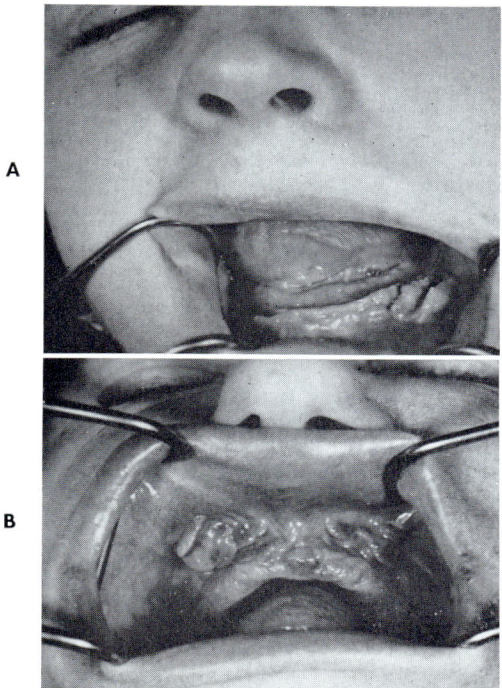

Fig. 7-14. **A,** Redundant folds in mandibular sulcus. **B,** Similar condition in maxillary sulcus. (From Goodsell, J. O.: J. Oral Surg. 13:8, 1955.)

patient's old irritating denture should not be worn for about 3 weeks prior to corrective surgery. It can be inserted, with surgical cement attached, to act as a tissue support after the operation is completed. On occasion it is necessary to perform more than one operation to attain the final desired result.

A technique that has been found useful in the elimination of single or multiple folds is accomplished by sharply dissecting the full thickness of the mucosa away from the fibrous bulges beneath it. These strands of fibrous tissue are then cut away until a smooth base is provided. (See Figs. 7-15 and 7-16.) The large mucosal flap is then shifted superiorly, the excess trimmed off, the midportion sutured as deeply into the sulcus as possible, the edges sutured with fine nonabsorbable sutures, and, finally, the cement-lined denture placed in the mouth as a tissue support. The cement should be very thick, reinforced by cotton shreds on the flanges, and the denture inserted just before the "setting" takes place so that the mucosa is firmly compressed into the cavity. Four days or more should elapse before the retainer is removed for any length of time. Smooth, deep sulci have been obtained more consistently with this technique than with any other.

Scar bands, frenums, and high muscle attachments

The most common buccal vestibule interferences are scar bands, frenums, and high muscle attachments, which have a tendency to mobilize dentures when the cheeks or lips move. Utilization of Z-plasty (Figs. 7-17 and 7-19, A) and sliding flaps of the Burow (Fig. 7-18) and V-Y (Fig. 7-19) types can lessen these deficiencies. Scar bands are amenable to the Z-plasty procedure. Frenums may be treated by a cross-diamond incision (Figs. 7-20 and 7-21) or by Z-plasty. Occasionally the labial frenum (usually the maxillary) will extend between the central incisors in the form of a dense fibrous band. This may be removed if it is believed that it will obstruct the orthodontic movement of the central incisors. High muscle attachments (that is, close to the ridge) may be treated by transverse incision to free them for repositioning at a lower level.

DEEPENING OF BUCCOLABIAL SULCUS: RIDGE EXTENSIONS*

The desirability of surgical intervention to aid the prosthodontist in instances of shallow mouth sulci has been established.

---

*The material on ridge extensions is adapted largely from Kruger, G. O.: Ridge extension: review of indications and technics, J. Oral Surg. 16:191, 1958.

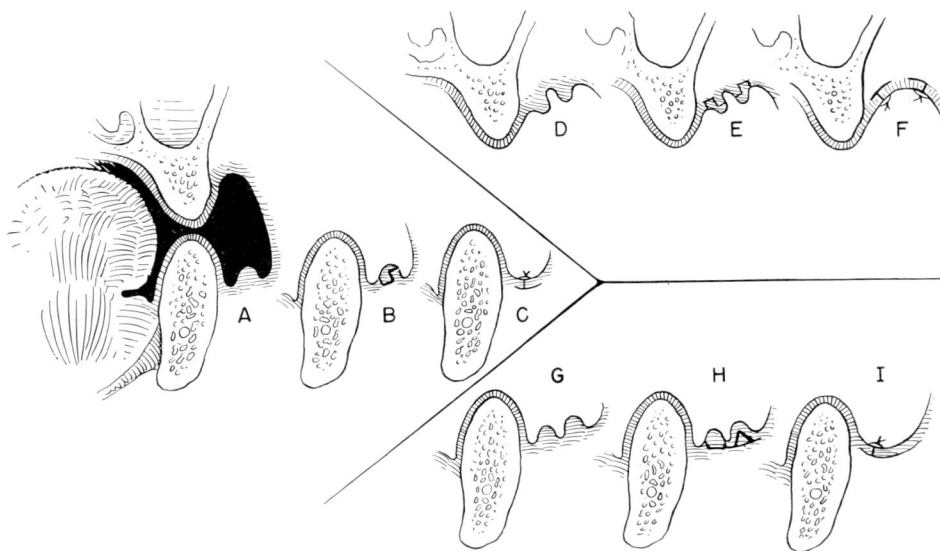

Fig. 7-15. **A**, Single fold in buccal sulcus. **B**, Edges undermined and section to be discarded outlined. **C**, Wound sutured. **D**, Two folds in sulcus. **E**, Tissue to be excised is outlined. Removal of both these folds in one piece without saving any of the inner fold membrane would result in serious loss of sulcus depth. **F**, Sutures applied. **G**, Alternate method of removing double fold. **H**, Medial fold is excised and mucosa is dissected from second fold. Fibrous tissue that underlies lateral fold is carefully dissected away and discarded. **I**, Flap has been slid across denuded area and is sutured in place. Patient's old denture with attached surgical cement periphery is now inserted as previously described.

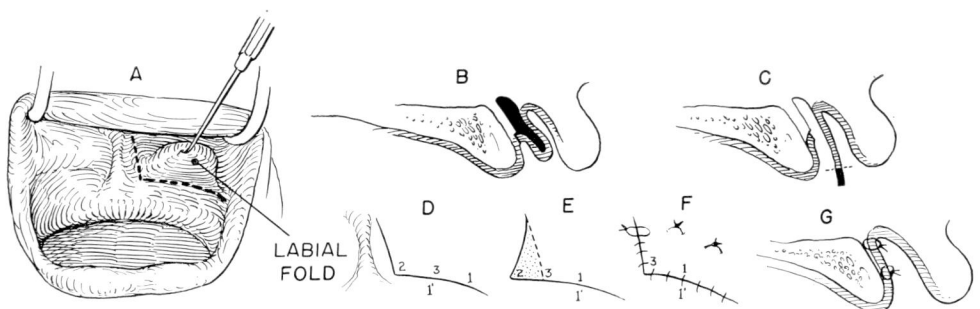

Fig. 7-16. Excision of large fibrous hyperplasia in labial sulcus. **A**, Dotted line shows line of incision. **B**, Shaded area of fibrous tissue is dissected from mucosa and periosteum and discarded. **C**, Excess is trimmed from large mucosal flap. **D**, Anterior view of flap shown in C. **E**, Shaded area of flap is excised and discarded. **F**, Flap is then advanced from position 3 to position 2 and sutured. **G**, Flap is sutured to periosteum as deeply into sulcus as possible. The wound is now ready for insertion of denture support.

Abnormalities of the mouth   113

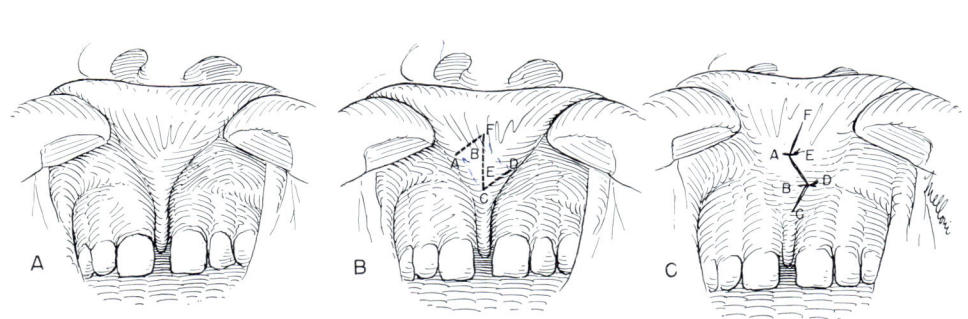

Fig. 7-17. Z-plasty. **A**, An interfering band, in this instance a tight frenum. **B**, Outline for Z-plasty technique. **C**, Angular flaps *B* and *E* transposed into their new positions.

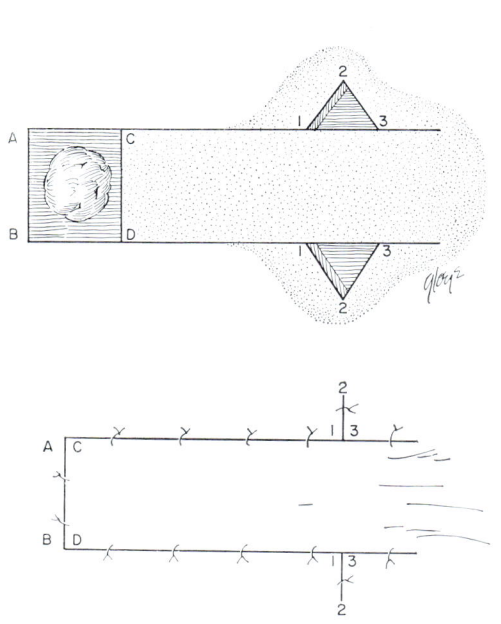

Fig. 7-18. Burow's principle of sliding flap advancement following excision of a large lesion. Incisions are made as shown in the upper diagram, and the dotted area is undermined. Tissue in the triangles *1-2-3* is removed to allow advancement of the flap without producing tissue folds. The lower diagram shows the flaps after advancement and edge-to-edge suturing. This principle can be used to cover bare spots in the mouth and old drainage sites and fistulas.

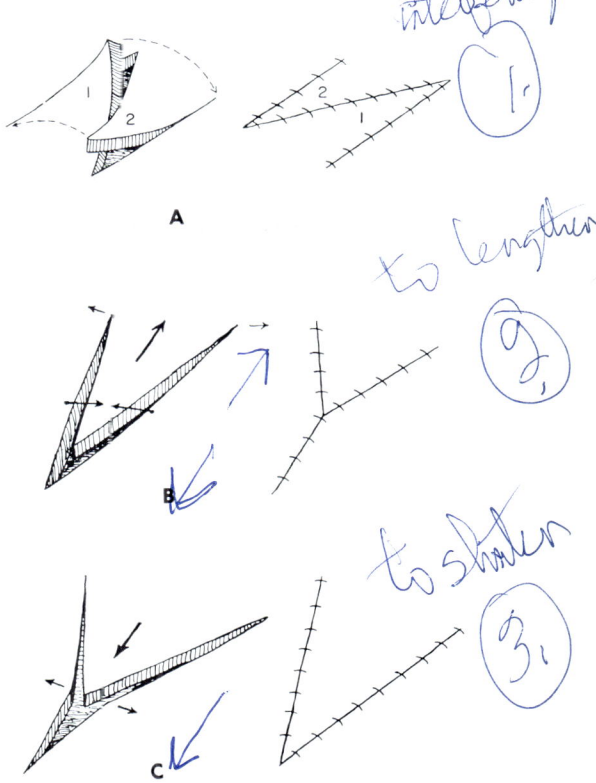

Fig. 7-19. Modification of local flaps. **A**, Z-plasty for breaking up linear scars or for releasing tension of scar band. **B**, V-Y procedure for lengthening localized area. **C**, Y-V procedure for shortening localized area of tissue. (Courtesy Dr. Edward C. Hinds.)

114 Textbook of oral surgery

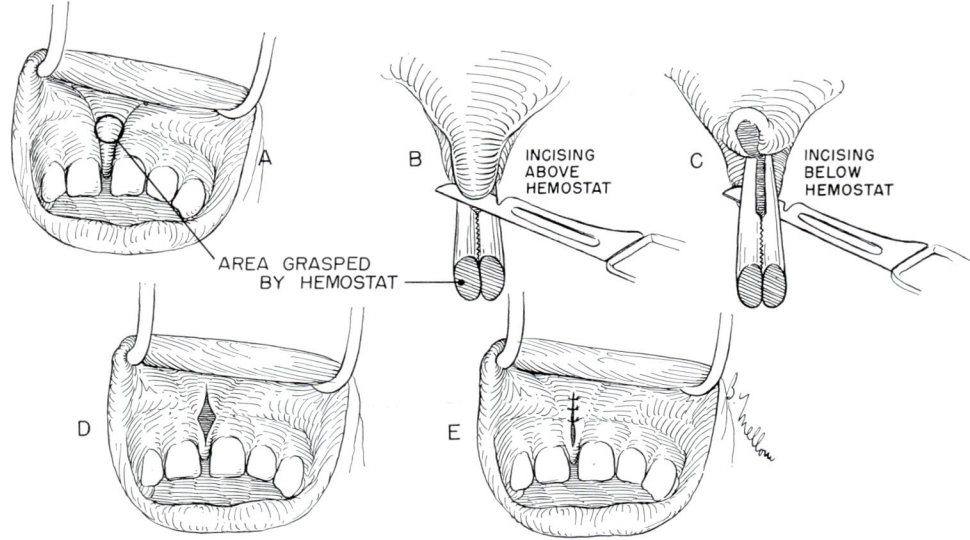

Fig. 7-20. Cross-diamond excision of labial frenum. **A**, Area grasped by hemostat. **B** and **C**, Incision above and below hemostat. **D**, Surgical defect produced by excision of fibrous band. **E**, Closure.

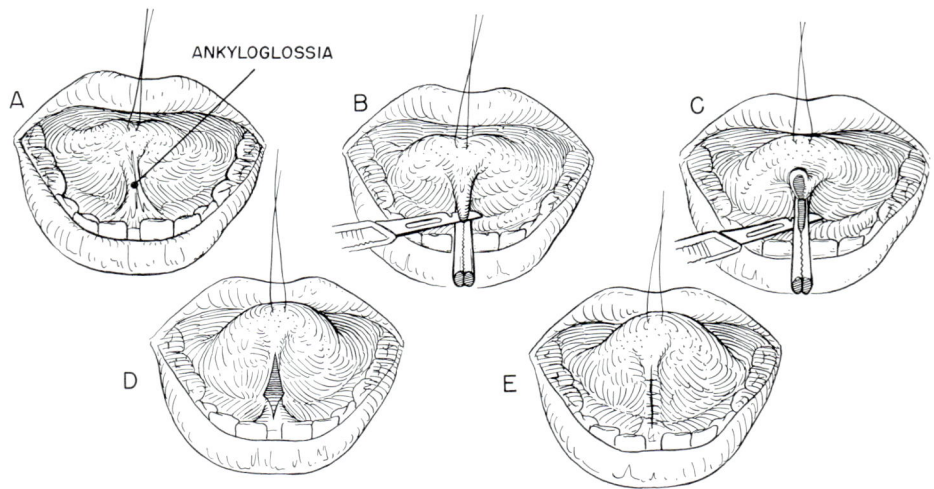

Fig. 7-21. Cross-diamond excision of lingual frenum for ankyloglossia. **A**, Area grasped by hemostat. **B** and **C**, Incisions above and below hemostat. **D**, Surgical defect prior to closure. **E**, Closure.

The techniques are concerned mainly with a repositioning of structures, including muscles, on the bone. Nothing much can be done if complete resorption of the alveolar bone has left an inadequate jaw. Even if it were feasible to reposition the structures to the inferior border of the mandible, there would still be no significant advantage in sulcus depth if the bone is too small. Moreover, such repositioning is limited by natural structures such as the mental foramen and the base of the malar process.

Implant dentures and onlay bone grafts to the ridges give some promise of assistance to edentulous patients with markedly atrophic ridges. However, these procedures are not proved yet as routinely accepted methods in most surgeons' hands.

Many methods have been advocated with varying theories behind them. Ridge extension techniques fall into two basic categories—those depending on secondary epithelization and techniques that provide for immediate epithelial covering to all denuded surfaces. These techniques involve different degrees of surgical difficulty, and they satisfy specific indications. A review of some of the commonly used methods follows; in some instances the techniques are modified by common usage.

Secondary epithelization technique using a labial flap (Kazanjian's technique)

The classic labial flap method starts with an incision just through the mucosa of the inner surface of the lip. This incision is extended parallel to the alveolar ridge, and the distance between it and the ridge crest is determined by the depth of the desired sulcus. A flap is then created by sharp dissection, undermining the mucosa from the incision to a base on the mucoperiosteum of the alveolar ridge (Fig. 7-22, A). The desired sulcus depth is obtained by sharp supraperiosteal dissection along the labial surface of bone (Fig. 7-22, B). As this dissection is carried posteriorly care should be given to the mental foramen area, where injury to the mental nerve will result in lip paresthesia. When sufficient vertical depth has been obtained, the mucosal flap is positioned over the periosteum-covered bone and sutured to the periosteum with interrupted sutures (No. 3-0 gut).

To ensure that the depth obtained is maintained during healing, pressure is

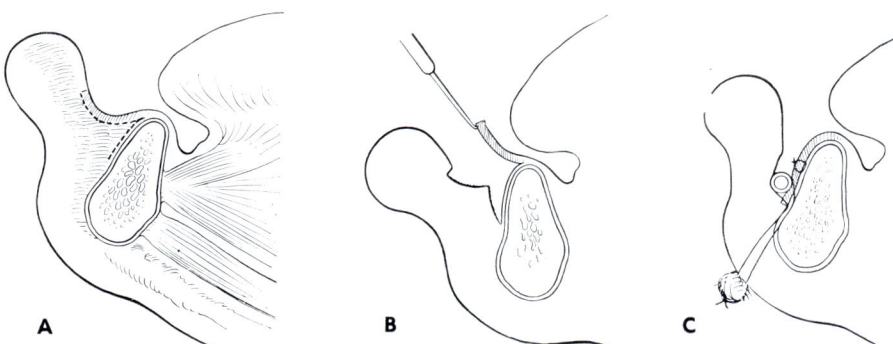

Fig. 7-22. Kazanjian's method. **A,** Incision is made through the mucosa of the inner surface of the lip. **B,** The mucosa is dissected back to a base on the crest of the alveolar ridge. The flap is held out of the way with an instrument while sulcus depth is obtained by supraperiosteal dissection. **C,** The mucosal flap is sutured to the periosteum. A rubber or polyethylene tube is held in place at the bottom of the new sulcus by circumferential sutures tied around cotton rolls. (Redrawn from Kruger, G. O.: J. Oral Surg. 16:191, 1958.)

brought to bear in the bottom of the wound with a rubber tube (size 16 Fr. urethral catheter) held in place by several nylon sutures. These are passed around the tube and through the tissue and tied over cotton rolls on the skin surface (Fig. 7-22, *C*). The use of nylon suture avoids the wick effect of silk or cotton, which may carry oral fluids into deep tissues and result in abscess formation. An external pressure bandage is worn for 3 days. The tube and sutures are removed in 7 days, after which the new denture should be inserted as soon as possible to avoid relapse.

In place of the rubber tube technique a denture, extended to maintain the new sulcus depth, can be used. This should be held in place with circummandibular wires until healing has occurred.

In recent years the Kazanjian technique has lost popularity since many prosthodontists believe that a scar-free peripheral seal is essential to denture retention. However, others find that in selected cases the scar band on the lip side is useful in preventing displacement of the denture by lip movements.

Secondary epithelization technique using an alveolar flap

The alveolar flap technique as described by Clark is especially adapted for the anterior part of the mandible in instances in which the mentalis muscle is involved. Incision is made over the crest of the ridge, and immediate sulcus depth is obtained by sharp and blunt dissection (Fig. 7-23, *A*). The dissection is carried down supraperiosteally. The lip mucosa is then undermined from the edge of the incision to the vermilion border. A monofilament nylon suture is placed through the mucosal flap in mattress style, and the two ends are carried out to the skin surface, where they are tied over a cotton roll (Fig. 7-23, *B*). Three such sutures are placed. The raw surface of the soft tissue is thus covered, leaving the periosteum-covered bone to

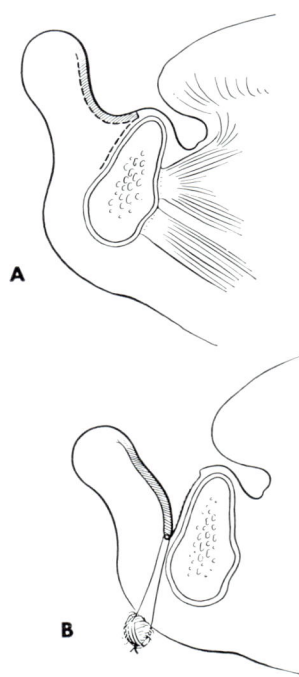

Fig. 7-23. Clark's technique. **A**, Incision is made slightly labial to the crest of the ridge. Sulcus depth is obtained by supraperiosteal dissection. The lip mucosa is undermined from the edge of the incision to the vermilion border. **B**, The mucosal flap is held over the wound by sutures placed to the skin surface. (From Kruger, G. O.: J. Oral Surg. **16**:191, 1958.)

granulate and epithelize. Clark based his alveolar flap ridge extension on a plastic principle, which states that raw areas on bony surfaces cannot contract. He noted, however, a tendency for relapse of any tissues undergoing plastic revision and recommended overcorrection and firm fixation to maintain depth in ridge extension procedures.

Spengler and Hayward[8] performed the Kazanjian and Clark procedures on dogs for purposes of comparing their relapse tendency. Results indicated that both techniques resulted in equal reversion. In the Clark procedure relapse occurred during the period of periosteal epithelization. The epithelium was pulled from both sides of the raw periosteal surface by the scar contracture. This resulted in diminished sulcus depth. Relapse occurred in the Kazanjian procedure because of contraction of the lip cicatrix rather than denuded periosteum. In both procedures contracture stopped after epithelization was complete, and no further reversion occurred.

Procedures employing an immediate epithelial covering

Other ridge extension techniques provide for an immediate epithelial covering to all raw surfaces in an attempt to avoid scar contracture. Split-thickness skin grafts can be taken from the buttocks or the undersurface of the arm. These areas are relatively free of hair, and the healed donor site, although usually pigmented differently than the surrounding skin, is seldom objectionable. Those patients needing ridge extension procedures are rarely at their best in abbreviated bathing costumes. Skin grafts are applied to the periosteal surface with the aid of an acrylic splint wired in place. After healing has occurred the skin-mucosal border is trimmed.

Submucous vestibuloplasty

Obwegeser[7] advocates a method of submucous vestibuloplasty that provides for

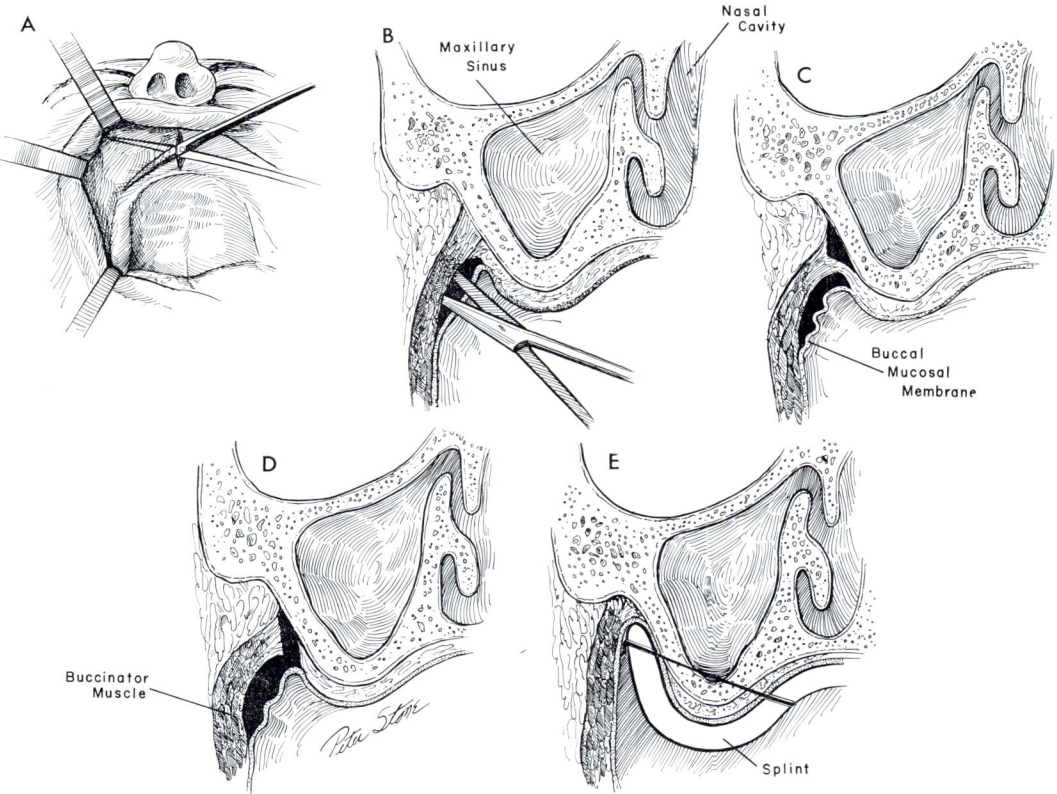

Fig. 7-24. Submucous vestibuloplasty. **A**, Vertical incision provides access for undermining the mucosa and severing the muscles from their attachment. **B**, Undermining of the mucous membrane. **C** and **D**, Supraperiosteal detachment of muscle. **E**, Retention of sulcus depth with acrylic splint. (Ends of the peralveolar wire should be tucked into a nearby hole.)

an immediate covering of the surgical area with oral mucosa. This procedure is particularly indicated for the labial and buccal regions of the maxilla, but can be used elsewhere with modification.

In the operation to deepen the labial sulcus the initial step is to make a single vertical incision near the midline. This is to provide access for undermining the mucosa and releasing muscle attachments. If necessary, additional vertical incisions can be made more posteriorly. The mucous membrane is separated from the submucosa by undermining with scissors (Fig. 7-24). The next step is to carefully sever the muscles from their bony attachments, leaving the periosteum intact. Because this is a relatively blind step, the surgeon should be cautious to avoid the infraorbital and mental foramina when in those areas. The muscles, along with the submucosa, are reflected away from the alveolar crest, and the elastic mucous membrane is adapted to the periosteum and maintained there by a preconstructed acrylic splint lined with surgical cement. This splint is removed in 1 week, and the new denture should be inserted immediately.

Because it provides for an immediate epithelial covering to all tissues, the submucous vestibuloplasty results in rapid healing and a lesser tendency to relapse than methods that depend on secondary epithelization. This technique should not be used if the labial mucous membranes are associated with tumors or are otherwise of poor quality.

DEEPENING OF LINGUAL SULCUS
Supraperiosteal method

When sufficient depth of sulcus is not obtainable by other techniques on the buccal and labial surfaces of the mandible, Trauner[9] has advocated a repositioning of the mylohyoid muscle (Fig. 7-25). A criterion for the operation is that the mylohyoid muscle attachment must be located at the level of the crest of the ridge.

Incision is made close to the crest of the ridge on the lingual side, extending from the second molar region to the cuspid region. Supraperiosteal blunt dissection is carried down to the mylohyoid muscle. A curved Kelly clamp is placed beneath the muscle, and the muscle is incised down to the clamp. The lingual mucosa and the muscle are caught with a monofilament nylon suture that is carried close to the bone to exit on the skin, where it is tied over cotton rolls. Three such sutures are

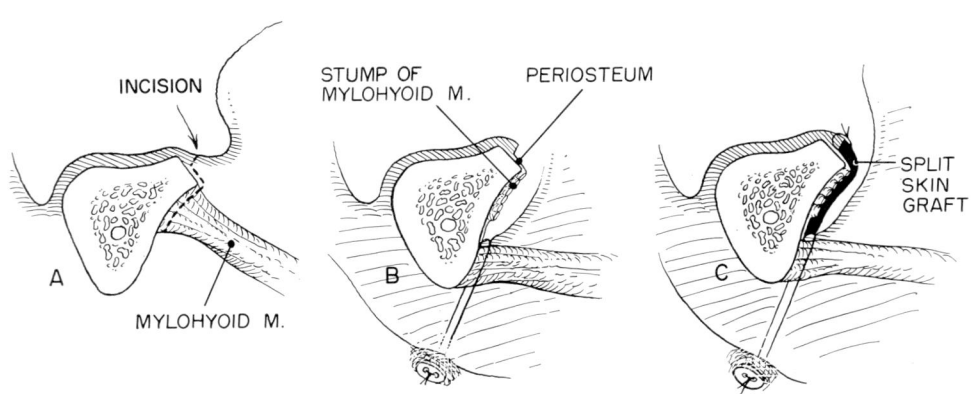

Fig. 7-25. Trauner's procedure. **A**, Line of incision through mucosa and mylohyoid muscle. **B**, Anchorage of mylohyoid muscle to floor of mouth by means of external sutures. **C**, Surgical defect on mylohyoid stump may be covered with split graft or allowed to heal by granulation.

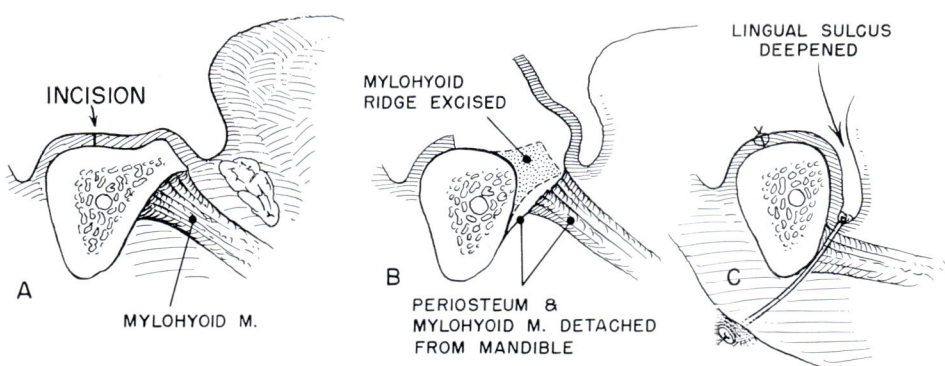

Fig. 7-26. Caldwell's procedure. **A,** Line of incision. **B,** Periosteum and mylohyoid muscle detached from mandible. **C,** Suturing and anchorage to floor of mouth.

placed; then a pressure bandage is applied. Both sides of the mandible are treated in one operation, usually in the hospital.

Subperiosteal method

A modification of the Trauner procedure has been suggested by Caldwell[1] to permit reduction of the bony internal oblique line; such reduction is often necessary (Fig. 7-26). Incision is made through the periosteum over the crest of the ridge. The mylohyoid muscle is detached from the mylohyoid ridge, and the ridge is removed with a chisel. A rubber catheter is transfixed in the lingual sulcus over the intact mucosa by means of sutures carried through to the skin. The ridge incision is then closed.

OTHER PROCEDURES

Electrocauterization has been used with good results for the removal of fibromatous hyperplasia and simultaneous deepening of the sulcus. The main advantages of this procedure are that the pendulous masses that present so little usable mucosa are removed entirely and the technique is direct, simple, and speedy. The possible disadvantages are those associated with electrocauterization—odor during burning, soreness that persists for some time, and scarring.

REFERENCES

1. Caldwell, J. S.: Lingual ridge extension, J. Oral Surg. **13:**287, 1955.
2. Clark, H. B., Jr.: Deepening of labial sulcus by mucosal flap advancement: report of case, J. Oral Surg. **11:**135, 1953.
3. Goodsell, J. O.: Surgical aids to intraoral prosthesis, J. Oral Surg. **13:**8, 1955.
4. Hayward, J. R., and Thompson, S.: Principles of alveolectomy, J. Oral Surg. **16:**101, 1958.
5. Kazanjian, V. H.: Surgery as an aid to more efficient service with prosthetic dentures, J. Amer. Dent. Ass. **22:**566, 1935.
6. Kruger, G. O.: Ridge extension: review of indications and technics, J. Oral Surg. **16:**191, 1958.
7. Obwegeser, H.: Surgical preparation of the maxilla for prosthesis, J. Oral Surg. **22:**127, 1964.
8. Spengler, D. E., and Hayward, J. R.: The study of sulcus extension wound healing in dogs, J. Oral Surg. **22:**413, 1964.
9. Trauner, R.: Alveoloplasty with ridge extension on the lingual side of the lower jaw to solve the problem of a lower dental prosthesis, Oral Surg. **5:**340, 1952.

Chapter 8

SPECIAL CONSIDERATIONS IN EXODONTIA

Donald C. Reynolds

REMOVAL OF TEETH FOR CHILDREN

The management of a child who must undergo dental extractions is based on (1) his age and maturity, (2) past medical and dental experiences that might influence behavior, (3) physical status, and (4) the length of time and amount of manipulation necessary to accomplish the surgery.

The age and maturity of the child often determine the type of anesthesia best suited for the intended procedure. Children below the age of reason generally are best managed under general anesthesia since a slight amount of discomfort is always associated with the administration of local anesthesia. During the extraction the child will experience pressures and noises associated with the necessary instrumentation. If these phenomena cannot be explained to the child, he will become anxious and rebellious. For these reasons general anesthesia is often used for the very young patient.

Good rapport must be established between the dentist and the pediatric patient. The dentist should be friendly, but firm. Short, simple explanations of the sensations the child will experience should be made. At the time of needle insertion he is told that he will feel a little "stick," and during injection of the solution he is told that he will feel pressure. The forces the child will experience during the extraction can be demonstrated by pushing gently, but firmly, on his shoulders. The child is told that he will feel the "pushing" in the area of surgery, just as he has felt it on his shoulders. It should be pointed out that "pushing" is the only sensation that will be felt. At no time should the word "pain" be mentioned.

The child should be verbally reprimanded for unwarranted actions. During and at the end of the procedure he should be praised for his cooperation. Speaking to the child in a friendly, understanding manner throughout the procedure will greatly enhance the efficacy of "verbal anesthesia."

Scheduling the pediatric patient in the morning is desirable. At this time he is less likely to be tired and difficult to manage. Delays should be eliminated as much as possible between the time the child enters the office and the initiation of treatment. Delays allow only for the development of apprehension. Premedication with a sedative is indicated if the child appears apprehensive. Such premedication will be helpful with the administration of local as well as general anesthesia. A sedative is indicated also if a lengthy procedure such as removal of supernumerary teeth is planned. A child will tend to become restless and unmanageable during prolonged procedures.

At no time should the child be allowed to see the instruments necessary for anesthesia and surgery. A Mayo stand is placed behind the chair and the instruments brought to the mouth from behind and below to keep them out of the child's visual field. Small syringes and extraction forceps are available, which can be more easily "hidden," but they are by no means necessary for the successful management of the pediatric patient. One example regarding the advisability of keeping instruments out of the child's view involves a youngster who became hysterical at the sight of a suture needle after having sat quietly throughout multiple extractions. Upon questioning the patient it was discovered that during the previous year the child had lacerated his scalp, which required suturing. The child associated the needle with the pain experienced during the suturing of his scalp and related it to the current operation.

In general, the removal of deciduous teeth is not difficult; it is facilitated by the elasticity of young bone and the resorption of the root structure. The children's upper and lower forceps can be used for the removal of all deciduous teeth (Fig. 8-1). These forceps have the basic design of the universal upper and lower forceps (Nos. 150 and 151). If children's forceps are not available, deciduous teeth can be removed with the forceps used for the removal of their succedaneous analogues. However, the "cowhorn" (No. 16) forceps is not used for the extraction of lower deciduous molars because the sharp beaks of this forceps could cause damage to the unerupted premolar teeth.

The maxillary and mandibular six anterior teeth are removed by luxation to the labial side, followed by mesial rotation and then pressure in the direction of removal. Because of the lingual position of the erupting permanent incisor teeth, very little can be gained by placing lingual pressure on these teeth. The maxillary and mandibular molars are luxated to the buccal and lingual areas and delivered to the lingual. Very often a mesial or distal path of exit is necessary because of the root formation.

Adequate radiographs are invaluable for the removal of any deciduous tooth. The presence and position of the permanent successor must be established as well as the status of the root formation of the

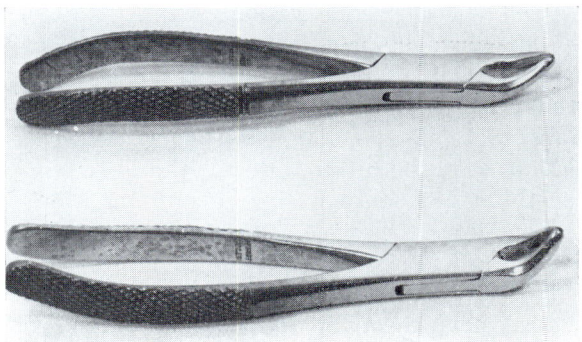

Fig. 8-1. Children's forceps.

122 *Textbook of oral surgery*

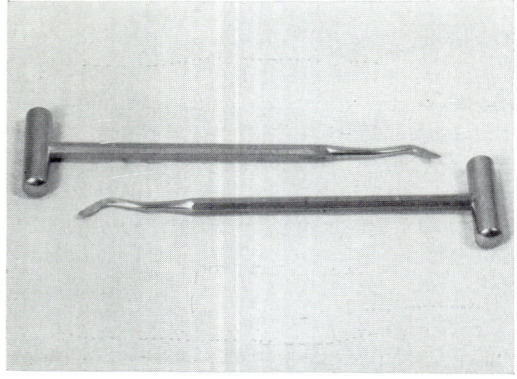

Fig. 8-2. Potts' elevators for removal of deciduous roots.

deciduous tooth that is to be removed. Many times the resorption of the deciduous root is unequal, leaving a long, thin root portion. If a root is fractured during the extraction, it should be removed by the judicious use of root exolevers or a small curet. The Potts elevators also are valuable here (Fig. 8-2). Care must be exercised not to injure the crown of the permanent tooth or its surrounding bony support. If the removal of the deciduous root tip jeopardizes the permanent tooth, it is better to leave the root tip intact. It will resorb or can be removed at a later date without jeopardy to the permanent tooth.

Occasionally the radiograph will demonstrate that the permanent premolar is wedged tightly between the bell-shaped roots of the deciduous tooth. This occurs most often in a deeply carious tooth of a young patient in which no deciduous root resorption has occurred. Care must be taken that the succedaneous tooth is not removed with the deciduous tooth because of the viselike grip of the roots. If the radiograph shows this condition, the deciduous crown should be sectioned into a mesial and a distal half before a forceps is placed on the tooth to remove the two portions separately. If at any time a permanent tooth is removed during the extraction of a deciduous tooth, it should be replaced in the alveolar bone with as little handling as possible, making sure that the buccal aspect of the tooth is placed on the buccal side of the alveolus.

SELECTION OF ANESTHESIA FOR EXODONTIA

The types of anesthesia available for exodontia are (1) regional or local anesthesia, (2) local anesthesia with heavy sedation or supplementation by light general anesthetic agents, and (3) general anesthesia, which can be given intravenously or by inhalation.

Factors that determine choice of anesthesia are (1) age and physical status of the patient, (2) infection, (3) trismus, (4) emotional status of the patient, (5) nature and duration of the procedure, (6) allergies, (7) wishes of the patient, and (8) training and office equipment of the operator.

As was stated previously, the very young patient is best managed under general anesthesia, usually of the inhalation type or in combination with small doses of intravenous barbiturates. The geriatric patient metabolizes barbiturates poorly and requires reduced dosages. Older patients are more likely to have systemic diseases that complicate the use of general anesthesia. The geriatic patient is often managed with local anesthesia with judicious use of sedatives, when necessary, to relieve apprehension.

In the presence of infection local anesthesia is not always profound. If local anesthesia is used, a nerve block is most effective and allows injection of the anesthetic solution in a noninfected area. Under no circumstances is a local anesthesia solution injected into or through an area of cellulitis. This serves only to spread the infection, with possible serious consequences. General anesthesia is often indicated in the presence of acute infection, except when the overall systemic condition of the patient precludes its use, or the patient is toxic and dehydrated because of the infection. After the toxic manifestations have decreased and the patient is well hydrated, general anesthesia may be given and the tooth removed. Before removal of any tooth during an acute infection, adequate blood levels of antibiotics should be obtained.

Trismus, or the inability of the patient to open his mouth, may make the administration of local anesthesia by the usual route difficult. Extraoral nerve blocks usually can be given. When the nerve block has alleviated the pain, the patient may be able to open his mouth so that the necessary extraction can be accomplished. Ethyl chloride sprayed on the skin overlying the muscles that are in spasm may enable the patient to open his mouth sufficiently to allow the surgeon to administer local anesthesia and to perform the extraction. Care must be taken not to freeze the tissue with the ethyl chloride spray. General anesthesia, if deep enough to obtain muscle relaxation, is valuable when the trismus is caused by infection or trauma. When ankylosis of the temporomandibular joint is present, anesthesia can be accomplished by extraoral blocks or by performing a tracheostomy and administering a general anesthetic. If a general anesthetic is given to a patient having this condition, a tracheostomy is performed so that a patent airway can be maintained. Even though adequate anesthesia can be obtained, this type of patient still presents many problems because of the inaccessibility of the teeth to be extracted.

The emotional status of the patient may determine the selection of anesthesia. Some people have a phobia regarding injections within the mouth. Because of the recent advances in general anesthesia, it is comparable in safety to local anesthesia. For this reason patients of this type are better managed under general anesthesia.

If the apprehensive patient must be treated under local anesthesia, sedation is necessary. The patient should receive a barbiturate at bedtime the night before surgery and again 1 hour prior to surgery. Intravenous barbiturates can be given at the time of surgery to augment those already administered. Any patient who receives a sedative should be accompanied by a responsible adult. The surgeon is responsible for his patient while the latter is under the influence of the drug. Under no circumstances should a sedated patient be allowed to drive an automobile.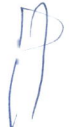

The nature of the procedure and the duration of time necessary to accomplish the exodontia can govern the anesthetic agent used. In general, procedures requiring more than 30 minutes are better managed under local anesthesia with premedication, or by admitting the patient to a hospital where adequate recovery facilities are available. With prolonged general anesthesia a prolonged recovery time is necessary.

All patients should be questioned with regard to drug allergies. Patients having a possible history of allergy to local anesthetics should be questioned as to the type of reaction experienced and referred to an allergist for evaluation. Patients who have a history of allergic reaction to procaine often are not allergic to lidocaine because of the different chemical configuration of the drug. Although lidocaine has a low incidence of allergic reactions, reactions to this drug have been reported. Infrequently, adverse reactions to barbiturates are found. Most of these are not true allergic reactions but are failures of the patients to respond to the drug in the normal fashion. Nausea, vomiting, or changes in the psyche are common reactions. In any office in which drugs are administered an emergency tray should be immediately available with the proper drugs necessary for treatment of allergic reactions. The treatment of these reactions will be described later in this chapter.

REMOVAL OF TEETH UNDER GENERAL ANESTHESIA

Organization and teamwork are essential when using general anesthesia. An efficient team is composed of three or four members: the surgeon, the anesthetist, the assistant whose duty is to use the suction apparatus and retract tissues, and sometimes an instrument nurse whose duty is to pass instruments or wield the mallet if a chisel technique is used. Every member of the team must know the technique and anticipate the needs of the surgeon and the patient. Unnecessary acts should be avoided. Each motion should be smooth and purposeful.

All of the instruments that may be needed for a procedure should be available so that a member of the team does not have to break scrub to get an instrument. The instruments should be on a tray and always be grouped in the same fashion, with the most frequently used instruments in the most accessible position.

For general anesthesia the patient may be supine or in a sitting position. Each position has its advantages.

The types of general anesthesia most frequently used are inhalation alone, barbiturates alone, barbiturates with oxygen and nitrous oxide, and barbiturates with oxygen and nitrous oxide in combination with a more potent agent such as fluothane. In addition, local anesthesia is sometimes administered for vasoconstriction and to decrease the amount of barbiturate used in lengthy procedures.

A mouth prop is inserted immediately prior to induction of the anesthesia. Two types of mouth props are used—either a solid rubber bite block or a ratchet-type prop. If the latter is used, it is inserted in a closed position, and the patient is instructed to close on the mouth prop to hold it in position. After induction the mouth prop is adjusted to the degree of opening desired.

Immediately after induction a mouth pack is positioned. The pack is placed in such manner as to hold the tongue and soft tissues of the floor of the mouth anteriorly to maintain an airway. Care must be taken not to place the pack so far posteriorly that the oropharynx is stimulated. When an inhalation anesthesia is used, an airtight pack is more important so that anesthesia may be maintained by use of a nasal mask. Extra sponges may be added over the pack to absorb secretions and blood. With general anesthesia more bleeding is experienced because of the lack of vasoconstrictive agents.

The surgical team should be ready to work as soon as the patient is anesthetized. Do not lose 2 or 3 precious minutes by not being prepared. The mouth prop is opened immediately and the mouth pack placed. The tooth is extracted and the socket compressed and covered with a gauze sponge. The mouth pack is removed and the mouth suctioned. The mouth prop is closed but left in place until the patient responds. The patient is transferred to a mobile chair or table and moved to a recovery room where he is watched carefully by an attendant.

During longer procedures a gauze sponge is placed over the mouth pack and changed as necessary. The assistant retracts and suctions in the most dependent portion of the mouth, not necessarily in a socket. A careful, efficient, unhurried technique is developed. Efficiency comes from precise instrumentation with few instrument changes. Accomplish all that is to be done with a given instrument before the instrument is exchanged for another (for example, curet around all teeth that are to be extracted before picking up forceps). In multiple extractions the maxillary teeth are removed in one quadrant first, and the necessary alveoloplasty there is finished and sutured. A gauze sponge is then placed over this wound to help control hemorrhage. The mandibular teeth are removed in the opposing quadrant. After completion of surgery in this area, a new gauze sponge is placed over the wound before the mouth prop is shifted so that extractions can be done in the two remaining quadrants. Many times when extracting a series of teeth, as each posterior tooth is removed the socket is covered with a sponge to help control hemorrhage while the next anterior tooth is removed.

A powerful suction apparatus is necessary. The greatest hazard when operating under general anesthesia comes from allowing blood, secretions, and debris to collect within the mouth. If these materials are allowed to descend, the larynx can be irritated to cause a laryngospasm, a lung abscess can be formed, or nausea and vomiting may follow entrance into the stomach. The average suction available in a dental unit is inadequate. Two types of suction tips should be available. A tonsillar suction tip is best adapted for handling a large volume of fluid efficiently, but is too bulky to allow for suctioning within a socket. A neurosurgical suction tip will enter a small area. It is helpful to have two suction tips on the table in case debris clogs one of the tips.

The art of exodontia is never one of force. This is particularly true when operating under general anesthesia. Because of the loss of subjective symptoms in the patient, it becomes easy for the novice to apply great force with an exolever or to retract soft tissue carelessly. Meticulous surgery under general anesthesia is important so that the postoperative healing will not be a painful experience for the patient.

REMOVAL OF TEETH IN THE HOSPITAL

Hospitalization of patients for exodontia should always be considered when medical management of the patient may be a problem or the postoperative course may necessitate special care.

Before a patient is admitted to a hospital, arrangements must be made with the admitting office so that a bed will be available. The operating room secretary is also called so that an operating room can be reserved for the procedure.

The dental staff of the hospital is obligated to observe the basic rules of the hospital and the American Hospital Association. While it is not the object of this text to outline hospital procedure, some of the basic rules should be noted. A patient who will undergo general anesthesia must have a physical examination, which includes a history. All patients admitted to a hospital for more than 24 hours should have the routine laboratory tests. These usually consist of a hematocrit (HCT), a white blood cell count (WBC), a differential white count, and a urinalysis. A chest radiograph and serological tests may be required by some hospitals. Patients over 45 years of age often are examined by an electrocardiogram (ECG) if general anesthesia is to be used. The dentist must write the necessary orders and an admission note, which includes the reason for the admission and the contemplated procedure. A dental history and oral examination should also be included in the dentist's note.

The dentist should check with the operating room personnel to be sure that all instruments necessary for the procedure will be available. In many hospitals the dentist must provide certain instruments.

In the operating room sterile precautions are followed. The surgeon is expected to scrub and to wear a cap, gown, mask, and gloves.

The area around the patient's mouth should be prepared with an antiseptic solution to remove surface contaminants. If a single extraction or a very minor procedure is to be performed, the simple placement of sterile towels to isolate the mouth is all the draping necessary. For multiple extractions or more extensive procedures, sterile sheets should be added so that the entire patient is covered to guard against contamination.

Upon completion of surgery a description of the operative procedure is dictated so that it may be added to the patient's chart. This note should include the following: date; names of the patient, surgeon, assistant, and anesthetist; type of anesthesia and agents used; surgical procedure and how it was accomplished; any complications (such as extensive hemorrhage); and condition of the patient at completion of surgery.

New orders are written since preoperative orders are usually cancelled by the operating room procedure. Orders suggested by the consulting physician have to be rewritten to be given. Routine postoperative orders include patient's ambulatory status (bed rest until recovered, then up and about), hot or cold applications for swelling, antibiotics if needed for infections, diet, and an order for an analgesic and a hypnotic, if needed. Daily progress notes are entered by the dentist.

At the time of discharge from the hospital a discharge summary of one paragraph is written, including reason for admission, surgical procedure, postsurgical course, and condition upon discharge.

MANAGEMENT OF ACUTELY INFECTED TEETH

With the advent of antibiotics the management of acutely infected teeth has changed. In the past it was necessary to treat the patient palliatively until the infection could be localized and drained and the tooth extracted. Today this sometimes long delay can be avoided by use of antibiotics. If the cause of the infection (that is, the tooth) can be removed, the resolution of the infection will be accelerated. The abscess formation may not have reached the stage at which tissue is broken down and pus formed. Antibiotics may control the acute infectious process so that pus formation does not take place. In any event a blood level of antibiotics should be established as soon as possible. Once this blood level is established the tooth should be removed if a surgical extraction is not deemed necessary. If a difficult extraction is anticipated, the patient should be placed on antibiotics until such time as a surgical flap can be raised and bone be removed without spreading the infection into the surrounding tissues. The patient should remain on antibiotics after removal of an acutely infected tooth until 3 days after all evidence of the infection has disappeared.

COMPLICATIONS OF EXODONTIA

Complications arise from errors in judgment, misuse of instruments, exertion of extreme force, and failure to obtain proper visualization prior to acting. The old adage that states "To do good, you must see good" is apropos to exodontia, and we might add "Do well what you see."

Because of the anatomy of the maxillary antrum and its proximity to the maxillary premolar and molar roots, the antrum should always be considered when extracting teeth in this area.

The methods used for removal of maxillary roots are described in the section on root removal.

Extreme force applied to upper molars can result in removal of the molar tooth along with the entire maxillary alveolar process and the floor of the antrum. The first, second, and third molars, along with the tuberosity, have been removed in one segment because of improper use of force in the maxilla. If during an extraction the surgeon feels large segments of bone moving with the tooth when pressure is applied, the forceps should be set aside and a flap raised. If judicious removal of part of the alveolar bone allows the tooth to be removed, then the remaining bone, which is attached to the periosteum, may be retained, and it will heal. This will minimize the bony defect. If the bone cannot be removed from the tooth, the mucosa should be incised and reflected so that the mucosa will not tear as the tooth and bone are removed. A laceration is much more difficult to repair than a well-planned incision.

Large antrum perforations resulting from exodontia should be closed at the time of the extraction. The bone in the area should be smoothed with a rongeur or bone file. The mucoperiosteal flap is returned to position and a water-tight closure should be accomplished without putting undue pressure on the flap. If this cannot be done, the flap should be freed by means of an incision extending vertically into the mucobuccal fold and the mucosa of the flap undermined to allow it to advance over the defect.

When the antrum is entered during exodontia, the patient should be made aware of the situation and asked not to blow his nose and also to refrain if possible from coughing or sneezing. Antibiotics and vasoconstrictive nose drops are prescribed to guard against infection of the sinus and to allow for emptying of the fluids that will collect within the sinus.

Occasionally, buccal roots of premolars and molars are pushed laterally through the wall of the maxilla and lie above the attachment of the buccinator muscle. When using root exolevers in this area, a finger of the left hand should be held against the buccal plate so that one can be aware of any movement of the root in this direction. If the root is dislodged into these tissues, a small incision is made in the mucosa inferior to the root tip and the root tip is removed by use of a small hemostat or similar instrument.

The infratemporal space lies directly posterior and superior to the tuberosity of the maxilla. Within this space lie many important neurovascular structures. In the elevation of third molars or third molar root tips and in the removal of supernumerary molars, care must be taken not to dislodge them posteriorly. If an object is to be removed from the infratemporal space, adequate visualization and careful dissection are necessary. The incision should include the entire tuberosity and extend posteriorly to the anterior pillar of the fauces. Blind dissection and groping for objects in this area can be complicated by massive hemorrhage or nerve damage.

In the third molar region of the mandible the lingual surface of the mandible curves laterally, close to the apices of this tooth. Therefore, it is not difficult to dislodge a root tip inferiorly into this space when the lingual plate is fractured. When a root tip is displaced in this area, a finger should be placed inferior to the root tip (in the mouth) so as to stabilize the tip against the lingual plate of the mandible. Access to this area is gained by making a mucoperiosteal flap on the lingual side of the mandible and extending anteriorly enough so that the tissues can be retracted lingually for good vision.

Recovery of a root tip into the mandibular canal is principally a problem of access and vision. Usually it is difficult to remove bone overlying the canal from within the depths of the wound, which is usually the third molar socket. Access may be gained by removal of bone from the buccal plate and by careful removal of bone that overlies the canal. If one of the vascular components of the canal has been injured, it may be necessary to pack the socket with gauze, allowing 10 minutes for control of the hemorrhage. If hemorrhage cannot be controlled in this manner, the injured vessel should be severed completely and allowed to retract into the canal. At this time the socket is again packed and hemorrhage control is usually accomplished.

POSTEXODONTIA COMPLICATIONS

Postoperative hemorrhage is the most common complication following exodontia. If the patient calls from home to report that hemorrhage has started again, he should be advised first to clear his mouth of any blood clots with a gauze sponge. The mouth is rinsed with warm salt water. All excessive blood clots should be removed from the vicinity of the socket, but the clot in the socket should not be removed. The patient is instructed to bite firmly on a sterile gauze sponge, which has been folded so that pressure may be exerted on the area of surgery. If a sterile gauze sponge is not available, the patient may use a tea bag that has been placed in cold water to soften the tea leaves. The patient is advised to bite (not chew) on the pad or tea bag for 20 minutes. If bleeding persists at the end of this period, the patient should be seen by the dentist.

In cases of persistent hemorrhage, gauze sponges and hemostatic agents such as Gelfoam, topical thrombin, and oxidized cellulose are necessary for the local control of hemorrhage, besides an adequate armamentarium (Fig. 13-11).

The patient is seated and local anesthesia administered. The clot that has formed within the socket is removed. Next the area of hemorrhage is located. If the hemorrhage is coming from a bone bleeder within the socket, the dull side of a curet is used to burnish the bone in the area of hemorrhage. If generalized bone bleeding is present, the socket is packed with a hemostatic agent such as Gelfoam soaked in thrombin, and a purse-string suture is applied to hold the hemostatic agent in place. The patient is asked to bite on a moist gauze sponge. If the hemorrhage is from the surrounding soft tissue, a tension suture is placed to apply pressure to the area (see Chapter 13).

Infection can occur as a postoperative complication. Treatment of such infection is managed by using the principles outlined in Chapter 13.

Dry socket (localized osteitis) is one of the most perplexing postoperative complications. The etiology of the dry socket is unknown, but the following factors increase the incidence of this painful postextraction sequela: trauma, infection, vascular supply of the surrounding bone, and general systemic condition.

This condition rarely occurs when minimal traumatic methods are employed during difficult or simple extractions. Meticulous debridement of all extraction wounds should be done routinely. The etiology may be related to factors that impede or prevent adequate nourishment from reaching the newly formed blood clot within the alveolus. Patients with dense, osteosclerotic bone or with teeth that have osteosclerotic alveolar walls because of chronic infection are predisposed to dry sockets. Excessive amounts of local anesthesia containing a vasoconstrictor infiltrated around the field of extraction may also be a contributing factor to an impeded blood supply to the wound.

Dry socket most commonly develops on the third or fourth postoperative day and is characterized by severe, continuous pain and necrotic odor. Clinically the condition may be described as an alveolus in which the primary blood clot has become necrotic and remains within the alveolus as a septic foreign body until it is removed by irrigation. This usually occurs a few days following extraction, leaving the alveolar walls divested of their protective covering. The denuded bone is accompanied by severe pain, which can be controlled only by local application of potent analgesics and oral or parenteral use of analgesics or narcotics.

To treat a septic alveolus properly the physiology of bone repair must be understood. If the loss of the primary blood clot is due to a sclerotic condition of the alveolar walls and the absence of nutrient vessels, then this must be viewed as any other denuded bone surface, and we must rely on nature's methods of bone repair for ultimate recovery and not employ any other methods, which would offend the healing process.

A septic alveolus is a denuded bone surface. Nature abhors denuded bone and responds to repair it. Behind this denuded and traumatized surface an immediate mechanism is set up to physiologically correct the defect. All denuded bone becomes dead bone and must be removed before it can be replaced by normal bone. During this period the contiguous region behind the alveolus is defended against invasion of pyogenic organisms within the septic alveolus, provided nothing is done to break through or violate this wall until the repair mechanism is ready to replace the nonvital structure. This process usually takes 2 to 3 weeks, depending upon the regenerative capacity of the individual. With the completion of this cycle the nonvital alveolar wall is sequestrated molecularly or en masse, and immediately behind it is a defensive and regenerative layer of juvenile connective tissue, which ultimately fills the void and undergoes osseous replacement. During this period treatment should be directed only to maintenance of wound hygiene and employment of antiseptic, analgesic dressings within the alveolus of sufficient potency to keep the patient comfortable. Nature must do the repairing. Curettage is contraindicated and will not only delay physiological healing and repair, but may also permit invasion of infection into and beyond the area of defense immediately behind the denuded alveolus.

Prevention, of course, is the best treatment. To this end atraumatic surgery, avoidance of contamination, and maintenance of a good level of general health are important. Antibiotics and sulfonamides placed in the socket after extraction are widely used in the belief that they help in preventing postoperative complications. Systemic antibiotics are used also and are certainly indicated in many cases, particularly when infection is present or severe trauma is unavoidable.

When a dry socket does develop, treatment should be palliative. The socket is gently irrigated with warm normal saline solution to remove all debris. After the socket has been carefully dried with cotton pledgets it is lightly dressed with ¼-inch plain gauze saturated with an obtundent paste such as equal parts of thymol iodide powder and benzocaine crystals dissolved in eugenol. The dressing may be changed as necessary until pain has subsided and granulation tissue has covered the walls of the socket.

EMERGENCIES IN THE DENTAL OFFICE

The number of emergencies that arise in a dental office is inversely proportional to the preventive measures taken by the dentist. Although dental emergencies are rare the dentist and his staff must be prepared to manage those that do arise. A well-organized plan of treatment should be worked out and rehearsed to cope with these situations. Emergency drills, just like fire drills, may save lives. The dental office should be equipped with oxygen that can be applied under positive pressure. An emergency tray containing all the necessary drugs should be readily available and checked from time to time to ensure completeness. Drugs should never be taken from an emergency tray for routine use. Emergency situations can be of a minor or a major nature, but in all instances if improper care is given the outcome can be disastrous.

Syncope (fainting) is probably the most common emergency and is usually associated with the administration of local anesthesia. The etiology is cerebral hypoxia resulting from disturbance of the normal mechanism of blood pressure control. Dilation of the splanchnic vessels causes a fall in blood pressure with a decrease in cerebral blood flow. The initiation of this reaction is of a psychic nature and should not be interpreted as a reaction to the drug administered. Symptoms include pallor, dizziness, light-headedness, clammy skin, nausea, and sometimes complete loss of consciousness. The treatment consists of placing the patient in a supine position with the head lower than the rest of the body. An airway is maintained, and oxygen should be administered. Mild respiratory stimulants such as spirits of ammonia can be used, but analeptics and other more potent agents are generally not used unless specifically indicated. Prevention of syncope can be accomplished by considering the psychic constitution of the patient. Measures should be taken to allay apprehension.

Reactions to local anesthetics, with the possible exception of lidocaine, are characterized by an initial excitatory phase followed by marked depression. The patient may become very talkative and anxious. Nausea and vomiting may occur. If the drug is given intravenously, the initial excitatory phase may be very brief, terminating in convulsions followed by marked depression. If any signs of reaction to the drug are noted during an injection, the needle should be withdrawn immediately.

Most reactions to local anesthesia are of a minor nature and can be treated palliatively. If convulsions occur and become increasingly intense, a short-acting barbiturate such as Nembutal or Pentothal should be given intravenously to control the convulsion. Oxygen should then be given to ensure adequate oxygenation. When the stimulatory phase is mild or of short duration, no sedative is given, but oxygen is administered and steps are taken to maintain adequate circulation.

In cases of severe central nervous system stimulation, depression, or cardiovascular collapse, the dentist should initiate treatment, but call for additional professional help. The calling of other professional personnel does not indicate inadequacy on the part of the dentist, but instead shows his good judgment.

To avoid reactions to local anesthesia an adequate history and evaluation should be completed before use of the drug. Always aspirate before injecting. Vasoconstrictors will help by decreasing the assimilation of the drug. Large quantities of any drug should not be used. Premedication with a barbiturate will guard against serious reactions in patients with a history of allergies to many drugs.

Allergic reactions to drugs can vary from delayed reactions that are more annoying than dangerous to anaphylactoid reactions that are severe and often lead to the death of the patient. Most drugs at one time or another have been associated with allergic reactions. Penicillin, sulfonamides, and other antibiotics are the most common drugs the dentist may use that are associated with allergic reactions.

The delayed or less severe reactions may be characterized by swelling at the site of injection, angioneurotic edema, pruritis, and urticaria. Treatment consists of antihistamines and palliative care.

Anaphylactoid reactions come on very quickly. The patient becomes very apprehensive, intensive itching occurs, and asthmatic breathing develops. Urticaria may develop rapidly, the blood pressure falls, and the pulse becomes weak or absent. The patient may lapse into an unconscious state with or without convulsions. Death may occur within a few minutes or several hours later.

Treatment of an anaphylactoid reaction consists of the immediate application of a tourniquet above the site of injection. Inject 0.5 ml. of 1:1,000 aqueous epinephrine subcutaneously or intramuscularly into the opposite arm. Aminophylline, 250 mg. in 10 ml., is given intravenously if epinephrine does not relax bronchial constriction. Artificial respiration with positive pressure oxygen is started as soon as possible. Epinephrine, 0.1 ml. of 1:1,000 aqueous solution, is given at the site of injection to delay absorption of the drug. Diphenhydramine, 50 mg., is given intramuscularly or intravenously for antihistaminic effect. Professional aid should be called as soon as possible to consult in the further treatment of the patient. If the symptoms continue, consider readministration of epinephrine or antihistamine. If the blood pressure is low, consider the use of a vasopressor drug such as phenylephrine, 1 to 5 mg. intramuscularly.

During exodontia teeth are sometimes inadvertently displaced into the oropharynx, larynx, trachea, and esophagus. Teeth in these positions can present serious problems, which could be avoided by simple precautions. A gauze screen should always be placed to block off the oropharynx from the mouth. This is true whether the exodontia is performed under general or under local anesthesia.

Teeth displaced into the oropharynx present no problem, provided they can be retrieved before they descend into the deeper structures. When a tooth is displaced in the oropharynx while the patient is under local anesthesia, the patient is instructed to hold perfectly still and not swallow or take a breath until the tooth can be retrieved. If this occurs under general anesthesia, everything stops until the tooth is retrieved. The assistant should be cautioned not to move the retractor or suction tip, as any movement may cause the loss of the tooth into the larynx or esophagus.

When a tooth is displaced in the posterior portion of the mouth, the natural reflex of the patient is to cough or swallow. In the majority of cases the patient will swallow, carrying the tooth into the esophagus. Regardless of the patient's reactions, radiographs should be taken to determine the exact location of the tooth. If the tooth is found to be in the gastrointestinal tract, a high bulk diet should be prescribed and the patient should contact the dentist if any gastrointestinal symptoms occur. Usually the tooth will be passed without incident.

In coughing, either the patient can cough up the tooth or it will be lodged in the larynx or aspirated into the tracheobronchial tree. In the case of teeth in the larynx a laryngeal spasm may occur, blocking the exchange of air. The tooth may be removed by means of a laryngoscope and a Magill forceps. If the tooth cannot be removed quickly, an airway must be established. This can be accomplished by placing a cricothyroid trocar through the triangularly shaped cricothyroid membrane and into the trachea. The cricothyroid membrane is located between the thyroid cartilage (Adam's apple), which is the largest of the tracheal cartilages, and the cricoid cartilage, which is the next inferior tracheal cartilage. Oxygen then should be given with positive pressure through the established airway until the tooth is removed and the laryngeal spasm is broken.

Teeth that are aspirated into the tracheobronchial tree present a serious problem. The removal of teeth in this position can be accomplished only by someone trained in methods of bronchoscopy. The patient will cough continuously and cyanosis may occur. Oxygen should be given until the patient can be transferred to an area where a radiograph of the chest and direct bronchoscopy can be accomplished. The aspiration of teeth and other debris during dental operations has been associated with a high incidence of lung abscesses.

Under all circumstances a radiograph of the chest and possibly of the abdomen must be taken to establish the exact location of any tooth that is displaced.

Chapter 9

SURGICAL BACTERIOLOGY

S. Elmer Bear

INFECTION

An ever-present problem in the field of oral surgery is infection. Under normal circumstances the oral cavity is never sterile, and if it were not for certain intrinsic and extrinsic factors, the care of a dental patient would be immeasurably more difficult.

The intrinsic factors include the normal regional immunity of the host to the bacterial flora of the mouth; the natural slough or desquamative function of the adjacent epithelium; the abundant blood supply present in the oral cavity; and the immediate response of the leukocytes when bacteria invade the host. In addition, saliva has been found to have an inhibitory effect on some bacteria, particularly those foreign to the normal flora. The normal flora also acts as a barrier to invading microorganisms.

The extrinsic factors that may aid in the control of oral infections are many, the most notable of which are the observance of good surgical and aseptic techniques and the use of antibiotics and chemotherapeutic agents, the former having been discussed in detail (Chapter 2). The philosophy behind the use of antibiotics and chemotherapeutic agents is very similar, and though the terms are not technically interchangeable because of their derivation, the former term shall be used henceforth for the sake of brevity and simplicity. Other factors aid in the control of infection, but a review of the source and physiological response, both local and systemic, should be evaluated before specific therapy is discussed.

In any discussion of surgical bacteriology applicable to the oral cavity and its adjacent structures, one must be aware of the existence of innumerable microorganisms, which are normal inhabitants of this region. The most common bacteria found in the mouth include the alpha and beta streptococci, nonhemolytic streptococci, *Staphylococcus aureus, Staphylococcus albus,* Vincent's spirochetes, and fusiform bacillus. Increasing numbers of antibiotic-resistant organisms have been noted in saliva, particularly those resistant to penicillin. The virulence and quantity of these bacteria are generally controlled in the oral cavity by the mild bactericidal effect of saliva and the deglutition of oral fluids into the stomach, where the pH level is sufficient to destroy the majority of the bacteria and digest the balance. These two factors are not always sufficient to abort an infectious process; therefore, those factors that contribute to an inflammatory reaction will be considered first.

Local factors

A mouth that is already chronically infected or contains large deposits of calculus and debris is a poor environment for a surgical procedure. Chronic irritation damages the tissues to the point where the normal resistance is markedly impaired, and the area is therefore more prone to infection. Invading bacteria will frequently destroy the protective reparative properties of the blood clot, preventing normal consolidation by the adjacent tissues. To operate in a mouth in which evidence of necrotic gingivitis is present is extremely hazardous. The gingival structures are necrotic, and a surgical procedure performed in this field places the general health of the patient in jeopardy not only because of localized infection and pain in the field of operation but also because the fascial spaces of the head and neck may be readily invaded, and a general septicemia may result if the bacteria are of sufficient virulence.

Systemic condition of the patient

Numerous factors of a systemic nature play a role in the predisposition to infection. Diabetes mellitus is one of the classical illustrations of a disease that, if uncontrolled, provides a poor environment in which to perform surgery. This is a disease of carbohydrate metabolism characterized by hyperglycemia and glycosuria and is directly related to insufficient insulin. One of the most characteristic features of diabetes is the fact that these individuals are more susceptible to infection and, once established, infection can proceed rapidly. Under these conditions insulin demand is increased enormously, leading to additional complications. The oral manifestations of the diabetic, such as dryness of the mouth, lingual edema, periodontal disease, etc., are well known, but may not be demonstrable on clinical examination if the disease is partially controlled. Surgical intervention, however, may precipitate an infectious process because of the lowered local and systemic resistance. Impaired healing may also occur, making the patient more prone to infection.

Patients who give any indication of diabetes, either by history or by clinical examination, should be evaluated carefully. If the patient is under a physician's care and is under control, surgery can be performed in the usual manner. If, on the other hand, some doubt exists about the diabetic status, treatment should be deferred until a physician has been consulted and a urinalysis and fasting blood sugar study completed.

It should be stressed that though surgery is sometimes more hazardous in the diabetic patient, the elimination of oral infections is most important. It should be done as soon as practical since the removal of an infectious process may aid in the control of the disease symptoms.

Blood dyscrasias

Several blood dyscrasias are predisposing factors of oral infection, the most notable of which are the leukemias. In acute leukemia and acute exacerbations of chronic leukemia, infections of the oral cavity are frequently seen, and they are difficult to treat. Surgical intervention in patients so afflicted is hazardous not only because of excessive hemorrhages so frequently seen in these patients, but also because of susceptibility to infection and poor healing qualities. The use of antibiotics is imperative if surgery must be done, and these drugs are often used to reduce the oral symptoms of the disease.

Agranulocytosis and the anemias cause a general lowering of the host's ability to resist infection, and serious consequences may result if the dyscrasia is marked. In the former disease spontaneous hemorrhages of the oral cavity are not unusual, and this condition may be accompanied by various ulcerations of the mucosa. The clinical picture of anemia in the oral cavity is exactly what one would expect to find in a situation in which either a decrease in the number of red cells or a decrease in the hemoglobin content of the cells is present. The lips and mucosa are pale in color and delicate in texture. The tongue is often smooth, glossy, and painful. This may be the first clue to the systemic problem and should never be ignored. The decreased number of leukocytes and the subnormal oxygen-bearing elements are the systemic manifestations and make the patient easily susceptible to infection.

Malnutrition

Malnutrition, or poor nutrition, is the physical state resulting from the failure to ingest, assimilate, or utilize any or all of the substances essential for the normal body metabolism. This disease entity is not necessarily confined to an inadequate caloric intake, but is found in those persons whose digestive tract fails to absorb or utilize the necessary elements for body metabolism.

The latter problem is, in fact, more common today than actual starving, primarily because of our increased geriatric population. Longevity, one of the accomplishments of modern science, has presented dentistry with many new problems—denture construction on atrophied ridges, treatment of markedly abraded dentition, treatment of chronic periodontal disease, etc. With increased longevity comes the problem of malnutrition caused by the inability of the digestive tract to function properly in the aged. When this happens, the patient is more prone to infection. In addition, malnutrition, regardless of etiology, slows and impairs healing, which is of major importance in the oral cavity. This is not meant to imply that surgical procedures should not be done on the elderly patient, but that attention should be given to specific supportive measures. Antibiotics and vitamin therapy should be routine if extensive surgery is to be done or if the patient gives a history of an unfavorable sequela during prior surgery.

Chronic alcoholism, unfortunately, is an increasing factor as a cause of malnutrition. This group of patients requires the same precautionary therapy as those who are subject to the normal deterioration of old age. Local factors, such as poor oral hygiene, and unsatisfactory postoperative care certainly contribute to the numerous oral infections that arise in this type of patient. Impaired metabolic function, from whatever cause, cannot be ignored and should be treated accordingly.

Miscellaneous systemic problems

Numerous other systemic diseases have some direct or indirect relationship to infections of the oral cavity and adjacent tissues either preoperatively or postoperatively. Any debilitating disease or affliction of the host can cause impairment of healing and decreased body resistance to infection.

Liver diseases. In the field of oral surgery one normally is concerned with cirrhosis of the liver, hepatitis, etc. because of the impaired clotting mechanism. A sufficient degree of liver damage can cause considerable impairment of the healing process due to the resultant anemia and poor metabolism. Any patient presenting with the obvious clinical manifestations of jaundice should be carefully evaluated before surgery is attempted.

Renal diseases. The kidneys are responsible, in part, for the elimination of the nitrogenous waste of the body, in maintaining the normal fluid and electrolyte balance, and in maintaining the proper level of plasma protein. Any disease or abnormality of these organs may well complicate the progress of a patient undergoing a surgical procedure and may in fact cause the demise of the patient if sufficient caution is not exercised. It is generally agreed that an abnormal immune response to the hemolytic streptococcus usually precedes glomerulonephritis. Though this disease entity usually gives a history of prior respiratory tract infection, the possible occurrence of hemolytic streptococcus in the oral cavity cannot be ignored by the dentist. A history of oral infections predisposing to nephritis, pyelitis, etc. is not uncommon, and one must be very careful about subjecting a patient with a history of kidney disease to reinfection. Patients with active renal disorders should definitely be protected with prophylactic antibiotics for two reasons. First, the renal function has been impaired by disease, and any blood-borne infection, however transient, may produce serious consequences. Second, local resistance and healing properties of the tissues operated upon have been reduced because of the increased uremia and other waste materials in the blood. Infection following surgery is not uncommon in patients so afflicted, and every supportive measure available must be instituted.

Cardiovascular diseases. All patients who have a history of cardiovascular disease should receive special attention at all times, but the treatment varies considerably, depending on the type of cardiac disease. In angina pectoris, coronary occlusion, hypertension, and congestive failure, the primary concern of the dentist is the control of pain and apprehension that may precipitate a relapse. A history of rheumatic fever, chorea, or congenital heart disease requires specific attention for an entirely different reason—infection. These cardiovascular problems are often aggravated by a transient bacteremia, however brief, and the literature is replete with cases showing the relationship of extractions and bacterial endocarditis. Alpha hemolytic streptococcus is the organism usually responsible for this cardiac complication. These organisms can be found almost routinely in a blood culture following an extraction or extensive periodontal therapy. Consequently, it is good medical and dental practice to protect patients with rheumatic or congenital heart disease by prophylactic measures.

The procedures that would fall within the scope of dental interest include root canal therapy, periodontal treatment regardless of its extensiveness, and, of course, all surgical procedures within the oral cavity. If uncertainty exists about the degree of gingival manipulation that may produce a transient bacteremia, then the antibiotics should be administered. Although the exact dosage and duration of therapy are somewhat empirical, it is generally agreed that high concentrations are desirable before any dental procedure is undertaken.

The American Heart Association recommends the use of penicillin as the drug of choice and suggests the following method of administration:

First choice: Intramuscular and oral penicillin combined
  For 2 days prior to surgery—200,000 to 250,000 units by mouth four times a day
  On day of surgery—200,000 to 250,000 units by mouth four times a day and 600,000 units aqueous penicillin with 600,000 units procaine penicillin shortly before surgery
  For 2 days thereafter—200,000 to 250,000 units by mouth four times a day

Second choice: If injection is not feasible—oral penicillin
  200,000 to 250,000 units four times a day, beginning 2 days prior to the surgical procedure and continuing through the day on which surgery or dental procedure is done and 2 days thereafter

The Association also suggests that patients be instructed to report to their physician should they develop fever within a month following the operation.

The importance of prophylactic antibiotics for patients who have rheumatic or congenital heart disease when undergoing a dental procedure is well established. Advances in the field of cardiovascular surgery have permitted the prosthetic replacement of damaged valves and surgical correction in congenital heart problems.

This has increased the obligations of the dental profession as more and more of these patients are being seen as patients both before and after surgery. Two major considerations have arisen as a result of these advances. Recent studies have shown the importance before heart surgery of complete examination and completion of all possible dental procedures to remove all sites of focal infection arising in the oral cavity. In addition, all patients who have had valvular surgery with or without the insertion of a valve prosthesis must have massive doses of antibiotics. Dosage levels normally administered for prophylaxis have been found totally inadequate. Prompt consultation with the cardiovascular surgeon or the patient's physician should be obtained before dental treatment is started, particularly when periodontal therapy or an oral surgery procedure is contemplated.

The physiology of infection

A frequent cause of acute inflammation is the invasion of microorganisms. This is usually the cause in the oral cavity and its adjacent structures. The response to infection of the host follows a relatively normal pattern. Accepting this premise, one can state that the physiological response to infection is inflammation. The nature of the inflammatory reaction is dependent in turn on the site, type, and virulence of the bacteria. In addition, the physical status of the host may determine the degree of inflammation, dependent upon the local and systemic factors that have already been discussed.

The response of the host to infection may be local and systemic. The local reaction is inflammation, which is defined by Moore as "the sum total of the changes in the tissues of the animal organism in response to an injurious agent, including the local reaction, and the repair of the injury. If the inflammatory reaction is adequate, it minimizes the effect of the injurious agent, destroys the injurious agent, and restores the part to as near normal structure and function as possible. If it is not adequate, there is extensive destruction of tissue, invasion of the body, and somatic death."* More briefly stated, one might say that inflammation is the reaction of the body to irritants, the most common of which are bacterial. The classical signs of inflammation are redness, swelling, heat, and pain. The degree and frequency of these signs vary considerably, depending upon the virulence of the bacteria and their location. For example, in the oral cavity one might find a mild gingivitis, which is a minimal inflammatory reaction, and at the same time find a fulminating cellulitis of the neck caused by the same microorganisms. The different response is dependent in part upon the location of the bacteria involved and may vary considerably if its environment is aerobic or anaerobic. In addition, the various body tissues respond differently to the same invading organism.

The signs and symptoms of inflammation can be explained when the tissue response to an irritant is understood. Initially a marked dilation of the vascular bed occurs, which is accompanied by a deceleration of the blood flow due to the greater volume of the vascular bed. The increased capillary volume is responsible for the cardinal signs of redness, swelling, and heat. As the rate of blood flow decreases, leukocytes begin to penetrate through the vessel walls into the surrounding tissues. This phenomenon is accompanied by an exuding of blood plasma through the walls, producing an inflammatory edema. The escape of the blood plasma may be due to the toxic reaction of the capillary walls to infection or to an increased osmotic pressure of the surrounding tissues. This tissue distention produces pressure against the neurogenic fibers and may actually cause the destruction of these fibers. This pressure phenomenon, along with the release of histamines from injured cells, plays a major role in the appearance of the fourth classical sign of inflammation—pain.

Varied types of inflammation are seen, depending upon the tissue involved, the type of bacteria, and the resistance of the

---

*From Moore, R. A.: A textbook of pathology, Philadelphia, 1948, W. B. Saunders Co.

host. The most important are pyogenic, serous, catarrhal, fibrinous, hemorrhagic, and necrotizing inflammation.

The type of inflammation encountered most frequently in the field of oral surgery is pyogenic, meaning "pus forming." Most infections in this region, if allowed to progress without treatment, will eventually produce pus. The invasive bacteria and/or their toxins may produce several different clinical entities, which will be covered in detail in a later chapter. They include lymphadenitis, cellulitis, abscess formation, phlegmon, and osteomyelitis. All may be either acute or chronic, and combinations of two or more of these clinical manifestations may be present. The pattern of infection is dependent upon the numerous factors discussed earlier, the length of time the infection has been present, and the mode of treatment.

Systemic effects of oral infection

In all infectious diseases except the most trivial, systemic manifestations of bacterial invasion are found. The reaction may be due to the actual destructive ability of the bacteria, as in an abscess, or to its toxins, as in diphtheria. When bacteria are present in the blood, the condition is known as "bacteremia." Most authors use the term "septicemia" when the bacteria and their toxins are found in large numbers, suggesting actual growth while in the bloodstream. Transient bacteremias are usually seen following the removal of teeth or periodontal therapy. This is generally of little consequence except when a cardiac valve deformity exists or the resistance of the host is impaired or the organism is highly virulent.

Fever is perhaps the most outstanding symptom of a systemic infection and probably results from the action of the bacterial toxins on the heat and regulating mechanism of the brain. As one might suspect, fever may vary considerably from one individual to another, though they may be afflicted with the same infectious process. The exact nature of temperature control is not clearly understood, but with sufficient fever an accompanying reduction in blood volume is caused by a shift of blood fluids to the tissues and extravascular spaces. This phenomenon, together with the loss of fluid caused by excessive perspiration, leads to decreased urinary output (oliguria) and retention of chlorides. An increase in the nonprotein nitrogen, both in the blood and urine, results from an increased metabolism, which is also a consequence of fever. If the kidneys are functioning properly, this is not a serious problem, but if marked dehydration goes uncorrected, the patient may be in real difficulty because of the abnormal electrolyte balance and retention of nitrogenous waste products.

The elevated metabolism resulting from a fever also causes an increased pulse rate, cardiac output, and respiratory rate. These clinical symptoms of a fever are invaluable in determining the progress of the disease and the effectiveness of the therapy used. Any marked deviation of these manifestations from normal would require an alteration of the therapy and increased supportive care.

Focus of infection

The principle of focal infection has been a controversial issue for many years. The pendulum of opinion has swung in both directions many times since the turn of the century. The modern concept of focal infection was given strong support by Billings and Rosenow so that in the 1920's considerable importance was placed upon this concept. Since that time many studies have been conducted to ascertain the validity of the earlier conclusions. Some have substantiated the principle of focal infection and some have not. Today the pendulum has gradually swung back to a more conservative concept. It is generally agreed that the principle of focal infection is valid and that a focus of infection should be eliminated when possible. However, the general concensus is that a minor focus is as a rule not capable of producing exacerbations of unrelated disease except in specific and occasional instances.

In the last half century thousands upon thousands of teeth have been condemned on the block of focal infection. Today with the aid of roentgenograms, vitalometer tests, and better clinical judgment the dentist is able to defend his position in attempting to salvage a patient's dentition. A focus of infection may act as a depot from which bacteria or their products may be disseminated to other parts of the body, or it may act as a site in which blood-borne bacteria may localize, setting up an acute inflammatory reaction.

The concept of elective localization of microorganisms is not fully understood, but it explains in part why certain bacteria have an affinity for one or more specific tissues of the body. Undoubtedly some close chemical interplay takes place between bacteria and the tissues. This would explain why most apical lesions do little damage elsewhere unless the body resistance is depressed or a specific area elsewhere has been damaged. An excellent illustration of this phenomenon is the effect of the alpha hemolytic streptococcus on a previously damaged mitral valve.

The practitioner must keep these possibilities in mind in making a decision concerning the preservation of a tooth or its supporting tissues. If a tooth is infected, the infection must be removed. Little controversy exists about this basic tenet of good dental practice. This does not necessarily mean the extraction of the tooth. One can and should do root canal therapy if indicated in relation to the remaining dentition and, in addition, a root resection should be performed if the apical lesion cannot definitely be eliminated by more conservative means. A root resection ensures a complete seal of the accessory canals and also eliminates the area of infected cementum. If the question of focal infection arises, it seems reasonable to accept the principle of root resection as being more reliable regarding the elimination of a focus of infection.

Periodontal disease of varying degrees has been accepted as a frequent site of focal infection. This disease, except for caries, is perhaps the most common chronic infectious process in man. Clinical evaluation regarding the presence of pus and inflamed gingiva is perhaps more reliable in determining if the disease is infectious than are roentgenograms. The latter may show bone loss, which may be persistent over a period of years though the surrounding tissues show no clinical evidence of infection. When the dentition is firm even in the presence of moderate bone loss and clinical evidence of infection is absent, conservatism is justified in considering the teeth as a possible focus of infection.

As mentioned above, specific diseases have been shown to have a direct relationship to oral foci of infection. Acute infections of the eyes, heart, kidneys, and joints have on occasion shown a direct correlation to oral infection. Some forms of optic neuritis and iritis have been traced directly to a chronic periapical or periodontal lesion. In the past it was not unusual to remove a chronically infected tooth and find a sudden exacerbation of a chronic iritis. The bacterium causing the initial eye condition, being suddenly released into the bloodstream in relatively large quantities, may produce an acute condition. Today this clinical observation is not as frequently seen since most patients with iritis are given some supportive therapy with antibiotics prior to extractions.

The arthritic patients as a group have in the past probably lost more teeth under the guise of focal infection than all other groups combined. Arthritis is a painful and debilitating disease, and everyone associated with the case makes every effort to leave no stone unturned in the hope of finding the etiological factor. Arthritis occurs in a number of different forms, dependent upon various etiological factors. In infectious arthritis, such as gonococcal and pneumococcal, and in degenerative arthritis the etiological factors are readily established. Thus no effort is made to establish an oral focus. In rheumatoid arthritis, however, the exact etiology is unknown, though it is thought to be infectious. For this reason the dentist invariably sees the patient to eliminate any possible focus of infection. This is not an unreasonable request since the patient is in desperate need of assistance. Any active infectious process of the oral cavity should be eliminated. Teeth that have root canals and no apical involvement, areas of condensing osteitis, etc. should not be removed unless the dentist is convinced that infection is present or unless the physician insists and has examined the patient for all other possible foci of infection. In this way it is possible to aid the patient and yet protect him in the retention of his dentition.

Recent studies have been reported that attempt to explain one of the disturbing aspects of focal infection. Some infectious processes in specific areas of the body are definitely felt to be secondary to a primary focus of infection, yet do not respond favorably when the primary focus is removed. These studies have shown that the secondary focus has been present long enough and the damage is of sufficient magnitude to be irreversible. The secondary site then is no longer dependent upon the primary focus. This would explain the absence of dramatic results in many cases where teeth are removed as a focus of infection. An illustration of this problem as it relates to dentistry is the presence of some long-standing apical infection. This infectious process might well be the primary focus for pyelitis, bacterial nephritis, etc. and yet, though the apical infection be eliminated, the secondary focus will not respond since the process is no longer reversible.

ANTIBIOTICS
Historical background

The antagonism of microorganisms to each other and the ability of various bacteria and fungi to produce antibacterial substances have been known since the late nineteenth century. Prior to 1938 this phenomenon was a scientific curiosity utilized only to separate various bacterial species from one another. Since that time, however, this well-known fact has all but revolutionized modern medicine. Fleming in 1928 reported the value of penicillin in the isolation of *Haemophilus influenzae*. It was not until 1940 that a group from Oxford was able to develop penicillin as a therapeutic agent. The investigation of Waksman and his associates and Dubos and his group at about the same time led to the development of numerous other antibiotic agents suitable for clinical use. Some time earlier, in 1935, Domagk observed the therapeutic value of Prontosil in the treatment of mice with streptococcal septicemia. This was only the beginning of a new era in the treatment of infection. Countless lives have been saved by sulfanilamide and related sulfonamide drugs. Though since 1944 the antibiotics have supplanted the sulfonamide drugs, the sulfonamides should not be ignored as excellent agents for the treatment of oral infections.

General considerations

The ideal antibiotic has not yet been found. If one is ever discovered, it would have to have numerous important attributes. (1) It should be antimicrobial and therapeutically effective in vivo in concentrations that would not injure the host. (2) It should be able to attack the pathogenic organisms regardless of their location within the host. (3) It should have consistant therapeutic value. (4) It should not impair normal antibody or phagocytic activity. (5) It should not readily induce the development of resistant strains of microorganisms. (6) Its effectiveness should not be impaired in the presence of other therapeutic agents that might be administered concurrently. (7) It should be stable and easy to administer. (8) It should be inexpensive.

Before an antibiotic can be administered safely and effectively, certain factors require careful consideration.

Nature of the lesion

The nature of the lesion caused by microorganisms commonly found in the field of oral surgery may fall into one of three categories. (1) The one encountered most often in general practice is wound contamination, as in a "dry socket." Though the clinical picture is not necessarily caused by infection, it is not uncommon when teeth have been removed in the presence of oral filth and chronic infection. The blood clot is delicate, and if bacterial enzymatic action occurs before vascularization from the side walls of the wound, the clot will be destroyed. The use of unsterile instruments and materials is likely to cause wound contamination since the bacteria are foreign to the oral flora and thus normal local tissue resistance is absent. (2) Abscess formation is the second most common bacterial lesion related to the oral cavity. These lesions may be chronic or acute, depending upon the virulence of the bacteria, resistance of the host, and location of the infectious process. Apical abscesses are generally chronic, as the microorganisms in this location are not particularly virulent and the normal body responses are able to build up a protective reaction as seen in a granuloma. Only when the body resistance is lowered or the environment altered to favor bacterial growth do these lesions become acute. (3) The third type of bacterial lesion is the invasive type of infection, which spreads through the soft tissues and usually results from an acute episode of an apical abscess. Until evidence of purulent material appears this clinical entity is known as a cellulitis. An inflammatory reaction occurs in response to the invading microorganism and/or its toxins. In the field of oral surgery it almost invariably involves the connective tissues and muscles adjacent to the mandible and/or maxilla since the lesion generally results from a breakdown of the periosteum. Unless prompt measures are taken to control the infection, abscess formation with necrosis of tissue, lymphadenitis, and bacteremia will occur.

The effectiveness of antibiotic therapy has a direct bearing on the nature of the lesion. If a wound is contaminated and is on a surface where the antibiotic can be applied topically and maintained in sufficient quantity without producing sensitivity to the drug, then topical administration may be the method of choice. However, in the majority of instances an infected oral wound cannot be treated topically, since the concentration of the drug is difficult to maintain because of saliva dilution. More important, however, is the fact that the oral mucosa is highly prone to producing a drug sensitivity in the host. For this reason alone the use of topical antibiotics is to be avoided and is contraindicated except in a few instances in which the more insoluble antibiotics may be beneficial. Before any type of antibiotic therapy is effective in wound contamination, it is usually necessary to debride the area of necrotic material. This will ensure a healthy wound periphery for healing and an adequate blood supply.

Extracellular microorganisms are most often responsible for acute infections, and unless an accumulation of pus has developed they can generally be destroyed by the phagocytic cells and the antibiotics. The absence of normal tissue structures in an abscess deprives the leukocytes of the surface upon which they operate effectively, and when deprived of oxygen, as in the case of an abscess, the leukocytes become nonmobile and lose their phagocytic properties. An antibiotic to be effective must come into direct contact with the infective agent. This is not possible in many abscesses since the only contact can come through the intact capillaries at the periphery of the lesion. The larger the abscess the less effective is the antibiotic. This fact alone illustrates the necessity for continued surgical intervention when fluctuant material is within a tissue space. A fact that has become quite apparent in recent years is the realization that the antibiotics are only adjunctive aids in the presence of pus and that the purulent material must be evacuated surgically.

A cellulitis, on the other hand, that has not undergone sufficient degenerative changes to produce pus may be amenable to antibiotic therapy alone. The rich blood supply, characteristic of early inflammation, provides optimal transport of the antibiotic to the involved tissues. In addition, the drug tends to accumulate in the infected area because of the increased vascular bed and permeability of the vessel walls. Antibiotic therapy, therefore, must be instituted promptly if surgery is to be avoided. Before therapy is discontinued it is advisable to remove the causative factor to eliminate the possibility of a relapse.

Sensitivity of microorganisms

An ever-increasing problem in the treatment of an infectious process is the response of the causative organisms to the antibiotics. When the antibiotics were first introduced and as each new one was placed on the market, the manufacturer could generally predict, on the basis of laboratory data, which of the species and strains of bacteria would be sensitive. This is no longer the case. True, the antibiotics are said to be effective against certain bacterial groups, but specific effectiveness is no longer the general rule. On the contrary, individual strains and species are showing wide variations in susceptibility to the same antibiotic. Making the treatment even more complex is the fact that initial susceptibility to an antibiotic by a specific strain of bacteria may change during treatment.

It is difficult to explain why microorganisms change in their response to an antibiotic. Most investigators feel that bacteria actually undergo sufficient change to be considered mutations. Some, however, feel that an organism initially sensitive to one or more antibiotics gradually builds up a resistance and is no longer affected by the bacteriostatic or bactericidal property of the drug. Though the exact rationale is still controversial, the problem is a serious one and promises to become even more difficult. For example, in numerous hospitals throughout the United States strains of staphylococcus are found that are resistant to all available antibiotics. Research installations are working overtime to produce new drugs that they hope will be effective.

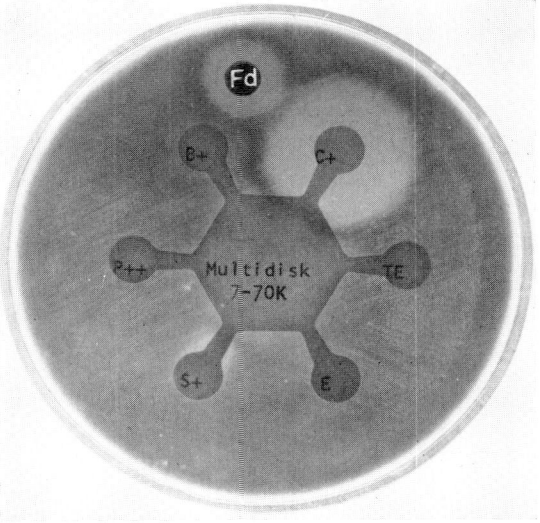

Fig. 9-1. Disk method for determining sensitivity of microorganisms to multiple antibiotics. The organism tested was inhibited by chloramphenicol and Furadantin, as shown by the lack of bacterial growth. The size of the clear area should not be taken as an indication of the relative degree of sensitivity. The center section is commercially prepared and contains a predetermined amount of drug on each segment. Key: C, chloramphenicol; TE, tetracycline; E, erythromycin; S, streptomycin; P, penicillin; B, bacitracin; Fd, Furadantin.

Because of the numerous deaths caused by this strain, it has been necessary in some hospitals to close their operating suites for long periods of time.

One of the most effective means of determining the antibiotic sensitivity of the causative microorganism is to test it in the laboratory. It is first necessary to secure some of the purulent material. This is usually accomplished early in the treatment of oral surgery cases since incision and drainage of the abscess, as stated earlier, is generally indicated promptly. An agar plate is inoculated with the freshly obtained material, and medicated disks, each containing a measured amount of antibiotics, are spaced over the plate. If the microorganism is sensitive to the antibiotic, it will fail to grow around the medicated disk (Fig. 9-1). Resistant organisms will grow to the disk, and gradations of sensitivity or resistance may be present that can be evaluated by an experienced observer. If, however, the degree of susceptibility is important or if a mixed infection (more than one organism) is anticipated, other laboratory aids such as the tube dilution method are available.

It should be pointed out that though the laboratory procedures are important and should be used whenever possible, antibiotic therapy should not be delayed until the results of the test are available. On the contrary, these drugs should be used and the antibiotic therapy altered if the laboratory studies warrant the change (Fig. 9-2).

Dosage and route of administration

When contemplating the use of an antibiotic, the dosage and route of administration are important considerations. The purpose of the therapy is to produce as promptly as possible an optimum concentration of the drug at the site of infection and to maintain it at an effective level. The causative bacteria must, of course, be sensitive to the antibiotic used. Each antibiotic has its own characteristics regarding rate of absorption and excretion, which in turn are dependent upon the mode of administration. For example, penicillin has a slower rate of absorption when administered orally as compared to parenteral injection, though some of the newer oral preparations have increased the rate of absorption considerably. The rate of absorption will also vary with the vehicle, whether oil or aqueous. In addition, penicillin combined chemically with a procaine radical has a

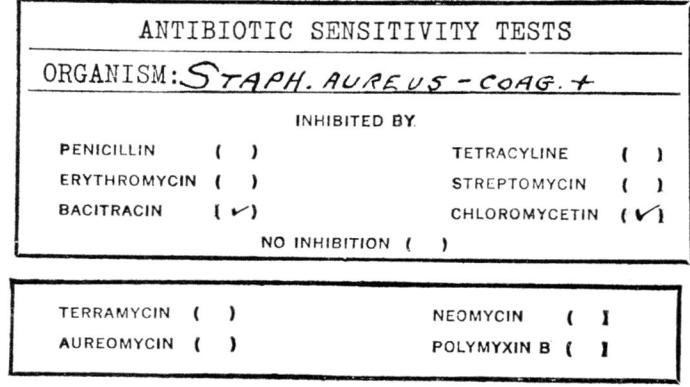

Fig. 9-2. Typical laboratory report sent by the bacteriologist following sensitivity test. This organism is a resistant strain of *Staphylococcus aureus* found in hospitals. A coagulase-positive test is presumptive laboratory evidence for pathogenicity of the genus *Straphytococcus*.

much slower rate of absorption than potassium penicillin alone.

Dosage is also determined by the rate of inactivation and excretion of the drug used. When administered orally, several antibiotics are destroyed readily by the lower digestive tract, whereas some are absorbed very slowly and may be excreted before therapeutic value can be obtained. At one time it was felt that the maximum tolerated dose was the only limitation on the amount given a patient. This has been found to be an erroneous conception and can cause untoward side effects in the host. The premise that if a little does some good then a lot will do better does not apply in the use of antibiotics.

Antibiotics may be administered intramuscularly, intravenously, orally, or topically. With the exception of the latter method, the antibiotics reach the area of infection via the bloodstream. When placed intramuscularly, the site acts as a depot from which the drug is taken slowly into the bloodstream.

Intravenous administration produces a rapid high level of concentration in the bloodstream, but the excretion rate is even more rapid. This method of administration is generally used when an acute fulminating disease must be treated with the utmost haste. To maintain an adequate level the intravenous method is often combined with one or more other routes of administration.

Originally the oral administration of some antibiotics was necessary since this was the only route available other than the intravenous. This is no longer true, but this mode of administration has become popular with the doctor and the patient. It is painless and convenient and particularly valuable when children are concerned. Palatable oral suspensions are most advantageous in treating children. Several disadvantages occur with the oral route of administration, the most serious being the reliability of the patient. Therapy depends on the cooperation of the patient, who is likely to be lax and forgetful about maintaining the dosage at regular intervals for as long as it is necessary. Some clinicians have taken the attitude that if a patient is ill enough to warrant an antibiotic, they would rather administer the drug themselves, thereby having the assurance that the patient receives the drug and also the added opportunity of evaluating the patient's progress more often.

One of the most controversial subjects with respect to antibiotics is the topical use of these drugs. Perhaps the greatest hesitancy has arisen because of the serious complications that have come about by the use of the sulfonamide preparations in topical form. It has been well established that the topical use of the sulfonamides often induces allergic reactions in the host. This has caused severe complications, even death, and is definitely contraindicated except in specific and rare instances under strictly controlled conditions.

Antibiotics have caused similar allergic responses in the host and also tend to produce resistant strains of bacteria. In addition, in the oral cavity the topical use of some of the antibiotics leads to partial destruction of the normal oral flora, permitting the rapid overgrowth of some of the fungi. This is particularly true of the prolonged use of lozenges. The normal antagonisms as well as the normal symbiotic associations are eliminated, and a flora that is naturally resistant to the drug becomes predominant. Thrush, cheilitis, and the production of resistant strains that can cause superinfections may be the result of the indiscriminate use of topical antibiotics.

Several antibiotics cannot be given systemically without hazard to the host because of toxic reactions to the drug. On occasion it is most beneficial to use this group topically, particularly when the offending organism is resistant to the drugs normally employed. Fortunately these topical agents (bacitracin, tyrothricin, neomycin, polymyxin) are rather insoluble, which is a distinct advantage when used topically, and relatively nontoxic. They seldom produce allergic manifestations and only occasionally produce resistant strains.

The therapeutic value of these drugs in the field of dentistry is still to be questioned except in isolated instances. Maintaining sufficient concentration for therapeutic efficacy in the oral cavity is well nigh impossible due to the constant dilution by saliva. They can be used effectively in ointment form on the lips and soft tissues outside of the oral cavity, primarily as a prophylactic agent. In the presence of a chronic osteomyelitis the topical antibiotics have been found most beneficial, particularly when one can be placed in a cavity of bone and maintained there in adequate concentration. Antibiotics administered parenterally do not diffuse into infected bone in therapeutic concentrations due to a variety of factors, including impaired circulation and fibrous barriers. When this is the case, the practitioner must resort to any method left open to him. Parenteral therapy is indicated to prevent the spread of the infection, and topical administration is indicated in an effort to control and abort the infective process within bone.

Indiscriminate use of antibiotics

Undoubtedly the discovery of the antibiotics as therapeutic agents must be considered among the greatest advancements of medical science, but with their discovery came the unnecessary, indiscriminate, and dangerous use of these drugs. Antibiotics have their therapeutic limitations and on occasion can produce toxic results far more serious than the initial disease for which a drug may have been given. On the basis of present-day knowledge the practitioner must make a new appraisal of the situation and use these drugs in a more reasonable manner.

The two most hazardous sequelae of antibiotic therapy are the toxic reactions exhibited by the host and the increasing problem of drug resistance by numerous microorganisms. Bacterial resistance can occur in two basic forms—the naturally insensitive strains, which are present to some degree in all bacterial populations, and, by far the most dangerous, resistant strains developed as a result of inadequate and indiscriminate use of antibiotics. Resistance to the drugs has been shown to develop when the bacteria are exposed to suboptimal concentrations. The practicing dentist must be made acutely aware of this problem since in some locales the habit of administering antibiotics in insufficient dosage has become common practice. Following the removal of an impacted tooth, for example, the operator gives the patient a "shot" of penicillin as a prophylactic measure and then does not see the patient for subsequent antibiotic therapy. This procedure is to be condemned since it has little therapeutic value and can produce resistant strains of organisms that may cause the patient considerable damage.

Drug resistance is not dependent on inadequate dosage alone. Antibiotics administered therapeutically for protracted periods of time and producing excellent results for a specific organism may still cause alterations of other bacteria, which can produce difficulty at a later date either for the host or by cross infection. As mentioned earlier, the problem of cross infection has become a serious one in hospitals throughout the country due to the production of resistant strains of staphylococcus. Rigid aseptic techniques must be adhered to in the dental office for this reason alone if for no other. Most of our population has received antibiotic therapy at one time or another and may be the carrier of a resistant strain of bacteria. It is imperative that those associated with the healing arts, as well as the lay public, be appraised of the ever-increasing problem of drug resistance since the incidence is related in large measure to the indiscriminate use of antibiotics.

A toxic reaction of the host to antibiotic therapy is another complicating factor in the use of these drugs. It is more prevalent when the drugs are used indiscriminately and may be produced in two ways. First, a sensitivity or allergic response of the host to the drug may be produced and, second, the alteration of certain normal physiological activities of the host may be disturbed either by prolonged or massive dosage. The incidence of allergic responses to the antibiotics is increasing primarly because of the repeated indiscriminate use of the drugs for trivial problems. As has already been pointed out, one of the best means of sensitizing a patient is by the use of topical preparations, particularly on the skin and oral mucosa. Erythemas, hives, exfoliative dermatitis, etc. are not uncommon and are being seen more frequently as the population becomes increasingly sensitive to the drugs. Having been forewarned by one of the relatively minor reactions or by the patient's history, the practitioner should avoid the use of the offending drug, or the results may be disastrous. Anaphylactoid reactions generally occur after the patient has had a minor reaction on a previous occasion. This reaction is characterized by the rapid onset of cyanosis, coughing, tonic spasm, a weak and thready pulse, and a marked drop in blood pressure. The incidence of serious and fatal results is increasing, and though more common, by far, following the use of penicillin, the problem cannot be ignored whenever any of the antibiotics are used.

Several of the antibiotics other than penicillin are capable of producing episodes of headaches, nausea, vomiting, and diarrhea. Most often these reactions are mild and can be controlled with adjunctive therapy, but occasionally the symptoms become acute and difficult to treat. Vertigo, nerve damage, renal disorders, blood dyscrasias, and resistant secondary infections are but a few of the additional complications that may evolve from the use of antibiotics. The specific toxic reactions and contraindications of each drug will be discussed independently.

Masking of the true clinical entity is another complication of the indiscriminate use of antibiotics. When a patient presents with symptoms that suggest infection, treatment must not consist of antibiotic therapy alone. It is equally important to establish the diagnosis before treatment is instituted. For example, if a patient gives symptoms of infection in the maxillary arch, an acute sinusitis and even a malignancy of the maxillary sinus might be masked if antibiotics are given on the premise that an acute apical abscess is the causative factor. Once the drug has been administered it is conceivable that the acute symptoms may subside and lie dormant only to arise again at some later date with more serious consequences. Antibiotics administered in the presence of pus may also complicate the problem. Surgery is still the best means of treating a fluctuant infected area, and it should be borne in mind that antibiotic therapy is only adjunctive therapy. Failure to evacuate pus might well produce what is known as a "sterile abscess," and though dormant for awhile it will be activated again with increased virulence.

Specific antibiotics

New antibiotics and modifications of old ones are being released frequently by various pharmaceutical houses. This is a natural by-product of active and competitive research and is to be encouraged. It is necessary if the increasing number of resistant strains and incidence of superinfections are to be combated. The antibiotics of today may be useless or outmoded tomorrow, though the ones that are to be discussed have stood the test of time reasonably well. An effort has been made to discuss the antibiotics on a generic basis rather than by proprietary names.

Penicillin

Penicillin, though the oldest, is still the most widely used antibiotic. Unlike most of the other antibiotics, it is both bactericidal and bacteriostatic. The exact mechanism of the bactericidal property is not well understood, but evidence indicates that it actually interferes with the metabolic processes of the sensitive bacteria. Penicillin is effective against the gram-positive streptococci and staphylococci, which are of particular interest to the oral surgeon. It is also effective against several gram-negative cocci, notably meningococci and gonococci, but most gram-negative rods are naturally resistant. In addition, most spirochetes are quite sensitive, making penicillin the drug of choice in syphilis. With the exception of the presence of resistant organisms, some gram-negative organisms, and the incidence of allergic responses, penicillin is still the desirable drug for the treatment of oral infections.

Preparation and dosage. Penicillin is available in numerous preparations for intramuscular, oral, and topical use and is combined with various chemical radicals and carrying agents to produce short or long effective doses.

Intramuscular. Because of the recent increase in allergic reactions to penicillin some clinicians have discontinued the use of intramuscular penicillin except when the patient is hospitalized. Treatment of allergic manifestations following intramuscular injection is more difficult than treatment of those reactions resulting from the oral route.

1. Procaine penicillin G is the preparation most frequently used today as a prophylactic and therapeutic drug. One milliliter contains 300,000 units, and the recommended dose is 600,000 units a day for moderately severe infections, with a reduction in dosage toward the end of treatment. When the patient requires hospitalization, it is practical and desirable to administer the drug every 12 hours.

2. Crystalline potassium penicillin G in aqueous suspension was one of the original preparations, but because of its rapid absorption it is used in combination with procaine penicillin G, except in intravenous therapy. The combining of these two penicillin preparations (referred to as fortified) permits a rapid high blood level (30 to 60 minutes) with a maintenance level. The usual dosage is 1 ml. (300,000 units of procaine penicillin and 100,000 units of crystalline potassium penicillin) given every 12 or 24 hours, depending on the severity of the infection.

3. Benzathine penicillin G is the newest long-acting preparation and has found favor with those who feel the need for a prolonged blood level in their patient. The average dose is 300,000 to 600,000 units every 10 days. Like procaine penicillin it can be combined with aqueous penicillin, thus giving a high level for 24 hours and a sustaining low blood level. Its most frequent use in oral surgery is as a prophylaxis against secondary infection or in a systemic condition such as rheumatic fever. It is not generally used in the treatment of acute infections and should not be used if the patient is sensitive to iodides.

4. More recently the semisynthetic derivatives methicillin, oxacillin, and nafcillin have become available. As noted previously, the indiscriminate use of antibiotics can produce resistant strains, and many infections today are caused by resistant penicillinase-producing staphylococci. These new semisynthetic penicillins may be used for this type of infection, in which resistant strains such as those of hospital-acquired infections are suspected. However, sensitivity of the bacterium should be determined by in vitro tests when possible.

Use of penicillinase-resistant drugs should be restricted to treatment of resistant staphylococcus infections since their extensive or indiscriminate use may produce more resistant strains of bacteria.

The intramuscular dosage and frequency of administration for the new semisynthetic penicillins vary from 250 mg. to 1.5 Gm. every 4 to 6 hours, depending on the drug used, size and age of the patient, and severity of infection. Before the dosage is established all pertinent factors should be evaluated and a review of the prescribed dosage studied.

Oral. The more recent preparations of oral penicillin have an excellent absorption ratio in the bloodstream. When one is assured of a cooperative patient, they are quite effective even for serious infections. It should be emphasized that the oral penicillins should be taken when the stomach is empty to minimize gastric retention, and preferably with an antacid.

1. Penicillin G as an oral preparation has been available for some time, but some hesitancy has prevailed about its use because the degree and rate of absorption are variable. In addition, one must depend on the patient to take the drug exactly as prescribed since a high blood level is not sustained for any length of time. When used, the average dose is 250 mg. (250,000 units) given four times a day. This is believed to be equal in effectiveness to one injection of 300,000 units intramuscularly.

2. Penicillin V is a more recent development and is being used rather extensively for the oral administration of penicillin. This drug has been found to be quite reliable in its rate of absorption and effective blood level. It is also compatible with penicillin G, which may have been given during the acute phase of an infectious process. It is generally administered three or four times a day and is available either in tablets or capsules containing from 125 to 300 mg. (200,000 to 500,000 units). Oral suspensions containing 125 mg. per teaspoonful are available for children.

3. As noted above, a number of new semisynthetic penicillins are available. Those that are prepared for administration by the oral route are ampicillin, cloxacillin, nafcillin, and oxacillin. Here, too, the exact dosage depends on the age and size of the patient and severity of the infection. The dosage for these drugs will vary from 250 mg. to 1 Gm. every 4 to 6 hours. A careful evaluation of the problem is imperative.

Topical. Penicillin has been prepared in various topical forms, including troches, aerosols, dusts, ointments, pellets, and toothpaste. Because of the uncertain degree of concentration and particularly because of the high percentage of sensitization that can result from this type of therapy, penicillin in topical form is contraindicated.

Precautions. As noted above, the route of administration must be carefully considered before penicillin is prescribed. In addition, all the precautions noted below must be prudently observed.

1. Penicillin should not be administered if the patient has a history of reaction, however mild, following previous use of the drug.

2. The administration of penicillin to patients with an allergic history, such as

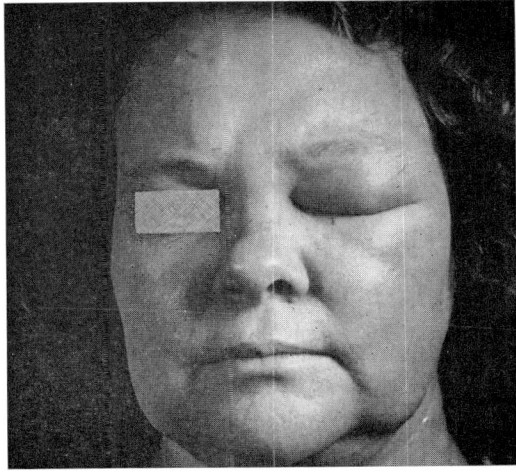

Fig. 9-3. Allergic response following the administration of penicillin.

hay fever, etc., should be viewed with caution since these individuals are more prone to sensitization.

3. Penicillin therapy should be discontinued at the first sign of allergic symptoms to the drug, including minor reactions such as itching and redness at the site of injection (Fig. 9-3).

4. When administered intramuscularly, extreme care should be taken to avoid an accidental intravenous injection.

5. If used intramuscularly, it is preferable to administer penicillin in the deltoid or triceps of the arm so that a tourniquet may be applied if the patient gives any indication of an anaphylactoid reaction.

6. Penicillin in any of its topical preparations is generally to be avoided.

Erythromycin

Erythromycin has a bacterial spectrum similar to that of penicillin and because of its unequaled safety record is used by many clinicians in preference to penicillin, particularly for oral infections. It is active against the gram-positive cocci and a few of the gram-negative rods. It has also been reported to be effective against some of the viruses, rickettsiae, and certain strains of the diphtheria bacilli. Like penicillin, it may be either bactericidal or bacteriostatic, depending upon the concentration of the drug and the organisms involved. Strains of *Staphylococcus aureus* that are insensitive to penicillin may be susceptible to erythromycin. This drug has its chief usefulness in the management of infections produced by staphylococci or other penicillin-resistant gram-positive organisms.

Erythromycin is indicated for treatment of a large variety of infections caused by a wide spectrum of susceptible microorganisms. Indications include cases in which use of other antibiotics is limited by undesirable or serious side effects. In cases in which organisms have become resistant to other antibiotics, particularly penicillin, erythromycin is often the drug of choice.

Side effects from the administration of erythromycin are rare. The oral administration may occasionally cause mild gastrointestinal disturbances, but the withdrawal of the drug is rarely necessary since the symptoms disappear promptly.

Serious complications are extremely rare, but several proprietary preparations should be used cautiously when liver function is impaired.

Preparation and dosage. The usual mode of administration of erythromycin is orally, but it is available for intramuscular or intravenous use if the infection is of sufficient magnitude. It is supplied in enteric-coated tablets of 100 and 250 mg. The usual dosage for an adult is one or two tablets every 6 hours, depending on the severity of infection. Pediatric oral suspensions are available that contain 100 mg. per teaspoonful (5 ml.) and should be given every 4 to 6 hours.

The tetracyclines

The tetracyclines are a group of antibiotics that has been developed over the past several years, and though they differ slightly chemically, the pharmacological and therapeutic actions are essentially the same. The most notable of this group are chlortetracycline, oxytetracycline, and tetracycline. Although they are dispensed under numerous proprietary names, they will be discussed together.

The tetracyclines belong to the so-called broad-spectrum antibiotics because they are effective against many gram-positive and gram-negative bacteria. They are primarily bacteriostatic in their action and normally are effective against all the pathogenic organisms arising from the oral cavity. They are also effective in the treatment of some rickettsia infections. These drugs are of considerable importance in that many gram-positive organisms resistant to penicillin and some of the gram-negative organisms resistant to streptomycin are susceptible to the tetracyclines.

Like most antibiotics, these drugs produce resistant strains, but fortunately the susceptible organisms do not develop resistance rapidly, with the exception of certain gram-negative strains.

Preparation and dosage. The tetracyclines are generally administered orally, but numerous topical and intravenous preparations are available if desired. The standard oral regimen for the average acute infection is 0.25 to 0.5 Gm. (250 to 500 mg.) every 6 hours for a total daily dose of 1 to 2 Gm. For children this dosage is reduced to 100 mg. every 6 hours. Most of the proprietary preparations are available in oral suspension in which 5 ml. (1 teaspoonful) contains 100 mg. of the antibiotic. This is a particularly effective mode of administration for children who are unable to tolerate a capsule. When the infection is of sufficient magnitude, the drug may be prescribed every 4 hours instead of every 6. Interestingly enough, to increase the antibiotic intake by increasing the dose is of little value, since the use of a dosage beyond the optimum amount fails to produce proportionately higher blood levels because of some limiting factor in the ability of the intestinal mucosa to absorb the antibiotics.

Intravenous preparations are available for those patients who require a rapid high blood level due to the severity of the infection. In instances in which the patient cannot take oral medications this mode of administration is most acceptable. Unconsciousness, trismus due to infection, and mechanical immobilization of the mandible are several instances that would warrant the use of the intravenous preparations. The dosage will vary from 500 to 1,000 mg. administered with 5% glucose intravenous solution every 12 hours. Injecting these antibiotics in concentration should be done with some hesitancy since they can produce a thrombus within the vessel. Intramuscular and subcutaneous injections are not recommended since they are quite painful and may cause tissue damage due to their irritating action. Several new preparations have eliminated this problem.

Topical preparations are available in multiple forms, including ointments, troches, powders, and tablets. The amount of drug contained in each preparation varies considerably with the manufacturer and the purpose for which it was prepared. In dentistry, topical preparations have been used in treating various manifestations of periodontal disease, postextraction wounds, etc. Some clinical evidence has supported their use, but systemic administration is undoubtedly more effective and less likely to produce resistant strains and host sensitivity.

Precautions. Signs that indicate discontinuance of the tetracyclines include the following:

1. Perhaps the most frequent untoward reaction of the host to the tetracyclines is the occurrence of nausea and diarrhea. These symptoms sometimes can be prevented by having the patient take the antibiotic with a bland drink such as milk. Should the diarrhea continue unabated the drug must be discontinued immediately to avoid severe complications. Discontinuing the drug will usually permit the gastrointestinal flora to return to normal, thus aborting a possible fatal outcome.

2. Glossitis, stomatitis, and skin eruptions are not unusual following the administration of one of the tetracyclines, particularly when a topical preparation has been employed. The appearance of these relatively minor allergic manifestations warrants the prompt discontinuance of the drug—they may be a warning of more serious manifestations of drug sensitivity.

3. Prolonged use of the tetracyclines may permit the overgrowth of organisms that are not susceptible to the antibiotic. The overproduction of *Monilia albicans*, for example, can produce symptoms that are painful and persistent. Oral discomfort and anal and vaginal itching are common manifestations of moniliasis and may be very

difficult to treat. The drug should be discontinued promptly if these symptoms arise.

4. When an infectious organism fails to show any clinical sensitivity to one of the tetracyclines, it is most unlikely that it will respond to one of the others in the group. Similarly, a patient with an allergic response to one is likely to have the same response to any of the tetracyclines.

5. The topical use of the tetracyclines, as suggested previously, should be viewed with caution since allergic responses are not unusual.

Streptomycin

Streptomycin and dihydrostreptomycin are effective against a number of gram-positive and gram-negative organisms. Like penicillin, these agents are bactericidal and bacteriostatic in their action. These drugs are ineffective in syphilis and in infections caused by clostridia, fungi, and rickettsiae. Due to their toxic side effects and the relative ease with which microorganisms become resistant, their general use for infections about the oral cavity is not recommended except as a last resort.

Preparation and dosage. Intramuscular injection of streptomycin (or dihydrostreptomycin) is the only effective means of administering the drug. Dosage ranges from 1 to 3 Gm. daily in divided doses of 0.5 Gm. Most of the preparations on the market today are combined with penicillin to treat chronic and persistent infectious processes.

Precautions. The complications that may accompany the use of these two drugs must be watched for carefully and use discontinued immediately should untoward symptoms appear.

1. The topical use of streptomycin is contraindicated because of the high degree of sensitization.

2. Both streptomycin and dihydrostreptomycin have been reported as producing vestibular and auditory damage even in small doses. Recovery of vestibular function may occur after the drug is withdrawn, but auditory damage may be irreversible.

3. Renal complications may occur after the use of these drugs, and when renal malfunction is present the drug is contraindicated.

Chloramphenicol

Chloramphenicol is one of the broad-spectrum antibiotics and is effective against most pathogenic organisms associated with the oral cavity. In addition, the rickettsiae and some viruses respond to this drug. It is a specific therapeutic agent for typhoid fever. The spectrum is not unlike that of the tetracyclines, and it is bacteriostatic in its action. Its molecular weight is lower than that of the other broad-spectrum antibiotics, and thus it is capable of producing a rapid high blood concentration, which is advantageous in severe infections. The drug's high diffusibility results in effective concentration in the cerebrospinal fluid. This attribute makes the drug particularly valuable in treatment of severe maxillary fractures complicated by cerebrospinal rhinorrhea. It is effective against many microorganisms that have developed a resistance to the older, more frequently used drugs. Chloramphenicol, like all antibiotics, produces resistant strains, and its indiscriminate use, particularly in minor infections, should be avoided, or its present advantage will probably be dissipated.

Preparation and dosage. The average adult daily dose of chloramphenicol is 1 to 2 Gm. in divided dosage, either four times during the day or every 6 hours, depending on the necessity of a constant blood level. The drug is dispensed for oral administration in 50, 100, and 250 mg. capsule form. For children an oral suspension is available that provides 125 mg. per teaspoonful (5 ml.).

For the average infectious process the oral administration is preferred, but when indicated it may be administered intravenously or intramuscularly. The adult dose for intravenous administration is 0.5 to 1 Gm. every 6 to 12 hours, either with a physiological sodium chloride solution or 5% dextrose in normal saline solution. This mode of administration should be discontinued as soon as the patient can take oral medication.

Chloramphenicol also may be administered intramuscularly in 1 Gm. doses and because of its repository quality can be given only every 12 to 24 hours. This generally sustains an adequate blood level to combat most infections.

Like the tetracyclines, chloramphenicol is available in several forms for topical application. Inadequate concentration and a tendency to allergic reactions are factors that must be considered. As a topical agent the drug seems to have little value in the field of oral surgery.

Precautions. Continuing and careful study of the patient who is taking this drug is necessary. Chloramphenicol should not be used when other and less potentially dangerous agents will be effective.

1. Chloramphenicol is a potent therapeutic agent, and certain blood dyscrasias have been associated with its administration, though to a lesser degree of frequency than was originally thought when the drug was first introduced. Depression of the bone marrow may result in neutropenia, agranulocytosis, or, in extreme cases, aplastic anemia. Prolonged administration is to be avoided, and blood studies should be made at regular intervals during treatment. It has been suggested that chloramphenicol not be administered longer than 10 days to an adult and 7 days to a child.

2. Like the tetracyclines, chloramphenicol is capable of producing nausea and diarrhea, but the latter complication occurs much less often since this antibiotic does not suppress the intestinal flora as readily. This is explained on the basis that it is absorbed more rapidly in the upper intestinal tract and does not reach the large bowel in any quantity.

3. Moniliasis, which occurs with the use of most of the antibiotics, may also result from prolonged or topical use of this drug.

Novobiocin

Novobiocin is an antibiotic that has been found to be effective in treating infections caused by both gram-positive and gram-negative bacteria. It has been quite effective against some strains of *Staphylococcus aureus* and is also used in infections caused by *Streptococcus hemolyticus, Diplococcus pneumoniae,* and *Proteus vulgaris.*

Preparation and dosage. The recommended dosage in adults is 500 mg. every 12 hours or 250 mg. every 6 hours, continued for at least 48 hours after the temperature has returned to normal and all evidence of infection has disappeared. In particularly severe infections it may be desirable to double the average dosage. The route of administration is orally in the form of capsules and a syrup for children. The syrup contains 125 mg. per teaspoonful.

Precautions. Novobiocin is capable of producing urticaria and maculopapular dermatitis. Reports have appeared of leukopenia following the administration of this drug, but it is reversible when the drug is discontinued.

As some other antibiotics are generally more effective against microorganisms causing oral infections, it is perhaps best to reserve novobiocin for resistant infectious processes of systemic character.

Lincomycin

Lincomycin has an antibacterial spectrum similar to that of erythromycin. In vitro it inhibits the growth of many gram-positive organisms, especially staphylococci, including penicillinase-producing staphylococci, pneumococci, and some streptococci. It appears to have little effect on enterococci, meningococci, and gonococci, and it is inactive against gram-negative bacilli.

Favorable responses have been reported from its use in cases of osteomyelitis. Lincomycin is useful in the treatment of infections caused by sensitive organisms when resistance to penicillin or erythromycin has developed or when these drugs cannot be used because the patient is allergic to them. The drug may be administered in combination therapy with other antimicrobial agents when indicated.

Preparation and dosage. Lincomycin is adequately absorbed either by the oral or intramuscular route. The oral dosage for adults is 500 mg. given three or four times daily. The intramuscular dosage is 600 mg. every 12 hours, more frequently in severe infections. Oral dosage for children is based on weight (15 to 30 mg. per pound).

Precautions. Since lincomycin is a relatively new drug, patients must be observed carefully for the appearance of unforeseen reactions. Patients receiving treatment for longer than 1 or 2 weeks should have liver function tests.

1. Because of the lack of adequate clinical data, use of the drug is not indicated in those patients with preexisting kidney, liver, or metabolic diseases.

2. Evidence of moniliasis or monilial infection necessitates prompt discontinuance of the drug.

3. Minor gastrointestinal disturbances such as nausea, vomiting, abdominal cramps, and diarrhea have been reported.

Kanamycin

Kanamycin sulfate is the salt of an antibiotic derived from strains of *Streptomyces Kanamycetius*. The antibacterial activity is similar to that of neomycin. It is active against many aerobic gram-positive and gram-negative bacteria. This drug is indicated for the treatment of serious infections caused by susceptible organisms. When osteomyelitis, bacteremias, and soft tissue have shown resistance to conventional antibiotics, Kanamycin may be used if the causative bacteria have been shown to be sensitive by in vitro studies.

Preparation and dosage. Kanamycin may be administered by the intramuscular, intravenous, or oral route. The oral administration of the drug should be reserved for those patients with gastrointestinal problems since the drug is poorly absorbed from the gastrointestinal tract and therefore not too effective in systemic problems. The intramuscular route is generally the route of choice, and the dosage is calculated not to exceed 0.7 mg. per pound of body weight in two or three divided doses.

Precautions. As noted previously, Kanamycin should be reserved for infections resistant to other antibiotics. Patients should be carefully evaluated during the administration of this drug and probably should be hospitalized.

1. The major toxic effect of parenterally administered Kanamycin is its action on the auditory portion of the eighth nerve. Excessive dosage seems to be a factor, and use of the drug should not be prolonged unnecessarily. Deafness may be partial or complete, and in most cases it has been irreversible.

2. Renal irritations frequently occur in those patients with prior kidney problems or in those patients who are not well hydrated.

Cephalothin

Cephalothin is a new broad-spectrum bactericidal antibiotic for parenteral administration. Its spectrum is comparable to that of certain penicillins, covering some gram-positive and gram-negative bacteria, including cocci and bacilli.

Because cephalothin is new and every effort should be made to avoid producing strains that will be resistant, its use should be restricted to the treatment of serious infection. It should be considered for use when penicillin is indicated but cannot be used because the patient is allergic to it. The drug is effective against penicillin-resistant organisms.

Preparation and dosage. Intramuscular injection of cephalothin is the most desirable route of administration. The drug must be reconstituted with 4 ml. of water and must be injected deep into muscle since it is irritating to tissues. Intravenous injections must be given with caution or thrombophlebitis may result. Dosage varies from 0.5 to 1 Gm. given four to six times a day.

Precautions

1. Cephalothin is not absorbed following oral administration and therefore must be given via a rather painful intramuscular route at fairly frequent intervals.
2. Patients having a history of allergic reactions, particularly to drugs, should receive this drug with the utmost caution.
3. Adverse reactions are similar to the penicillins, including urticaria, skin rash, fever, eosinophilia, and rarely neutropenia.

Polymyxin B

Polymyxin B has its principal effect upon gram-negative bacteria (except *Proteus* species) and should be reserved for this group. It has been used primarily as a topical drug, but the incidence of gram-negative strains has forced clinicians to resort to polymyxin B for systemic use.

Topical polymyxin is usually nontoxic and nonsensitizing. It has been combined in complex preparations for use as troches and ointments.

Systemic administration must be carefully controlled since the drug may induce nephrotoxic and/or neurological disturbances (dizziness, facial paralysis). The problems are not pronounced when the recommended dosage range is not exceeded.

Preparation and dosage. The suggested route of administration is by intramuscular injection at intervals of 8 hours. The total daily dose is from 1.5 to 2.5 mg. per kilogram of body weight. The maximum dosage must not exceed 200 mg.

Precautions. In those patients who exhibit any impairment of renal function, the use of polymyxin should be avoided. If the patient has normal renal function, the nephrotoxic effects of the drug may become evident in the fourth or fifth day of treatment, but these can generally be controlled if the recommended dosage is not exceeded. The same is true regarding the neurological disturbances.

It should be emphasized that polymyxin B must be reserved for those patients afflicted with an infection caused by organisms proved to be sensitive to the drug.

Local antibiotics

Antibiotics that are not normally used as systemic drugs because of their toxicity, but have some benefits when used topically, are referred to as local antibiotics. Used systemically, they produce untoward complications and are therefore contraindicated except under dire circumstances. One common characteristic is their ability to be used topically with allergic reactions held to a minimum. These agents do have a place in dentistry, but it should be borne in mind that the concentrations employed are insufficient to control the infection and should be used as adjunctive therapy. These local antibiotics have been prepared commercially in various combinations and concentrations. Only a brief résumé of their specific characteristics seems indicated.

Bacitracin

Bacitracin is active against fusiform bacilli and some spirochetes and has a similar range to that of penicillin. Because of this relationship in activity it may be effective when employed with systemic penicillin in combating Vincent's infection. The effectiveness of bacitracin is not altered by serum, pus, or necrotic tissue. This characteristic makes it valuable in the treatment of osteomyelitis when the infected area can be approached directly and an adequate concentration maintained. To be effective the drug must be in contact with the pathogenic organisms.

Neomycin

Neomycin is bactericidal in vitro against both gram-negative and gram-positive or-

154   *Textbook of oral surgery*

ganisms. Though occasionally administered parenterally it has no general application because of the toxic effect on the kidneys and on the eighth nerve. Topically it is effective in skin infections and has been combined with other local antibiotics in the preparation of troches and ointments. The troches have been of value in controlling secondary local infection, particularly in those persons who are allergic to a number of the parenteral antibiotics.

Tyrothricin

Tyrothricin, like bacitracin, is particularly effective against the gram-positive organisms. It is made up principally of two active ingredients, gramicidin and tyrocidine. It is most effective when in direct contact with the offending microorganisms. Applied in compress form to open wounds it has been effective, and infected bone lesions have responded favorably when the drug, in solution, is carried directly to the injured part. The usual concentration is 0.01% to 0.05% in isotonic solution irrigated directly into the wound through a drain two or three times daily. Tyrothricin is also prepared in troche form particularly to combat streptococcal oral infections.

SULFONAMIDES

As a group the sulfonamides have been replaced in the last decade by the antibiotics primarily because of the dramatic effect of the newer agents and the toxicity of the older drug. Now, however, the antibiotics are producing resistant organisms that can be treated with the sulfonamides, and improvements have been made in these drugs that make them less toxic.

The primary toxic complication of the sulfonamides when they were first introduced was crystalluria, resulting in renal shutdown. Drug fever, dermatitis, and alterations in the blood-forming organs, with resultant hemolytic anemia, leukopenia, and agranulocytosis, were additional complications (Fig. 9-4). Most of these complications have been eliminated or at least minimized by proper controls during administration and the combination of three of the sulfonamides into one medication. The combination of sulfadiazine, sulfamerazine, and sulfamezathine into a triple sulfonamide preparation has reduced toxic reactions considerably. Sulfisoxazole and sulfadimetine are also well tolerated when properly administered and controlled.

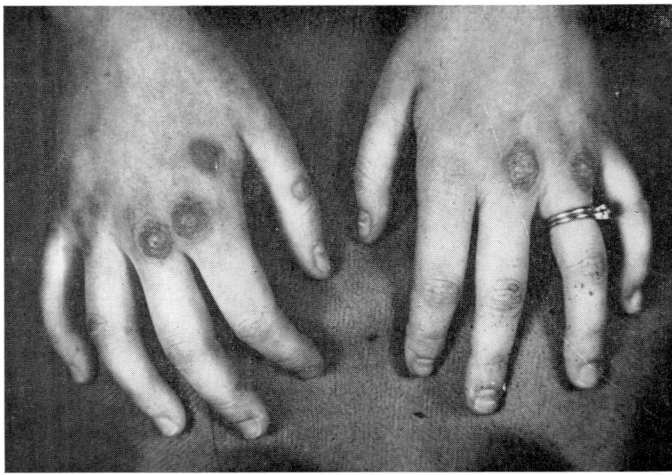

Fig. 9-4. Skin reaction following the administration of sulfadiazine.

Triple sulfonamides are prepared in 0.5 Gm. tablets, and the dosage is generally 2 Gm. initially, to be followed by 1 Gm. every 6 hours. Oral suspension for children is also available in concentrations of 0.5 Gm. in each teaspoonful. Dosage for a child is usually one half that of the adult dose. Most authorities recommend that an equal amount of sodium bicarbonate be given with each dose of the sulfonamides. This will reduce the incidence of urinary complications.

Precautions. The following factors are considered in the safe use of the drugs:

1. A history of previous sulfonamide sensitivity would normally contraindicate the further use of these drugs unless the exact sensitizing drug could be ascertained.

2. Daily supervision of the patient and constant observation for signs of toxicity are imperative in sulfonamide therapy.

3. High fluid intake is mandatory to avoid renal complications, and urinary output should be above 1,200 ml. per day.

4. Sulfonamide blood concentrations are indicated in severe infections to maintain a sufficient therapeutic level.

5. A complete blood count and urinalysis should be done every other day to ascertain any early toxic reaction.

6. Patients should be advised to avoid any unnecessary exposure to ultraviolet rays since photosensitivity may result.

ADJUNCTIVE THERAPY

In the use of antibiotics the practitioner is often confronted with the necessity of using other drugs as supportive therapy or to combat the complications of the antibiotic. To discuss the relative merits and defects of each drug would be impossible, but an awareness of what agents are available seems appropriate.

Vitamins

Vitamins are well established as an effective group of drugs in the treatment of dental problems; they have been useful in treating gingival disorders, cheilitis, impaired healing, etc. In the use of antibiotics they are valuable in supplementing the dietary intake, particularly when the antibiotics are administered orally. Several of the broad-spectrum drugs cause a decrease in the intestinal flora, which may produce an avitaminosis. Numerous vitamins are dependent upon the intestinal bacteria for their production, and in the prolonged use of antibiotics, supportive vitamins should be administered. A therapeutic vitamin preparation that includes the B complex, ascorbic acid, and various minerals is usually adequate. A recent study indicated that tetracycline therapy is more effective and rapidly induced with minimum dosage when administered with ascorbic acid. The recommended dosage is 500 mg. of ascorbic acid for every 250 mg. of the tetracyclines.

Antihistamines

Allergic reactions to antibiotic therapy make it imperative to have some effective means of treating these untoward manifestations. The antihistamines are very useful in treating urticaria, itching, allergic rhinitis, serum sickness angioneurotic edema, etc. Penicillin is undoubtedly the antibiotic that produces most of the local reactions, and should mild symptoms appear, antihistamine therapy is indicated to keep the reaction to a minimum. Prompt therapy will make the patient more comfortable and may prevent more serious complications.

Many antihistamines are available in the form of elixir, tablets, nasal sprays, and in combinations with other drugs. Intravenous and intramuscular preparations are also available when a rapid high level is necessary. Most of these drugs currently available may produce drowsiness or vertigo in some patients. Less frequently encountered is nausea. The advantages, disadvantages, and dosage of each antihistamine are not within the scope of this text. A pharmacology reference provides an excellent source in the selection of the proper drug and dosage.

Cortisone, hydrocortisone, and epinephrine are used when the allergic manifestations become marked. Administered in suitable formulations and by the appropriate route, these drugs usually give dramatic relief. They should be used judiciously and in consultation with the patient's physician if the symptoms are severe or therapy is prolonged.

Penicillinase

An enzyme, penicillinase, has been introduced for the specific purpose of combating allergic reactions to penicillin. It catalyzes the hydrolysis of penicillin to penicilloic acid, which is nonallergenic. Whereas the antihistamines and steroids treat the effects of an allergic response to penicillin, this specific enzyme counteracts the cause of the reaction by neutralizing the penicillin itself.

The drug is administered intramuscularly as soon as signs and symptoms of a reaction appear. It may be repeated daily if needed and should be given intravenously in the presence of an anaphylactoid reaction to penicillin.

SEQUELAE

The use of antibiotics as a prophylaxis against possible infectious complications has become fairly common practice. It is now clear on the basis of recent studies that in most situations such prophylaxis is of no value and in many cases superinfections result. It appears that the unnecessary and prolonged use of antibiotics may induce, rather than prevent, infection. One recent assessment on a general surgical service showed that when antibiotics were used arbitrarily the incidence of infections in the group receiving systemic prophylactic antibiotics following clean surgery was three times higher than in the group receiving none.

These findings do not preclude the necessity of administering antibiotics in selected cases, giving them to the patient with rheumatic fever, severe facial injuries, etc., but one should develop a cautious approach to the use of these drugs.

REFERENCES

1. Appleton, J. L. T.: Bacterial infections in dental practice, ed. 4, Philadelphia, 1950, Lea & Febiger.
2. Billings, F.: Chronic focal infections and their etiological relations to arthritis and nephritis, Arch. Intern. Med. 9:484, 1912.
3. Burnett, G. W., and Scherp, H. W.: Oral microbiology and infectious disease, Baltimore, 1957, The Williams & Wilkins Co.
4. Copeman, W. S. C.: Textbook of rheumatic diseases, ed. 2, London, 1955, E. & S. Livingstone, Ltd.
5. Dobbs, E. C.: Pharmacology and oral therapeutics, ed. 11, St. Louis, 1956, The C. V. Mosby Co.
6. Friedberg, C. K.: Diseases of the heart, ed. 2, Philadelphia, 1956, W. B. Saunders Co.
7. Leevy, C. M.: Practical diagnosis and treatment of liver disease, New York, 1957, Hoeber-Harper.
8. Meakins, J. C., editor: Practice of medicine, ed. 6, St. Louis, 1956, The C. V. Mosby Co.
9. Moore, R. A.: A textbook of pathology, Philadelphia, 1948, W. B. Saunders Co.
10. Pulaski, E. J.: Surgical infections, Springfield, Ill., 1954, Charles C Thomas, Publisher.
11. Rosenow, E. C.: Studies on elective localization of focal infection with special reference to oral sepsis, J. Dent. Res. 1:205, 1919.
12. Smith, D. T., and Conant, N. F.: Zinsser's bacteriology, ed. 11, New York, 1957, Appleton-Century-Crofts, Inc.
13. Traut, E. F.: Rheumatic diseases, diagnosis and treatment, St. Louis, 1952, The C. V. Mosby Co.
14. Welsh, H., and Marti-Ibanez, F., editors: Antibiotics annual 1957-1958, New York, 1958, Medical Encyclopedia, Inc.
15. Pulaski, E. J.: Antibiotics in surgical cases, Arch. Surg. 82:545, 1961.
16. Cullen, J. C., Roberts, C. E., Jr., and Kirby, W. M.: Clinical evaluation of dimethroxyphenyl-penicillin, Antimicrobial agents annual, 1960, New York, 1961, Plenum Press.
17. Johnston, F. R. C.: An assessment of prophylactic antibiotics in general surgery, Surg. Gynec. Obstet. 116:1, 1963.
18. King, G. C.: The case against antibiotic prophylaxis in major head and neck surgery, Laryngoscope 71:647, 1961.

19. Archard, H. O., and Roberts, W. C.: Bacterial endocarditis after dental procedures in patients with aortic valve prosthesis, J. Amer. Dent. Ass. **72:**648, 1966.
20. Holloway, W. V., and Scott, E. G.: Clinical experience with lincomycin, Amer. J. Med. Sci. **249:**103, 1965.
21. New drugs, Chicago, 1966, American Medical Association, pp. 1-70.
22. Physician's desk reference to pharmaceutical specialties and biologicals, ed. 21, Bradell, N. J., 1967, Medical Economics, Inc.
23. Accepted dental remedies, Chicago, 1967, American Dental Association, pp. 114-136.
24. Dipalma, J. R., editor: Drill's pharmacology in medicine, ed. 3, New York, 1965, McGraw-Hill Book Co., pp. 1279-1414.
25. Krantz, J. C., Jr., and Carr, C. J.: Pharmacological principles of medical practice, ed. 6, Baltimore, 1965, The Williams & Wilkins Co., pp. 82-126.
26. Prevention of bacterial endocarditis, 1965, American Heart Association.
27. Goodman, L. S., and Gilman, Alfred: The pharmacological basis of therapeutics, ed. 3, New York, 1965, The Macmillan Co., pp. 1242-1259.

Chapter 10

SPECIAL INFECTIONS AND THEIR SURGICAL RELATIONSHIP

George E. Morin

Patients who seek dental care sometimes harbor organisms that are different from the bacteria that cause ordinary infections. These organisms may secondarily complicate a traumatic or surgical wound, or they may have caused the primary oral disease for which the patient seeks relief.

Diagnosis can be a problem when dealing with anaerobic bacteria, fungi, and viruses. Special culture techniques are necessary. Biopsy is often necessary to establish the presence of the organism in the tissues. The clinical picture of these more rarely encountered infections is frequently variable, and since they are not seen frequently in an office practice, they may often go unrecognized.

Special care is strongly indicated for the rare infections. The usual antibiotics are not often beneficial, but when they are, many times the usual dose may be necessary.

In the established case that has been diagnosed and is being treated the problem of an intercurrent acute dental infection can present itself. For example, the patient with active pulmonary tuberculosis is permitted by the chest physician to have necessary extractions done under proper precautions. This combination of circumstances can cause a real problem in the uncontrolled rare infections.

Tetanus and gas gangrene are not seen often today, the former because of active prophylactic measures for each patient after an accident involving broken skin, and the latter because it does not often attack oral tissues. Tuberculosis is being treated more effectively. Syphilis was not seen often after the advent of penicillin, but now a sharp increase in incidence is reported by the Public Health Service.

The fungi that live in endogenous saprophytic balance with the bacteria in the healthy person now seem to be responsible for more diseases. The antibiotics, which are being used universally for the treatment of diseases as well as prophylactic feeding in dairy and beef cattle, fowl, and hogs, serve to upset the ecology of the organisms. The study of viruses is a relatively new field that is providing more and more information in areas formerly unknown.

Consultation with the family physician, internist, dermatologist, and bacteriologist is extremely beneficial in the management of the oral lesions of these conditions.

TETANUS

Tetanus, commonly referred to as lockjaw, is a severe systemic infection caused by an anaerobic bacillus, *Clostridium tetani*. The pathogenicity of this organism results from the production of a powerful exotoxin that, when carried to the central nervous system by lymphatics and the bloodstream, acts upon motor nerve cells to produce powerful spasm of muscular tissue. Although tetanus infection is relatively infrequent, spores of the organisms are widely distributed in nature, being commonly found in soil and in the gastrointestinal tract of horses, cattle, and human beings. Wounds and lacerations contaminated with these spores provide a portal of entry for these microorganisms. The relative infrequency of tetanus infection is attributed to phagocytosis of the spores. The incubation period varies from 5 to 21 days.

Signs and symptoms. The most frequent initiating symptoms are stiffness and trismus of the mandible. At times this may be accompanied by restlessness, irritability, dysphagia, and neck rigidity. Later the patient may demonstrate headache, fever, chills, exaggerated reflexes, and convulsions. Spasm of the facial muscles may cause a fixed smile with raised eyebrows (risus sardonicus). Spasm of the chest wall and glottis may lead to cyanosis and death from asphyxia.

Diagnosis. Diagnosis is made on the basis of signs and symptoms. Tetanus should be considered in the differential diagnosis of all cases of trismus with a recent history of injury or laceration.

Prophylaxis. All patients with contaminated lacerations, abrasions, puncture wounds, compound fractures, etc. should receive adequate tetanus immunization. The previously immunized person should receive booster doses of toxoid (1 ml. intramuscularly). For those persons not previously immunized, passive immunity should be instituted immediately by the subcutaneous or intramuscular injection of tetanus antitoxin in doses of 500 to 5,000 units, depending on the extent of the injury. A second injection after 6 to 8 days is generally advised. Before antitoxin is administered the patient should be tested for serum sensitivity to avoid anaphylaxis. Local prophylaxis consists of thorough cleansing and debridement of wounds. Severe, grossly contaminated wounds may require anesthesia for proper cleansing. For the closure of such wounds care must be taken to provide for irrigation and drainage.

GAS GANGRENE

Gas gangrene, a severe necrotizing infection, is caused by the exotoxin of the genus *Clostridium*, including *Clostridium perfringens (welchii), novyi (oedematiens), septicum,* and *bifermentans*. Each member of this family can produce gas gangrene independently, but generally mixtures of all of these can readily be cultured from a gas gangrene infection. These spore-forming organisms are gram-positive, strictly anaerobic saprophytes that liberate powerful hemolysins, fibrolysins, hyaluronidase, and lecithinase.

The infection, when it manifests itself, becomes evident in from several hours to 3 days after the occurrence of the wound, laceration, or compound fracture. Tissues in the area of the wound become swollen, yellowish gray, and tense because of underlying pressure. The wound or surrounding skin may rupture, with a scanty serosanguinous exudate demonstrating numerous gas bubbles. The tissue soon becomes greenish black and foul smelling. In severe cases death may rapidly ensue as a result of the systemic action of the powerful hemolytic exotoxin liberated. This condition is rare in the areas of the jaws.

Treatment. Therapy consists of the administration of polyvalent antitoxins and massive antibiotic treatment. Penicillin appears to be especially effective. Local therapy includes generous debridement and, if practicable, total excision of infected tissue.

SYPHILIS

A detailed description of syphilis with its etiology, ramifications, and manifestations is obviously not within the scope of this text. Accordingly, the discussion of this pathological entity will be limited to those manifestations of the disease that are pertinent to dentists in general and specifically to the practice of oral surgery.

Primary chancre. The usual primary manifestation of syphilis is the chancre. It usually involves the genitalia, but on occasion its initial appearance may be on the lips. On occasion the gingiva, tongue, and tonsils may be infected. These are solitary ulcerations with thick, dark encrustations. Induration is a prominent feature. This lesion is highly infectious and not an uncommon source of infection for the dentist. Diagnosis is made by dark-field microscopic examination since the serology is negative at this stage. The differential diagnosis of such lesions should include herpes labialis, chancroid, and squamous cell carcinoma.

Syphilitic mucous patches. A manifestation of the secondary stage of the disease and homologous to the macular and papular skin rashes seen at this stage are slightly raised, grayish erosions of the mucosa surrounded by an area of erythema. They may be painful and have a tendency to bleed easily. Common sites of occurrence are the tongue, buccal mucosa, inner surface of the lips, tonsil, and pharyngeal mucosa. These lesions are also highly infectious and a potential source of infection for the dentist. Diagnosis is established by means of serological and dark-field microscopic examination.

Syphilitic gummas. The gumma is a manifestation of late or tertiary syphilis. It begins as an erythematous macule, which progresses to a nodule, which then ulcerates after undergoing central necrosis. These slow-healing lesions are painless and may involve any part of the skin, mucous membranes, or viscera. The tongue and palate are commonly affected. Perforation of the palate and nasal septum is not uncommon. Syphilitic interstitial glossitis or healed gummatous lesion of the tongue simulates the appearance of advanced leukoplakia and is considered precancerous. Diagnosis of these lesions is dependent upon biopsy since the serology is frequently negative in tertiary syphilis.

Syphilitic periostitis and osteomyelitis. Syphilitic involvement of bone is seen in both congenital and tertiary syphilis. The infection may be limited to a painful periostitis or progress to a diffuse osteomyelitis difficult to differentiate radiographically from purulent osteomyelitis. The early bone change following the periostitis is essentially one of osteoporosis, but later central osteosclerosis with peripheral osteoblastic activity may simulate the roentgenographical appearance of osteogenic sarcoma.

Diagnosis. The diagnosis is made by biopsy and serological examination. This bone infection usually responds readily to systemic antibiotic treatment.

ORAL TUBERCULOSIS

Tuberculous infection of the lips, tongue, palate, buccal mucosa, and pharynx is relatively rare. It manifests itself in the form of indolent, chancrelike, sharply defined purulent ulcers with undermined, scalloped edges. The ulcers result from secondary inoculation from another focus, usually advanced pulmonary tuberculosis, with sputum being the vehicle of transmission. The lesions are painful and extremely slow in healing. Diagnosis is dependent on biopsy examination. The clinical appearance is suggestive of chancre and squamous cell carcinoma. The treatment is essentially the treatment of pulmonary tuberculosis, such as streptomycin, isoniazid, and para-aminosalicylic acid.

MONILIASIS (THRUSH)

Oral moniliasis is characterized by single or multiple white, loosely adherent patches on the oral mucosa. These patches have a tendency to slough, leaving raw, denuded areas of mucosa. The lesions occur in all portions of the oral cavity and pharynx.

The upper portions of the trachea and esophagus may become involved.

Etiology. This condition is generally caused by a fungus, *Candida albicans*. It occurs spontaneously in infants, possibly from nipple infections. Monilial vaginitis in the mother has also been suggested as a factor in its transmission. It is also frequently seen in elderly and debilitated patients. Here a vitamin deficiency, especially riboflavin, is considered important as a predisposing factor. It is also frequently seen in normal adults following the administration of antibiotics, especially broad-spectrum troches, because of a disruption in the relative balance of the oral flora.

Moniliasis is also seen under old or ill-fitting dentures. This condition is sometimes referred to as denture sore mouth. Here the occurrence of the infection does not present the usual white plaque, but rather a fiery red appearance limited to the outline of the prosthetic appliance. The palate may assume a verrucous or papillated appearance.

Diagnosis. Diagnosis is easily made by direct smear or culture on Sabouraud's medium. The fungus can also be demonstrated in a biopsy section. The differential diagnosis includes diphtheria, secondary syphilis, lichen planus, and Vincent's stomatitis.

Treatment. Moniliasis responds readily to topical applications of a fresh solution of 2% gentian violet, three to four times a day. More recently, excellent results have been obtained by the topical application of nystatin suspension three to four times daily. In the case of chronic moniliasis under an old denture, nystatin ointment placed on the denture has been found to be effective. However, construction of new dentures prior to treatment is advised.

ACTINOMYCOSIS

Actinomycosis is primarily a disease of animals (lumpy jaw in cattle), but it does manifest itself with some frequency in human beings, causing a chronic granulomatous reaction with multiple abscess and fistula formation. The area of the head and neck (cervicofacial actinomycosis) is involved in about 60% of cases, with 25% involving the abdominal area and 15% the thoracic area.

Etiology. Several forms of the disease are caused by different fungi. In man the *Actinomyces bovis* is responsible for about 90% of the cases. This organism is acid-fast, gram-positive, nonsporulating, and microaerophilic. It is found commonly in the soil and grows readily on vegetation; hence a greater incidence of the disease is noted in the plains and cattle-raising areas. It also occurs fairly frequently in the metropolitan areas, and some believe that the organism may be part of the normal oral flora, becoming a pathogen under special circumstances.

Findings. Actinomycosis frequently occurs following tooth extraction or a break in the oral mucous membranes. It develops slowly. Central involvement of bone with gradual enlargement and central osteolysis may occur. The infection may be peripheral, primarily involving the soft tissue. The submaxillary space is most commonly involved (90% of cases), but the tongue and maxillary area may be primarily involved. The infection develops slowly with the formation of a hard, tumorlike swelling. Trismus may be a prominent finding, but usually lymphadenopathy is not a prominent feature in the early stages of the swelling. As the swelling progresses, central necrosis leads to multiple fistula formation and drainage of yellowish pus. Drainage may occur intraorally or extraorally. Pain is not a prominent part of the clinical picture.

Diagnosis. Several of the typical symptoms of this infection are valuable in arriving at a diagnosis. The presence of multiple draining fistulas surrounded by areas of purplish discoloration is highly suggestive of actinomycosis. The presence of sulfur granules in the exudate may be considered pathognomonic. The granules are weblike mattings of the mycelial filaments of the fungus. The typical ray fungus may be demonstrated on tissue section. On occasion the organism may be cultured on Sabouraud's glucose agar medium.

Treatment. Actinomycosis is most difficult to eradicate. Broad-spectrum antibiotics have been utilized successfully in some cases. Massive doses of penicillin in the order of 2 to 4 million units a day for several months have been advocated recently. Complete surgical drainage with excision of fistulous tracts is indicated. Roentgen therapy and potassium iodide have been beneficial in some instances, but are rarely used at the present time.

BLASTOMYCOSIS (NORTH AMERICAN BLASTOMYCOSIS)

Blastomycosis is a specific infection caused by the fungus *Blastomyces dermatitidis*. The infection is exogenous, producing cutaneous lesions by inoculation or pulmonary lesions by inhalation, the latter terminating fatally. The cutaneous lesions may involve all portions of the oral cavity. Invasion of bone, with loosening and exfoliation of teeth, has been reported. The oral lesions consist initially of multiple, small, elevated abscesses, which may enlarge to an abscess several centimeters in diameter. Each abscess is said to contain a single fungus cell characterized by prominent capsule and budding. This infection attacks men over women in a ratio of 9:1 and may run a protracted course of several years before a fatal systemic dissemination.

Diagnosis. The causative organism may be identified by tissue microscopic examination and culture of the organism on Sabouraud's medium. Skin tests with vaccines or extracts of *Blastomyces dermatitidis* may reveal a sensitivity to the fungus.

Treatment. No truly effective systemic treatment for blastomycosis is known. Cutaneous and muccocutaneous lesions respond to roentgen therapy.

HISTOPLASMOSIS

Histoplasmosis is a cutaneous mycotic infection that frequently involves oral mucous membranes and the lungs. In the latter case pyrexia, cachexia, and the x-ray appearance of the lungs may be suggestive of tuberculosis with an associated splenomegaly, hypochromic anemia, and leukopenia. Oral manifestations consist of gradually enlarging, painful granulomatous ulcers that have a tendency to bleed easily. Fetid breath is a prominent feature.

All portions of the mouth may be affected, with a predilection for the tongue and pharynx.

Etiology. This infection is caused by the fungus *Histoplasma capsulatum*. The disease affects all age groups, with some predilection for children and adult males, particularly on farms and rural areas. The disease is believed to be contracted through breaks in the skin and by aspiration into the respiratory and the alimentary tracts.

Diagnosis. The organism can be identified by culture on Sabouraud's medium or by biopsy.

Treatment. No effective treatment is known for histoplasmosis.

ORAL HERPES
Herpetic ulcers

Typical herpetic lesions consist of small, painful, eroded ulcers having a bright red, raised border. They vary in size from 2 to 25 mm. or more. The lips, face, chin, and oral mucous membranes are primarily affected. The lesions are most frequently solitary, but may occur in small clusters, especially on the lips (cold sore), where they have been mistaken for squamous cell carcinoma. The etiology is generally ascribed to the herpes simplex virus. Gastrointestinal upsets and hormonal disturbances during menstruation may be predisposing factors.

Treatment. These lesions do not respond to specific therapy and are treated symptomatically. The exquisite pain associated with intraoral craters may be controlled by mild caustics such as negatol or 7% chromic acid. The lip and facial lesions should be protected with medicated ointments to prevent secondary infection.

Herpetic (aphthous) stomatitis

Since considerable disagreement exists on whether aphthous and herpetic stomatitis are separate entities, they will be discussed simultaneously in view of the fact that the symptomatology and clinical course are essentially similar. The etiological agent of herpetic stomatitis is generally considered to be the herpes simplex virus. Some authors prefer the term aphthous stomatitis for those cases in which the herpes virus cannot be conclusively implicated. This disease affects both sexes equally, but is more common in children and young adults. It frequently follows an upper respiratory infection. It has been seen in elderly individuals with serious nutritional deficiencies. It is considered to be communicable.

The condition appears as a general involvement of the oral mucosa with edematous craters resembling those seen in solitary herpes. The lesions vary in size and tend to coalesce. The gingiva may become markedly edematous and inflamed. An accompanying elevation of temperature, lymphadenopathy, and malaise may appear. Fetor oris is also a prominent feature. The mouth becomes extremely painful, and swallowing and feeding become a serious problem, especially in children.

Treatment. The disease is self-limiting (10 to 14 days), and treatment is symptomatic with precautions against secondary infection. Alkaline mouthwashes and anesthetic trouches are helpful in maintaining oral hygiene and controlling pain. Beneficial results have been reported with the use of high vitamin therapy, especially B complex and C. Broad-spectrum antibiotics such as the tetracyclines should be employed to control secondary infection. A bland liquid diet during the more acute phase facilitates feeding.

Repeated cowpox vaccination has been reported as helpful in controlling the recurrent forms of this disease.

ERYTHEMA MULTIFORME

Erythema multiforme is a self-limiting skin disease of rapid onset that occurs in many forms. It frequently involves the face and oral mucous membranes, particularly in the form of erythema bullosum and vesiculosum. The skin lesions are large, crimson, polymorphous macules that have a tendency to be located bilaterally symmetrical on the dorsum of hands, feet, legs, forearms, face, and neck. The macular stage is followed by vesicle and bulla formation. Oral lesions occur as papules and vesicles, terminating in ulcer formation. Pain is not a distinctive feature although gross involvement of the lip may result in considerable discomfort due to encrustation and bleeding. The symptoms develop rapidly in from 12 to 24 hours. An accompanying sore throat, malaise, and elevated temperature may be present. The disease usually heals spontaneously after 2 to 3 weeks, but in occasional severe cases fatal termination due to secondary nephritis, carditis, and arthritis may result.

Etiology. The cause is unknown. However, all the following agents have been implicated in its etiology by various workers in the field: viruses; administration of antisera; drugs such as sulfonamides, quinine, arsenic, belladonna, iodides, salicylic acid; arthritis; endocrinologic and allergic disorders.

Treatment. The treatment is nonspecific and chiefly symptomatic. Oral hygiene and proper feeding are of particular concern with oral involvement. Alkaline mouthwashing with bland liquid feedings are advised. Systemically, chlortetracycline,

ACTH, cortisone, antihistamines, and massive B complex vitamins have been used with varying degrees of success.

Stevens-Johnson syndrome

Stevens-Johnson syndrome (erythema multiforme exudativum major) is believed to be a variant of erythema multiforme in which a triad of symptoms appears, including conjunctivitis, oral lesions, and urethritis.

Behçet's syndrome

Behçet's syndrome is believed to be a variant of erythema multiforme, having the symptoms iritis, oral lesions, and cutaneous genital lesions.

HERPANGINA

Herpangina is a syndrome of virus etiology occurring chiefly in epidemic form among children. It is characterized by fever, anorexia, dysphagia, and sore throat. Oral symptoms consist of grayish papules and vesicles, each with a red areola, on the uvula, soft palate, pillars of the fauces, and tonsils. The organism responsible for the disease has been identified as the Coxsackie or group C virus.

Treatment is symptomatic, and recovery is usually uneventful within a week or two.

PEMPHIGUS

Pemphigus in its various forms is a serious and frequently fatal disease of the skin and mucous membranes. Several forms of the disease are recognized: pemphigus acutus, pemphigus vulgaris, pemphigus vegetans, pemphigus foliaceus, and pemphigus erythematosus. The basic lesion in all forms is the vesicle or bulla. All forms have been reported to involve oral mucous membranes with the initial lesion frequently appearing orally in the acutus, vegetans, and vulgaris forms.

Etiology. The cause of the disease is unknown, but a viral or streptococcal infection has been suspected.

Findings. Oral aspects of the disease are of interest because of the frequent initial appearance of the disease at this site. Oral bullae of various sizes, depending on the type, form painlessly, but become acutely painful upon eruption, leaving a shallow crater with ragged edges. These craters may become infected and necrotic, giving the breath a fetid odor. Excessive salivation is also frequently noted. Oral lesions may be located on the tongue, palate, lips, mucosa, and gingivae.

Diagnosis. The diagnosis of pemphigus may be rather difficult. A differential diagnosis should include herpetic stomatitis, syphilitic mucous patches, erythema multiforme, fusospirochetal mucous patches, and allergic reactions to drugs. Nikolsky's sign is considered an aid in diagnosis. This consists in forcibly stroking the skin or mucosa of a suspected case with a blunt instrument. The formation of a small bleb is considered a positive reaction. The Pels-Macht test is now considered by many to be of doubtful value.

Treatment. The treatment of pemphigus is not uniformly successful. ACTH and cortisone have been used with varying degrees of success. Dental aspects of treatment consist of controlling oral pain and maintaining oral hygiene. Alkaline mouthwashes and anesthetic troches are beneficial. Aniline dyes (2% to 4%) have been suggested to help control secondary infection of oral ulcers.

REFERENCES

1. Agastas, W. N., Reeves, N., Shanks, E. P., and Sydenstricker, V. P.: Erythema multiforme bullosum (Stevens-Johnson syndrome), New Eng. J. Med. **246**:217, 1952.
2. Allen, A. C.: The skin, St. Louis, 1954, The C. V. Mosby Co.
3. Anderson, W. A. D.: Pathology, St. Louis, 1961, The C. V. Mosby Co.
4. Appleton, J. L. T.: Bacterial infection, Philadelphia, 1950, Lea & Febiger.
5. Bell, W. H., and Arnim, S. S.: Periostitis ossificans of the mandible secondary to congenital syphilis, Oral Surg. **10**:1254, 1957.

6. Bernier, J. L.: The management of oral disease, St. Louis, 1959, The C. V. Mosby Co.
7. Bruce, K. W.: Oral tuberculosis, Chron. Omaha Dist. Dent. Soc. 20:49, 1956.
8. Burket, L. W.: Oral medicine, Philadelphia, 1952, J. B. Lippincott Co.
9. Cheraskin, E., and Langley, L. L.: Dynamics of oral diagnosis, Chicago, 1956, Year Book Publishers, Inc.
10. Herzog, W., and Conrad, F. W.: Pathology of tracheal syphilis; penicillin therapy of syphilis in the oral cavity, Dent. Abst. 1:217, 1956.
11. Lever, W. F.: Pemphigus, Medicine 32:1, 1953.
12. Lorenz, O.: Cervicofacial actinomycotic mixed infection; report of 120 cases, Dent. Abst. 2:629, 1957 .
13. Robinson, I. B., and Laskin, D. M.: Tetanus of oral origin, Oral Surg. 10:831, 1957.
14. Smith, D. T., and Martin, D. S.: Zinnser's textbook of bacteriology, New York, 1948, Appleton-Century-Crofts, Inc.
15. Stark, M. M.: Recurrent aphthae and herpetic infections; their etiology, prognosis and treatment, Acad. Rev. 5:119, 1957.
16. Stephenson, J. W., and Blackey, B.: Tetanus infection causing dysphagia; report of case, Dent. Abst. 1:332, 1956.
17. Thilander, H., and Wennstrom, A.: Tuberculosis of the mouth and surrounding tissues, Oral Surg. 9:858, 1956.
18. Thoma, K. H.: Oral pathology, St. Louis, 1960, The C. V. Mosby Co.
19. Zylka, N.: Tetanus after tooth extraction, Dent. Abst. 2:682, 1956.

Chapter 11

ACUTE INFECTIONS OF THE ORAL CAVITY

Sanford M. Moose

The subject of acute infections of the oral cavity could in itself occupy a sizeable volume if descriptions of diagnosis and treatment procedures for all the acute infections that are found in the oral cavity were included.

Many of the acute inflammatory processes that are manifested in the oral cavity may at some period during their course give evidence of acute infection. If a text on dermatology is examined, it will be found frequently that oral manifestations of infection are among the cardinal symptoms of dermatological disease. The same may be said of many other systemic diseases too numerous to mention. At some period during the course of a disease certain visible signs may appear on the mucous membrane surfaces of the body. The oral cavity is the area that is most frequently invaded. Many of the acute exanthematous diseases of childhood have primary lesions in the oral cavity, which under certain circumstances become acutely inflamed or even infected. Any primary systemic condition that is capable of rendering the oral mucosa less resistant to infectious invasion is capable of producing a lesion that is extremely vulnerable to a secondary infection. This, of course, then appears as an acute infection of the oral cavity.

Patients who are allergic to one or several extraneous agents may also have visual lesions of the oral cavity that, although primarily the result of an allergy, may on occasion become infected by some secondary invader.

Nutritional and deficiency diseases have a great tendency to form oral lesions, which often appear as infectious ulcers. These lesions can defy the most astute diagnostician's ability to arrive at the etiological factor. Several types of stomatitis, lucidly described in the texts on this subject, appear as spectacular and classical acute infections of the oral cavity, usually confined to the oral mucosa.

Chemical poisonings capable of producing oral lesions and ultimately secondary infections occur most frequently from certain occupational hazards and are described in minute detail in bulletins that may be obtained from the United States Department of Labor and the United States Department of Agriculture.

Many of the odontogenic tumors or cysts are first discovered by the appearance of an acute inflammatory lesion, ultimately resulting in an acute infection in some part of the maxilla or mandible, but not infrequently invading the soft tissues of the cheek, lip, tongue, or soft palate through a fistula.

Several of the blood dyscrasias and blood-borne diseases have oral manifestations of acutely infected lesions. The terminal symptoms of some blood dyscrasias are acutely ulcerative gingival and buccal lesions that resemble, in many respects, several other types of stomatitis.

Many cancers have manifested themselves by their first objective symptoms as an acute inflammatory lesion of the oral tissues. They frequently start in the retromolar region, where in early stages they could be confused with an ulcerative pericoronitis of the third molar.

Metastatic cancers from primary breast or prostate cancers have given their first secondary objective symptoms in acute inflammatory lesions of the oral tissues. They resemble many other abscesses or ulcers that form in the jaws and are temporarily relieved by excision and drainage or other palliative treatment.

Considering the realm of etiological factors capable of producing acute infections in the oral cavity, the practitioner must ever be on the alert for the more obscure causes rather than jumping at some obvious conclusions simply on the basis of what appears to be apparent. The astute diagnostician immediately sees the most obvious; but he must always be conscious of the possibility of "not seeing the forest on account of the trees." Your ears are frequently of more value in arriving at a diagnosis than are your eyes and nose. A carefully elicited history is often the only thing that reveals the missing link needed to reach a conclusion on a diagnosis.

ACUTE INFECTIONS OF THE JAWS
Periapical abscess

The periapical abscess, commonly called an acute alveolar abscess, usually begins in the periapical region and usually is the result of a nonvital or degenerative pulp. It may occur almost immediately following injury to the pulpal tissues, or after a long period of trauma it may suddenly flare into an acute condition with the symptoms of acute infection such as pain, swelling, and systemic reactions.

Factors that cause some of these periapical lesions to suddenly become acute are not understood, although many theories have been advanced regarding this transition. The fact simply remains that a nonsymptomatic tooth today may cause extreme distress requiring definitive treatment by tomorrow.

Though the symptoms producing distress are often confined to the immediate region of the tooth, occasions arise when the toxins released from the infectious process produce a systemic reaction sufficient to render a patient generally ill. Periapical abscesses may confine themselves to the osseous structures and during the transitional periods of abscess formation may cause excruciating pain without any outward evidence of edema. However, just as many cases may start primarily in this manner, but the abscess finally burrows through the cancellous and cortical bone until it reaches the surface and invades the soft tissues in the form of either a subperiosteal or supraperiosteal abscess.

Prior to this actual abscess formation, however, the infection is capable of producing a general cellulitis in the tissues of the region involved (Fig. 11-1). Until it becomes well circumscribed and forms a true abscess the patient is usually in extreme discomfort. When an abscess invades the soft tissue, it is generally preceded by a period prior to abscess formation in which the cellular structures of that region appear dense and hard. During this period when the infection is infiltrating the soft tissues this hard, brawny condition is known as induration.

It is during the period of induration that all treatment should be directed toward

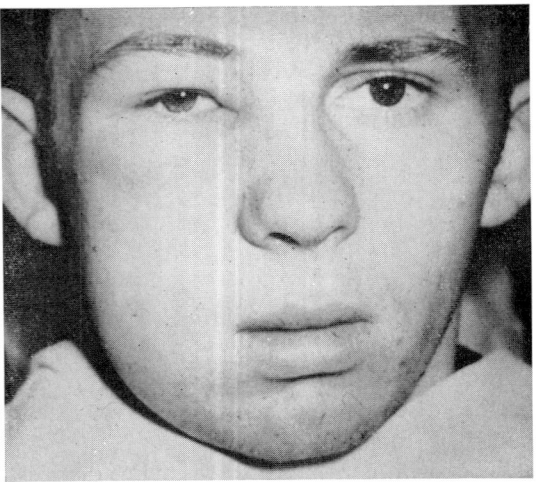

Fig. 11-1. Infraorbital cellulitis from infected tooth. (Walter Reed Army Hospital.)

localization of the infection and all efforts should be directed at confining the infection to the region of onset. This can be done by the use of warm compresses and the use of warm mouth rinses at frequent intervals. The primary objective at this time is localization. It is only when localization takes place that an abscess should be drained. Physiologically it is at this time that nature has thrown up a barrier around the abscess, walling it off from the general circulation and making it possible to palpate the presence of fluid purulent material within the abscess cavity. The deeper the abscess forms in the tissue, the more difficult it is to palpate.

An early decision should be made on the most desirable disposition of the tooth. The tooth in question should be studied and the pulp canal opened in an effort to quickly drain the periapical abscess through the root canal. If this fails to accomplish the desired relief, the decision to extract the tooth should be made. The sooner this is done, the quicker the symptoms may be expected to subside.

The philosophy of never extracting a tooth during an acute exacerbation of an abscess has long been abandoned. It should be realized that frequently the only route through which the abscess can be drained is through the alveolus from which the tooth is extracted. The alveolar bone in such cases is so dense and resistant to further penetration of the abscess that all of the infectious process is confined, increasing the symptoms until extraction is the only recourse. Under such circumstances pus is usually observed flowing from the alveolus immediately following the extraction. If the extraction is delayed under such circumstances, a later possibility exists of the infection being diffused into tissues remotely located from the original site with toxic systemic involvement and/or osteomyelitis.

When definitive action is indicated in the presence of acute infection, the patient should be protected by the administration of adequate doses of an antibiotic to ensure a rapid and sustained blood level. Multiple extractions or extensive surgery should be postponed until the remission of acute symptoms.

When an abscess has formed or is induced to localize and the infectious process invades the extra-alveolar tissues, it should be incised simultaneously with the extraction of the tooth. If the tooth is to be retained, the palpable abscess should be incised and drained simultaneously with the opening of the pulpal chamber. If a fluctuant localized abscess is palpable intraorally, then the choice of drainage incision should be at a point below the most fluctuant portion of the abscess if in the region of the maxillary or mandibular buccal vestibule. On the other hand, if the abscess should localize or point subperiosteally or supraperiosteally on the palate or on the lingual surface of the mandible, then the site of incision should be chosen in deference to the neurovascular structures found on these surfaces.

If the presence of important anatomical

structures becomes a hazard, then the incision should be made with a sharp scalpel through only the superficial tissues, followed by blunt dissection with a hemostat into the abscess cavity and down to the bony surface. With the hemostat closed, the point is forced through the incised surface into the abscess cavity and then opened and the aperture dilated to permit the installation of an adequate-sized drainage material. Small openings for the purpose of draining abscesses are entirely unsatisfactory and do not permit adequate drainage. A large opening for the drainage of most abscesses should permit the end of the gloved index finger to be admitted to the bony surface from which the abscess has emerged.

Pericoronal infections

A pericoronal infection may occur at any time throughout life. The most usual periods for a pericoronal type of infection to occur are during infancy, childhood, and young adulthood. Pericoronal infection in infancy is associated with the eruption period, at which time the supradental tissue involving the superior portion of the follicle and mucoperiosteum overlying it may become chronically inflamed and ultimately develop into an actual fluctuant abscess. Occasionally these abscesses may develop into a cellulitis, causing not only local but systemic reactions associated with high temperatures. When fluctuance can be visibly and digitally ascertained, incision and drainage followed by warm saline mouth rinses held over the area at frequent intervals usually gives prompt relief so that no further treatment is necessary. Similar conditions may occur at any time during the eruption period of permanent teeth and should be managed in the same manner.

The type of pericoronal infection less frequently encountered is the one that occurs in late adult life in an edentulous ridge. For some reason a tooth has failed to erupt and a denture has been constructed for the patient, either because the existence of the unerupted tooth was not known or in the belief that the tooth could remain asymptomatic in the edentulous jaw.

It is generally believed that the cause of the acute infection of such teeth is the result of pressure from the denture over a period of years. At the onset of a patient's wearing of dentures such embedded teeth are in all probability a sufficient distance from the surface to be unaffected by the pressure reaction from the denture. However, as time goes on, with the resultant resorption of the ridge, the embedded tooth is ultimately subjected to the inflammatory reaction of the denture pressure as a result of the resorption of the overlying bone between the tooth and the denture.

When an acute infection occurs under these circumstances, a different course of treatment is indicated. If a fluctuant abscess occurs overlying the crown of this embedded tooth, it should be incised and drained and a sufficient time allowed to pass for the acute condition to become subacute. At this later time surgical removal of the unerupted tooth is indicated.

The most common type of pericoronal infection is the one found around the

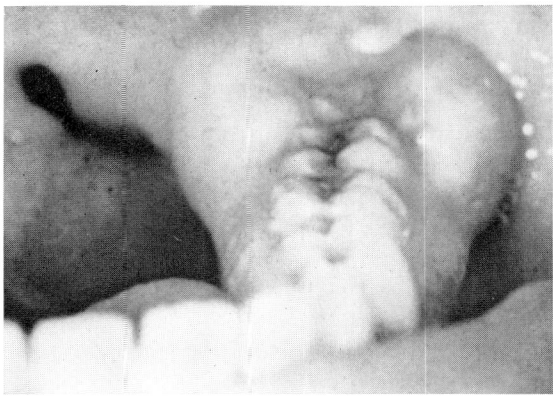

Fig. 11-2. Pericoronal abscess around third molar. (Walter Reed Army Hospital.)

mandibular third molar (Fig. 11-2). This occurs most frequently during the adolescent period of life. The symptoms accompanying this type of pericoronal infection are variable, and it is not unusual for patients to experience their only symptoms in the peritonsillar region. For this reason they seek the services of a physician, believing they have a sore throat or tonsillitis. The interesting aspect of this type of pericoronal infection is that they actually do have peritonsillar symptoms marked enough that visual symptoms lead to the diagnosis of peritonsillar abscess or streptococcal sore throat, for which the patient is not infrequently hospitalized and treated accordingly. Repetition of these symptoms may occur for several years before an unerupted third molar is finally diagnosed as the offender.

The most typical symptoms of pericoronal infection of the third molar are submandibular adenitis, trismus, pain in the region of the third molar, and a general condition of malaise not infrequently attended with a moderate elevation of temperature. These symptoms vary in degree from mild to extreme, to a point at which the patient may suffer extreme pain and may develop a cellulitis capable of producing difficulty in swallowing, extreme tenderness to palpation extraorally and intraorally, and edema visible both in the submandibular and pharyngeal regions. At a time when symptoms of this type occur, the tooth or one of the surfaces of the unerupted tooth is usually close to the surface. A visible surface of the tooth may be exposed to the oral cavity. The communication to the oral cavity may be so obscured by edema and the general inflammatory process that this communication may be ascertained only by the use of a rounded silver probe.

More frequently than not this communication permits the probe to be advanced along the buccal aspect of the unerupted tooth. Careful palpation with the probe permits entry into an expanded follicular space. After dilation of the aperture of entrance, the evacuation of pus and other septic material is made possible. If the aperture can be dilated sufficiently to permit drainage, the installation of a folded ¼-inch strip of rubber dam, ⅛-inch wide piece of rubber band, or ¼-inch strip of iodoform gauze immersed in an analgesic, antiseptic, therapeutic agent (equal parts of guaiacol and olive oil) into the aperture should induce continuous drainage and provide a suitable analgesic to relieve pain. The patient should be instructed to use warm saline mouthwashes for 5 minutes at intervals of every half hour until retiring. Antibiotic therapy is indicated immediately in sufficient dosage to assure a rapid, adequate blood level. This should obtain prompt relief from the acute symptoms, and as soon as a subacute condition exists, definitive treatment may be instituted.

Definitive treatment, of course, will depend upon the judgment on the final disposition of the unerupted tooth. If the third molar is impacted, surgical removal should be performed as soon as the symptoms become subacute. If the tooth is not impacted, but has been recurrently troublesome without eruption, and it is ascertained that insufficient room exists for adequate eruption space in the patient's mouth, then extraction is also indicated.

If, however, carious first and second molars are present, or molars that have been filled to such an extent that the pulps are in great jeopardy and early loss may be expected, then the third molar may be permitted to erupt in anticipation of its need as an abutment should the loss of the molar teeth anterior to it become necessary. If the latter course is decided upon, then an evaluation should be made of the persistence and recurrence of these unpleasant infectious episodes. Consideration should be given to an adequate excision of the overlying soft tissues, which by this time have become fibrotic as a result of the chronic inflammatory condition that has persisted.

If excision of the overlying tissues is decided upon, it should be done adequately. All of the overlying tissues should be thoroughly excised, and the occlusal portion of the unerupted tooth should be completely exposed. After excision has been completed the wound should be packed with a surgical dressing, which will harden. This should be allowed to remain at least 7 days.

The time for the employment of a definitive surgical procedure has been a controversial subject for a number of years; but since the advent of the chemotherapeutic and antibiotic era, patients can be protected from violent postoperative systemic reactions, acute cellulitis, and bone infection by the use of these therapeutic agents. Delay in the employment of definitive surgical procedures is believed to be a predisposing factor in permitting an osteomyelitic infection to become established. Consequently, discretion should be employed in the selection of a suitable time for definitive action. In the presence of acute, fulminating infection the author believes that primary incision and drainage is the method of choice, followed by an early definitive surgical treatment of the condition as soon as it becomes subacute, employing antibiotics simultaneously.

The maxillary third molar can be a contributing factor to pericoronal infections of an unerupted mandibular third molar. In the primary examination of a patient with a pericoronal infection of the mandibular third molar, it is imperative that we examine the region of the maxillary third molar to see whether or not it has erupted, whether it is in malocclusion, or whether it has elongated as a result of the delayed eruption of the mandibular third molar. It must be determined whether or not room is present in the patient's jaw, in the mandibular retromolar area, for the eruption of the mandibular third molar and if the presence of the maxillary third molar is a continuous source of trauma to the expanding tissue in the mandibular retromolar area during the eruption period of the mandibular third molar.

On occasion it is found desirable to retain the mandibular third molar even when recurrent infectious episodes persist from the traumatic influence of the erupted maxillary third molar. In such cases it is desirable to remove the maxillary third molar if its presence is a continual source of trauma. Pericoronal infections occur less frequently around an erupted or unerupted maxillary third molar, but when they do, the same procedure should be employed as the one described in the management of the mandibular third molar.

Dissecting subperiosteal abscess (Fig. 11-3, A). A certain type of subperiosteal infection may occur several weeks following an uneventful healing of a mandibular third molar wound. This may present itself primarily as an indurated swelling in the mucoperiosteal tissue as far forward as the first molar or second bicuspid. It may become progressively edematous and indurated and finally develop into a fluctuant, palpable, and visible subperiosteal abscess that has migrated from the original third molar wound beneath the periosteum to the point of fluctuance. When this is observed, antibiotic therapy should be employed immediately, and as soon as fluctuance is palpable the abscess should be incised and drained. This type of abscess may be visible and palpable as a swelling in the cheek in this region.

The drainage incision should start from the point of origin, which is the third molar region deep in the buccal vestibule, and extend anteriorly to the point of fluctuance. The incision should be made through the mucoperiosteum down to the bone. The tissues on either side of the incision should then be expanded by use of a hemostat and the wound, along the length of its entire course, packed open with iodoform

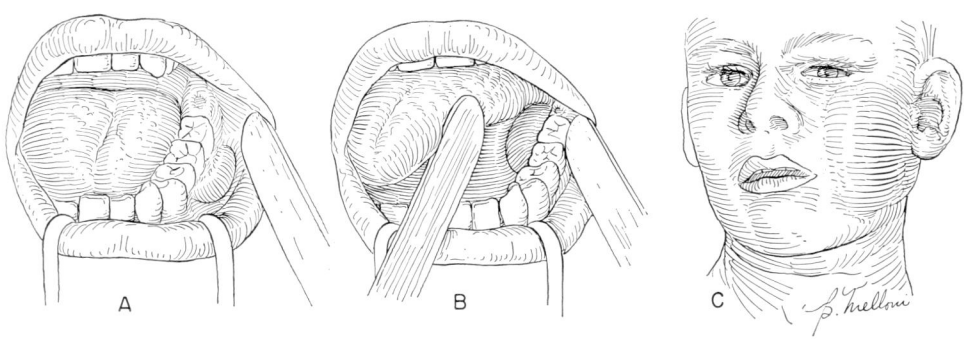

Fig. 11-3. **A,** Dissecting subperiosteal abscess. **B,** Medial mandibular angle postoperative abscess. **C,** Acute infected emphysema.

gauze impregnated with a suitable analgesic, antiseptic, lubricating agent (equal parts balsam of Peru and castor oil) or other suitable agent having similar properties. This type of packing material should not be changed daily, but should be allowed to remain, thereby keeping the wound expanded and permitting the purulent material to drain out around it. It should be observed at 48-hour intervals, and the dressing should be allowed to remain in place for at least 6 days. If the dressing is expelled from the wound during this period by action of the muscles of mastication, it should be replaced so that the wound remains saucerized and therefore will heal by granulating from the bottom.

Medial mandibular angle postoperative abscess (Fig. 11-3, *B*). A medial mandibular angle postsurgical abscess may occur several days following the surgical removal of a third molar. It is accompanied by extreme discomfort, trismus, and difficulty in swallowing. The symptoms become progressively worse until it is with great difficulty that the patient is able to open his mouth for adequate examination. Whenever symptoms of this type are present and no symptoms are visible on the facial or occlusal surface of the wound, one may suspect this lingual type of abscess. It therefore becomes necessary either by persuasion under adequate sedation or by force to open the mouth sufficiently to permit digital examination of the medial surface of the angle of the jaw.

At this point edema will be observed and an extremely tender bulging of the tissues. The pain is excessive. When fluctuance is determined, a small, curved, closed hemostat should be forced down through the wound of the third molar. It is introduced between the periosteum and the lingual surface of the bone, and, sliding along the bone, it is advanced inferiorly and posteriorly until an abscess cavity is encountered. At this point the hemostat should be opened widely to dilate the track through which the infection has descended into this region. If the diagnosis is correctly timed for definitive action, pus will immediately be seen emerging from the cavity following the withdrawal of the hemostat. A small, round-tipped Adson brain-type aspirator may now be inserted into the cavity to aspirate additional amounts of pus that may be present. A gentle compression of the soft tissue under the angle of the jaw may also expel pus through the intraoral aperture.

Following this, a ½-inch piece of folded rubber dam or a small Penrose drain may be inserted deep down into the region of the abscess, with the end protruding slightly into the third molar wound. Antibiotic therapy should be employed simultaneously.

Acute infected emphysema (Fig. 11-3, C). Acute infected emphysema is usually caused by the indiscreet use of air-pressure syringes or atomizing spray bottles activated by compressed air. In drying out a root canal with a compressed air syringe it is possible to force septic material through the apical foramen into the cancellous portion of the alveolar process and ultimately out through the nutrient foramina into adjacent soft tissues, with the ultimate formation of a septic cellulitis and emphysema.

A similar condition can be induced by the use of a compressed air spray bottle for irrigation of wounds, particularly in the retromolar region. If enough pressure is applied, it is possible to force air and septic materials through the fascial planes into the surgical spaces, which, after being forced open, remain in communication with this septic region. It is safer to use a hand-activated syringe when irrigating wounds or drying root canals since it is unlikely that an emphysema would be produced under these circumstances.

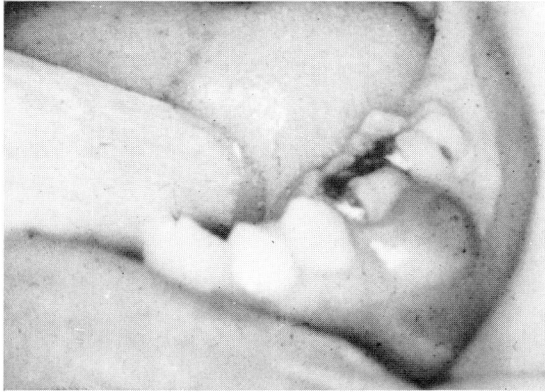

Fig. 11-4. Periodontal abscess.

Peridontal abscess

Acute periodontal abscesses (Fig. 11-4) are usually the culmination of a long period of chronic periodontitis. This type of infection usually starts in the gingival crevice at the surface and extends down one or more surfaces of the roots, frequently as far as the apical region. The acute episodes usually have a sudden onset with extreme pain and expansion of the periosteal and mucosal tissues overlying the surface of the infected root. For some unknown reason the tissues apparently seal themselves off at the gingival surface, impeding the drainage of the abscess and causing the ultimate distention and discomfort, which is usually the patient's first indication of this condition.

A periodontal abscess may or may not be associated with nonvital teeth or traumatic factors, either external or occlusal. It may, however, be induced by the traumatic influence of a partial denture. The primary treatment for relief of acute symptoms is incision of the fluctuant abscess from the bottom of the abscess cavity to the gingiva. The incision should extend through the soft tissues to the root surface, which has been previously denuded by the presence of the infectious process. If one or more surfaces of the root of such a tooth have been denuded to a point beyond the apical third of the tooth, extraction is indicated. If a third or more of the investing bone appears normal, then an evaluation of the potential usefulness of such a tooth should be made by a consideration of all the factors involved, including the general condition of the patient's health and his regenerative and resistance capacity.

Definitive treatment by debridement of root surface, removal of granulation tissue, and treatment for new attachment and tissue regeneration should be deferred until the infection has become subacute.

A lateral periodontal abscess is able to produce a subacute infection capable of diffusing from the original offending tooth through the alveolar bone to involve several teeth on either side of the offender, rendering them extremely mobile and tender. Frequently this can baffle the most astute diagnostician and make the identification of the primary offending tooth difficult. Radiographs are, of course, a primary aid to diagnosis. Frequently, however, the lateral surface of the root involved is so obscured by the tooth structure that a radiograph contributes nothing in the ultimate diagnosis.

ACUTE CELLULITIS

When infection invades tissues, it may remain localized if the defensive factors in the region are capable of walling off the infection and preventing it from spreading. In such cases a physiological barrier is formed around the nidus of infection, and it is either resolved and drained off in the lymphatic circulation or suppuration occurs, at which time surgical drainage is indicated.

Occasionally the bacterial infection is overwhelming, or the bacteria are either extremely virulent or resistant to antibiotic therapy. The resistance of the host tissues may be minimal, and bacterial invasion under these circumstances is unimpeded as it progresses through surrounding tissues to areas remote from the original site of infection. When physiological response fails to control the invasion of infection through anatomical barriers and therapeutic agents prove futile, then death ensues.

An acute cellulitis of dental origin usually is confined to the general area of the jaws. The tissues become grossly edematous and often hard in palpation. At this period the infection has not localized, and during this stage suppuration has not occurred.

The patient may show a severe systemic reaction to the infection. The temperature is usually elevated, the white cell count is increased, and the differential count may be altered in severe cases. The sedimentation rate is also usually increased, and the pulse rate is accelerated. The electrolyte balance is changed, and the patient frequently experiences malaise.

When the invasive process is overwhelmed by the physiological defense, the resolution is achieved. Frequently a specific antibiotic can complete resolution of the process, and either no pus is formed or the small amount present can be removed by the lymphatic circulation. Usually, however, a massive cellulitis will ultimately suppurate, particularly if the bacteria are staphylococci or other pus-producing organisms rather than streptococci. Since pus indicates localization of the infection, the old literature referred to it as "laudable pus."

Purulent material may burrow its way toward the surface, where it will evacuate spontaneously or be intercepted by surgical intervention (incision and drainage). Depending upon its location and the proximity of anatomical structures that guide its progress, pus may evacuate into the nose, maxillary sinus, oral vestibule, floor of the mouth, face, or the infratemporal fossa (Fig. 12-2). It can burrow into the cranial vault by bony resorption or it can go through the numerous foramina into the base of the skull.[1] Haymaker[2] reported cases in which fatal termination followed extension of infection into the cranium, usually by means of a bacteremia. Progress in this direction is difficult to diagnose, and neurological signs form the basis for such diagnosis. Every deep infection of long standing must be observed closely for such signs.

TREATMENT

Surgical evacuation of pus will eliminate the absorption of toxic products, thereby allowing the patient to recover. It will prevent further burrowing of the purulent mass in an attempt toward spontaneous evacuation. Antibiotics may control further infection, but they will not evacuate pus.

Acute infections of the oral cavity 175

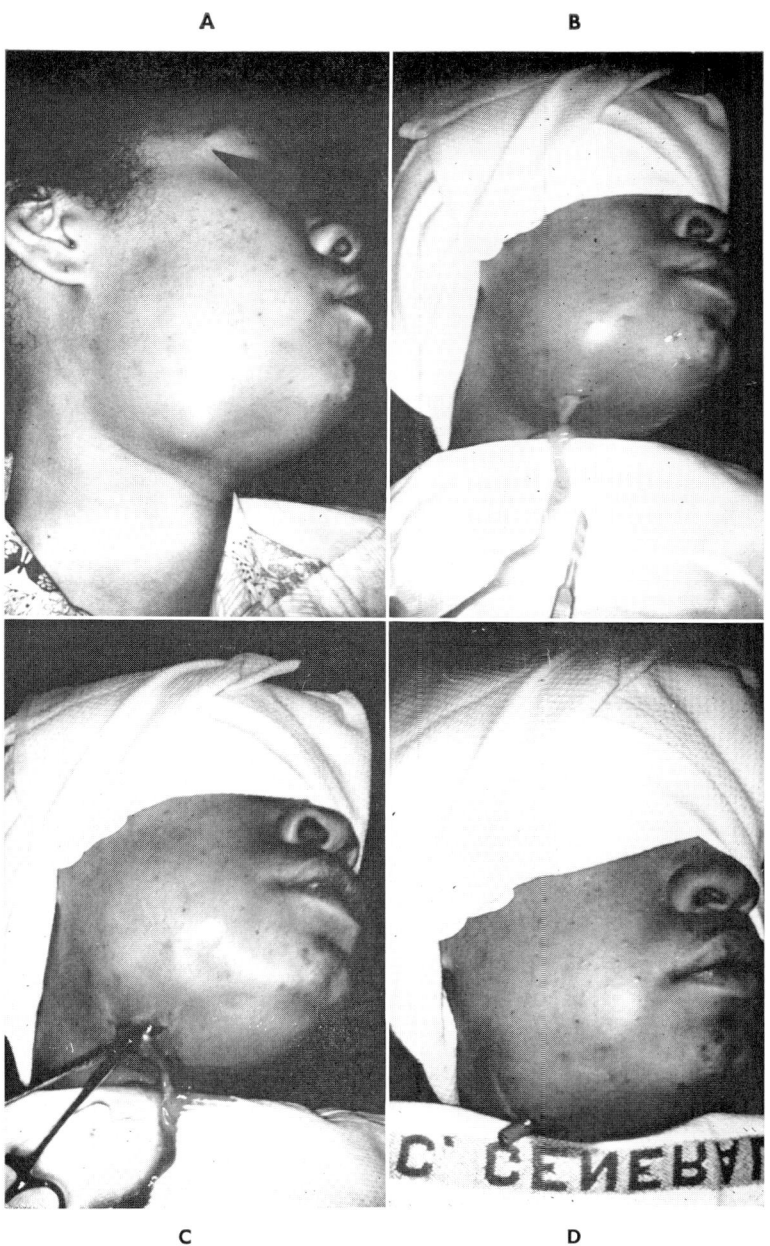

Fig. 11-5. **A,** Fluctuant cellulitis. Note shiny area (which is red), indicating that the abscess is ready for incision. **B,** Incision. **C,** Hemostat opened in abscess cavity. **D,** Rubber tube affixed in wound by skin suture to maintain drainage. (Courtesy Dr. Arthur Merril.)

The optimum time for incision and drainage may be difficult to determine. No difficulty in timing is encountered when a large cellulitis develops a superficial erythematous spot, which is pathognomonic of pus near the surface. Bimanual palpation will reveal a body of fluid material. One finger pressing down on one side of the mass will convey a fluid movement to a finger placed on the other side of the mass. This mass should be incised immediately and a drain inserted. When no superficial red spot is present, fluctuance is more difficult to determine, particularly if deep pus is suspected, and the palpation must be accomplished through superficial indurated tissues. Incision into an unlocalized cellulitis in an erroneous search for pus can disrupt the physiological barriers and cause diffusion and extension of the infection.

It is often difficult to determine by manual palpation the presence or localization of fluid. Under such indefinite circumstances, aspiration may prove a valuable diagnostic aid. Needle aspiration may be used as a diagnostic aid or to evacuate deep fluctuant areas. A large 13- to 16-gauge needle is used to penetrate the area after the superficial skin or mucosa is properly prepared. Pus is aspirated into a glass Luer-Lok syringe. The pus is sent to the laboratory for culture and antibiotic sensitivity tests. Successful early evacuation of deep pus will circumvent days and perhaps weeks of treatment. This procedure is primarily used for diagnostic purposes.

Surgical incision and drainage is performed when the presence of pus is diagnosed (Fig. 11-5). Surgical drainage of deep fascial spaces is usually done in the hospital under general anesthesia. However, large fluctuant masses can be incised for an ambulatory clinic or office patient under either general or local anesthesia. The skin is prepared in an aseptic manner, and the prepared area is draped with sterile towels. If local anesthesia is used, a ring block of peripheral skin wheals is made for skin anesthesia. No attempt is made to make a deep injection. The knife is introduced into the most inferior portion of the fluctuant area. A small hemostat is introduced into the wound in closed position and then opened in several directions when introduced into the abscess cavity. A rubber drain is placed in the deepest portion of the wound so that ½ inch remains above the skin surface. This is sutured in place, and a large dressing is applied.

In areas involving considerably more infection a through-and-through Penrose drain is introduced. A skin incision is made near the anterior extension of the mass. A large Kelly clamp is used to traverse the fluctuant area to its posterior border. Another skin incision is made over the emerging point of the clamp. The rubber drain is placed in the jaws of the clamp, which is withdrawn to the primary incision, leaving the drain in the tissue tunnel. One inch of drain is left on each end outside of the tissue. A sterile safety pin is placed on each end of the drain so that it cannot be lost, and a heavy dressing is applied.

Fascial planes

Another problem of surgical evacuation of pus (after timing) is to determine its exact location and extent. The region of the jaws and mouth is well compartmented by fascial layers. Shapiro[3] states that "The fascial spaces are potential areas between layers of fascia. These areas are normally filled with loose connective tissue, which readily breaks down when invaded by infection."

Infection started in any area is automatically limited by tough fascial layers, although it may extend by lymphatic or blood vessel routes. The infection fills the immediate fascial space and is contained therein unless physiological factors cannot limit its activity. If the infection becomes massive, it breaks through a nearby fascial barrier into the next fascial space. It can be contained here, or it can erode through into contiguous spaces until it reaches the carotid space or the mediastinum, which is infrequent.

To understand and treat acute invasive infections it is necessary to have a thorough practical understanding of these anatomical routes.[4] A systematic survey of the various potential spaces will determine the extent of the infection, and from this knowledge and a knowledge of the optimum place of incision for the evacuation of each fascial space the location of the incision is determined (Fig. 11-6).

An excellent discussion of the fascial compartments of the head and neck in relation to dental infections, taken from an article by Solnitzky,[5] follows:

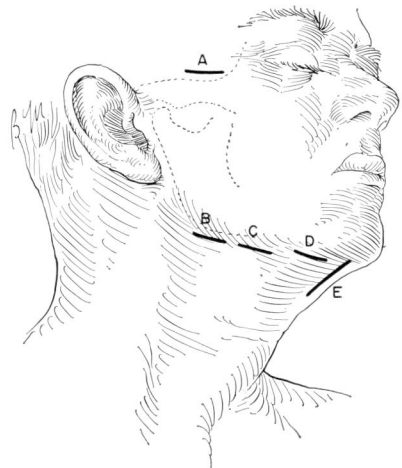

Fig. 11-6. Incisions for drainage of various fascial spaces. **A,** Temporal pouches. **B,** Masticator space. **C,** Submandibular space. **D,** Sublingual space. **E,** Submental space.

The most common dental sources of infection are infections of the lower molar teeth. Such infections tend to spread particularly to one of the following compartments: the masticator space, the submandibular space, the sublingual space and temporal pouches [Fig. 11-7]. Infections of the maxillary teeth are less frequent and tend to spread to the pterygopalatine and infratemporal fossae. In either case the spreading suppurative process may involve secondarily the parotid space and the lateral pharyngeal space. In fulminating cases the infection may spread through the visceral space into the mediastinum.

THE DEEP CERVICAL FASCIA

The deep cervical fascia consists of the following parts: (1) a superficial or investing layer;

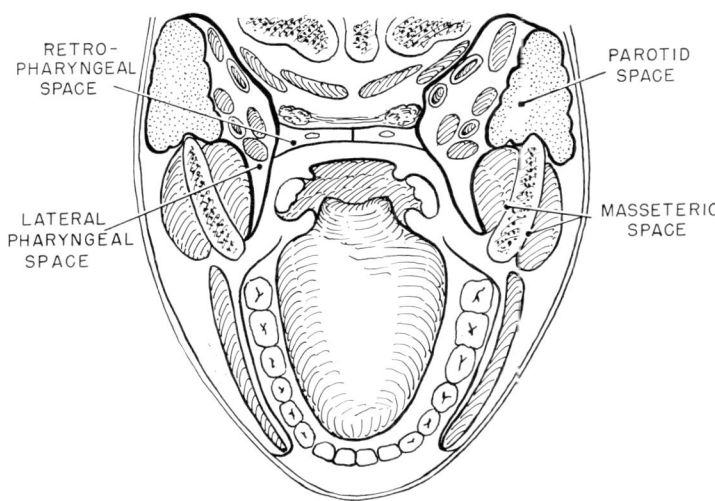

Fig. 11-7. Fascial spaces situated near the jaws. (Courtesy Dr. O. Solnitzky.)

(2) the carotid sheath; (3) the pretracheal layer; and (4) the prevertebral layer.

The superficial or investing layer surrounds the whole neck. It is attached above to the mandible, zygomatic arch, mastoid process, and the superior nuchal line of the occipital bone. Inferiorly it is attached to the spine of the scapula, the acromion, the clavicle, and the sternum. Anteriorly it blends with the same layer of the opposite side and is attached both to the symphysis menti and the hyoid bone. Posteriorly it is attached to the ligamentum nuchae and the spine of the seventh cervical vertebra. This layer splits to enclose two muscles; the sternocleidomastoid and trapezius; and two glands, the submandibular and parotid. It also splits above the manubrium sterni to form the suprasternal space. The investing layer is associated with three fascial compartments important in the spread of dental infections: the submandibular, the submental, and the parotid spaces.

The carotid sheath is a tubular sheath surrounding the common and internal carotid arteries, the internal jugular vein, and the vagus nerve. It blends with the investing layer where the latter splits to enclose the sternocleidomastoid. Near the base of the skull the carotid sheath is especially dense and is here also attached to the sheath of the styloid process.

The pretracheal layer extends across the neck from the carotid sheath of one side to that of the opposite side. It forms an investment for the thyroid gland. It is attached above to the thyroid and cricoid cartilages of the larynx. Inferiorly it continues into the thorax, where it becomes continuous with the fibrous pericardium.

The prevertebral layer lies in front of the vertebral column and the prevertebral muscles. Laterally it blends with the carotid sheath and also forms the fascial floor of the posterior triangle of the neck lying between the trapezius and the sternocleidomastoid muscles. Inferiorly it sends a tubular prolongation about the axillary vessels and the brachial plexus into the axilla.

Between the pretracheal and prevertebral layers is a large space, the visceral space, which is directly continuous with the mediastinum of the thorax. In the upper part of this space are the pharynx and the larynx; in the lower part are the esophagus and trachea, which of course are continued downward into the mediastium. This space can be reached by dental infections, with a resulting mediastinitis.

THE MASTICATOR SPACE

Anatomy. The masticator space includes the subperiosteal region of the mandible and a fascial sling containing the ramus of the mandible and the muscles of mastication. This space is actually formed by the splitting of the investing layer of the deep cervical fascia, the splitting occurring as the fascia becomes attached to the lower border of the mandible. The outer sheath of the fascia covers the external surface of the mandible, the masseter and temporal muscles, while the inner sheath covers the internal surface of the mandible and the medial and lateral pterygoid muscles. The fascial sling is not only attached to, but also reinforces, the periosteum of the mandible along its inferior border. Anterior to the masticator space the deep cervical fascia also helps to form the space for the body of the mandible. Hence the space of the body of the mandible and the masticator space are continuous with each other subperiosteally. Due to the fact that the mandibular periosteum is firmly attached inferiorly, infection follows the line of least resistance, which is posteriorly from the molar region into the masticator space. The firm periosteal attachment also prevents extension of infection inferiorly into the neck.

Posteriorly the masticator space is bounded by the parotid space laterally and the lateral pharyngeal space medially. Superiorly it is continuous with the superficial and deep temporal pouches.

Infections. Infections of the masticator space are practically always of dental origin, particularly the lower molar region. It is the masticator space that is involved in the well-known phlegmonous swelling of the lower jaw following dental extraction, which subsides within a few days without suppuration, the swelling resulting from an inflammatory reaction of the contents of the masticator space [Fig. 11-8].

It is important to remember, both from the standpoint of diagnosis and treatment as well as prognosis, that abscesses of the masticator space often simulate infection of the lateral pharyngeal space. As a matter of fact, abscess of the masticator space is not infrequently mistaken for abscess of the lateral pharyngeal space. It is very important to differentiate these two conditions since both the prognosis and treatment are different.

Infections of the masticator space have a great tendency toward localization. Unless properly drained such infections may spread to the superficial and deep temporal pouches, the parotid space, and even to the lateral pharyngeal space. Masticator space infections usually result from one of the following:

(1) Infections of the last two lower molars, especially the third molar
(2) Nonaseptic technique in local anesthesia of the inferior alveolar nerve
(3) Trauma to the mandible: external, or fracture into the socket of diseased third molar

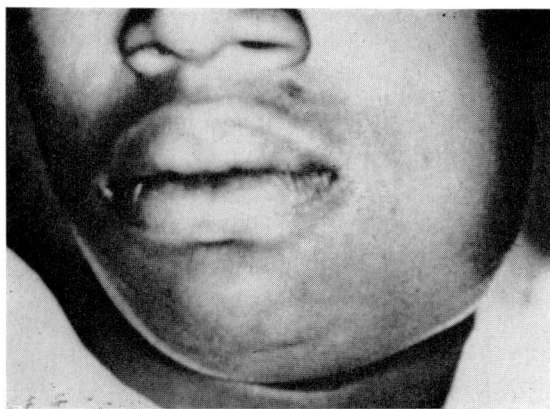

Fig. 11-8. Masticator space infection. (Walter Reed Army Hospital.)

Pathologically, infection of the masticator space is characterized by mandibular subperiosteal abscess and cellulitis of the mandible. The masseter and medial pterygoid may also be involved. If the abscess lies more anteriorly, it may involve also the body of the mandible. In some cases osteomyelitis of the ramus of the mandible may set in, particularly if proper drainage of the abscess is not instituted in time.

Clinically the picture of masticator space infection is dominated by trismus, pain, and swelling occurring within a few hours following a molar extraction or trauma to the mandible. The clinical signs increase rapidly to reach a peak in 3 to 7 days. The trismus is likely to be particularly severe because of irritation of both the masseter and internal pterygoid. It may be so intense that the incisors can be opened only to the extent of about half a centimeter. The pain may be excruciating and radiate to the ear. While some rise in temperature is present, chills do not occur as a rule. Dysphagia may be present.

The swelling associated with masticator space infections may be internal, external, or both. As a rule the swelling is both external and internal. The external swelling consists of a brawny induration over the ramus and angle of the mandible. The swelling may extend below the mandible and cross the midline to the opposite side. The subangular space is usually at least partially obliterated to palpation. At the same time constant tenderness occurs along the ramus of the mandible and in the subangular space. In the case of external swelling the mandibular subperiosteal abscess has reached the masseter along the lateral border of the mandible. Internal swelling may predominate in some cases. Such swelling involves the sublingual region and the pharyngeal wall. The pharyngeal swelling pushes the palatine tonsil toward the midline. However, the lateral pharyngeal wall behind the palatine tonsil is not swollen. This feature is important in differentiating a masticator space infection from an infection of the lateral pharyngeal space. In the latter the lateral pharyngeal wall is swollen also behind the palatine tonsil. The pharyngeal swelling in masticator space infection is somewhat lower and more anterior than in lateral pharyngeal or peritonsillar infections. The sublingual region adjacent to the involved portion of the mandible is also swollen and prevents satisfactory depression of the posterior portion of the tongue. The sublingual swelling may give the impression that the condition is a beginning Ludwig's angina.

Since masticator space infections tend to become localized, it is wisest to treat the condition conservatively for several days. If spontaneous drainage has not occurred, surgical drainage should be employed. Spontaneous drainage is apt to occur if the swelling is exclusively or predominantly internal and if dysphagia is a prominent symptom. Spontaneous intraoral drainage when it occurs usually takes place between the fourth and eighth day. The point of spontaneous drainage is consistently from the lingual border of the mandible near the base of the tongue. Chemotherapy alone is of no avail in the presence of a suppurative process.

The surgical approaches to the masticator space are both internal and external. The internal approach is not satisfactory except in cases where the swelling is exclusively internal.

The internal approach consists of an incision in the mucobuccal fold opposite the third molar, which is extended posteriorly to the ascending ramus of the mandible. The incision is made down to bone. A curved hemostat is then introduced into the incision and directed medial to the ramus into the masticator space behind the angle of the mandible.

The external surgical approach to the masticator space is essential if the swelling is external or both external and internal. The incision for drainage should be made just below and parallel to the angle of the mandible [Fig. 11-9]. As a result of brawny induration it may be difficult to determine the exact line for incision. Because of the swelling, the distance between the angle of the mandible and the skin may be greatly increased above normal. In any case the incision must be carried deeply until the bone is actually reached. Since the pus lies subperiosteally, it is imperative that the incision be carried through the periosteum to the bone. Through the external incision at the

180 *Textbook of oral surgery*

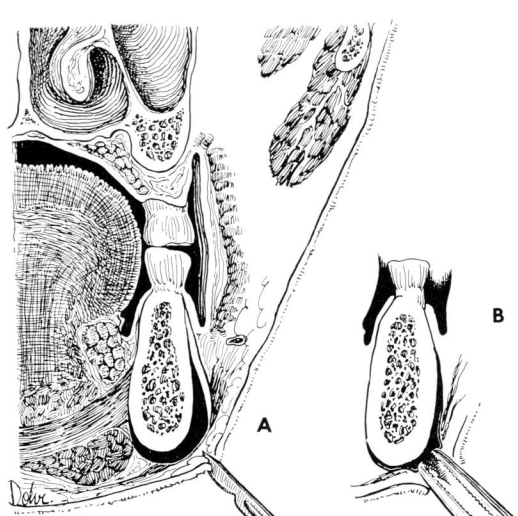

Fig. 11-9. **A**, External incision for drainage of pus in masticator space. **B**, After incision through skin and superficial fascia. A blunt dissection with hemostat is the safest method of avoiding important structures while advancing until bone is contacted for drainage of a subperiosteal abscess.

mandibular angle both the lateral as well as the medial aspects of the ramus of the mandible can be explored for pus.

If surgical drainage is postponed, osteomyelitis of the mandible is apt to occur. At the same time the danger is present of extension of the infection from the masticator space to the temporal pouches, parotid and lateral pharyngeal spaces. Osteomyelitis of the mandible may occur following curettage of the tooth sockets. In the presence of osteomyelitis, drainage may continue for months. It must also be remembered that osteomyelitis of the mandible may set in before the invasion of the masticator space becomes evident.

THE TEMPORAL POUCHES

Anatomy. The temporal pouches are fascial spaces in relation to the temporalis muscle. They are two in number: the superficial and deep [Fig. 11-10].

The superficial temporal pouch lies between the temporal fascia and the temporalis muscle. The temporal fascia consists of a very strong aponeurotic layer, which is attached above to the superior temporal line. Below, it splits into two layers, which are attached to the lateral and medial margins of the superior border of the zygomatic arch. The temporalis muscle arises from the whole of the temporal fossa. Its fibers pass downward, deep to the zygomatic arch, through the gap between

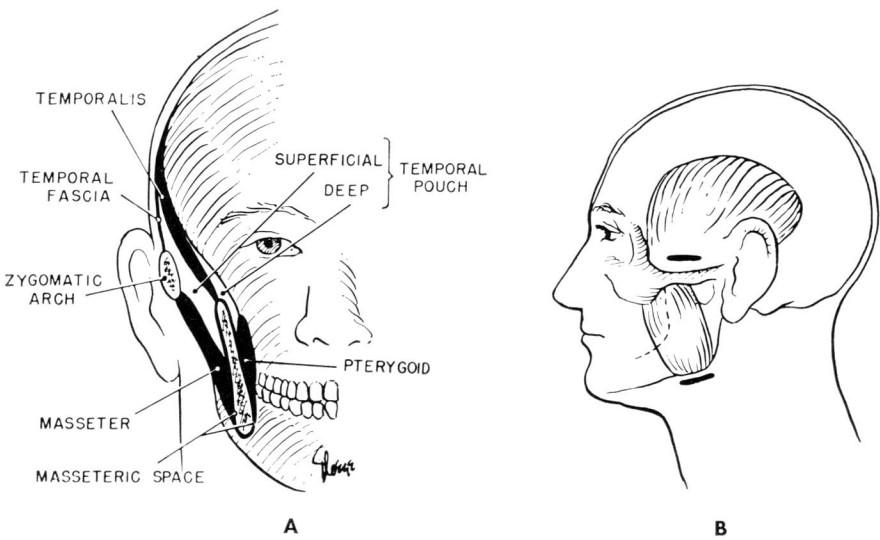

Fig. 11-10. **A**, The temporal pouches. **B**, Incisions for drainage of the temporal pouches and the masticator space. (Courtesy Dr. O. Solnitzky.)

the zygoma and the side of the skull, and insert into the coronoid process and ramus of the mandible. The deep temporal pouch lies deep to the temporalis muscle, between the latter and the skull. Below the level of the zygomatic arch the superficial and deep temporal pouches communicate directly with the infratemporal and pterygopalatine fossae.

Infections. Infections of the temporal pouches are usually secondary to primary involvement of the masticator, pterygopalatine, and infratemporal spaces.

Clinically, pain and trismus are present. Externally, swelling over the temporal region may or may not be apparent.

Surgical drainage of the temporal pouches is effected through an incision above the zygomatic arch, carried through skin, superficial fascia, and the temporal fascia. This incision reaches the superficial temporal pouch. To reach the deep temporal pouch the incision is then carried through the temporalis muscle.

THE SUBMANDIBULAR AND SUBLINGUAL SPACES

The term submandibular space includes the submandibular and submental spaces. Since these spaces communicate with each other, they will be described together.

Anatomy. The submental space lies in the midline between the symphysis menti and the hyoid bone [Fig. 11-11]. It is bounded laterally by the anterior belly of the digastricus. Its floor is formed by the mylohyoid muscle, while its roof is formed by the suprahyoid portion of the investing layer of the deep cervical fascia. In this space the anterior jugular veins originate. It also contains the submental lymph nodes that drain the median parts of the lower lip, tip of the tongue, and floor of the mouth.

The submandibular or digastric space lies lateral to the submental space [Fig. 11-12]. It is bounded posteroinferiorly by the stylohyoid muscle and the posterior belly of the digastricus, anteroinferiorly by the anterior belly of the digastricus, and above by the lower border of the mandible. Its floor is formed by the mylohyoid and the hyoglossus muscles. This space is enclosed by the investing layer of the deep cervical fascia, the superficial layer being attached to the inferior border of the mandible and the deep layer to the mylohyoid line. Elsewhere the two layers fuse around the periphery of the submandibular gland and become continuous with the fascia covering the mylohyoid and the anterior belly of the digastricus. The submandibular space contains as its major structure the superficial part of the submandibular gland, the deep portion of the gland continuing around the posterior border of the mylohyoid into the sublingual space. Deep to the gland is the facial artery, the nerve to the mylohyoid and the mylohyoid vessels. The facial artery gives off the following branches in this space: the ascending palatine, the tonsillar, the glandular, and the submental. Superficial to the gland is the facial vein. This space also contains the submandibular lymph nodes.

The sublingual space lies above the mylohyoid. Its roof is formed by the mucous membrane of the floor of the mouth. Laterally it is bounded by the inner surface of the body of the mandible

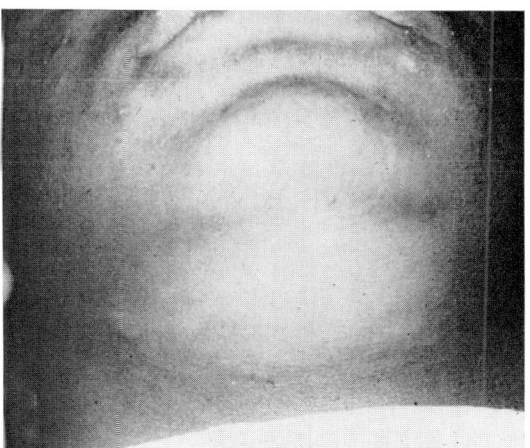

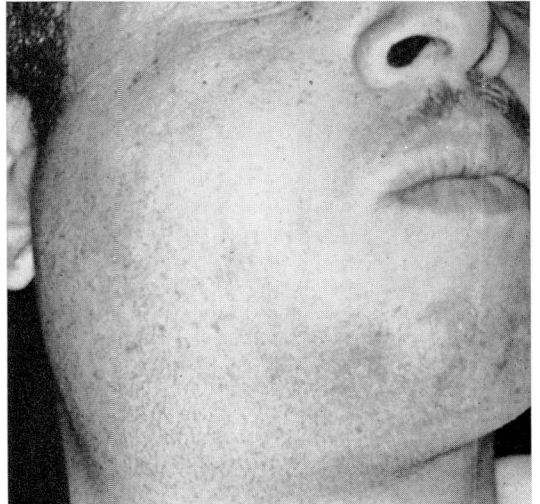

Fig. 11-11. **A,** Submental abscess. (Walter Reed Army Hospital.) **B,** Parotid space abscess. (Courtesy Dr. George Morin.)

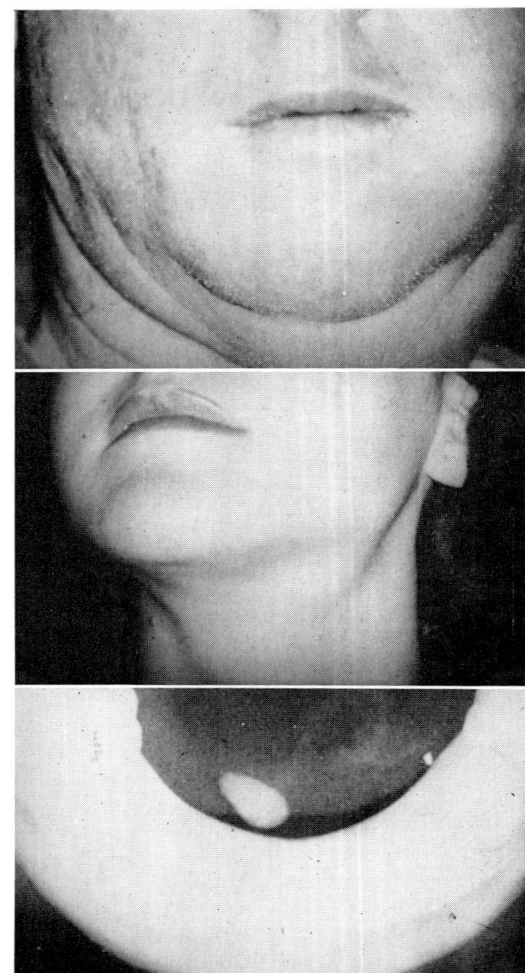

Fig. 11-12. A, Submandibular space abscess. B, Swelling of the submandibular salivary gland secondary to calculus in the duct. Salivary gland involvement must be differentiated from fascial space involvement. (Walter Reed Army Hospital.)

above the mylohyoid line. Medially it is limited by the geniohyoid and the genioglossus muscles. The floor is formed by the mylohyoid muscle. It contains the sublingual gland, the submandibular duct, the deep portion of the submandibular gland, the lingual and hypoglossal nerves, and the terminal branches of the lingual artery.

Infections. The most serious infection involving the sublingual, submandibular, and submental spaces is Ludwig's angina. . . .

THE LATERAL PHARYNGEAL SPACE

Anatomy. The lateral pharyngeal space is also known as the parapharyngeal space. . . . It is a deeply situated fascial space lying lateral to the pharynx and medial to the masticator, submandibular, and parotid spaces. It extends from the base of the skull to the level of the hyoid bone. It is bounded medially by the superior constrictor muscle of the pharynx, laterally by the mandible, medial pterygoid muscle, and retromandibular portion of the parotid gland, anteriorly by the pterygomandibular raphe, posteriorly by the apposition of the prevertebral and visceral layers of the deep cervical fascia, superiorly by the petrous portion of the temporal bone with the foramen lacerum and jugular foramen, and inferiorly by the attachment of the capsule of the submandibular gland to the sheaths of the stylohyoid muscle and posterior belly of the digastricus.

This space is subdivided into two compartments by the styloid process: an anterior and a posterior compartment. These two compartments are not completely separated from each other. However, infections can and do involve each compartment singly. Often the two compartments are involved simultaneously. The anterior compartment contains lymph nodes (part of the deep cervical group), the ascending pharyngeal and facial arteries, and loose areolar connective tissue. The posterior compartment contains the carotid sheath with the internal carotid artery, internal jugular vein, and vagus nerve as well as glossopharyngeal, accessory, and hypoglossal nerves and the cervical sympathetic trunk. No lymph nodes are found in the posterior compartment.

Infections. Infections of the lateral pharyngeal space are very serious and often are a direct threat to life. While this space is most often involved by infections of the palatine tonsil, mastoid air cells, parotid gland, the retropharyngeal space, and deep cervical lymph nodes, it may also be involved directly or indirectly by infections of dental origin. . . .

This space is most often involved in dental cases by the spread of infection from the masticator space.

Pathologically, most often infections of the lateral pharyngeal space are represented by abscesses. However, sometimes the infection is a rapidly spreading cellulitis similar to that of Ludwig's angina. Fortunately this latter pathological picture is not frequently seen.

The clinical picture is marked by a rapid onset following infections of the upper third molar, accompanied by a rapid rise in temperature. Chills occur if septicemia exists. Marked trismus is present from irritation of the internal pterygoid muscle as well as severe pain resulting from the great tension produced by the accumulation of pus between the internal pterygoid and the superior constrictor muscle of the pharynx. Dysphagia may be marked. Dyspnea, while not so prominent a feature as in Ludwig's angina, may be present.

If the infection is confined to the anterior compartment, external swelling occurs anterior to the sternocleidomastoid muscle. This swelling is first seen at the angle of the mandible and in the submandibular region. It may obliterate the angle of the mandible. The external swelling also extends upward over the parotid region. Internally the anterior part of the lateral pharyngeal wall is swollen and pushes the palatine tonsil together with the soft palate toward the midline. The trismus and pain are particularly severe in infections of the anterior compartments. On the other hand, usually no evidence of septicemia is present.

With infections of the posterior compartment the clinical picture is apt to be dominated by septicemia. Usually little or no trismus and little pain are present. External swelling is apt to be less extensive than with involvement of the anterior compartment. The internal swelling involves the lateral wall of the pharynx behind the palatopharyngeal arch.

As previously mentioned, the lateral pharyngeal space may be the site of a rapidly spreading cellulitis. The clinical picture is grave, being marked by evidence of septicemia and respiratory embarrassment due to edema of the larynx. Externally there is a brawny induration of the face above the angle of the mandible. This induration may extend downward to the submandibular region as well as upward to the parotid region and the ipsilateral eye.

The complications of lateral pharyngeal space infections are particularly serious, especially if the infection involves the posterior compartment. These complications include:

(1) Respiratory paralysis resulting from acute edema of larynx
(2) Thrombosis of the internal jugular vein
(3) Erosion of the internal carotid artery

Of these complications perhaps the most dramatic is erosion of the internal carotid artery. Occasionally the erosion may involve the ascending pharyngeal or facial arteries. Such hemorrhages may prove rapidly fatal unless heroic measures are promptly taken.

Since most infections of the lateral pharyngeal space, secondary to dental conditions, have a tendency to localization with abscess formation, it is wisest to wait for such localization before instituting surgical treatment. Prompt surgery is always indicated in the presence of septicemia or hemorrhage.

The surgical incision for drainage may be external or internal.

The external incision is to be preferred for easy access to the carotid arteries in case of hemorrhage. The incision is made along the anterior border of the sternocleidomastoid muscle, extending from below the angle of the mandible to the middle third of the submandibular gland. The fascia behind the submandibular gland is incised, and a curved hemostate is then introduced and carefully directed medially behind the mandible as well as superiorly and slightly posteriorly until the pus cavity is reached. A drain is then inserted.

The internal surgical approach is to be avoided as much as possible since in the presence of erosion of the internal carotid artery the resulting hemorrhage may be massive and uncontrollable. However, if no evidence of such a contingency is found, the internal approach consists of passing a curved hemostat through the pterygomandibular raphe along the surface of the mandible, medial to the medial pterygoid and just lateral to the superior constrictor of the pharynx. The instrument is then directed posteriorly into the pus pocket. . . .

Edema of the larynx is a complication that may arise with great suddenness with lateral pharyngeal space infections. Unless treated promptly by tracheostomy, the issue may be fatal. Hence preparations for immediate tracheostomy should always be made in the presence of such an infection.

THE PAROTID SPACE

Anatomy. The parotid space is a compartment formed by the splitting of the investing layer of the deep cervical fascia. It contains the parotid gland as well as extraglandular and intraglandular parotid lymph nodes. The fascia covering the external surface of the gland is very thick and sends septa into the interior of the gland, subdividing it into lobules. The internal layer of the fibrous capsule is thin and often incomplete superiorly where it may communicate with the lateral pharyngeal space. Posteriorly the parotid space is also in close relation with the middle and external ear. Inferiorly the fascia is reinforced, presenting a strong band called the stylomandibular ligament, which very effectively separates the parotid from the submandibular space.

Infections. While this space is not usually involved by infections of dental origin, sometimes dental infections may extend up the ramus of the mandible and invade it. This may occur particularly in improperly treated masticator space infections.

In the presence of infection in this space a

hard, smooth swelling occurs over the parotid region in front of and below the external ear. The swelling gradually becomes more intense. This may be accompanied by fever and chills. The swelling may extend over the entire side of the face with edema and closure of the eye on the affected side.

The surgical approach to the parotid space is made by an incison in front of the external ear, extending from the level of the zygoma to the angle of the mandible. The skin and subcutaneous fascia are reflected over the external surface of the gland. Since the parotid fascia is firmly attached to the skin, this reflection must be done carefully. After exposure of the gland transverse incisions are made into the gland superficially. The gland and abscess should then be opened by blunt dissection in a direction parallel to the branches of the facial nerve. However, since the branches of the facial nerve lie deep to the superficial part of the parotid gland, they are not very likely to be injured by this procedure. Drains are then inserted.

THE PTERYGOPALATINE AND INFRATEMPORAL FOSSAE

These two spaces are usually involved by infections of the upper molar teeth.

Anatomy. The pterygopalatine fossa lies behind the maxillary sinus, below the apex of the orbit, lateral to the muscular plate of the pterygoid process of the sphenoid bone and deep to the temporomandibular joint. The pterygopalatine fossa communicates with the infratemporal fossa through the pterygomaxillary fissure. At its upper end the pterygomaxillary fissure is continuous with the inferior orbital fissure, which leads from the pterygopalatine fossa into the orbit. The inferior orbital fissure contains the infraorbital nerve, the continuation of the maxillary nerve. The infraorbital nerve gives off the anterior and middle superior alveolar nerves, which pass through canals in the bony wall of the maxillary sinus to be distributed to the upper incisor, canine, and premolar teeth, and the mucous membrane of the upper gums. The pterygopalatine fossa also communicates with the pterygoid canal, which transmits the nerve of the pterygoid canal (Vidian). The Vidian nerve is made up of the great petrosal nerve from the facial, transmitting preganglionic parasympathetic fibers to the pterygopalatine ganglion, and the deep petrosal nerve conveying postganglionic sympathetic fibers from the superior cervical sympathetic ganglion by way of the internal carotid artery. The pterygopalatine fossa contains part of the maxillary nerve, the pterygopalatine ganglion, and the terminal part of the maxillary artery. Superiorly the pterygopalatine fossa is closely related to the abducens nerve and the optic nerve. Both of these nerves may become involved in infections of the pterygopalatine fossa.

The infratemporal fossa lies behind the ramus of the mandible below the level of the zygomatic arch. It is bounded medially by the lateral plate of the pterygoid process and the lateral wall of the pharynx, represented here by the upper part of the superior constrictor, and the auditory tube covered by the tensor veli palatini muscle. Posteriorly the fossa is limited by the parotid gland, which overlaps here into it. Anteriorly the infratemporal fossa is limited by the maxilla, superficial to which the fossa extends forward into the cheek superficial to the buccinator muscle. The buccal pad of fat plugs this space and extends for some distance between the buccinator and the ramus of the mandible. Superiorly the roof of the infratemporal fossa is formed, as far as the infratemporal crest, by the infratemporal surface of the greater wing of the sphenoid, perforated by the foramen ovale, which transmits the mandibular nerve, and the foramen spinosum, which transmits the middle meningeal artery. Lateral to the infratemporal crest the infratemporal fossa is continuous with the temporal pouches. Inferiorly the infratemporal fossa is continuous with the region deep to the body of the mandible that above the mylohyoid line forms part of the wall of the mouth and below the mylohyoid line constitutes part of the submandibular region.

Infections. Infections of the pterygopalatine and infratemporal fossae are comparatively rare.

Primary infections of these fossae usually result from:

(1) Infections of the molar teeth of the maxilla, especially the third molar
(2) Local infiltration of the maxillary nerve

Clinically, marked trismus and pain occur. Externally, swelling is evident in front of the external ear over the temporomandibular joint and the zygomatic arch. The swelling soon extends to the cheek. In severe and untreated cases the swelling involves the whole side of the face. The eye is closed and proptosed. Abducens paralysis may be present. The swelling may also extend into the neck. In such severe cases optic neuritis may also develop.

At the same time osteomyelitis of the maxilla may set in. The osteomyelitis is usually confined to the alveolar process. The osteomyelitis of the maxilla may lead to secondary involvement of the maxillary air sinus.

The pterygopalatine and infratemporal fossae may also become involved secondarily from infections of the masticator, parotid, and lateral pharyngeal spaces.

Infections of the pterygopalatine and infratemporal fossae have a great tendency to later abscess formation.

These spaces may be reached surgically by two approaches. The external approach consists of an incision made just above the zygomatic arch. The underlying fibers of the temporalis muscle are then spread and a curved hemostat is introduced and directed downward and medialward beneath the zygomatic arch into the abscess cavity. The internal approach consists of an incision made in the buccolabial fold lateral to the upper third molar. The incision is made down to, but not including, the periosteum of the maxilla. A curved hemostat is then introduced carefully behind the tuberosity of the maxilla and then directed medially and superiorly into the abscess cavity. A drain is then inserted.

Surgical drainage should not be delayed if sepsis is present.*

Ludwig's angina

Ludwig's angina may be described as an overwhelming, generalized septic cellulitis of the submandibular region (Fig. 11-13). Although not seen often, when it does occur it usually is an extension of infection from the mandibular molar teeth into the floor of the mouth since their roots lie below the attachment of the mylohyoid muscle. It is usually observed following extraction.

This infection differs from other types of postextraction cellulitis in several ways. First, it is characterized by a brawny induration. The tissues are boardlike and do not pit on pressure. No fluctuance is present. The tissues may become gangrenous, and when cut, they have a peculiar lifeless appearance. A sharp limitation is apparent between the involved tissues and the surrounding normal tissues.

Second, three fascial spaces are involved bilaterally: submandibular, submental, and sublingual spaces. If the involvement is not bilateral, the infection is not considered a Ludwig's angina.

---
*Reprinted with minor changes (approved by author) from Solnitzky, O.: Bull. Georgetown Univ. M. Center 7:86, 1954.

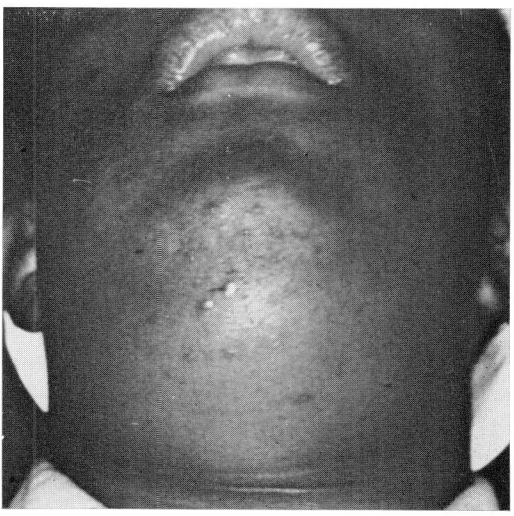

Fig. 11-13. Ludwig's angina. (Courtesy Dr. Arthur Merril.)

Third, the patient has a typical openmouthed appearance. The floor of the mouth is elevated and the tongue is protruded, making respiration difficult. Two large potential fascial spaces are at the base of the tongue, and either or both are involved. The deep space is located between the genioglossus and the geniohyoid muscles, and the superficial space is located between the geniohyoid and mylohyoid muscles. Each space is divided by a median septum. If the tongue is not elevated, the infection is not considered a true Ludwig's angina.

The infection is often caused by a hemolytic streptococcus, although the infection may be a mixture of aerobic and anaerobic organisms, which accounts for the presence of gas in the tissues. Chills, fever, increased salivation, stiffness in the tongue movements, and an inability to open the mouth herald the infection. Thickness is found in the floor of the mouth, and the tongue is elevated. The tissues of the neck become boardlike. The patient becomes toxic, and respiration becomes difficult. The larynx is edematous.

Treatment consists of massive antibiotic therapy. In the acute stage tracheostomy must be considered, and if the respiration becomes embarrassed, this procedure should be done to maintain an airway. If the signs do not change for the better in a matter of hours, surgical intervention is necessary for two reasons: the release of tissue tensions and the provision for drainage. Although in the classic case little pus is present, in other cases quite a bit is found, even though fluctuance cannot be palpated through the induration. The small pocket of pus is usually found not in the midline but near the medial aspect of the mandible on the side where the infection originated.

The radical surgical approach in acute cases takes the form of an incision under local anesthesia parallel and medial to the lower border of the mandible, which may be difficult to find. The incision is extended upward to the base of the tongue in the submandibular area. In the submental area the incision extends through the mylohyoid muscle to the mucous membranes of the mouth. The tissues are probed for a pus pocket. To obtain maximum release of tissue tension no attempt is made to suture.

Cavernous sinus thrombosis

Infections of the face can cause a septic thrombosis of the cavernous sinus that was almost always fatal before the advent of antibiotics. Furunculosis and infected nose hairs are frequent causes. Extractions of maxillary anterior teeth in the presence of acute infection and especially curettage of the sockets under such circumstances can cause this condition. The infection is usually staphylococcal. The antibiotic to which the organism is most susceptible is given in large doses. Occasionally the antibiotics will not adequately resolve the septic thrombus, and death ensues (Fig. 11-14).

The infected thrombus ascends in the veins against the usual venous flow. This is possible because of the anatomical variant of the absence of valves in the angular, facial, and ophthalmic veins.

The diagnosis of cavernous sinus thrombosis is made in the presence of the following six features, according to Eagleton[6]: (1) a known site of infection, (2) evidence of bloodstream infection, (3) early signs of venous obstruction in the retina, conjunctiva, or eyelid, (4) paresis of the third, fourth, and sixth cranial nerves, resulting from inflammatory edema, (5) abscess formation in the neighboring soft tissues, and (6) evidence of meningeal irritation.

Clinically one eye experiences early involvement. Later the other eye may be involved. Empirical antibiotic therapy followed by specific antibiotic therapy based

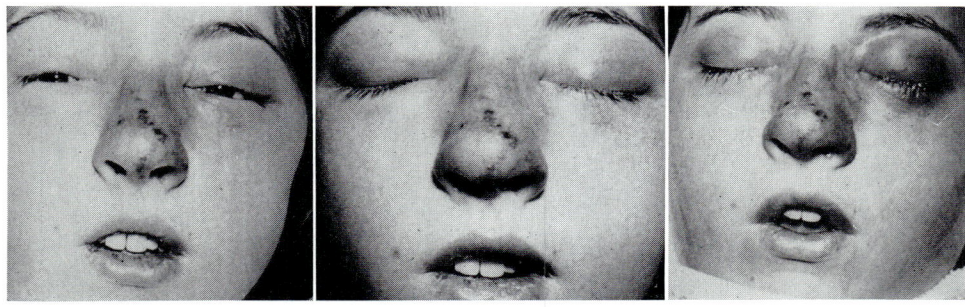

Fig. 11-14. Cavernous sinus thrombosis with fatal termination in spite of massive antibiotic therapy. (Courtesy Dr. I. D. Fagin.)

on blood or pus culture is the treatment. Surgical access through eye enucleation has been suggested.

GENERAL MANAGEMENT OF PATIENT WITH ACUTE INFECTION

The care of the patient with an acute infection is directed toward two ends—to destroy or inhibit the bacterial growth and to encourage the defense mechanism through active attention to the patient's physiological needs.

Immediate empirical use of an indicated antibiotic in adequate doses is the preferred treatment for bacterial infections unless contraindicated by a history of allergy.

In severe or fulminating infections blood should be drawn for a blood culture for later laboratory diagnosis, followed by immediate empirical antibiotic therapy after the blood is drawn. In general, the broad-spectrum antibiotics should be used for more specific treatment after bacteriological diagnosis and sensitivity tests have been made. If the patient does not respond within 48 hours to the drug that is used empirically, then in the average case increasing the dose of penicillin for 24 hours should be considered, or another drug may be tried empirically, although blood culture is often done at this time.

For hospitalized patients intravenous drip therapy may be used to produce high therapeutic levels of antibiotic drugs in short order and to maintain them effectively during the acute phase.

Patient care is important. Dehydration alone can account for a degree or two of increased temperature. Fluid in several forms should be continually urged upon the patient. In severe cases an input-output record is kept. Hospitalized patients benefit from intravenous fluid therapy and other aids to help them achieve an adequate fluid balance. Adequate nourishment is essential, in liquid or soft form if necessary. A laxative can be suggested if needed.

Complete rest is necessary. Analgesics and sedatives will relieve pain and anxiety.

The use of heat and cold applications has been predicated upon tradition. In general, moderate heat has been found to supply an analgesic effect and is beneficial in localizing infection.[7] Ice compresses applied intermittently for short intervals in an early postoperative period may inhibit the edema following traumatic operative procedures, but they have no other therapeutic value. Excessive or prolonged use of ice compresses may impede healing by inhibition of the normal defense processes, which function best at normal body temperature. When heat is used for therapy, it should be in the form of moist dressings. A washcloth placed under tap water as warm as the wrist can stand, wrung out, and folded in fourths is applied to the face, which has been protected from dehydration with cold cream. The face with washcloth is covered with a dry turkish towel and a hot-water bag placed over this. The compress is maintained for 30 minutes, removed for 30 minutes, and then reapplied. Flaxseed poultices hold the heat better.

OSTEOMYELITIS

Acute osteomyelitis occurs more frequently in the mandible than in the maxilla. It starts with an infection of the cancellous or medullary portion of the bone, which usually enters by way of a wound or an opening through the cortical plate of bone (for example, the alveolar socket), admitting an infection into the central structure. This infection may enter as a result of a periapical or pericoronal infection prior to any surgical intervention, or it may be introduced through a needle puncture, particularly if pressure methods have been employed or interosseous anesthesia has been a method of choice.

The infection may be localized or it may diffuse through the entire medullary structure of the mandible or maxilla, and it may be preceded by an acute infection. It can be preceded by septic cellulitis, or it can follow what was apparently a simple extraction of an infected tooth.

The onset of an osteomyelitis is evidently associated with the lack of resistance of an individual patient to the particular organisms that invade the osseous structure.[8] Prior to the advent of chemotherapeutic and antibiotic agents, osteomyelitic infection was not uncommon. It most frequently followed an invasion through a third molar wound. Since the employment of antibiotic therapy upon the first sign of septic postoperative sequelae, osteomyelitis is rarely seen. On infrequent occasions, however, this disease still occurs, and the use of antibiotics has but little impeding effect on its progress.

The symptoms include a deep persisting pain, occasionally accompanied by intermittent paresthesia of the lip. An edema of the overlying soft tissues and an accompanying periostitis is usually present. The patient may ultimately give evidence of malaise and an elevation in temperature. The condition may persist to a state at which the infection breaks through the cortical bone and invades the soft tissues, and induration followed by abscess formation becomes evident (Fig. 11-15).

Since wide variations in radiographic evidence or clinical symptoms occur, early diagnosis sometimes is quite difficult. The osteomyelitic process originates within the cancellous structure of the bone, and destruction of the cancellous structure takes place with much less resistance than that of the cortical bone. The cortical bone is very dense, and the destructive process may progress before it can be revealed in the radiograph because of the superimposition of the denser cortical bone. In the more aggressive or rampant types destruction may occur quite rapidly, and the cortical bone may be invaded so that radiographic evidence becomes visible at an early date. This destructive process has no definite pattern. A radiolucent area seen in the radiograph is often described as having a wormy appearance.

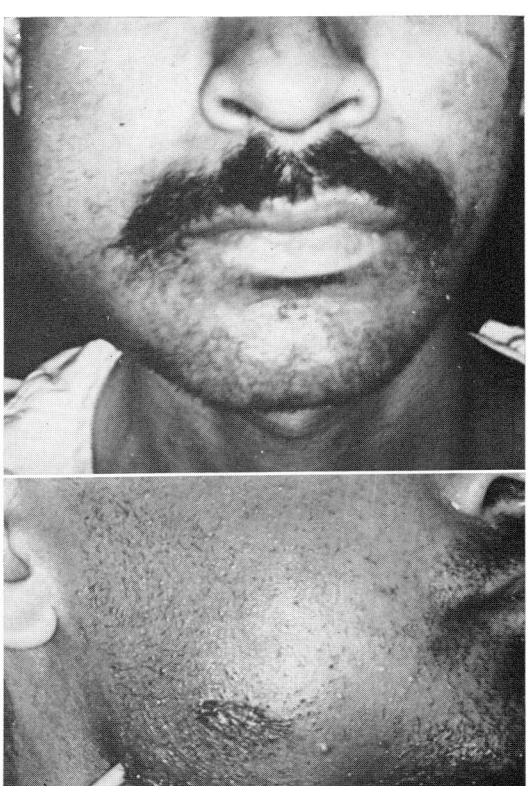

Fig. 11-15. A, Acute osteomyelitis. B, Drainage tube in position. The portion of the tube lying in the tissues is perforated by a series of holes for irrigation and drainage. (Courtesy Dr. Arthur Merril.)

In the invasive or rampant nonlocalized type all of the teeth in the section of the mandible or maxilla may become mobile or tender, and pus may be observed around the necks of the teeth and interproximal spaces. Multiple perforating sinuses may be draining pus into the oral vestibule or burrowing into the overlying musculature and forming abscesses, which, if not incised and drained, will spontaneously rupture to the surface. If this latter condition is permitted, an ugly, indented scar results.

Treatment. The earlier a diagnosis can be made and definitive treatment started, the greater is the opportunity of impeding the progress of the infection. Even before purulent material can be obtained for culture it is advisable to start with an antibiotic in high doses. Of course this may make it difficult to obtain a culture when suppuration begins, but time is the important factor, and the earlier antibiotic therapy can be started, the better is the chance of therapeutic control. As soon as it is possible to obtain a culture the antibiotic that the laboratory finds to be most efficacious may be given.

Edema and induration should be observed closely for the first indication of fluctuance so that at the earliest possible moment a liberal incision can be made down to the bony surface for the early evacuation of pus, thereby preventing the pus from elevating the periosteum. If induration extends beyond the limit of the incision after the primary drainage, then the incision should immediately be extended.

The destructiveness of osteomyelitis is caused by the pressure and lysis of suppurative material in a confined space. A staphylococcus is usually the cause. If the bacteria are killed or their growth is stopped by the antibiotic, resolution of the infection occurs without the need for surgery beyond the extraction of the etiological tooth (if the infection is odontogenic in origin). If the bacteria are resistant to all antibiotics (for example, a "hospital staphylococcus"), or if a massive collection of pus has formed before effective antibiotic therapy can be instituted, then portions of the bone become devitalized because their blood supply has been cut off by thrombosis of the vessels. The island of dead bone thus formed becomes a convenient place for precipitation of the ionized calcium that has been mobilized by the surrounding osteolytic process, and therefore this sequestrum appears as a radiopaque shadow on the radiograph (Fig. 11-16). Nature tends to expel the seques-

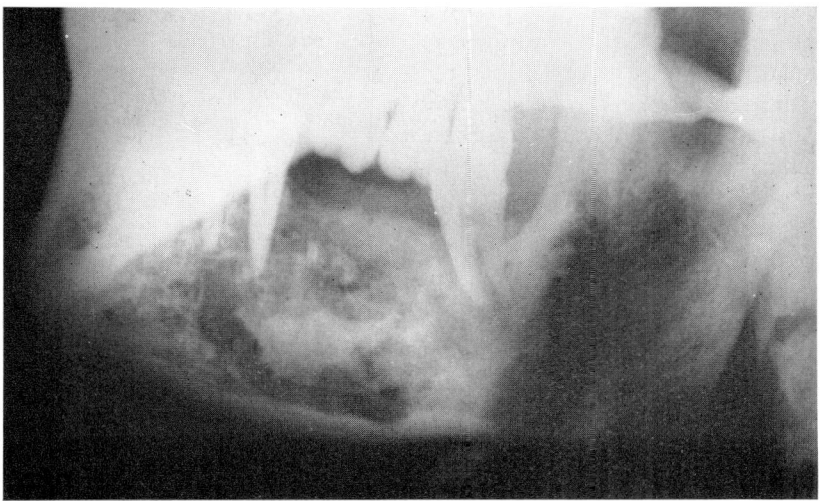

Fig. 11-16. Chronic osteomyelitis. Note sequestrum surrounded by radiolucent involucrum.

trum, although occasionally a small sequestrum is lysed during long, effective antibiotic therapy.

The pattern for treatment, then, is (1) effective antibiotic therapy, (2) drainage of purulent material if and when pus forms in spite of antibiotic therapy, (3) a period of supportive therapy during which the drainage area is kept open by dressings and the antibiotic therapy is continued, and (4) sequestrectomy.

The sequestrum should not be removed too early. It should be clearly outlined on the radiograph. If the infection has been controlled, the sequestrum is lifted gently out of its soft tissue bed, or involucrum. This bed is not curetted. Occasionally the overhanging margins of cortical bone are ronguered back to cortical bone that rests on intact medullary bone. This is called saucerization.

The treatment pattern can be interrupted at any of the four stages if normal healing occurs. The antibiotic should be continued for a minimum of 4 to 6 weeks after drainage has ceased.

If clinical and radiographic evidence of rampant invasion of the medullary structure of the bone is found and the cortical plate has not been perforated by the infectious process, holes may be drilled through the inferior border of the mandible to permit drainage of the cancellous structure. This latter procedure is controversial and depends upon the judgment and discretion of the surgeon who will have to evaluate the case according to its behavior pattern. The decision whether or not to extract excessively mobile teeth in the segment of the jaw where suppuration is visible around the gingiva is another point of controversy, one that requires the keenest discretion and judgment. Some of the most spectacular suppurative and rampant cases can apparently reach a crisis at which point symptoms will subside and regeneration begin without the extraction of mobile teeth. The etiological tooth, of course, is always extracted.

Drainage incisions for osteomyelitis have a tendency to proliferate large amounts of granulation tissue, which will expel artificial drains from the wounds. Unless retained with mattress sutures over the dressings, drainage gauze that is packed into the wound may become extruded. Suturing of the drainage material may be necessary to maintain its position so that the wound remains saucerized. This procedure pertains to both intraoral and extraoral wound dressings. I advocate the retention of dressings that maintain saucerization of the wound for intervals of 5 to 7 days without replacement unless clinical symptoms indicate intervention.

REFERENCES

1. Hollin, S. A., Hayashi, H., and Gross, S. W.: Intracranial abscesses of odontogenic origin, Oral Surg. 23:277, 1967.
2. Haymaker, W.: Fatal infections of the central nervous system and meninges after tooth extraction, Am. J. Orthodontics & Oral Surg. (Oral Surg. Sect.) 31:117, 1945.
3. Shapiro, H. H.: Applied anatomy of the head and neck, Philadelphia, 1947, J. B. Lippincott Co.
4. Spilka, C. J.: Pathways of dental infections, J. Oral Surg. 24:111, 1966.
5. Solnitzky, O.: The fascial compartments of the head and neck in relation to dental infections, Bull. Georgetown Univ. M. Center 7:86, 1954.
6. Eagleton, W. P.: Cavernous sinus thrombophlebitis and allied septic and traumatic lesions of the basal venous sinuses. A clinical study of blood stream infection, New York, 1926, The Macmillan Co.
7. Moose, S. M.: The rational therapeutic use of thermal agents with special reference to heat and cold, J. Amer. Dent. Ass. 24:185, 1937.
8. Killey, H. C., and Kay, L. W.: Acute osteomyelitis of the mandible, J. Int. Coll. Surg. 43:647, 1965.

Chapter 12

CHRONIC PERIAPICAL INFECTIONS

Leslie M. Fitzgerald and James A. O'Brien

When trauma or caries causes a tooth to die, the pulp cavity and canals become repositories for necrotic pulp tissue. This degenerating tissue (with or without bacteria) produces periapical irritation through the apical foramina. The body attempts to combat this irritation by an inflammatory response. If a virile organism is responsible for the infection, the process is likely to be acute. On the other hand, if the organism is not virile or if the irritation is produced by toxins of the necrotic pulp, the process is likely to be chronic. (See Fig. 12-1.)

TYPES OF CHRONIC PERIAPICAL INFECTION
Chronic alveolar abscess

An abscess, by definition, is a localized collection of pus in a cavity formed by the disintegration of tissues. The chronic alveolar abscess may be the aftermath of an acute periapical infection, or it may be produced by a chronic periapical infection. In either case periapical bone is destroyed by a localized osteomyelitis, and the resultant cavity is filled with pus. The inflammatory process walls off the area. If the chronic irritation continues, the abscess will expand until it drains itself by perforating the gingiva ("gumboil") or the skin (Fig. 12-2).

If the source of the irritant is removed, either by extraction of the tooth or by means of a root canal filling, the abscess cavity will drain itself and be replaced by granulation tissue, which then will form new bone.

Granuloma

A granuloma is, literally, a tumor made up of granulation tissue. However, the term dental granuloma is used to designate the situation in the periapical region in which an abscess or a localized area of osteolysis is replaced by granulation tissue.

The chronic irritation from the dental pulp has resulted in destruction of periapical bone. The body's attempt to repair the defect consists of an ingrowth of capillaries and immature connective tissue that, were it not for the continued irritation from the dental pulp, would rebuild the bone tissue. However, the continued irritation causes a mixture of this reparative tissue with the inflammatory exudate, and this makes up the dental granuloma.

Microscopically, the granuloma is made up of organizing connective tissue with numerous capillaries, with a fibrous capsule that has collagenous fibers running parallel to the periphery, and with evident inflammatory exudate (principally lymphocytes and plasma cells). The radiograph usually demonstrates a discrete, rounded lesion,

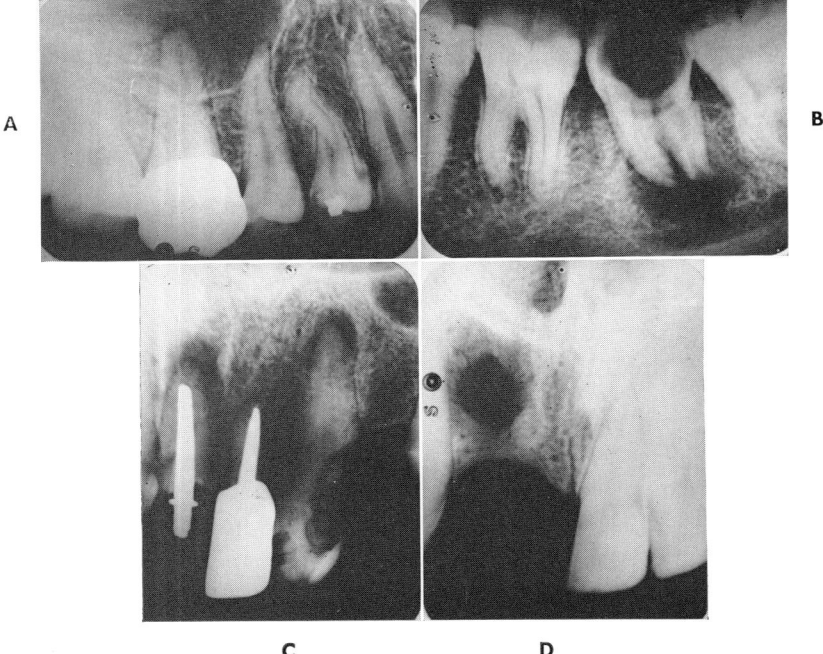

Fig. 12-1. **A,** Break in lamina dura at apex of lingual root, first molar. This disturbance can lead to an acute infection or grow slowly into a chronic lesion without an acute phase. **B,** Chronic alveolar abscess. The margins of the lesion are indistinct, the roots show slight resorption, and a condensing osteitis is demonstrated. **C,** Granuloma. The lesion on the cuspid, in particular, is rounded. Frequently the granuloma stays attached to the extracted tooth. **D,** Residual defect of bone following loss of both palatal and labial plates of bone through surgery or disease. In the absence of clinical symptoms this defect should not be reopened.

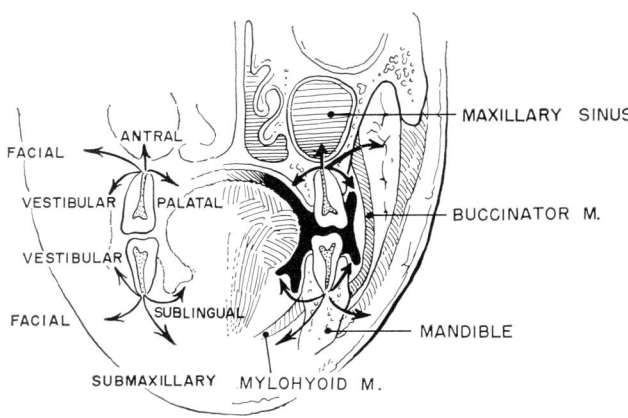

Fig. 12-2. Possible pathways for spontaneous eruption of pus from dental infections. Note that the buccinator and mylohyoid muscle attachments determine whether the pus will erupt intraorally or through the skin.

which is difficult, if not impossible, to differentiate from a cyst.

A granuloma may contain epithelial cell rests of Malassez. These cell rests have the potential to form a cyst if the granuloma remains in the bone, even if the tooth is removed.

Periapical cyst

A cyst is defined as a sac that contains a liquid or semisolid. The periapical cyst is an epithelium-lined sac containing liquid or semisolid inflammatory exudate and necrotic products. The periapical cyst is considered to originate from the dental granuloma. The epithelial cell rests of Malassez entrapped in the granuloma are stimulated to proliferate. A central area of breakdown forms, and the proliferating epithelium becomes an encapsulating membrane. Cellular disintegration within the cyst causes diffusion of additional fluid into the cystic cavity and resultant pressure. This increased pressure causes the peripheral bone to resorb and the cyst to enlarge. An inconstant radiographic finding is a radiopaque line around the cyst cavity (Fig. 12-3). The mechanism of cyst growth or the reason one cyst becomes larger than another is still not clearly understood. As a rule, the periapical cysts, which are always considered to be infected, do not grow as large as the follicular cysts, which are not infected unless contamination occurs.

A periapical lesion may be quite large without showing radiographic evidence of bone destruction. This is because osteolytic lesions in cancellous bone cannot be detected radiographically; it is only when a portion of cortical bone is destroyed that the radiograph demonstrates it.[1-3]

TREATMENT

Chronic periapical pathology may be subject to acute exacerbations. The treatment of the acute phase is similar to that for primary acute infections, described in Chapter 11. Chronic infections are complicated, however, by the presence of the original organized pathological lesion. Several working rules apply here.

1. If the patient is acutely ill, with elevated temperature, swelling, and malaise, it is desirable to establish a therapeutic antibiotic level for 4 to 6 hours before removing the responsible tooth. This allows

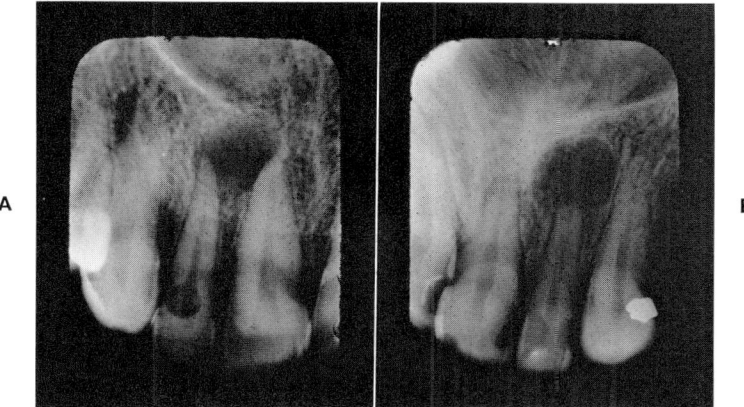

Fig. 12-3. A, Periapical cyst. No white line encircles it, and therefore it cannot be differentiated radiographically from a granuloma. B, Periapical cyst, well defined. (From Stafne, E. C.: Oral roentgenographic diagnosis, Philadelphia, 1958, W. B. Saunders Co.)

time for deposition of the antibiotic in the tissues. A concomitant incision and drainage may be necessary.

2. In the presence of acute infection the alveolar socket and the periapical area should not be curetted following extraction. To do so might disrupt the walling-off process of inflammation.

3. The periapical pathology should be curetted following tooth extraction if no acute infection is present.

4. If the radiograph demonstrates an area of periapical pathology and a root canal filling will be performed, this should be followed by curettage of the periapical area if it is suspected that the area is a cyst or if it will be impossible to follow the progress of the case postoperatively. The reasoning here is that if healing occurs promptly following endodontic therapy alone, periapical curettage is unnecessary. However, if the area cannot be reexamined by a radiograph in 3 months, it is wiser to do the periapical curettage at the time the root canal is filled and know that any cystic tissue is removed. Since periapical curettage is not a complicated procedure, many operators find it preferable to do the curettage (and apicoectomy, if necessary) at the same time the root canal is filled, even when no radiographic evidence indicates a cyst is likely.[4-7]

5. If the root canal is underfilled or overfilled, correction through a surgical window is made. The unfilled apical end of the canal acts as a breeding place for bacteria, and therefore it will continue as a source of irritation. Overfilling of the canal may produce a foreign body reaction in the area. If it is overfilled, the excess silver point or gutta percha is removed. If it is underfilled, an apicoectomy or a retrograde filling may be indicated.

6. If the root canal filling is accurately done, apicoectomy is not essential, but it often facilitates access for complete removal of any remnants of the periapical cyst or granuloma.

Technique of apicoectomy

1. Make a radiograph after the root canal filling has been completed to determine the level at which the root should be amputated. This level should be such as to remove any unfilled portion of root canal, and it should also facilitate access to the periapical cyst or granuloma to ensure its complete removal.

2. Design the mucoperiosteal flap with three considerations in mind (Fig. 12-4): (a) Be sure blood supply and tissue mass are adequate to avoid necrosis and poor healing. Incisions sharply made perpendicular to bone are important. (b) Make the

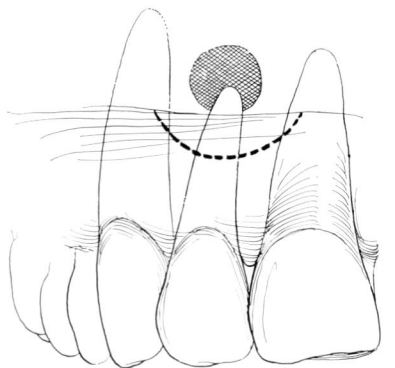
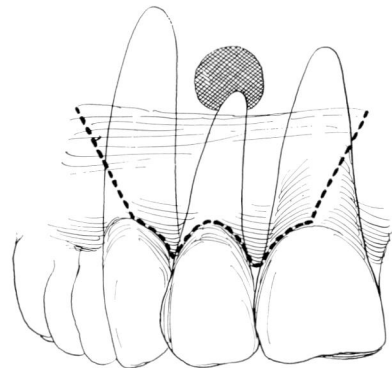

Fig. 12-4. Two types of incision for apicoectomy.

flap large enough to provide good access. (c) Make the flap extend well beyond the bony defect so that the soft tissue will be supported by bone when it is replaced.

3. After the mucoperiosteal flap has been raised, make an opening into the periapical bony defect, using a surgical bur or chisel if the granuloma or cyst has not already perforated the labial plate of bone. Extend the opening in the labial plate with bur, chisel, or rongeurs to obtain good access to the limits of the defect.

Then, using a fissured cylindrical bur, amputate the root at the level determined with the aid of the radiograph. The cyst or granuloma should be enucleated, preferably in toto, by means of small curets.

In the technique of retrofilling a root canal, the apex of the root is cut off on a bevel so as to provide access to the canal from the labial side.

4. Control hemorrhage within the defect by crushing bleeding points in bone, by pressure, or by Adrenalin-dipped cotton pledgets.

5. Suture the mucoperiosteal flap by using a small cutting needle with No. 4-0 silk or catgut.

6. After closing, maintain firm pressure over the area for 10 minutes to avoid formation of a hematoma.

7. Obtain an immediate postoperative radiograph for checking the level of root amputation and for future comparison.

Technique of removal of periapical cysts

Recognition of periapical cysts is dependent primarily upon radiographs and the vitality tester. A cardinal point is this—it is not a periapical cyst if the tooth is vital. If the tooth is vital, the periapical radiolucency has some other basis, and the fact that the root of a tooth lies within the apparent cyst is no indication for extracting it.

Two considerations are primary in the removal of periapical cysts:

1. Every remnant of the cyst must be removed or it may form a nidus for reformation of the cyst.

2. Damage to the roots of the adjacent teeth should be avoided.

If the tooth is extracted, the small periapical cyst usually can be enucleated through the socket. A small curet is inserted with the sharp edge against bone and the convex surface against cyst membrane (Fig. 12-5). By careful dissection the cyst can be separated from the bone and lifted out in toto. If it fails to come out intact, the wall of the defect must be curetted carefully to remove all remnants of the cyst.

For larger cysts the technique consists of

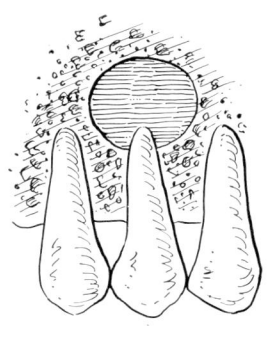 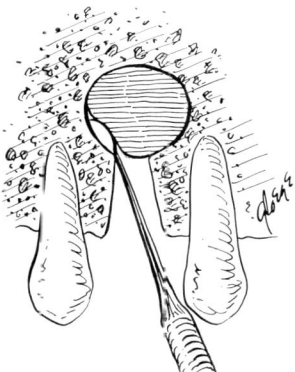

Fig. 12-5. The back of the curet is employed to remove a small periapical cyst through the socket.

raising a mucoperiosteal flap similar to the apicoectomy flap, removing the overlying bone by means of bur, chisels, or rongeurs, and enucleating the cyst by means of curets. Again, "shelling-out" a cyst is best accomplished by using the back side of the curet. That is, the concave side of the curet is toward bone and the convex side is against the cyst. In this way, the cyst is removed without tearing the cyst wall, and therefore the chance of leaving epithelial cells that might reproduce the cyst is lessened. After the cyst has been removed the mucoperiosteal flap is replaced and sutured, and pressure is maintained on the area for 10 minutes.

If a large periapical cyst is accessible and does not involve vital teeth or the maxillary sinus, it is usually best treated by enucleation. Primary closure of a large defect, however, can result in the accumulation of a pocket of necrotic material if the large, unsupported blood clot breaks down. Therefore, if the defect is more than 15 mm. in diameter, it is good practice to pack the void with petrolatum gauze (¼ or ½ inch) or Adaptic strip, bringing the end out through the line of closure. This packing prevents the accumulation of a pool of blood in the defect. The packing is removed after approximately 5 days.

When a large periapical cyst involves the roots of adjacent vital teeth or approximates the antral wall, treatment consists of exteriorizing the cyst, thus removing the central pressure that causes the expansion of the cyst. With this central pressure removed the periphery will slowly fill in, gradually decreasing the size of the defect. This process can be allowed to continue until the defect is obliterated, but this may take many months. The period of treatment can be shortened by enucleating the cyst after it has been reduced to a size that does not threaten the adjacent teeth and the antrum.

Two basic methods of exteriorizing a cyst are available:

1. The entire cyst can be unroofed. The epithelialized cystic membrane lining the cavity is then sutured to the mucosa immediately adjacent to it around the periphery. In effect the cyst wall is made a part of the oral mucosa. This is the Partsch procedure of marsupialization.

2. The other method of exteriorizing is based on the same principle, but differs in practice. Instead of removing the entire roof of the cystic cavity, a window is cut into the cavity. The fluid contents of the cyst are removed by aspiration. No attempt is made to remove the cyst wall. The cavity is then packed with iodoform gauze. The end of the gauze is brought out through the window in the mucoperiosteum. The iodoform gauze is removed after 5 days. Then an obturator is constructed to fit the window. The patient is instructed to remove the obturator daily and to irrigate the defect. Frequently the obturator can

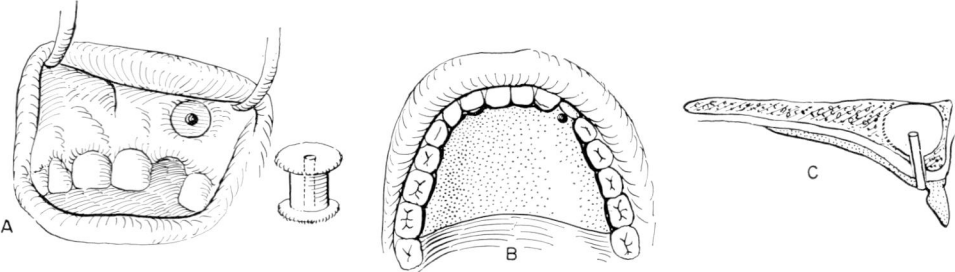

Fig. 12-6. Obturators used for exteriorizing a cyst. **A**, Acrylic button placed through labial wall. **B** and **C**, Plastic tube attached to acrylic partial denture, acting as obturator as well as prosthesis. See also Fig. 14-20, p. 233.

be constructed so that irrigation can be carried out with it in place. As the defect fills in it is necessary to reduce the size of the obturator periodically. A piece of rubber or plastic catheter or tubing makes a useful obturator; the external end is simply ligated to an adjacent tooth with wire. (See Fig. 12-6.)

Chronic periodontal infection

Someone has estimated that if the total area of actively suppurating granulation tissue in a generalized chronic case of periodontitis were placed in a single plane it would measure approximately 4 inches square. The person who ignores this amount of chronic infection in the mouth because it is not severely painful would certainly not ignore a similar patch of suppuration on the skin of his chest. Mastication massages the gingival tissues so that a demonstrable bacteremia is present after each meal. The continual introduction of bacteria, toxins, and suppurative material can have no beneficial effect, and perhaps the bacteria and their toxins can localize electively in an area of damaged tissue elsewhere to form one type of focal infection.

The removal of periodontally involved teeth ordinarily allows the surrounding tissues to heal. Several precautions should be observed. A small curet should be passed firmly down the root surfaces of the involved tooth before extraction to detach the tooth. The overlying tissue can be torn severely if the tooth is not separated from it. It is a good precaution to have the teeth scaled at least 7 days before extraction to eliminate the possibility of implanting crushed calculus in the wound during removal. This space of time allows the white blood count to return to its original level following manipulation. The surrounding alveolar bone is conserved as much as possible so that an alveolar ridge can be formed by the healing process. Isolated horizontal or vertical bony extensions can be removed to form an even ridge, and obviously wide alveolar sockets should be reduced for more comfortable healing, but conservatism should be paramount. If a question of judgment arises regarding alveoloplasty, the area can be allowed to heal without further surgery for 3 weeks. At that time the need for alveoloplasty, if present, will become more apparent, and it can be done then.

Removal of broken needles

In spite of all precautions a needle may break and disappear in the oral tissues. The removal of a broken needle may be a difficult procedure and should not be attempted unless the operator is thoroughly familiar with the technique and anatomy involved.

Location of the needle by means of radiographs made from several different angles is an important aid, particularly after insertion of another needle, which can be detached from the syringe and left in the tissues for purposes of orientation. The technique in locating the needle varies with the anatomical site, but one principle holds true for all—do not search in the direction that the needle was inserted but, rather, in a direction perpendicular to the direction of insertion. For example, if the needle was broken while blocking the mandibular nerve via an insertion near the pterygomandibular raphe, the incision for searching is not made at the site of insertion of the needle, but a vertical incision is made just medial to the anterior border of the ramus, and then the dissection is carried medially and posteriorly; that is, the needle is approached from a direction perpendicular to it (Fig. 12-7). If the anesthesia technique consisted of insertion immediately adjacent to the ramus rather than at the pterygomandibular raphe, the incision for searching should be made near the raphe, and the dissection then carried laterally. When the blade of the scalpel or blunt dissector comes in contact with the needle, it can be readily felt. The tissues are retracted to this depth, and when the needle comes into view it can be grasped with a hemo-

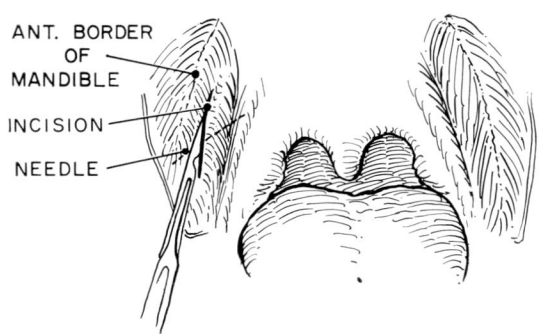

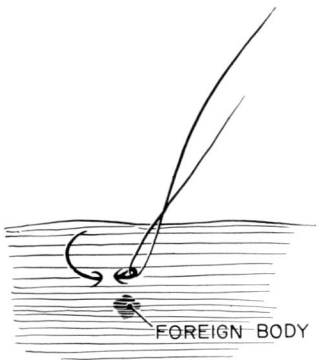

Fig. 12-7. Incision for removal of broken needle.

Fig. 12-8. Localization of a foreign body.

stat and removed. It is important in this procedure that good assistance be available so that it is unnecessary for the operator to look away from the operative site (for example, to pick up an instrument) once dissection has started.

The removal of a broken needle is not an acute surgical emergency. However, it is advisable to remove it as soon as possible to relieve the patient's anxiety. Actually, broken needles have been left in place permanently without complication, so failure to retrieve one is not a catastrophe.

The removal of other foreign bodies from the oral tissues presents problems in localization. If teeth are present in the area, localization is simply a matter of obtaining radiographs on which one can measure the distance from tooth to foreign body. In addition to the ordinary lateral radiograph a vertically directed view, such as an occlusal film, is often helpful.

Where no other landmarks are available for reference, a threaded suture needle can be placed through the mucosa in the approximate area (Fig. 12-8). After the radiographs have been taken the needle is pulled on through the tissues and the suture loosely tied to show the former position of the needle.

Once the foreign body has been localized on radiographs, its removal is exactly the same problem as the removal of a root tip.

A question of whether foreign bodies should be removed sometimes arises. If the patient is completely asymptomatic and no radiographic evidence of tissue reaction is found in the area, small fragments of amalgam and other metallic foreign bodies may be ignored. However, if pain or any other symptom appears that might be produced by the foreign body, removal is advised. In general, it is also good practice to remove any foreign body if a denture is to be placed over the area.

REFERENCES

1. Wuehrmann, A. H., and Manson-Hing, L. R.: Dental radiology, St. Louis, 1965, The C. V. Mosby Co., p. 264.
2. Bender, I. B., and Seltzer, B.: Roentgenographic and direct observation of experimental lesions in bone, J. Amer. Dent. Ass. 62:26, 1961.
3. Priebe, W. A., Lazansky, J. P., and Wuehrmann, A. H.: The value of the roentgenographic film in the differential diagnosis of periapical lesions, Oral Surg. 7:979, 1954.
4. Patterson, S. S., Shafer, W. G., and Healey, H. J.: Periapical lesions associated with endodontically treated teeth, J. Amer. Dent. Ass. 68:191, 1964.
5. Healey, H. J.: Endodontics, St. Louis, 1960, The C. V. Mosby Co.
6. Grossman, L. I.: Endodontic practice, ed. 5, Philadelphia, 1960, Lea & Febiger.
7. Sommer, R. F., Ostrander, F. D., and Crowley, M. C.: Clinical endodontics, ed. 2, Philadelphia, 1961, W. B. Saunders Co.

See also references of Chapter 14.

Chapter 13

HEMORRHAGE AND SHOCK

R. Quentin Royer

PREOPERATIVE EXAMINATION AND PREPARATION

The preoperative examination of the patient before oral surgery should include the taking of an adequate history, which may provide clues that the patient is a "bleeder." The patient should be asked whether he has ever had any episodes of bleeding, such as prolonged bleeding from cuts, sites of dental extraction, or other wounds. A history of unusual bleeding following childbirth or surgical procedures may be significant. The patient should be asked if he is currently taking anticoagulant drugs. The preoperative examination may reveal a state of significant hypertension, which can produce operative or postoperative bleeding problems.

If the history suggests a deficiency in the clotting mechanism, further investigation may be carried out. It is doubtful whether routine determination of bleeding or clotting time is necessary prior to minor oral surgical procedures. If the patient is currently taking Dicumarol or other anticoagulants, the prothrombin time should be determined. If the prothrombin time exceeds 30 seconds, postoperative bleeding may be a problem. The patient usually knows whether he suffers from hemophilia; if he does, great care must be exercised. The coagulation time must be determined in all patients suspected of having hemophilia. If an oral operation in the hemophiliac is imperative, preoperative and postoperative transfusion of AHG-positive blood should be carried out. Developments over the past few years have shown that certain blood fractions and certain agents are useful in the management of hemophiliacs. It is now possible by the use of these fractions and pharmaceutical agents to treat hemophiliacs without the dire outcome that has been noted in the past. Specifically, lyophylized plasma (Irradiated Human Antihemophilic Plasma) and cryoprecipitates rich in antihemophilic globulin[1] are used. Protein fractions of the blood that are necessary for coagulation may be deficient.[2] These include plasma thromboplastin antecedent and plasma thromboplastin coefficient. Laboratory tests that reveal such deficiency states are available. It is not within the realm of this chapter to discuss all the systemic diseases that contribute to prolonged bleeding. If such states are suspected, a competent internist should be consulted.

If major oral surgical procedures are contemplated, certain examinations should be carried out that will prepare the patient for transfusion if necessary. Blood typing, cross matching, and Rh determinations should be done.

ORAL HEMORRHAGE

The prevention, control, and treatment of oral hemorrhage require the constant attention of the dentist who engages in oral surgical procedures. The operative procedure itself can be conducted to diminish the necessity of treating postoperative bleeding. However, regardless of the attention given to control of hemorrhage during the operation, postoperative hemorrhage can occur, and the dentist must be able to control it. Proper measures locally applied will, at least temporarily, control nearly all hemorrhage of oral origin. However, in certain circumstances, such as those encountered in the surgical treatment of such telangiectatic lesions as hemangiomas or aneurysms, major vessels supplying arterial blood to the jaws must be ligated. Ligation of the external carotid artery is often necessary in major oral surgical procedures. Hollinshead[3] provides an excellent description of the surgical anatomy of the region of the external carotid artery.

Types of hemorrhage. Profuse oral hemorrhage can occur from various types of vessels that lie within either soft tissue or bone. Arterial hemorrhage is diagnosed by the bright red color of the blood as compared to the dark red color of venous blood. Arterial bleeding is characterized by its pumping, intermittent flow that corresponds to the contraction of the left ventricle of the heart. Blood flow from a severed vein exhibits a steady flow. Capillary hemorrhage evidences itself by a steady oozing of bright red blood. Oral surgeons occasionally encounter bleeding from a cavernous vascular bed, such as from a hemangioma.

Common sites of hemorrhage. The most severe hemorrhage of dentoalveolar origin is either from the inferior alveolar canal or

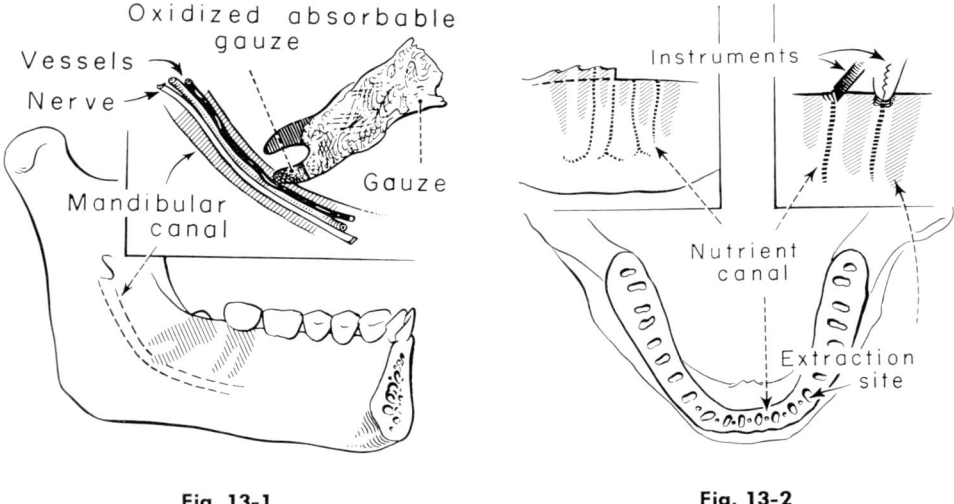

Fig. 13-1. Fig. 13-2.

Fig. 13-1. Proximity of the apical portions of the sockets of a mandibular third molar tooth to the mandibular canal. If one of the vessels contained in the canal is torn, oxidized cellulose (absorbable gauze) can be packed into the socket against the torn vessel. Pressure can be applied by means of an overlying sponge.

Fig. 13-2. Intrabony vessels in nutrient canals in the region of the mandibular incisors. Crushing, cauterization, or insertion of oxidized absorbable gauze into the severed ends of these canals will arrest bleeding. (See Fig. 13-3.)

from vessels of the palate. Usually the inferior alveolar vessels are encountered during surgical procedures in the vicinity of the mandibular third molar (Fig. 13-1). Large intrabony vessels are located in the interseptal bone between the mandibular incisors (Figs. 13-2 and 13-3). Profuse bleeding often is encountered as alveoloplasty is performed in this region.

Vessels of the palate, such as the greater and lesser palatine arteries and those of the incisive canal, sometimes are encountered when impacted maxillary canines are removed or when a pedicle flap from the palate is used to close an oroantral fistula (Fig. 13-4). Other operations on the palate, such as excision of torus palatinus, also predispose to bleeding from the palatal vessels.

Occasionally, profuse bleeding occurs when vessels of considerable size in the lingual mandibular periosteum are severed

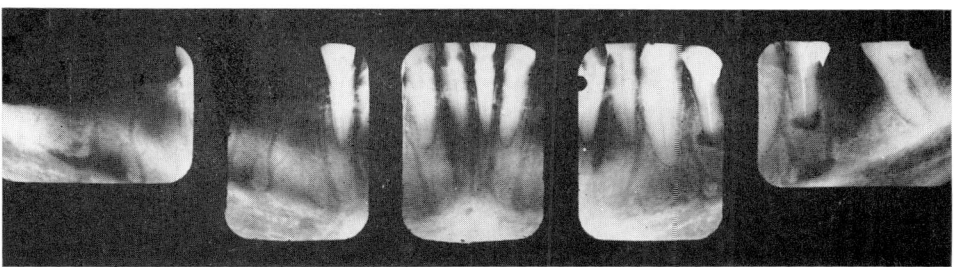

Fig. 13-3. Roentgenograms of the mandible show the presence of nutrient canals. (See Fig. 13-2.)

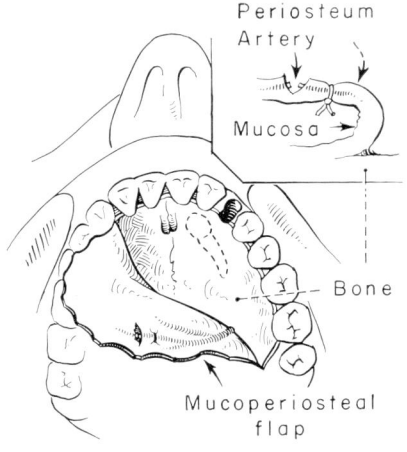

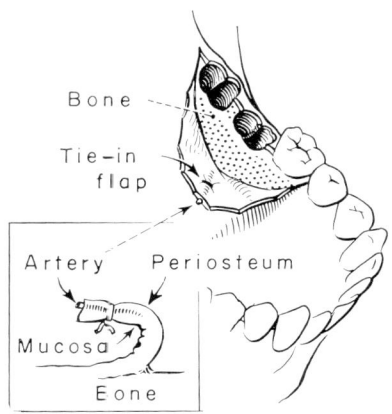

Fig. 13-4.   Fig. 13-5

Fig. 13-4. Vessels of the palate that can be severed during operations in this region. Ligation of the vessel by means of a "stick tie" through the entire mucoperiosteum will arrest bleeding.
Fig. 13-5. A vessel located in the mucoperiosteum covering the lingual surface of the mandibular alveolar ridge. The "stick-tie" method will arrest bleeding from a torn vessel in this region.

(Fig. 13-5). These are encountered when exostoses or bony irregularities are excised in these regions.

Occasionally a rather large artery is encountered on the flat, tablelike bone in the retromolar region of the mandible at its inner angle (Fig. 13-6). This vessel can be severed during the preparation of a mucoperiosteal flap when an impacted mandibular third molar is being uncovered.

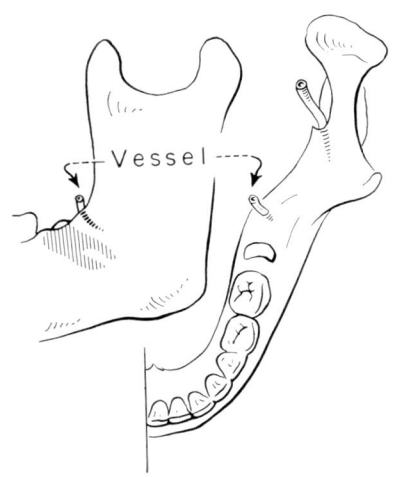

Fig. 13-6. An infrequently described intrabony vessel that often is severed during procedures in the retromolar region of the mandible.

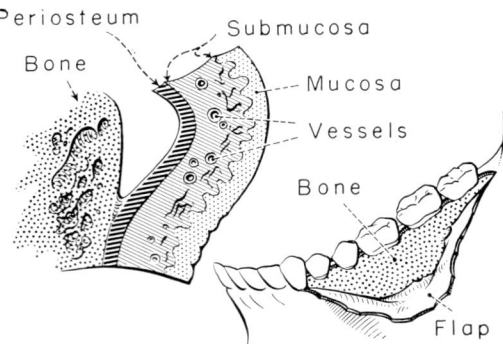

Fig. 13-7. The position of vessels within the mucoperiosteal flap. These vessels are not damaged if the periosteum is separated from the bone. If laceration occurs between mucosa and periosteum, ecchymosis will ensue.

Prevention or arrest of hemorrhage by surgical measures taken during operation. Clean and careful dissection will avoid postoperative hemorrhage in most instances. "Treat the tissues with loving kindness and they will heal in the same manner" is a maxim quoted by Berman.[4] This is true. Sharply prepared incisions and avoidance of tissue tears and fragmentation of bone are extremely important in this respect.

Proper preparation of mucoperiosteal flaps will reduce bleeding both during the operation and afterward. Incisions should be made through the entire mucosa and periosteum. As the flap is raised the periosteum should be lifted cleanly from the bone. Although the major vessels that supply the mucoperiosteum are small, they lie within the submucosa between the lamina propria and the periosteum (Fig. 13-7). If laceration of this layer occurs, more bleeding and ensuing ecchymosis will occur. If possible, incisions used in the preparation of oral mucoperiosteal flaps should be made through the "attached" gingiva—through that which overlies the alveolar bone near the crest of the ridge. The submucosal connective tissue in this region is composed of firm fibrous tissue, and postoperative ecchymosis will be minimal when these tissues are cut. The submucosal connective tissue that underlies

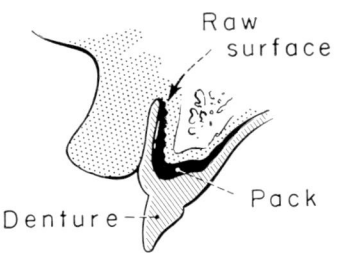

Fig. 13-8. Placement of denture containing a "pack" of modeling compound, zinc oxide cement, or soft, quick-curing acrylics upon a raw surface of the maxillary labial alveolus after excision of an epulis fissuratum.

the "unattached" mucosa found at the buccal sulcus is composed of soft areolar tissue. Incisions through the latter type of mucosa will inevitably be followed by submucosal bleeding, and ecchymosis will be evident. Thus, flaps should be prepared by stripping the mucoperiosteum away from the alveolar bone at the gingival crevice rather than by incisions through the unattached gingiva.

Extremely vascular soft tissue with an abundant supply of both medium-sized vessels and many capillaries often is encountered. For example, removal of an epulis fissuratum usually entails careful control of hemorrhage. The cut ends of larger vessels and capillaries can be cauterized. The application of pressure devices such as the placement of soft modeling compounds, zinc oxide cements, or soft, quick-curing acrylics within the denture is effective (Fig. 13-8). The denture can be inserted, and these materials as they harden serve as pressure agents to arrest bleeding.

Both the tongue and cheeks have a rich vascular supply. Operations on these structures, as well as on the floor of the mouth and the soft palate, entail the risk of gross hemorrhage. Bleeding vessels encountered within these structures can best be controlled by clamping and tying the vessel. The clamped vessel (Fig. 13-9) can be tied in a routine manner in many instances, but frequently the "stick-tie" method (Fig. 13-10) must be used because the severed vessel lies within a deep recess.

Roots of mandibular third molars, especially when impacted, often lie close to the inferior alveolar vessels. If these vessels are ruptured during removal of these teeth or roots, severe hemorrhage ensues. A gauze pack should be inserted immediately into the socket and pushed against the vessel with considerable pressure. The pack can be left in place for 5 minutes and then carefully withdrawn. One can proceed to another surgical site and complete

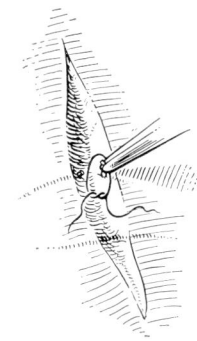

Fig. 13-9. Placement of a gut ligature around a clamped vessel.

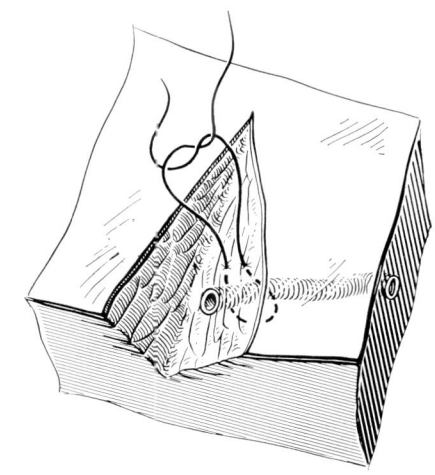

Fig. 13-10. Use of the "stick-tie" method of ligating a vessel that lies within a deep recess and cannot be clamped. The vessel and surrounding tissue are ligated.

it in the 5-minute interim and then return to the pack that has been originally placed upon the bleeding vessel. Frequently this controls the bleeding. If this procedure fails, a small portion of oxidized absorbable gauze (Oxycel or Hemopak) can be placed directly over the vessel and held there by pressure exerted against it and the vessel by means of a gauze pack placed and held as already described. The gauze may be removed in 5 minutes. If the oxi-

204 *Textbook of oral surgery*

dized absorbable gauze comes out with the gauze pack, a bit more may be added before closure of the wound.

Control of postoperative bleeding. Frequently the dentist is confronted with the problem of controlling postoperative bleeding. A well-organized, well-planned procedure carried out in a quiet, efficient manner is of utmost importance. Usually the patient appears with the mouth full of blood, and blood may be exuding from the mouth. He usually is excited and apprehensive, or he may be in shock. The first step is to assure him that the situation can be controlled and quickly place him in a comfortable, preferably a supine, position.

Proper equipment should be ready. The following must be at hand (Fig. 13-11): (1) light to illuminate the oral cavity, (2) adequate suction apparatus, (3) copious supply of gauze sponges, (4) cheek retractors, scissors, and hemostatic and gauze forceps, (5) sutures, (6) hemostatics, and (7) local anesthetic drug and syringes.

Isolation of bleeding site. First the mouth should be freed of all blood clots. This is done by wiping with gauze sponges and by aspiration. If bleeding is severe, it is frequently difficult to obtain this result because of the massive amount of blood that is constantly forthcoming. If so, one must quickly ascertain the exact location of the source of bleeding and place sponges that act as pressure packs over this region. By so doing, the remainder of the mouth can be freed of blood and saliva.

After the pressure packs have been in place for a few minutes, they can be carefully lifted and the type of bleeding determined.

The bleeding is usually from one of the sites already mentioned. The type of bleeding should be determined. Is the hemorrhage arterial, venous, or capillary in nature? Does it come from intrabony vessels or from soft tissue?

General care of patient. After the site of bleeding has been determined and pressure packs have been applied temporarily

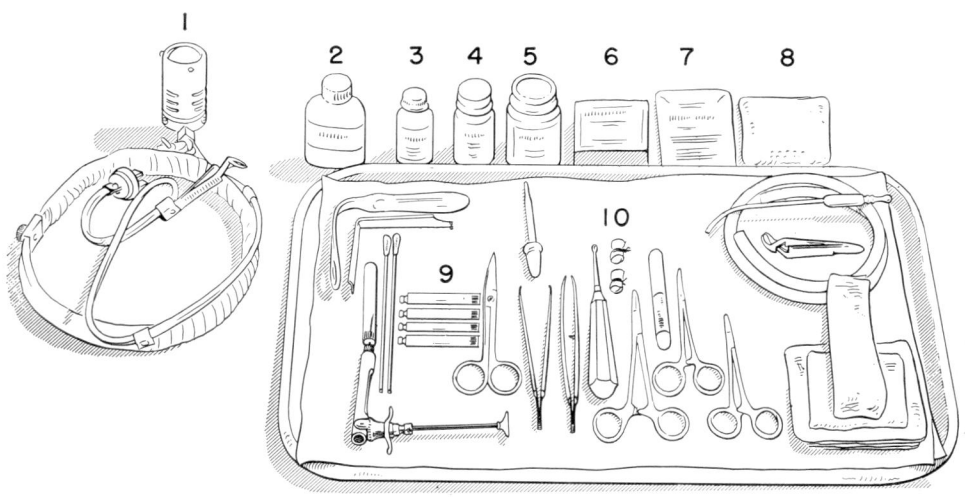

Fig. 13-11. Equipment used to control bleeding from the mouth and adjacent structures. **1,** Head light. **2,** Solution of ferric subsulfate (Monsel's solution). **3,** Solution of epinephrine hydrochloride (1:1,000). **4,** Oxidized cellulose (absorbable). **5,** Plain or iodoform gauze. **6,** Thrombin (topical). **7,** Absorbable gelatin sponge (Gelfoam). **8,** Gauze dressings. **9,** Carpules of local anesthetic solution. **10,** Silk or gut sutures.

to the site, attention must be directed immediately to diagnosis and to general care of the patient. This is especially so if signs of shock are present. The patient is observed for pallor, cold, sweating skin, rapid thready pulse, and diminished blood pressure. If the systolic pressure is less than 80 mm. of mercury, intravenous administration of fluids should be started. For further information on diagnosis and treatment of shock, consult the section on shock.

Measures to arrest flow of blood.* After the temporary arrest of hemorrhage and the general care of the patient, attention should be directed to the permanent control of bleeding.

To facilitate the surgical procedure for the arrest of oral hemorrhage, whether it be packing, tying, or suturing, it is well to anesthetize the region with a local anesthetic agent. Otherwise the pain of such procedures frequently is so severe that adequate measures cannot be carried out. If bleeding is from soft tissue and is either arterial or venous in origin, the vessel should be clamped and tied.

Capillary hemorrhage from soft tissues can be treated by various methods. Sponges that have been immersed in a solution of epinephrine hydrochloride, 1:1,000, and then wrung free of excess solution, can be inserted with pressure upon the bleeding site. An absorbable gelatin sponge (Gelfoam) or fibrin foam soaked in thrombin can be placed into the region. The method of choice is the placement under pressure of oxidized absorbable gauze into the bleeding capillary bed. Monsel's solution (solution of ferric subsulfate) is an excellent hemostatic for capillary bleeding but is difficult to manipulate because of its tendency to spread through the mouth. This produces clotted blood wherever the solution contacts fresh blood. This reaction discourages many surgeons, and the solution is condemned. However, Monsel's solution is a most useful agent when a small amount is carefully placed.

Frequently it is possible to arrest capillary or venous hemorrhage by closing the wound tightly with sutures. If soft tissue capillary hemorrhage originates from the superficial edges of a wound, this method is of value. This site must be carefully predetermined, however, because if hemorrhage is from a deeper source, the method is doomed to failure, and ecchymosis in the tissue will ensue.

Capillary bleeding from intrabony vessels can be arrested by applying the same principles as have been described for control of capillary bleeding from soft tissues.

Hemorrhage from larger intrabony vessels (veins or arteries) can be controlled by crushing the nutrient foramen that houses the vessel. The point of a small, blunt hemostat or a small Molt curet is an excellent instrument for this purpose. Hemorrhage from vessels such as these can also be well controlled by the use of electrocautery. A Bovie electrosurgical unit set at a cauterizing current, or a Hyfrecator, can be used to touch these bleeding vessels. This is an excellent method, which in most circumstances can be accomplished without postoperative complications. The coagulation of large amounts of bone will produce nonhealing of the soft tissues over the wound, and perhaps a small sequestrum will evolve. However, if only the small vessel is touched with the cauterizing unit, and if the gross amount of coagulated bone is scraped away with a curet, the instances of postoperative nonhealing will be most minimal. If the nutrient canal is large or is encased in a soft bone marrow, a very small piece of oxidized absorbable gauze can be rolled into a small spiral and inserted into the intrabony region.

The most important factor in the con-

---

*The measures to arrest the flow of blood as described here are as useful during the operative procedure as during the postoperative emergency.

trol of hemorrhage, regardless of the type or site, is the application of pressure pads over the site of bleeding. This is true regardless of the hemostatic agent utilized, and often the pressure itself suffices to control hemorrhage.

Temporary and sometimes permanent arrest follows infiltration or block anesthesia of the region involved if the anesthetic solution contains a vasoconstrictor drug as, for example, epinephrine hydrochloride, 1:50,000.

SHOCK*

In general, shock may be of three types: (1) primary or neurogenic, (2) cardiac and central nervous system, and (3) hypovolemic. It is the last type that is of concern here since it is the one usually seen after trauma, operations, burns, or hemorrhage.

In hypovolemic shock the circulating blood is reduced as a result of frank hemorrhage, loss of plasma by extravasation into injured parts, or dehydration. This type of shock is reversible if therapy is instituted swiftly to restore the intravascular blood volume. If this is not done, a chain reaction of cardiac, vascular, and other physiological dysfunctions is set up, the shock becomes irreversible, and death ensues.

Restoration of blood volume. In the treatment of hypovolemic shock, blood volume is best restored by transfusion of whole blood. Substitutes for blood are not as satisfactory as blood itself. It is usually not necessary to determine the blood volume to estimate the amount of blood required to restore normal circulating volume. The amount of blood transfused should equal the estimated amount lost or enough to return the blood pressure to normal levels and to maintain it there; possibly an additional 500 ml. of blood should be given after severe loss.

---

*The author is indebted to Dr. O. H. Beahrs for his valuable suggestions on this subject.

Blood of the same type should be given whenever possible, and cross matching of the blood of the donor and recipient is desirable. In an emergency, if the blood type of the patient is not known, type O (universal donor) with a low titer of agglutinins may be used.

Control of blood loss. As important as blood replacement in the management of hypovolemic shock is the control of the blood loss. (See section on control of postoperative bleeding.) If hemorrhage is occurring from inside the oral cavity or from the skin surface of the head or neck, then pressure or direct ligation of the vessel can be used. Also important in the control of shock is the relief of pain and the alleviation of fear. A temperate environment, not too cold and not too hot, is best. Placing the patient with his head down has been preferred to ensure better cerebral circulation. However, the horizontal position may offer the greatest safety for the patient in shock.

If red blood cells have not been lost, as in burns, or concentrated, as in dehydration, blood substitutes may be preferred to whole blood. Blood plasma was used extensively during the recent wars, but it has fallen into disuse because of the high (approximately 20%) incidence of serum hepatitis in patients receiving it. If plasma that has been stored at room temperature for 6 months is used, the incidence of hepatitis is much less. If plasma is being used to replace blood, the amounts used should correspond to the amounts of blood that would be used. Serum albumin also may be used to replace blood; it withstands heat and can be sterilized. Because of this it does not carry the risk of causing serum hepatitis; however, for common usage it is extremely expensive and therefore is used only when specifically indicated.

In recent years plasma volume expanders have become available for use as substitutes for blood and plasma. However, they are not to be considered as replacement for whole blood. The ideal plasma volume expander has a high molecular weight so that it will remain in the vascular compartment, is nontoxic, and is slowly metabolized. Plasma expanders that have been used clinically include 6% solution of dextran, 6% solution of ossein gelatin, and 3.5% solution of polyvinylpyrrolidone. Dextran, especially, has been used widely and can be transfused safely in amounts of 1,000 to 1,500 ml. Approximately 50% of dextran remains in the circulation after 12 hours. If large amounts are given, the bleeding time is prolonged. Plasma expanders, because of their retention in the vascular compartment, increase cardiac output and aid in stabilizing the blood pressure, but this is done at the expense of dilution of the red blood cells. If hemorrhage is not controlled when an expander is being used, dilution of blood could drop below the critical level. Circulating hemoglobin can be permitted to decrease to 50% safely, as a rule. If it is necessary to give more than 1,500 ml. of fluid to manage the shock, then whole blood should be administered in a ratio of 2:1 to plasma expander.

Vasoconstrictor drugs. Vasoconstrictor drugs are of value in the treatment of shock, but must be used with caution in the presence of hemorrhage. Norepinephrine is the most satisfactory one. It raises the blood pressure, but it is no substitute for transfusion. It may be given intravenously at the rate of from 8 to 10 micrograms per minute until the blood pressure is within normal limits and then reduced to from 2 to 4 micrograms per minute. Levarterenol bitartrate is also of value in maintaining blood pressure in a similar manner.

Adrenal insufficiency. Adrenal insufficiency has become an increasing factor in shock, especially since cortisone and corticotropin have become available for clinical use in a wide variety of conditions. The adrenal glands atrophy in patients who have been treated with corticotropin or cortisone, especially with high dosages and for long periods. Other causes of adrenal insufficiency are Addison's disease, tumors and dysfunction of the pituitary gland, and adrenalectomy. Patients having these are unable or less able to withstand the stresses and alterations in physiology following trauma, surgical procedures, hemorrhage, and disease. Under normal circumstances the insufficiency may not be apparent, but under added stress and strain it becomes apparent and shock occurs.

Adrenal insufficiency should always be suspected when shock occurs without hemorrhage. Other symptoms of postoperative adrenal failure, in addition to hypotension, are excessive fever, drowsiness, stupor, and finally coma.

The history obtained at the time of trauma or preoperatively should always indicate whether or not the patient has had adrenal disease or has received corticotropin or cortisone so that, when needed, adequate replacement therapy can be given to support the patient during and immediately after the stress. Patients with insufficiency should be given 100 to 200 mg. of hydrocortisone daily for 24 to 48 hours before operation. Patients not prepared before operation or trauma should receive 100 mg. intravenously and 200 mg. intramuscularly. Therapy should be continued as long as the patient is under increased stress.

FLUID AND ELECTROLYTE BALANCE IN ORAL SURGERY*

The locale of the operative field in oral surgery influences the intake of fluids and electrolytes. Certain factors may alter the intake of water. Curtailment of food and liquids for 6 hours before operation, preoperative limitation of intake of food and water because of anxiety, predisposing pathological conditions that produce pain,

---

*The author is indebted to Dr. K. G. Wakim and Dr. R. T. Oliver for their valuable suggestions on this subject.

and postoperative pain, swelling, trismus, malaise, or nausea are all factors that may lead to fluid imbalance.

If these factors supervene for more than 24 hours, the normal daily intake of 2,500 ml. is diminished, and the patient becomes moderately dehydrated. Dehydration is a state in which the output of water exceeds the intake. Intake is reduced when the patient is unable or unwilling to drink. Excessive loss in surgical patients can result from hemorrhage, vomiting, sweating, hyperventilation, diarrhea, or polyuria. Dehydration may be detected clinically when fluid equivalent to about 6% of the body weight has been lost. A loss of 8 to 9 pounds in the average adult would represent about 6% of the body weight in fluid, or mild dehydration.

This is not a serious problem if the period of alteration does not continue for more than 24 hours, because the dehydration can be compensated if the fluid intake can be restored to normal during this period. If, however, the alteration continues, intravenous administration of fluids should be started. If dehydration is the result of diminished intake of fluids, the administration of saline and dextrose solutions is indicated. Usually 0.5 to 1 liter of fluid is sufficient in moderate dehydration. If dehydration is caused by loss of blood, whether from operation or trauma, the best fluid for replacement is whole blood.

Often the amounts of blood lost during oral surgical procedures exceed the estimates. For example, 100 to 800 ml. of blood may be lost during operations involving multiple extraction and alveoloplasty.[5]

Dehydration disturbs the acid-base balance. Whether acidosis or alkalosis develops depends upon how the dehydration develops and whether the loss of sodium is greater or less than the loss of chloride. Often acidosis develops.

If the dehydration is caused by stoppage of oral intake, usually acidosis is present. This is thought to be the result of anhydremia with depression of oxidative processes leading to an accumulation of acid metabolites. Also, slower renal circulation favors retention of acid metabolites. These patients have a dry mouth, and they are thirsty. Thirst is the cardinal symptom of this type of dehydration. If dehydration is caused by excessive loss of fluid from the skin, the losses of sodium and chloride are about equal, and usually the acid-base balance is not disturbed. The important point in this event is to be aware that these losses are taking place and to see that the lost fluid is replaced in volume and in electrolytic composition.

Loss of fluid from the gastrointestinal tract in oral operations results from vomiting, and chiefly gastric juice is lost. Gastric juice contains normally 20 mEq. of sodium and 145 mEq. of chloride per liter. If the loss is severe enough, chloride is depleted more rapidly than sodium, and alkalosis develops. Under these circumstances, blood chemical studies show low levels of both sodium and chloride, but the level of chloride is much lower. Carbon dioxide is retained by the body in an attempt to make up for this inequality, and hence the carbon dioxide–combining power increases.

If dehydration occurs because of prolonged diarrhea, more sodium than chloride is lost, the carbon dioxide–combining power is reduced, and acidosis results.

The fluid and electrolyte needs of oral surgical patients may be considered in three categories.

Categories of patients. The first category consists of patients who have normal fluid and electrolyte balance before operation and suffer no significant loss of fluid at operation. Patients undergoing a general office procedure would probably fall into this category. Also, almost all patients who undergo minor operations not involving the viscera fall into this group. Since their loss of fluid is not significantly more than that of normal persons, their requirement for fluid is 2,000 to 2,500 ml., the normal daily requirement. The loss of salt is usually negligible. If these patients are unable to take fluids by mouth, 2,000 ml. of 5% solution of dextrose in water can be given intravenously daily until they are able to drink.

A second category consists of patients whose fluids and electrolytes are in balance before operation, but who lose appreciable amounts of fluid at operation or postoperatively. From the viewpoint of oral surgery, patients requiring hospitalization for long operations, such as the removal of all teeth with alveoloplasty, some fractures, and some severe infections, would generally fall into this category.

The well-dehydrated patient who is subjected to a prolonged operation may lose from 500 to 700 ml. of body fluid and also a considerable amount of blood. The blood loss should be carefully estimated, and it should be replaced by transfusion of blood. If the amount of blood loss is small, it may be replaced by isotonic saline solution. The normal daily requirement for fluid plus the amount of fluid lost at operation should be given.

These patients frequently lose fluids from excessive sweating or vomiting or both, and, in addition, may be unable to take food or water by mouth for several days. Actually, correction of the fluid and electrolyte loss in these cases is not difficult. The normal daily requirements can be met by giving 2,000 ml. of 5% solution of dextrose in water. The loss of salt from excessive sweating or vomiting can be corrected by an appropriate amount of physiological saline solution after the volume lost has been estimated.

Work by Coller and associates[6] indicates that the kidney does not work efficiently for 24 hours or more postoperatively. In general, it handles excesses of sodium poorly but excesses of water well. To be safe the saline solution administered during this period should be kept at a minimum.

A third category consists of patients who from the start have severe metabolic disturbances and severe acidosis or alkalosis and who experience difficult imbalances. Patients with severe, complicating systemic disturbances and those suffering from chronic debilitating diseases meet the requirements of this category. Treatment varies from group to group.

Rarely should the oral surgeon be called upon to assume full responsibility for the maintenance of fluid and electrolyte balance of patients in this last category. Patients suffering from severe metabolic disturbances and debilitating diseases have special problems of fluid balance that require special knowledge and experience. Usually such patients are already under treatment by an internist or family physician when the need for oral operation arises. All members of the patient's medical team must cooperate closely in planning operations on patients in this category.

Fluid needs in the young and the old. Fluid needs in the very young and the very old present special problems and warrant some separate consideration. The very young may need three or four times as much fluid per kilogram of body weight as an adult needs, because a higher metabolic rate and a greater surface area in proportion to body mass increase the rate of fluid loss.

As for the very old, too much fluid must not be given, and fluid must not be given too rapidly. They need less than normal adults, and their cardiovascular system may not tolerate fluids given too fast. Saline solutions must be given judiciously to elderly persons because their renal function may be poor.

Methods of administering fluids. The oral route is the best and most natural route for administration of fluids, when possible. It is surprising how often this route is overlooked. The rectal route can be used, but it is not the best because of the uncertainty of how much fluid is absorbed. Solutions given rectally do not have to be sterilized. Fluid can be given rectally by the drip method at the rate of 30 to 50 drops per minute. Sometimes 300 to 500 ml. can be given in 4 hours by this route.

The subcutaneous route is undesirable, but can be used. Pain is the chief drawback. This can be partially controlled by adding 2 ml. of a 1% solution of procaine hydrochloride to each 1,500 ml. of fluid given. The fluid should be isotonic and at body temperature. Frequent moving of the injection site favors more rapid absorption. Sloughing and infection are dangers at the injection site.

The intravenous route is used most frequently (Fig. 13-12). The normal rate of administration is 200 to 500 ml. per hour (3 to 8 ml. per minute). At this rate the body will utilize most of a 5% solution of dextrose in water.

Fluid can be given intrasternally if no other route is available. It may be given rapidly into the sternal marrow space. The skin and periosteum are first anesthetized, and then a 14-gauge needle with a guard is plunged into the sternum until the marrow cavity is entered.

Solutions used to replenish water and electrolytes. Basically, four solutions probably will suffice for replenishing body water and electrolytes in most cases: (1) dextrose solution (5% or 10%), (2) physiological saline solution (0.9% sodium chloride), which contains the principal extracellular ions, (3) potassium lactate, also known as "Darrow's solution," which is available under several trade names, and (4) blood and blood substitutes.

POSTOPERATIVE CARE

The most important factors in postoperative care that are of concern in this chapter are (1) control of hemorrhage, (2) reinstitution of normal intake of fluids, and, if necessary, (3) replacement of fluids that have been lost.

As has already been stated, the placement of pressure dressings is of extreme importance. Following the extraction of teeth, sterile gauze that has been saturated with water and wrung as dry as possible should be placed over the wounds and held here by gentle biting pressure. The following instructions can be printed and a copy given to each patient after the extraction of teeth.

Instructions to patients:

1. Leave the gauze in place for at least 30 minutes.

2. Place an ice bag or cold towels to your face for 6 to 12 hours. The earlier this is started the more effective it will be.

3. Do not rinse your mouth until the following morning. Rinsing may dislodge the blood clot and interrupt the normal process of healing.

4. In the morning rinse the mouth gently with a glass of hot salt water (½ teaspoonful of salt in the glass of hot water). Repeat three or four times during the day.

5. Follow your own natural inclination as to diet, but for your own comfort, soft foods are indicated for the first 24 hours. Drink plenty of fluids, but avoid drinking through a straw.

6. If abnormal bleeding occurs, fold a sponge, wet it, place it over the socket, and bite down on it for 20 minutes.

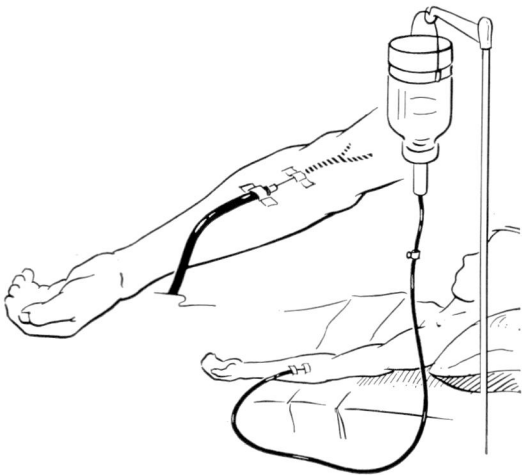

Fig. 13-12. Intravenous administration of fluids.

7. The teeth should be given their usual care, except in the region of the operation.

In case of emergency call the oral surgeon.

For the postoperative dressing of extraoral wounds about the face, drains and pressure dressings should be used. For deep wounds a Penrose drain should be sutured into the wound to prevent hematoma. After skin closure an abundant amount of gauze should be placed over the wound and tightly taped to exert pressure upon the wound.

As soon as possible after recovery from general anesthesia the intake of fluids by mouth should be encouraged. Dehydration often causes a postoperative rise in temperature that frequently is mistakenly attributed to infection. If vomiting or nausea prevents reinstitution of fluid intake by the oral route, an effective antiemetic should be prescribed. Several of the tranquilizing drugs (for example, chlorpromazine) have been useful as antiemetics. A combination of pentobarbital sodium, hyoscine, and atropine has been efficacious in this respect. Sipping of carbonated beverages or ice has also proved effective.

The replacement of fluids lost during operation is discussed in the section on shock.

REFERENCES

1. Pool, J. G., and Shannon, A. E.: Production of high-potency concentrates of antihemophilic globulin in a closed bag system, New Eng. J. Med. 273:1443, 1965.
2. Stegelske, R. F., Gores, R. J., Hurn, Margaret M., and Owen, C. A., Jr.: Bleeding from deficiency of plasma thromboplastin antecedent (PTA) coagulation factor: report of a case, Oral Surg. 10:225, 1957.
3. Hollinshead, W. H.: Anatomy for surgeons: the head and neck, vol. 1, New York, 1954, Paul B. Hoeber, Inc.
4. Berman, J. K.: Synopsis of the principles of surgery, St. Louis, 1940, The C. V. Mosby Co.
5. Gores, R. J., Royer, R. Q., and Mann, F. D.: Blood loss during operation for multiple extraction with alveoloplasty and other oral surgical procedures, J. Oral Surg. 13:299, 1955.
6. Coller, F. A., Campbell, K. N., Vaughan, H. H., Iob, L. Vivian, and Moyer, C. A.: Postoperative salt intolerance, Ann. Surg. 119:533, 1944.

Chapter 14

CYSTS OF BONE AND SOFT TISSUES OF THE ORAL CAVITY AND CONTIGUOUS STRUCTURES

Leroy W. Peterson

A cyst is a cavity occurring in either hard or soft tissue with a liquid, semiliquid, or air content. It is surrounded by a definite connective tissue wall or capsule and usually has an epithelial lining. The contained substance is a predominant feature in proportion to the size of the entire mass of tissue.

CLASSIFICATION

Congenital, developmental, and retention types of cysts occur within the oral cavity and about the face and neck. Cysts of dental origin are by far the most common. In the combined grouping of these cystic lesions, the following classification, modified from that given by Robinson and Thoma and others,[4] is offered for discussion.

- A. Congenital cysts
    1. Thyroglossal
    2. Branchiogenic
    3. Dermoid
- B. Developmental cysts
    1. Nondental origin
        a. Fissural types
            (1) Nasoalveolar
            (2) Median
            (3) Incisive canal (nasopalatine)
            (4) Globulomaxillary
        b. Retention types
            (1) Mucocele
            (2) Ranula
    2. Dental origin
        a. Periodontal
            (1) Periapical
            (2) Lateral
            (3) Residual
        b. Primordial (follicular)
        c. Dentigerous

Neoplasms that may appear to be cystic are not included in the above classification. These tumors are discussed elsewhere, but the most common ones encountered are the ameloblastoma and the mixed salivary gland tumor. The ameloblastoma, a true dental neoplasm, may have no clinical characteristics other than appearing to be a cystic lesion. This neoplasm involves bone primarily, with displacement of the adjacent soft tissue by erosion and expansion.

Other than the parotid area the mixed cell salivary neoplasms appear more often on the hard and soft palates than in any part of the oral cavity except perhaps the cheek. Rarely, they occur in the lips, where they form a palpable swelling and appear similar to a mucocele.

Various benign tumors of the soft tissues of the oral cavity that may have a clinical appearance of a cyst include the fibroma, lipoma, myoma, hemangioma, lymphangioma, and papilloma.

Additional neoplasms and dysplastic conditions of bone may appear roentgenographically as a cystic lesion. These neoplasms include the giant cell tumor, fibrous dysplasia, ossifying fibroma, metastatic and invasive carcinoma, osteolytic sarcoma and other rare primary bone tumors, and multiple myeloma.

Metabolic or systemic dysfunctions that may give rise to lesions having the radiographic appearance of a cyst are osteitis fibrosa cystica (hyperparathyroidism) and the diseases of the reticuloendothelial system (histiocytosis X).

Hemorrhagic or traumatic bone cavities (Fig. 14-14, A) as well as the idiopathic bone cavities (Fig. 14-14, B), described by Stafne and others, may also enter into the differential diagnosis of true cysts of the jaws.

Congenital cysts

Thyroglossal duct cysts. Thyroglossal cysts (Fig. 14-1) may arise from any portion of the thyroglossal duct. They are therefore in a midline position and are usually of dark color. They may be so vascular as to resemble hemangiomas. One frequent important symptom is hemorrhage into the mouth resulting from the rupture of the overlying veins.

The thyroglossal duct lies in the line between the thyroid gland and the foramen cecum on the tongue. A cyst or sinus tract derived from this structure is located in the midline at any point between the thyroid isthmus and the base of the tongue. The tract is usually attached to or in close relationship with the hyoid bone. The cyst may be asymptomatic or may cause symptoms as a result of pressure on other structures. Swallowing will cause the mass to move upward.

Because of the thyroglossal duct the cyst may become infected. If so, the lesion may drain spontaneously, but also may be incised. Ideally, it should be removed before infection occurs or after acute symptoms have subsided. Complete excision of the tract to the base of the tongue, frequently including a portion of the hyoid bone, is necessary for a cure.

Branchiogenic cysts. Several theories have been advanced concerning the origin of branchiogenic cysts (Fig. 14-2), but most of the evidence supports the belief that they arise from persistencies of the second branchial cleft. They are characteristically located along the anterior border of the sternocleidomastoid muscle at any level in the neck. A fistulous tract may extend up to the digastric muscle and terminate in the tonsillar fossa. These cysts or tracts are lined with ciliated and stratified squamous epithelium, which contains a milky or mucoid fluid. An external fistula may be present. Treatment consists of complete surgical excision.

Dermoid cysts. Dermoid cysts (Fig. 14-3) are relatively uncommon in the oral cavity. The dermoid cyst consists of a fibrous wall lined with stratified squamous epithelium. The cyst frequently contains hair, sebaceous and sweat glands, as well as tooth structures. They may occur on the

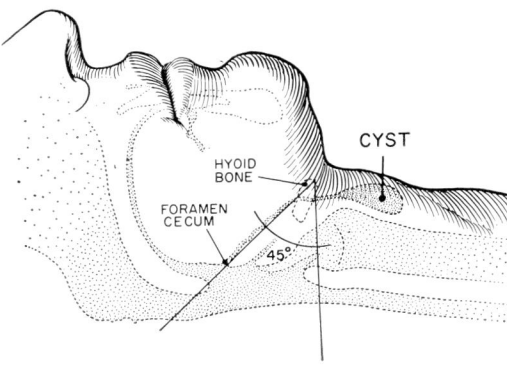

Fig. 14-1. Thyroglossal cyst. (From Copeland, M. M., and Geschickter, C. F.: Amer. Surg. **24**:321, 1958.)

214 *Textbook of oral surgery*

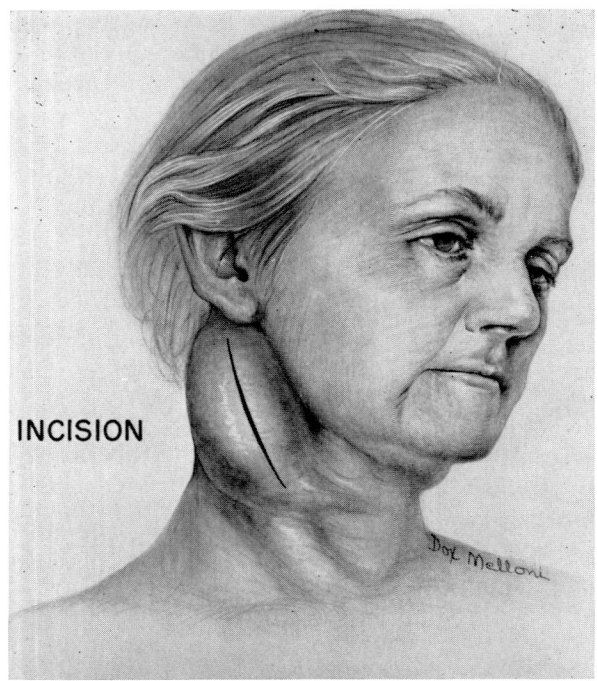

Fig. 14-2. Branchiogenic cyst. (From Copeland, M. M., and Geschickter, C. F.: Amer. Surg. **24:**321, 1958.)

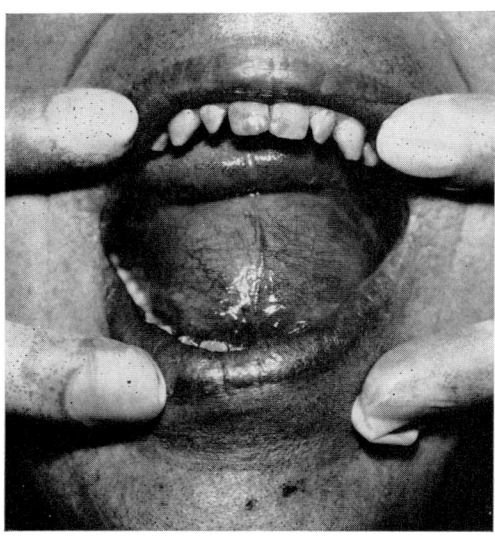

Fig. 14-3. Dermoid cyst. (Courtesy Dr. Frederick A. Figi.)

hard and soft palates, on the dorsum of the tongue, or more commonly in the floor of the mouth. They cause a swelling in the same location as the sublingual retention cysts and must be differentiated from them. They do not give the vesicular appearance of the ranula. The dermoid cyst may be located either above or below the geniohyoid muscle. Dermoids usually occur in the midline, but may be displaced laterally during development and, as such, must be differentiated from cysts of branchial origin.

Dermoid cysts are not easily discovered unless they cause swelling beneath the chin or up into the floor of the mouth. On palpation, these cysts give a rubberlike sensation. They generally contain a yellow cheesy material. This yellow color aids sometimes in differentiation of the dermoid cyst from the ranula, which has a bluish hue. X-ray examination may be helpful in distinguishing a dermoid cyst from other lesions of similar nature because of their contents, which frequently include radiopaque objects.

Treatment is the surgical removal of the entire tumor.

Developmental cysts
Nondental origin

Nasoalveolar cysts. A nasoalveolar cyst (Fig. 14-4) forms at the junction of the globular, lateral nasal, and maxillary processes. It produces a swelling at the attachment of the ala of the nose, and as it expands it encroaches upon the nasal cavity. Since these cysts are not central bony lesions, x-ray findings are negative. The cysts are usually lined with nasal-type epithelium but may also contain some stratified squamous cells. On clinical observation they may be mistaken for cysts of dental origin or dental alveolar abscesses on the maxillary anterior teeth.

Treatment consists of complete surgical excision. The nasoalveolar cyst is usually removed intraorally by carefully incising the overlying mucous membrane and enucleating the cyst.

Median cysts. The median cyst (Fig. 14-5) is a bone cyst that forms in a median fissure of the palate from embryonic remnants. Median alveolar cysts have also been described. Robinson[4] maintains that these are not true median cysts since the bones uniting in these areas have their origin deep within mesenchymal tissue with no chance for inclusion of epithelial rests. Robinson presumes that they are primordial cysts of supernumerary tooth buds. Median cysts of the mandible have been described; they are extremely uncommon.

Median cysts are differentiated from incisive canal cysts primarily by their location since they usually occur more posteriorly in the palate. X-ray findings are often misleading because of the overlapping shadows of the paranasal sinuses. Injection of a radiopaque material will definitely outline this cyst.

Surgical excision of these cysts is the preferred treatment, although the Partsch method may be used. Very frequently these cysts have to be approached by reflecting a mucoperiosteal flap from the labial aspect of the maxilla as well as from the palate. These cysts are in close proximity to the floor of the nose and bulge into the nasal cavity. The median cyst has a connective tissue sac lined by squamous epithelium. Like other cysts, cholesterol crystal spaces may be surrounded, in some instances, by foreign body cells.

Incisive canal cysts (nasopalatine cysts). Cysts located in the center of the bone are named incisive canal cysts (Fig. 14-6). Occasionally a soft tissue cyst forms in the palatine papilla. These cysts do not expand inside the bone, nor do they alter significantly the overlying mucosa. They are called cysts of the papilla palatini and are differentiated from a bone cyst by x-ray and surgical examination.

The radiograph is of great value in diagnosis of incisive canal cysts. However, the size of the incisive canal is by no means constant, and many a large canal and fora-

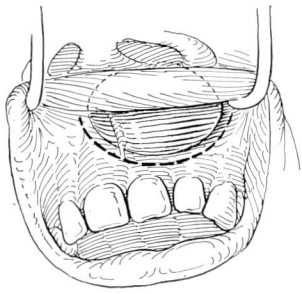

Fig. 14-4. Nasoalveolar cyst. This cyst presents no radiographic change. It usually bulges into the floor of the nose. It is removed intraorally.

216 *Textbook of oral surgery*

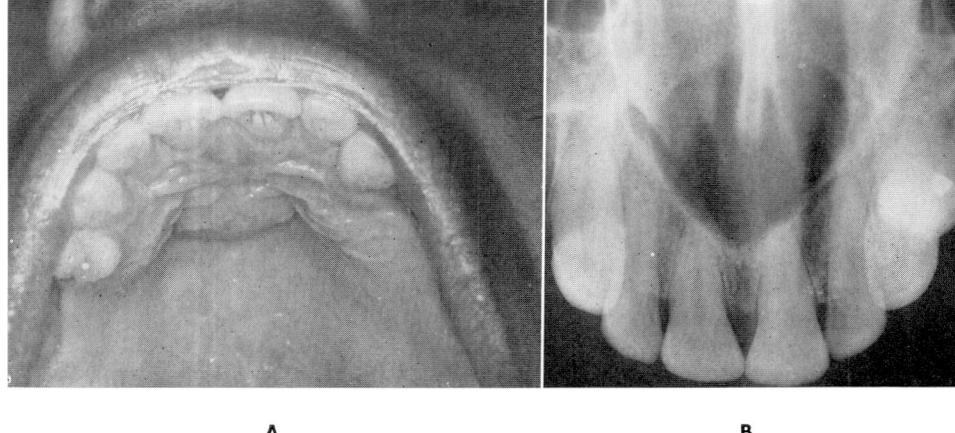

Fig. 14-5. Median cyst of palate. **A,** Clinical view showing expansion through palatal bone. **B,** Radiographic view.

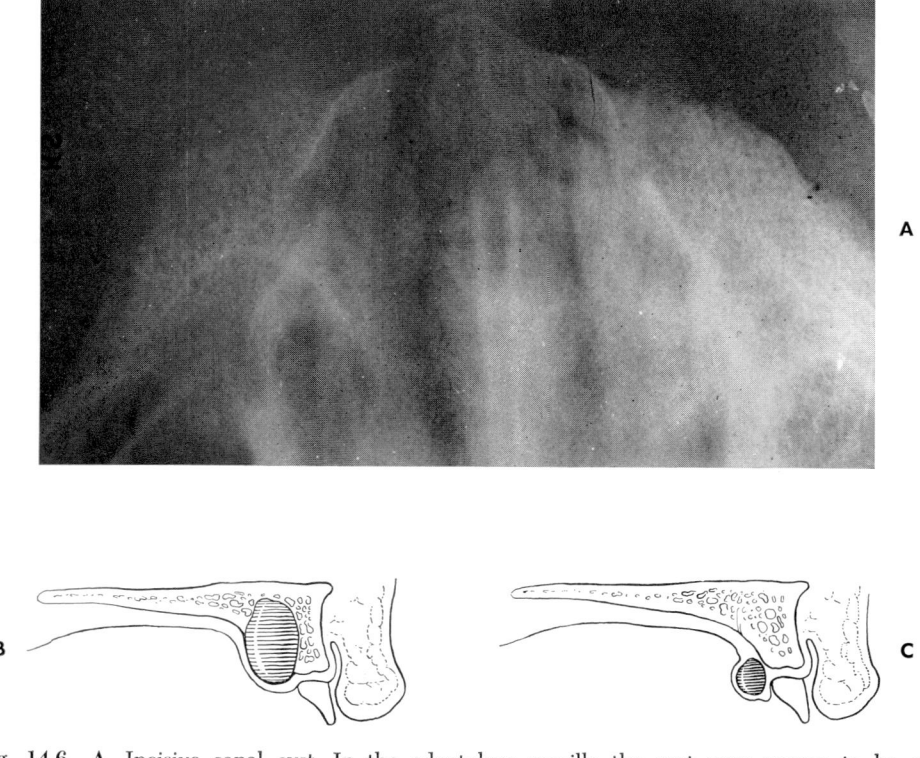

Fig. 14-6. **A,** Incisive canal cyst. In the edentulous maxilla the cyst may appear to be at the crest of the alveolar ridge. **B,** Diagram of cross section of incisive canal cyst. **C,** Diagram of cross section of cyst of the palatine papilla. Although a similar amount of clinical enlargement of the palatine area may be present, this cyst does not involve bone. This cyst is rare.

men may give the appearance of a cyst. In edentulous jaws, because of resorption, the cyst may appear closer to the surface. Differential diagnosis from radicular cysts is necessary to prevent devitalization or extractions of these teeth.

These cysts usually give no clinical symptoms unless they become secondarily infected. A persistent discharge, or pus escaping under pressure, may be noted. Probing or puncturing the area will usually allow the accumulation of fluid to escape, but swelling will recur unless the cyst is removed surgically. For the surgical approach to these cysts a palatal flap is usually retracted after incising along the lingual gingival margins. By careful elevation of the flap, the continuity of the nerves and vessels, which lie in the foramen and emerge at the papilla, can be preserved. Frequently the nerves and vessels must be interrupted for better access to the cystic tissue. This does not cause any undesirable sequelae. Usually the cyst can then be teased away gently from the soft tissue or the bony bed, as the case may be. The nasopalatine cysts usually contain a thick membrane of connective tissue. The lining of the lumen varies in type from squamous to transitional to ciliated columnar epithelium. In many cases marked inflammatory infiltration takes place as a result of secondary infection from the oral cavity.

Globulomaxillary cysts. Globulomaxillary cysts (Fig. 14-7) are epithelial-lined sacs formed at the junction of the globular and maxillary processes between the lateral incisor and canine teeth. They usually cause a divergence of the roots of these teeth and appear as pear-shaped radiolucencies on x-ray film. As is true with other cysts of the oral cavity, they become secondarily infected and undergo acute inflammatory changes.

Diagnosis of the globulomaxillary cyst depends almost entirely on its location between the lateral incisor and canine plus a clinical evaluation of the adjacent teeth to

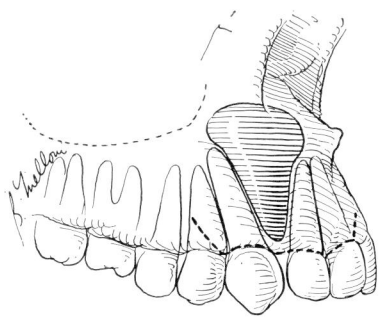

Fig. 14-7. Globulomaxillary cyst. Typical pear-shaped appearance on the radiograph. The adjacent lateral incisor and canine teeth, which have been pushed aside by the cyst, are vital. The wound is closed with drainage if it is secondarily infected.

differentiate it from one of dental origin. These teeth usually respond favorably to vitality tests. The cyst consists of a connective tissue membrane lined with stratified squamous epithelium. Treatment is surgical and consists of careful excision, although the Partsch method may be used. Generally the adjacent teeth need not be disturbed if the operation is planned and carried out properly. A mucoperiosteal flap must be reflected from the labial bone so that adequate access to the pathology may be obtained and the cyst carefully enucleated. The majority of these heal by first intention, and primary closure can be obtained without the use of dressings or other substances to obliterate the cavity.

Mucoceles. Mucocysts or mucoceles (Fig. 14-8) result from the obstruction of a glandular duct and are commonly located in the lip, cheek, and floor of the mouth. They may also be found on the anterior portion of the tongue, where glands are located at the inferior surface. These are small, round or oval, translucent swellings, sometimes having a very bluish color, and may be mistaken for a hemangioma. The mucocele is freely movable and usually found right underneath the mucosa.

218 *Textbook of oral surgery*

Occasionally it may be punctured accidentally or will rupture spontaneously, only to recur. The preferable treatment is complete excision. If it is incompletely removed, it has a marked tendency to recur, but the lesion is not known to become malignant.

Ranulas. A ranula (Fig. 14-9) is a cyst forming in the floor of the mouth, generally from a sublingual gland. The ranula forms in a manner similar to the mucocele, but develops to a much larger size.

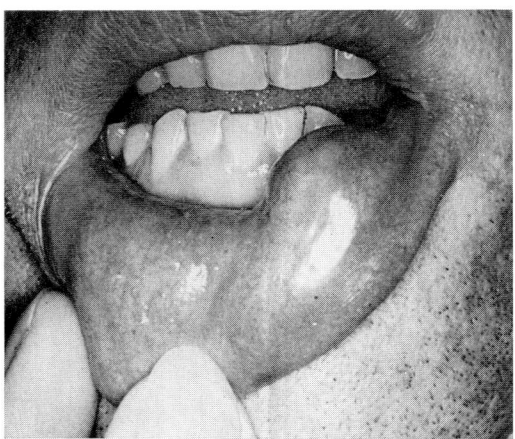

Fig. 14-8. Mucocele.

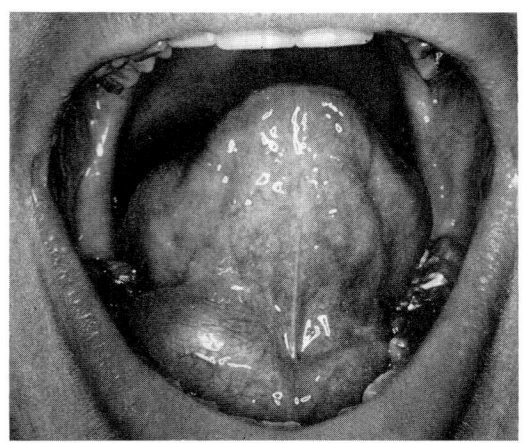

Fig. 14-9. Ranula.

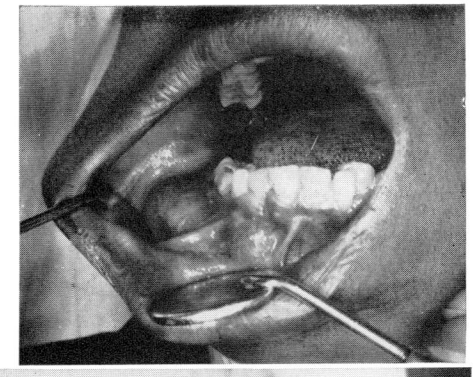

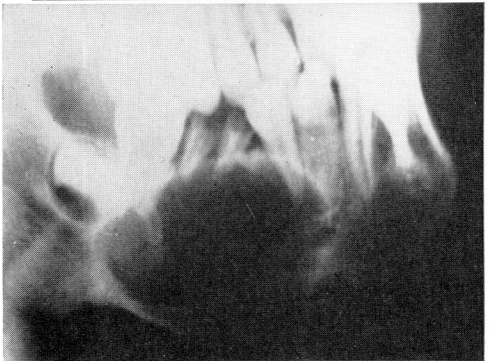

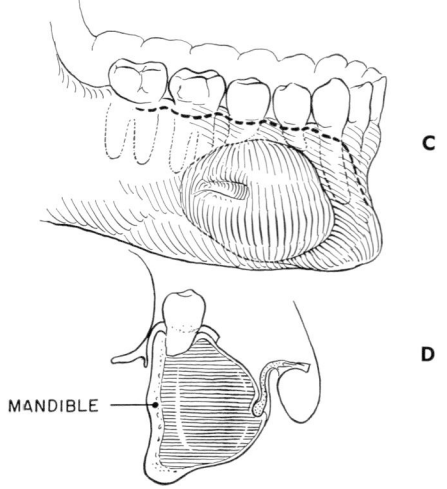

Fig. 14-10. Periodontal cysts. **A,** *Periapical (radicular) cyst.* Clinical appearance. **B,** Radiographic appearance. **C,** Incision for reflecting mucoperiosteal flap. The buccal cortical plate is thin because of the expansion of the cyst. **D,** The continuity of the mental nerve is preserved within the flap during the surgical dissection.

When it attains a large size, the mucosa is thinned out and the cyst assumes a bluish color. It is a nonpainful lesion, but the tongue might be raised and its motion hindered, thus impairing mastication and speech. The ranula is subject to rupture when injured, with escape of a mucoid fluid which reaccumulates as the area heals.

The size of the ranula cannot be determined from the appearance within the mouth. It is tense and fluctuant, but does not pit on pressure. It seldom causes any external swelling and rarely becomes infected. It is painless and contains a stringy, mucoid fluid. A ranula is much more firm than the angioma occasionally found in the

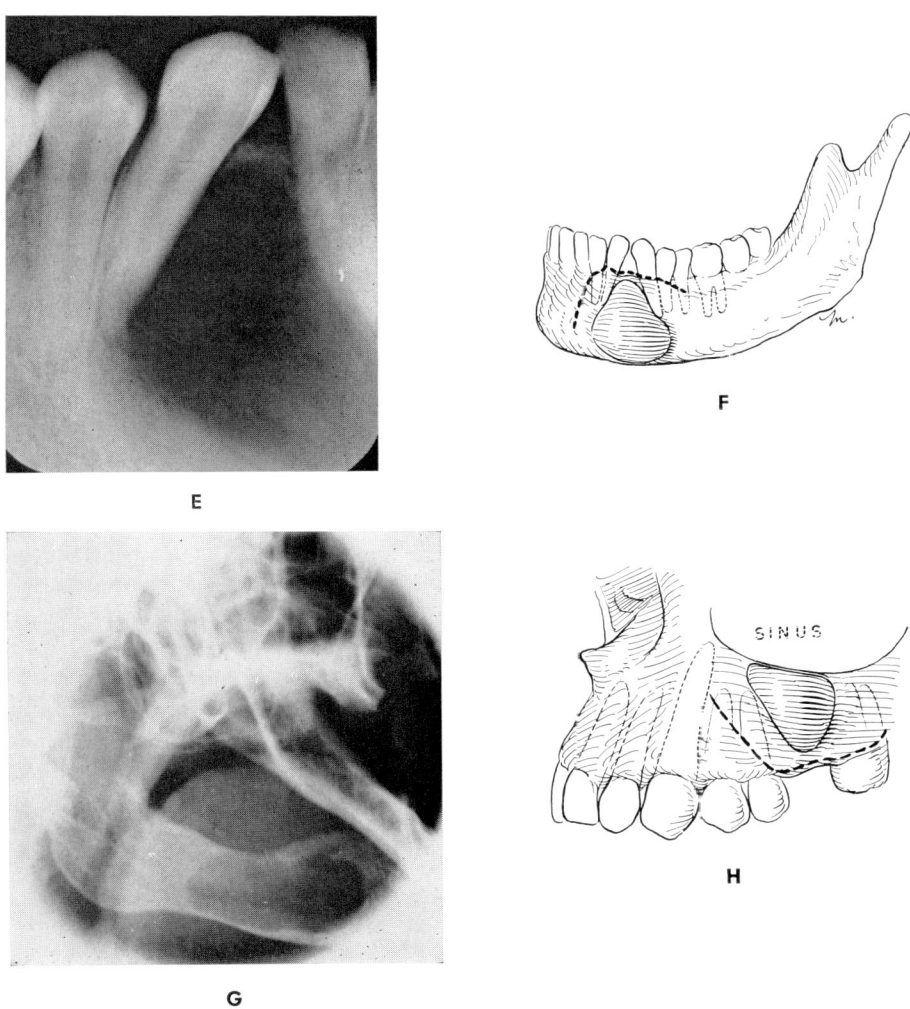

Fig. 14-10, cont'd. E, *Lateral cyst.* In this particular case the adjacent teeth are displaced. F, Incision for removal of lateral cyst. G, *Residual cyst.* The cyst may be treated by enucleation or the Partsch method. The continuity of the mental foramen structures can be preserved either way. H, Residual cyst from previous extracted first molar tooth. Radiopaque material could be injected to confirm the fact that the maxillary sinus is not involved if differential diagnosis is doubtful. The cyst should be enucleated carefully.

floor of the mouth. Dermoid cysts have a doughy feeling on pressure and occur more often in the median line. Lipomas are more firm. Cysts of the submandibular duct usually cause swelling in the gland. They develop more rapidly than the true ranula and are associated with pain and other symptoms of inflammation.

The best treatment for a ranula is surgery in the form of marsupialization.

Dental origin

Periodontal cysts. A periodontal cyst (Fig. 14-10) is formed from epithelial rests or remnants in the periodontal membrane. These cysts are all of inflammatory origin. The usual location is at the apex of the tooth, where they are termed radicular cysts, but they also may be formed along the lateral surface and are then termed lateral cysts. Cysts of inflammatory nature in edentulous areas are termed residual. These result from incomplete surgical removal of pathological tissue at the time an infected tooth is extracted.

Inflammatory cysts are a result of dental infection, with necrosis of pulpal tissue and resultant degeneration into granulomas or cysts. All epithelial granulomas do not develop into cysts. The formation of a cyst depends, first, upon the dissolution of the central part of the granuloma and, second, on transudation of fluid through the epithelial-lined connective tissue sac into the lumen. These cysts are commonly lined by stratified squamous epithelium. Round cell infiltration and other signs of chronic inflammation are usually found. The periodontal cyst, being primarily inflammatory in nature, will not show any progression toward neoplastic formation of the epithelial cells lining the cyst wall.

The small periodontal cyst can often be enucleated through the alveolar socket following removal of the involved tooth. However, it is frequently much better to elevate a surgical flap and remove the cyst by the labial or buccal approach. This ensures better visibility of the pathological region and allows for more definite removal of all the cyst tissue.

Large periodontal cysts usually appear to involve several teeth, and it is extremely important that vital teeth not be removed unnecessarily. This overlapping, as visualized on the x-ray film, may extend buccally, labially, or palatally to the apparently involved teeth and, as such, access and removal of the cyst can be gained by sacrificing sound dental structures. In these large cystic areas the Partsch method of treatment is preferred if adjacent teeth are in danger of damage.

Many of these inflammatory cysts become chronically infected and form fistulas through the alveolar bone to the overlying mucoperiosteum. In some instances expansion of the cyst is great enough that all overlying bone has disappeared and the cyst wall is adherent to the mucoperiosteum. In these instances the dissection involved in reflecting a mucoperiosteal flap becomes somewhat tedious, and care must be taken to strip the cystic lining cleanly from the soft tissue covering the bone.

Tooth roots that protrude into a bone cavity following enucleation of a cyst should be amputated after proper root canal therapy has been instituted, or the teeth should be extracted. Complete removal of cystic tissue in inaccessible areas is difficult since frequently the involved region cannot be too clearly visualized or approached surgically with tooth roots interfering.

Residual periodontal cysts cannot be diagnosed from x-ray findings alone and are often verified only on microscopic examination. Treatment in all cases, however, is either by enucleation or marsupialization.

Primordial cysts (follicular). Primordial cysts (Fig. 14-11) differ from periodontal and dentigerous cysts in that they contain no calcified structures. The term follicular has often been applied to this type of

Cysts of bone and soft tissues of oral cavity and contiguous structures 221

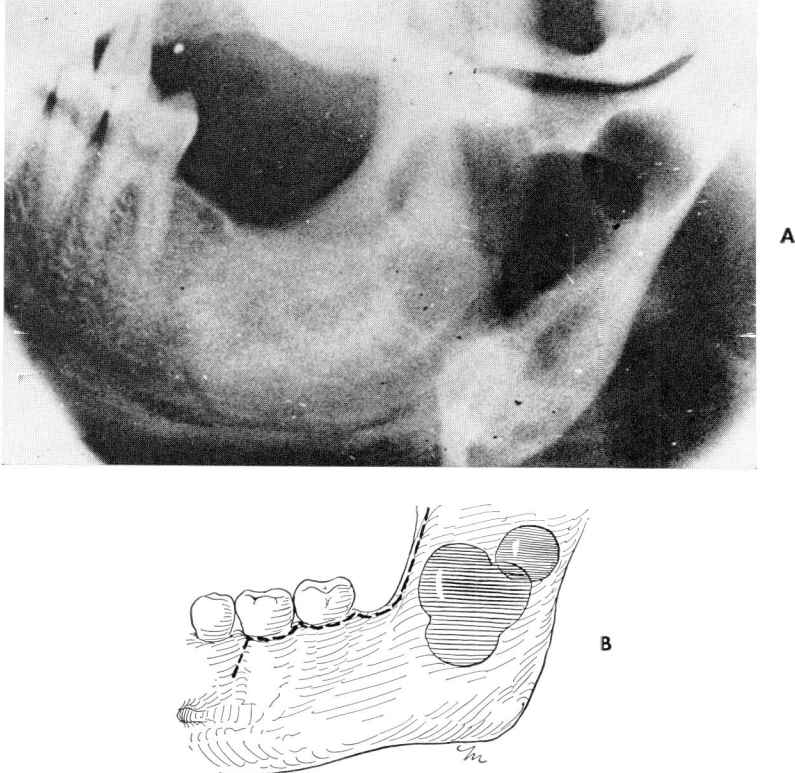

Fig. 14-11. **A,** Multilocular primordial cyst forming from tooth bud of third molar that never developed. **B,** Incision for intraoral removal of cyst.

lesion and can be used synonymously with it. In primordial cysts the retrogression of the stellate reticulum in the enamel organ takes place before any calcified tooth structure is formed. The word primordial means simplest and most undeveloped in character. These cysts are lined by stratified squamous epithelium and may be either locular, multilocular, or multiple. Odontogenic cysts, such as the primordial and dentigerous cysts, are formed from primitive oral epithelium and are therefore closely related to each other and to the ameloblastoma, a true dental neoplasm. In these cysts the epithelial cells have a definite potential of developing into a neoplasm.

Except for the absence of dental structures, resulting from the period in development when cystic changes took place, these primordial and dentigerous cysts are basically identical in all respects so far as surgical treatment is concerned, and their differential diagnosis, to a large degree, is purely academic.

Dentigerous cysts. A dentigerous cyst (Fig. 14-12) contains a crown of an unerupted tooth or dental anomaly such as an odontoma. These cysts develop after deposition of enamel and are probably a result of degenerative changes in the reduced enamel-forming epithelium. The fact that the epithelium of a dentigerous cyst is attached to the neck of the tooth is fairly strong evidence that in most cases the cyst

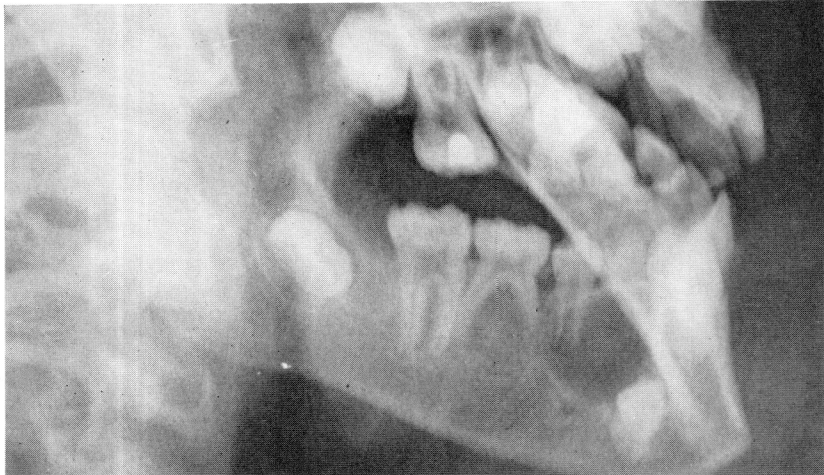

Fig. 14-12. The dentigerous cyst was removed and the unerupted tooth retained in this case. The tooth should continue to erupt. The Partsch method of treatment may be used because sometimes it is difficult to dissect the cyst free without displacing the unerupted tooth.

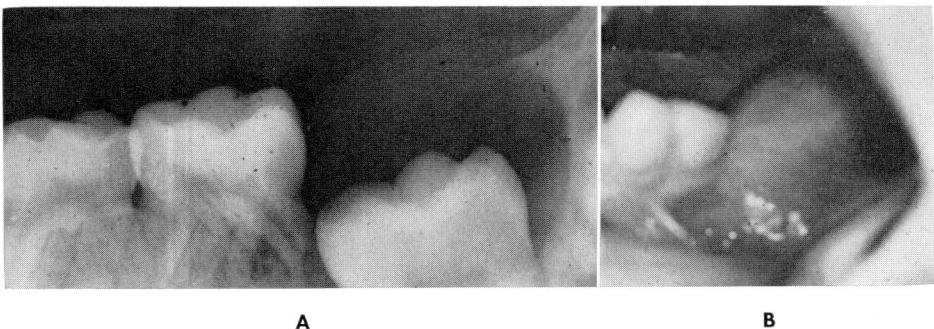

Fig. 14-13. A, Eruption cyst associated with a permanent first molar tooth. B, Intraoral swelling associated with eruption cyst.

is formed by the enamel organ and not independently of it.

If cysts form when a tooth is erupting, they are called eruption cysts (Fig. 14-13). These cysts interfere with normal eruption of the teeth. Eruption cysts are more commonly found in the child and young adult and may be associated with any tooth. If treatment is indicated, simple incision or "deroofing" is all that is needed.

Enlarged dentigerous cysts can cause a marked displacement of teeth. Pressure of the accumulated fluid usually displaces the tooth in an apical direction, and frequently the root formation becomes stunted. Dentigerous cysts may be found anywhere in the mandible or the maxilla, but are more frequently located at the angle of the jaw, the cuspid regions, maxillary third molar areas, the antral cavity, and also in the floor of the orbit.

Cysts may be produced by several tooth

germs acting together in their formation, giving a multiple follicular-type appearance. The tooth bud, given off from the dental lamina or outer epithelial layer of the enamel organ of the tooth, may branch and form a number of follicles. Each follicle may form a cyst, causing a formation of so-called daughter cysts, which necessitate careful exploration at the time of surgery. It should be remembered that the primordial or dentigerous cyst is a potential ameloblastoma. The formation of buds at the basal layer of the epithelium and papillary outgrowth into the lumen may be the beginning of this dental tumor.

These developmental cysts have a marked tendency to recur. Frequently, cysts with thickly epitheliated linings are more likely to recur than cysts with a thin layer of epithelium, especially if they are multiple.

Complete enucleation of the cyst sac is indicated in this type of developmental dental cysts. A partial excision is dangerous, and any small part left behind may contain the potential of developing into a true dental tumor. When, because of anatomical considerations, combined Partsch and enucleation techniques are used, multiple biopsy should be taken from the area and the postoperative course thoroughly followed with x-ray examination every 6 months. Any pathological tissue that is removed should not be discarded. It should be placed in a bottle of 10% formalin and prepared for complete microscopic examination. Carcinomas have been reported as developing in the epithelial cells of this type cystic lesion.[8]

Many of these cysts give no clinical symptoms until noticeable asymmetry of the face develops. These cysts can reach rather large proportions to involve the entire body or ramus of the mandible as well as a large portion of the maxilla, displacing the orbital and paranasal sinus cavities rather than invading them. Many times radiographs will show marked expansion of bone so that the overlying cortical plate is paper thin.

Treatment of choice, even in the extremely large cystic lesions, is careful enucleation. If one cortical plate of bone is entirely destroyed by expansive pressure, the periosteal tissue is left intact, which serves as an excellent aid for regeneration of bone. When marked expansion and asymmetry have occurred, in the repair process nature will reestablish normal jaw contour and complete regeneration of bone if the surgery is adequate and no recurrence of the cystic lesion takes place.

Each case presents its own individual problems in diagnosis and treatment, but if both are adequate the prognosis should be excellent and complications kept to a minimum. The patient must be given every consideration, and he should have as good an understanding of the surgeon's problems as the surgeon has of the patient's concern for a satisfactory prognosis.

GENERAL CONSIDERATION OF CYSTIC LESIONS

This discussion will include problems in differential diagnosis, x-ray examination, surgical technique, postoperative treatment, and complications of surgery.

Diagnosis

Diagnosis in each individual case should rest upon a combination of physical findings, history, x-ray evaluation, and tissue biopsy. Histological examination is desirable and often essential to establish a correct diagnosis, but other clinical laboratory studies are often necessary. A patient should not be subjected to biopsy immediately to eliminate other studies; biopsy should be deferred until indications for it are very clear. Clinical symptoms are generally absent unless the cyst reaches large proportions and causes a facial deformity. Pain may be caused by the pressure of a cyst on a nerve and, likewise, paresthesia or numbness may be a clinical complaint. Cysts may be multiple, each from a separate anlage, but, conversely, multiple cysts may be indicative of systemic disease.

Because cysts of the soft tissues in the neck are often very tense, the differentiation between cystic and solid tumors may be difficult. The presence of inflammation and tenderness on pressure is a better sign of a cyst than of a tumor because cysts become secondarily infected more frequently. However, the tenseness of a cyst and mobility of the neck structures frequently make fluctuation an unreliable sign of fluid. The location, mobility, fixation, consistency, regional changes, and associated diseases are the most important factors in diagnosis.

In large cystic, bony defects that produce facial asymmetry, expansion takes place usually along the line of least resistance in bone and generally in one direction. A true neoplasm will usually grow and expand in and through bone in any and all directions. Structures such as nerves, blood vessels, and paranasal sinuses are usually displaced by the pressure exerted by the fluid contents of the cyst in contrast to a neoplasm, which invades and surrounds these tissues.

X-ray findings

The x-ray examination gives information about the location and extent of a bone cyst and involvement of other teeth. Overlying shadows may be misleading when many teeth appear involved in a cystic area, and a thorough clinical examination, including vitality tests, should be made. Pressure of the cystic fluid within the cavity may cause the formation of a compact layer of bone in which the cyst sac is contained. This dense lamina is seen on the x-ray film as a thin white line outlining the area containing the radiolucent cyst. A diagnosis can never be made positively from the x-ray findings since many neoplastic and metabolic diseases appear radiographically cystic. The jaws have been frequently referred to as an area of surgical romance because of the complexity of disease entities they contain, all of which present a problem in differential diagnosis. (See Fig. 14-14, A and B.) Cysts usually have a very smooth, rounded, lobular outline and may be multilocular in appearance (Fig. 14-14, C). However, if secondary infection exists, the margins can be quite irregular.

Cysts occurring in the maxilla are often difficult to visualize because of the overlapping shadows cast by the paranasal sinuses on x-ray examination. A radiopaque substance such as Lipiodol may be injected into the cystic cavity (Fig. 14-14, D). The radiopaque material is injected into the cavity after aspiration of the cystic contents. A large 19- or 20-gauge needle is used on a 3 or 5 ml. Luer syringe. After the fluid is aspirated from the cyst the syringe is removed from the needle, which is left in place, and another Luer syringe, containing the Lipiodol, attached to it. The opening made for entry into the cavity must be immediately stopped with a hemostat or sponge and the x-ray picture taken as soon as possible to avoid escape of the fluid. This technique can also be used to visualize soft tissue cysts and sinus tracts that otherwise would not be outlined on the x-ray film. Dermoid cysts may contain radiopaque objects.

Occasionally a radiolucent, irregularly outlined, small, punched-out type of area seen radiographically is mistaken for a recurrence of a cystic lesion. This radiographic appearance results when both cortical plates of bone are involved in the cystic defect or else removed during surgical excision of the lesion (Fig. 14-14, E). Complete regeneration of these cortical plates rarely follows, and the defect will always be seen on the x-ray film. Here history is important, and it is wise to inform a patient of this finding so that it can be explained if he is examined by another dentist, thereby avoiding further and needless operations on these areas.

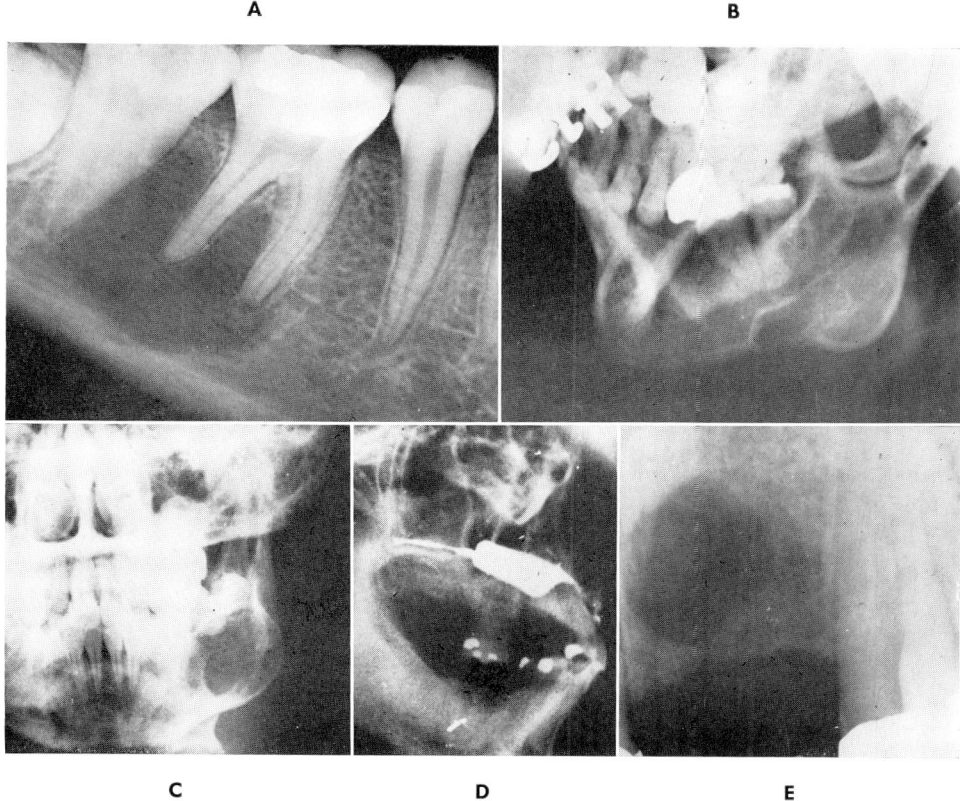

Fig. 14-14. **A**, Idiopathic bone cavity. The presence of an intact lamina dura and a positive vitality test indicate that the lesion is not of odontogenic origin. **B**, Lateral jaw radiograph showing latent bone cavity near inferior border of mandible. **C**, A characteristic cystic lesion showing expansion and thinning of the cortical bone. **D**, Maxillary cyst outlined by the injection of a radiopaque material. **E**, Radiographic appearance of a healed postoperative defect in which both labial bone and palatal cortical bone were lost in the removal of the original cystic lesion.

Surgical technique

Regardless of the etiology, nature, or location of the cyst, two methods of treatment are generally accepted:

1. Enucleation of the cystic sac in its entirety
2. The Partsch operation or marsupialization, by which the cyst is uncovered or "deroofed" and the cystic lining made continuous with the oral cavity or surrounding structures

In either case the surgical procedure must be based on sound fundamental principles. These principles include preservation of the blood supply to the area, avoidance of undue trauma to nerve filaments and nerve trunks in the region, control of hemorrhage, aseptic technique, atraumatic handling of the soft tissues, planning of a surgical flap so that adequate relaxation may be obtained to allow good access to a cystic area, avoidance of important anatomical structures such as muscle attachments and large blood vessels, and proper suturing and readaptation of the soft tissues. A sharp, clean incision planned so that soft tissues are readapted over a firm bony bed will always heal better with less postoperative discomfort than when tissue is torn, lacerated, or sutured directly over a bone defect.

The discussion on surgical technique will include the treatment of both soft tissue and bone cysts.

Soft tissue cysts

The soft tissue cysts include those of congenital origin, which occur primarily in the neck, and the retention-type cysts, mucoceles and ranulas, which occur primarily in the oral cavity. The surgical techniques described for the treatment of congenital cysts are presented primarily to indicate correct procedure rather than to describe the detailed dissection frequently necessary in the structures of the neck.

Congenital cysts. Congenital cysts occur usually in the neck, submandibular, and submental regions. They are benign entities, but thorough dissection and excision are necessary for a cure.

Thyroglossal cysts. Thyroglossal duct abnormalities should be treated by surgical excision. Repeated lancing of the cyst, except to alleviate an acute inflammatory condition, is ineffective. The use of sclerosing agents and irradiation is also contraindicated.

Surgical excision is accomplished through a transverse incision over the cyst (Fig. 14-1). Overlying tissues are carefully separated and the fibrous tract identified and followed by further dissection. Injection of a dye to more definitely outline the sinus tract has one disadvantage—the dye frequently spills over and stains other tissues, obscuring the operative field. Usually the fibrous tract can be followed without this additional aid. To facilitate exposure the hyoid bone is separated to aid in dissecting above this point and allow excision of the foramen cecum, which is the terminating point of the thyroglossal duct.

In closing the wound the musculature of the tongue is brought together with interrupted silk or chromic sutures, the severed edges of the hyoid bone are approximated with sutures through periosteum or adjacent fascia, and a small rubber tube drain is placed deep in the muscles of the tongue and through the skin incision.

Branchiogenic cysts and fistulas. In excising branchiogenic fistulas, a radiopaque substance such as Lipiodol or Pantopaque is used to identify the extent and location of the fistula and sinus tract. A probe may also be passed in the tract to aid in identification as the dissection proceeds. A stepladder technique, as developed by Hamilton Bailey, aids in following the sinus tract to its termination in the pharyngeal wall. This two-step procedure minimizes resultant scar formation.

The tract is ligated with fine silk or catgut at its entrance into the pharynx, and the wounds are closed in the usual manner with dependent drainage. The drain is usually removed in 2 or 3 days.

The best approach to a branchiogenic cyst is through an incision centered over the most prominent part of the cyst and parallel to the anterior border of the sternomastoid muscle (Fig. 14-2). The cyst may have attachments to important nerve trunks and vessels, and it is therefore necessary to have adequate exposure in visualizing the cyst. Care must be taken to prevent rupture of the cyst during the dissection. Any epithelium left behind will give rise to a recurrence. The wound is closed in layers and skin sutured in such a manner as to give the best cosmetic result. A small drain is left in the wound for 1 or 2 days.

Dermoid cysts. Dermoid cysts (Fig. 14-3) are, as a rule, more superficial to branchiogenic cleft cysts and are not attached to the lateral pharyngeal wall. Frequently it is rather difficult to make a careful distinction between these cysts as they occur in the neck prior to operation, but surgical removal is the treatment of choice in either case. The sublingual dermoid cysts, seen in

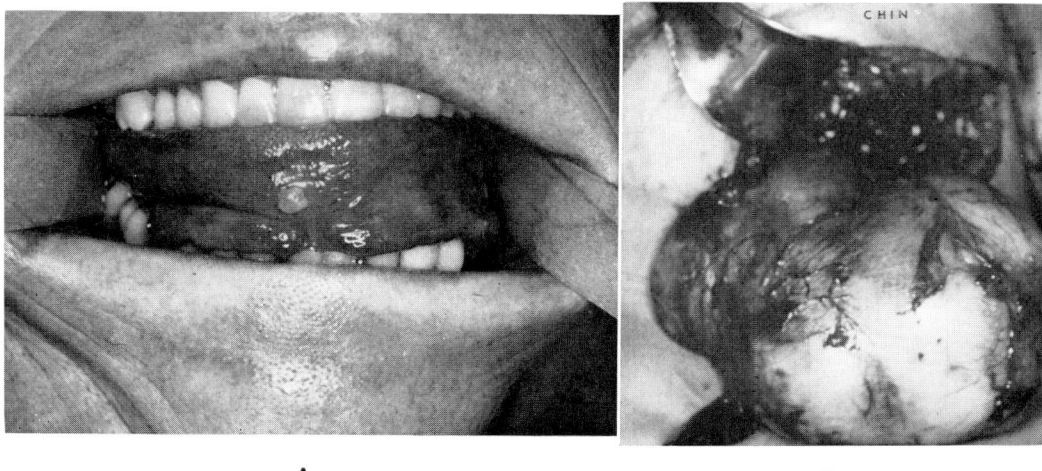

Fig. 14-15. A, Large dermoid cyst of floor of mouth. B, Removal through extraoral incision. (Courtesy Department of Oral Surgery, Henry Ford Hospital, Detroit, Mich.)

the floor of the mouth, are excised intraorally. (See Fig. 14-15.)

Retention cysts. Retention cysts are generally located in the oral cavity and are treated by simple excision or marsupialization, depending upon their size and location.

Mucoceles. The preferable treatment is complete surgical excision (Fig. 14-16). A very careful incision must be made through the thin overlying epithelium, which is usually stretched tight over the underlying mucous cyst. An alternate incision (Fig. 14-16, C) preserving the overlying mucous membrane, to aid in grasping tissue during enucleation of the mucocele, sometimes facilitates dissection. Usually the mucous cyst will tend to pop out of its soft tissue bed and can be carefully teased free, using blunt dissection with a small curved hemostat, curet, or periosteal elevator. Care must be taken not to rupture the sac since then the dissection becomes more difficult and one cannot be positive that the cyst has been removed in its entirety. Recurrence of these lesions is quite common. Shira[11] has described a technique in which he aspirates the contents of the mucocele and injects a thin mix of alginate or rubber-base impression material. This hardens and clearly outlines the entire extent of the lesion and aids in the dissection.

Ranulas. Simple incision and drainage of the ranula always results in its recurrence. Enucleation of a ranula without rupturing the thin cystic wall is practically impossible and fraught with considerable complications. Once a cyst ruptures it is very difficult to pick up the continuity of a lining, and if all is not thoroughly removed, the ranula is likely to recur. A seton in the form of a wire loop may be used to attempt to reestablish an epithelial-lined duct opening, but this frequently fails. Radium for the treatment of ranula is known to be effective.* The contents of the cyst are aspirated, and a Crowe nasopharyngeal applicator with 50 mg. of radium is inserted into the cyst cavity and held in place, usually ligated to the teeth, for 25 minutes. Some blanching of tissue follows treatment, but no undue sloughing occurs if the correct exposure time and dosage are used.

---

*Rex B. Foster, D.D.S., Waterloo, Iowa, personal communication.

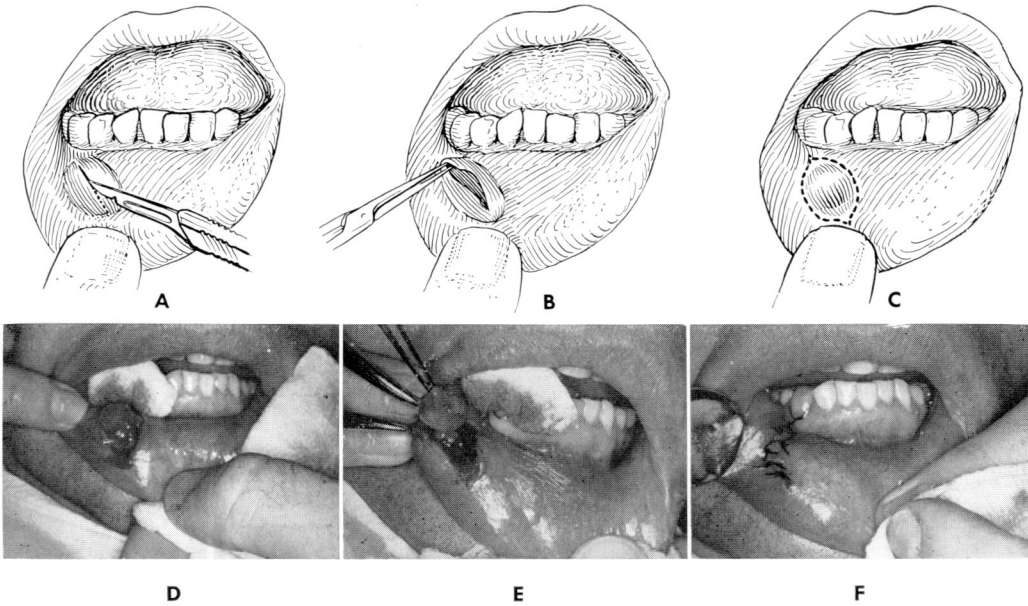

Fig. 14-16. **A,** Removal of mucocele, showing scalpel making light incision through the overlying mucous membrane. **B,** Fine scissors to free cyst wall from surrounding tissues. **C,** Alternate method: an eliptical incision leaving the mucous membrane intact over the cyst membrane may aid in dissecting the mucocele. **D,** Mucocele "popping out." **E,** Cyst grasped with tissue forceps and dissected free. **F,** Bleeding controlled and incision sutured.

The Partsch operation or marsupialization of a ranula is generally agreed upon as the best surgical procedure. This consists of excising the superior wall of the ranula and suturing the cystic lining to the mucous membrane of the floor of the mouth to make it continuous with the oral cavity.

The following technique is used (Fig. 14-17). A series of sutures is placed around the peripheral margins of the cyst. The sutures go through the normal mucosa of the floor of the mouth and the cyst lining. When the cyst outline is well marked with sutures, the superior wall is excised just inside the sutures. The bottom of the cyst then elevates into a normal position with escape of the fluid contents and becomes continuous with the floor of the mouth. The cystic membrane undergoes transformation and assumes the characteristics of the adjoining structures.

Some operators like to remove a small portion of the superior wall, aspirate the contents of the cyst, and outline the defect by filling it with sterile, selvedge-edged gauze. The dissection of the superior cyst wall is then completed, and peripheral sutures are placed. This procedure is best done under a local anesthetic with lingual nerve block. Supplemental local infiltration is generally unnecessary. If the swelling occurs across the midline, bilateral block is necessary.

Bone cysts

Access to a bone cyst must be gained by incising and reflecting the mucoperiosteum. The nature of the surgical approach is governed by the location and extent of the cyst. Whether a bone cyst is completely enucleated or treated by the Partsch method or its modifications depends more

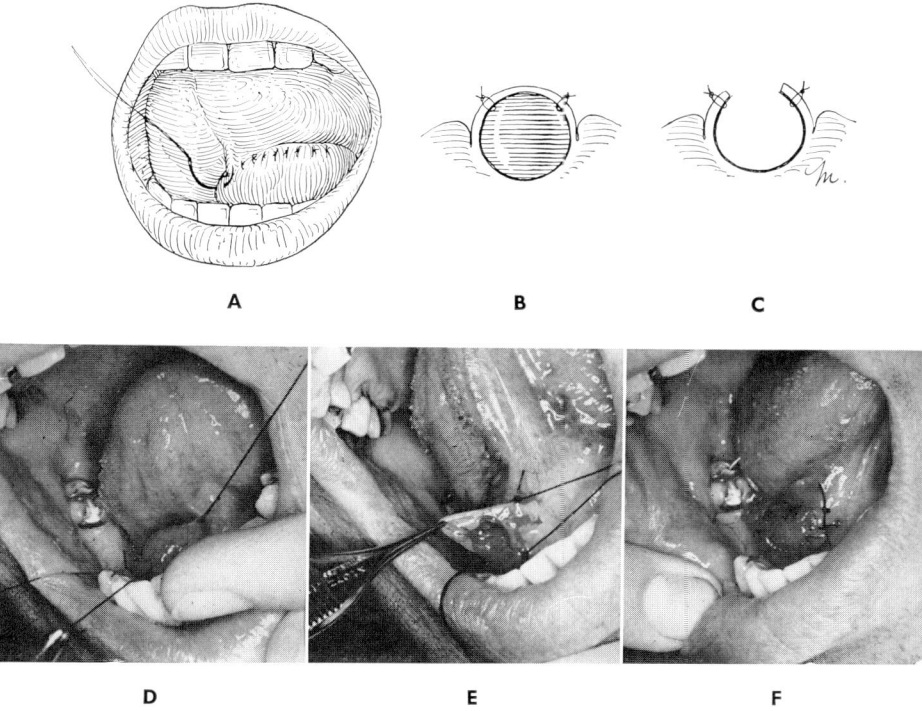

Fig. 14-17. **A,** Marsupialization of a ranula, showing sutures being placed through mucous membrane and underlying cyst wall. **B,** Cross section. **C,** Window cut and contents of cyst aspirated. The floor of the cyst becomes part of the floor of the mouth. **D,** Clinical view of first stage, showing placing of sutures. **E,** Mucous membrane overlying cyst, and superior wall of cyst grasped with tissue forceps and cut free with scissors inside of sutures. **F,** Additional sutures placed. The floor of the cyst, which is now a portion of the floor of the mouth, can be seen.

on its size and location than on the actual diagnosis of the cyst.

When enucleation is the method of choice, overlying bone must be removed with chisels, rongeur forceps, or bone bur. Many times the bone is of tissue-paper thickness and can be removed readily with a hemostat. Frequently the bone is entirely eroded through, and the cystic membrane becomes attached to the periosteum or soft tissue covering and has to be cleanly dissected from it. This is further complicated by secondary infection on occasions, with the formation of a fistulous tract and considerable scar tissue. The cystic sac must be well exposed so that it can be carefully teased from its bony bed (Fig. 14-18).

Mocse[7] has advocated the use of an osteoperiosteal flap in operating upon large tumors and cysts of the jaw that exhibit thin cortices (Fig. 14-19). This technique consists essentially of incising through the mucoperiosteum and the thin cortical plate of bone at the same time. This may be done with a knife if the bone is thin or by placing a sharp chisel on the flap outline and carefully tapping it so that the chisel penetrates the bone. The bone is then reflected, adherent to the mucoperiosteum, to expose the cystic area. This procedure is best carried out on the labial and buccal sides

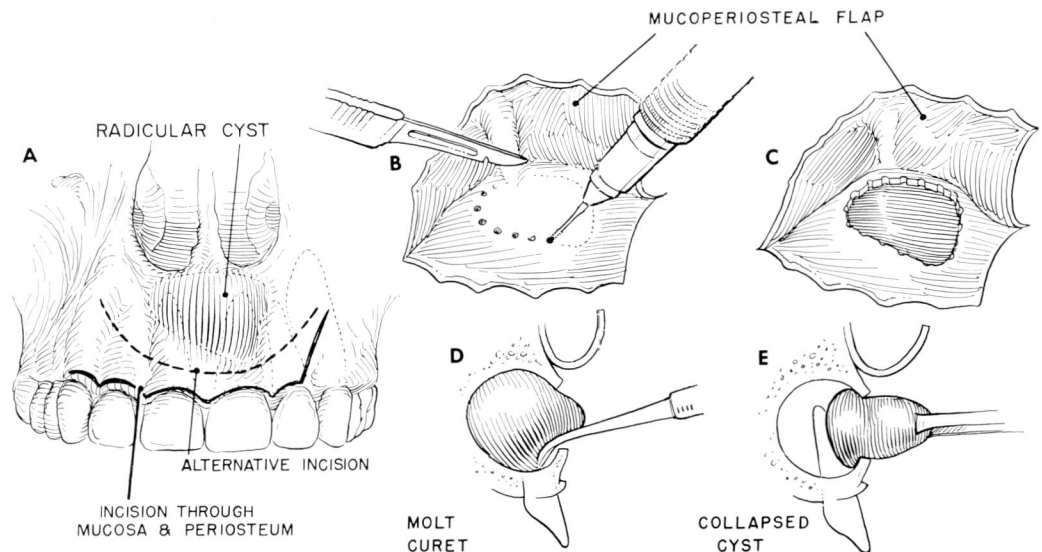

Fig. 14-18. Cyst enucleation. **A,** Incision is made either at the gingival margins or in semilunar form above the margins, and a large mucoperiosteal flap is raised. The central incisors are nonvital in this case. **B,** Note the fibrous attachment of the cyst wall to the mucoperiosteum because of a chronic fistula. The attachment must be dissected free. Perforations may be made carefully with a bone bur through the cortical plate to outline the cystic cavity. The bone chisel can be used equally well, or a rongeur will suffice if the bony perforation is large enough for initial entrance. **C,** The overlying bone has been removed. The anterior portion of the cyst wall is seen. **D,** The back of a curet is used to lift the cyst wall from the sides of the bony cavity. **E,** Gentle traction on the cyst wall with tissue forceps and concomitant release of the deeper portion of the cyst wall from the bone with the curet will deliver the cyst. The devitalized teeth must have root canal therapy with apicoectomy or else be extracted. A gauze dressing is placed in the defect and brought out through the alveolar socket, or through a stab incision in the flap if the teeth are retained. The wound is sutured.

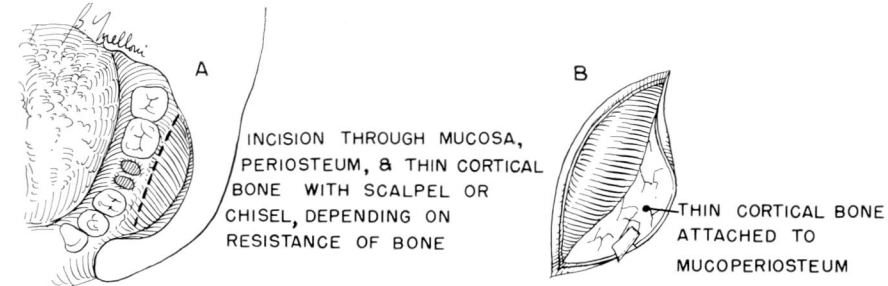

Fig. 14-19. Osteoperiosteal flap. **A,** Line of incision. **B,** Flap retracted. The underlying cyst wall can be seen.

of the maxilla and mandible. After removal of the lesion the flap is returned to its original position and sutured. The preservation of this bone attached to the periosteum increases the osteogenic surface of tissues surrounding the blood clot filling the cystic cavity. This enhances the possibility of primary healing and also forms a better nucleus for regeneration of bone. Fractures occurring in this thin bone as the flap is reflected are not important as long as the pieces do not become entirely detached from the periosteum. If they do become detached, they are removed and discarded.

A thin-blade curet is a very suitable instrument for removing a cystic lining from bone. The largest curet that can easily be placed in the defect should be used. The concave side of the curet is usually placed against the bone as the thin blade is teased in between the cyst wall and the bone cavity (Fig. 14-18, D). Care must be utilized to avoid tearing the cystic sac and allowing escape of the fluid contents if possible. Good lighting and direct vision are essential so that it can be determined that the entire cystic sac is removed from bone. Frequently in large cysts a suction tip can be used in dissecting the cyst free from its bony bed. In the large defects nerves and vessels are usually found pushed to one side, and they should not be traumatized unduly. The bony edges of the defect should then be saucerized and smoothed before the soft tissues are reapproximated with sutures and the wound is closed. This may be done with a rongeur, antrum bur, or bone file. Local antibiotic therapy in the form of dusting the walls lightly with topical drugs may aid in wound healing. Systemic antibiotic medication is favored in the presence of inflammation or infection. Any local use of an antibiotic drug should be augmented by systemic therapy.

The size and location of a cyst would govern whether or not a dressing in the form of gauze packing, Gelfoam, or bone chips may be placed. These dressings all tend to control bleeding, prevent hematoma formation with resultant breaking down of the blood clot and septic drainage, and also promote healing.

In the smaller cysts, up to 15 to 20 mm. in size, usually no dressing is necessary since the wound will heal by primary intention. This is particularly true in the maxilla. An organized blood clot forms in the cavity, which leads to proliferation of young connective tissue and ultimate new bone formation. In the larger cavities the wound heals by secondary intention with gradual apposition of tissue obliterating the defect. Here the original blood clot has no chance of surviving, and necrosis will occur before secondary proliferation of new vascular supply can form to preserve the center of the clot.

When a gauze dressing is used, ½ or 1 inch selvedged iodoform or plain gauze with a medication such as balsam of Peru incorporated in it is quite satisfactory. This gauze is well placed in the cavity to exert pressure against any points that may show some tendency toward bleeding and is usually removed, either entirely or partially, on the fifth to seventh postoperative day. If considerable bleeding is encountered at the time of surgery, it is usually best to loosen the dressing gradually and remove it in sections over a period of from 10 to 12 days. The defect can be carefully irrigated when the dressing is removed, and these areas are usually redressed twice a week until healing takes place over the bony walls where the cyst has been removed. This time interval usually involves 15 to 20 days.

The large cystic area may also be packed with bone chips obtained from the bone bank. Freeze-dried bone in small fragments suitably prepared from cancellous or cortical bone can be packed into the bony crypt.[5] Cancellous bone is preferred. Topical antibiotics or sulfa drugs may be incorporated into the mass before replacing the soft tissue flap and suturing the wound, closing the wound carefully. Occasionally some of the small chips may act as foreign bodies and be exfoliated. However, the great majority of the chips will remain to serve as a supporting structure for the blood clot. Also, some stimulation of the young connective tissue seems to occur, increasing fibroblastic and osteoblastic activity and further enhancing the rate of healing.

Various bone substitutes have been used to obliterate cystic cavities following removal of the pathological tissue. For instance, heterogenous processed bone has been given extensive trial.[10] Plaster of paris has been used to obliterate bone cavities.[13] Bahn[12] has published a review of the literature and reported many clinical cases in which results have been favorable. The search continues for a suitable bone substitute that can be used to fill large cystic cavities in bone so that the overlying tissues can be sutured tightly without the need for packing and removing gauze strips. The substitute ideally should be made from lower species tissue to be commercially available. It should be treated in such manner that the immune reaction will not cause graft rejection, and still it should be capable of stimulating host osteoclastic and osteoblastic activity.

The marsupialization technique as previously described for surgical treatment of ranula is also applicable to bone cysts. This cyst is "deroofed" and the surrounding mucoperiosteum sutured to the margins of the cyst wall or held in place with dressings. This, in effect, makes the cyst wall continuous with the oral cavity. (See Fig. 14-21.)

After reflecting the oral mucoperiosteal flap the bone overlying the cyst is carefully removed, taking care not to penetrate the cyst. When the periphery of the cavity is reached, a sharp pair of scissors can be used to cut out the exposed membranous wall. This tissue is sent to the laboratory for histological examination. After the contents of the cyst are evacuated the mucoperiosteum is allowed to fold into the defect and is sutured to the lining of the cyst. Apposition is maintained by pressure, using gauze dressings.

If gauze dressings are used, they may be removed in about 7 to 10 days, although it may be necessary to change the dressings in the interim. If a large opening has been made in the marsupialization of the cyst, usually nothing more is necessary as healing progresses. If only a small window is made to gain access to the cystic cavity, it sometimes becomes necessary to construct an acrylic plug, which can be drilled and made hollow to maintain drainage in the area and also keep the opening patent as healing progresses (Fig. 14-20). The wound can be kept irrigated and clean through this opening.

With the release of fluid pressure in bone, regeneration occurs beneath the defect and the cystic epithelial lining is transformed into normal mucous membrane by evagination from the adjacent areas. The tube drainage technique of treating large cysts, as advocated by Thomas, is also a modification of the Partsch method. (See Figs. 14-20 and 14-21.) A small opening is made into the defect, and a soft metal or polyethylene tube is inserted and held in place by ligation to adjacent teeth to maintain drainage. Either is easily adapted to the cyst opening. This relieves pressure from inside the cyst, and gradual obliteration of the cavity occurs by apposition of soft and bony tissue to close the defect. Periodic irrigation of the cavity is accomplished through the tube. The tube may be shortened as healing progresses.

Indications for marsupialization of a cyst include those conditions in which adjacent vital structures such as teeth may be involved if the cystic contents are completely enucleated, or danger exists of entering adjacent paranasal sinuses, or a marked bone defect is to be avoided. The possible occurrence of paresthesia from sur-

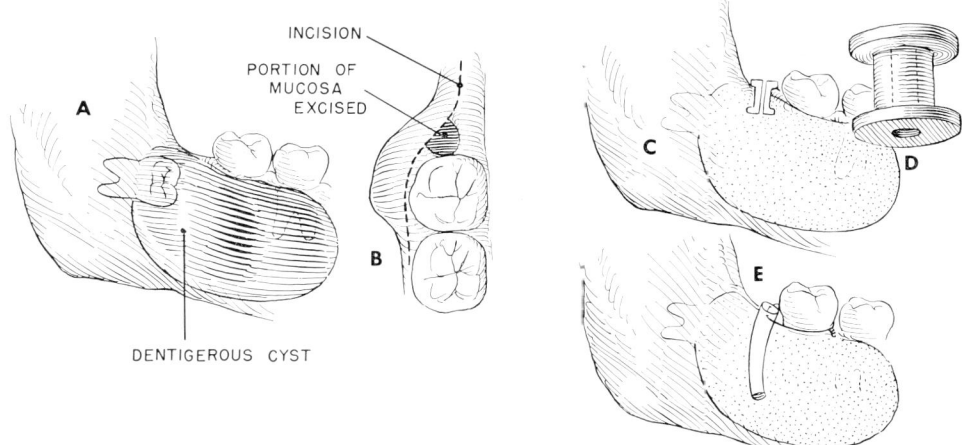

Fig. 14-20. Modified marsupialization technique. **A**, Dentigerous cyst around unerupted third molar. **B**, A window is cut in the mucosa to receive the obturator. The third molar is removed and a portion of the cyst wall is removed for microscopic study. Developmental cysts that have the potential of histological cell change must be carefully followed postoperatively. **C, D, E**, An acrylic button or a plastic or metal tube is used to keep the wound open, maintain drainage, and provide access for irrigating the cystic defect to keep the wound clean. These devices are removed when radiographic examination shows that new bone has formed up to them.

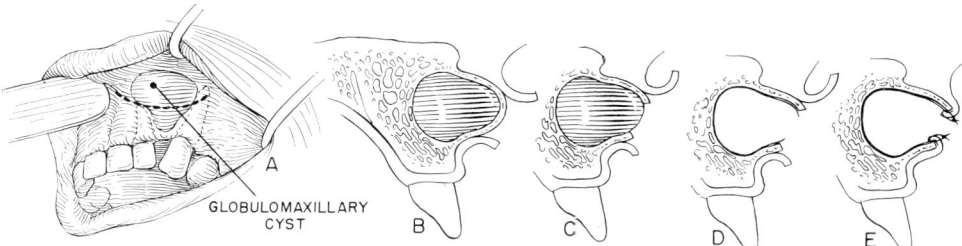

Fig. 14-21. Marsupialization technique. **A**, Enucleation of the globulomaxillary cyst in this case might endanger the adjacent teeth. **B**, Incision made through mucoperiosteum. The central portion of the flap is removed. **C**, The bone overlying the cyst is removed generously to correspond with the outline of the underlying cavity. **D**, The exposed portion of the cyst wall is excised and submitted for microscopic examination. **E**, The mucosa is sutured to the cyst wall, with the mucoperiosteal flap folded in. The cavity is packed with selvedged gauze for 5 days. The gauze may be changed once or twice before removing it entirely.

gical trauma or severance of a nerve is also eliminated.

This technique is applicable to a large number of cysts occurring in the oral cavity. However, it must be used with some reservation in those cystic lesions that have potentialities of developing into tumor. In these instances adequate exposure should be made so that the cyst lining can be thoroughly examined clinically, and in many cases biopsy should be taken from any suspicious section. This type lesion should be followed very closely postoperatively with clinical and x-ray examination.

Some operators will remove the cystic or epithelized lining as a second operation after enough bone apposition has occurred following relief of pressure from the cystic lesion. This eliminates the danger sometimes encountered in primary enucleation, but submits the patient to a second surgical procedure and does not materially affect the final outcome of treatment.

In the Partsch operation the actual filling in of a bone defect may take a longer period of time. However, in most instances no contraindication exists for not going ahead with whatever prosthetic restoration might be necessary. Maintenance of good oral hygiene and care in keeping the area clean should be all that is necessary after normal epithelization of the defect has occurred.

Postoperative complications

The complications that may result following enucleation or marsupialization of congenital and developmental cysts include swelling, infection, hematoma formation, sensory and motor nerve injury, primary or secondary hemorrhage, oral fistula, fracture of bone, and obstruction of the airway. Motor nerve injury and airway obstruction occur primarily in removal of lesions involving dissections in the neck and submandibular areas.

The best way to avoid complications is to prevent them by thorough diagnostic study, good surgical judgment, and proper surgical technique. However, complications will occur, and it is well to know how to treat them when they develop.

Postoperative edema is normal and physiological following most surgical procedures on the jaws. Most of this surgery is of a traumatic nature, and prolonged retraction of tissues adds to the interference of normal lymphatic drainage of the area. This, coupled with inflammatory reaction, is bound to produce edema and swelling. The patient should be advised of this beforehand. The height of the swelling should be reached about the second postoperative day, with gradual subsidence if no secondary infection or hematoma formation develops. The immediate application of cold is of doubtful benefit, but may be used for the first 8 to 10 hours postoperatively. Antiinflammatory agents such as corticosteroid drugs and animal and plant enzymes may in certain instances be helpful in controlling postoperative edema. These agents must be administered with a complete knowledge of possible side effects and contraindications.

The possibility of infection can be minimized by antibiotic therapy, good surgical technique, and strict adherence to rules of asepsis. Any acute infection occurring in these lesions should be well controlled before surgical intervention is done. Antibiotics must be carefully chosen and administered in therapeutic dosage, either empirically or by organism sensitivity tests.

Hematoma formation can be prevented by controlling the bleeding initially and by the additional use of dressings and applied pressure. Large blood vessels should be tied off, but most of the bleeding that might be encountered comes from areas inaccessible for ligation, and pressure is utilized for its control. Soft tissue flaps should be well sutured and adequate external pressure placed on the operative area for the first few postoperative hours.

A persistent hematoma that is readily accessible should be aspirated and drained. Otherwise a breakdown of the blood clot will occur, with septic drainage. The use of enzyme therapy, such as hyaluronidase, might be of some value in early hematoma formation, but should be avoided if any question of secondary infection is present. This substance, injected into the tissues, opens up the interstitial spaces and promotes a more rapid absorption and diffusion of fluids from an involved area.

Sensory nerve trunks are usually displaced by cystic lesions, and many times the cyst linings are stripped free of this nerve by careful dissection. When a sensory nerve trunk is exposed in a cavity, a paresthesia usually results. This may be of unknown duration since the rate of recovery to nerve injury varies considerably. However, large nerve trunks are usually not severed in careful surgical procedures, and return of sensation almost universally occurs. Small nerves that are sacrificed in these surgical areas usually have some cross innervation so that the immediate effect is not noticed by the patient. The patient should be thoroughly forewarned of this complication; he then is able to accept the resultant numbness much more graciously. One should carefully explain that possible fifth nerve injury involves sensation only and not any motor function, so that no outward changes to the appearance of the face will occur. However, in soft tissue dissection the anatomy of the facial nerve must be thoroughly understood. Injury to this motor nerve will result in muscle paralysis.

Primary hemorrhage must be controlled at the time of surgery. Secondary hemorrhage usually occurs in those cases in which injury to a large vessel has occurred at the time of surgery. It can also occur by inadvertent trauma of newly proliferated blood vessels during removal of surgical dressings. This complication is usually again controlled by pressure. Care should be taken to remove large blood clots and determine the site of bleeding before applying pressure in the correct manner. Occasionally a blood vessel can be identified and tied off with a ligature.

Oronasal or oroantral fistulas sometimes result from injudicious choice of surgical procedure or human error in surgical technique. It can also result from a normal anatomical relation of pathology to existing structures. This complication can often be avoided by careful dissection, and frequently cystic linings can be carefully peeled from other membranous linings without penetrating into nasal or antral cavities. Use of the Partsch method of treatment, if applicable, may be helpful. If small openings occur, proper healing can usually be attained by careful attention to wound closure and detailed instructions to the patient. Postoperative care is of paramount importance in many instances in preventing permanent fistula formation, which necessitates secondary closure. Secondary infection should also be prevented. The patient should be cautioned about excessive sneezing and coughing and instructed to keep his mouth open should these episodes occur, to equalize the pressure in the paranasal sinuses and prevent undue force on the area where the wound communicates with the oral cavity.

Bone is weakened by the presence of a cyst, with the exact amount of weakening dependent upon the size and extent of the pathology. Usually the possibility of fracture occurring during surgery is quite remote unless undue trauma is exerted upon the jaw or both cortical plates are excessively thin. Trauma in the form of a twisting movement producing torque is much more likely to fracture bone than is direct pressure. Because of the nature of a cyst, which expands primarily in a single direction, one cortical plate of bone is likely to be intact. This preserves the continuity of the jaw. Prevention again is the best form of treatment, and careful surgical technique must be used, particularly in those cysts in which unerupted teeth are present and difficult to remove. Should a fracture occur, proceed with the enucleation of the cyst and then pack the defect well with suitable gauze dressings or bone chips to maintain the position of the fragments and prevent unnecessary displacement. The jaw should also be immobilized. A patient with a large cystic involvement of the jaws should be cautioned to avoid any undue trauma, both preoperatively and postoperatively, since a blow is more likely to cause fracture in a weakened jaw than in a normal one.

Postoperative airway obstruction may follow surgical procedures involving the jaws, tongue, and tissues of the neck. Massive edema, hematoma formation, and infection are contributing factors. Should signs of labored breathing and inadequate respiratory exchange be evident, tracheostomy must be done. This should, so far as possible, be an elective procedure rather than an emergency one.

Proper postoperative care is just as important a part of the patient's over-all problem as the diagnosis and surgical treatment.

REFERENCES

1. Thoma, K. H.: Oral pathology, ed. 5, St. Louis, 1960, The C. V. Mosby Co.
2. Martin, H.: Surgery of head and neck tumors, New York, 1957, Hoeber-Harper.
3. Ward, G. E., and Hendrick, J. W.: Diagnosis and treatment of tumors of the head and neck, Baltimore, 1950, The Williams & Wilkins Co.
4. Archer, W.: Oral surgery, ed. 4, Philadelphia, 1966, W. B. Saunders Co.
5. Boyne, P. J.: Clinical use of freeze dried homogenous bone, J. Oral Surg. 15:236, 1956.
6. Kreuz, F. P., and others: Preservation and clinical use of freeze dried bone, J. Bone Joint Surg. 33A:803, 1951.
7. Moose, S. M.: Osteoperiosteal flap for operation of large tumors and cysts of jaws, J. Oral Surg. 10:229, 1952.
8. Pindborg, J. J., and James, P.: Variations in odontogenic cyst epithelium, Trans. 2nd Cong. Int. Assoc. Oral Surg., pp. 121, 127, 135-140, Munksgaard-Copenhagen, 1967.
9. Thomas, E.: Saving involved vital teeth by tube drainage, J. Oral Surg. 5:1, 1947.
10. Lyon, H. W., and Boyne, P. J.: Host response to chemically treated heterogenous bone implants, J. Dent. Res. I.A.D.R. Abstracts, 42:83, 1963.
11. Shira, R. B.: Simplified technic for the management of mucoceles and ranulas, J. Oral Surg. 20:374, 1962.
12. Bahn, S. L.: Plaster, a bone substitute, Oral Surg. 21:682, 1966.
13. Calhoun, N. R., Neiders, M. E., and Greene, G. W., Jr.: Effects of plaster of paris implants in surgical defects of mandibular alveolar processes of dogs, J. Oral Surg. 25:122, 1967.

Chapter 15

DISEASES OF THE MAXILLARY SINUS OF DENTAL ORIGIN

Phillip Earle Williams

DESCRIPTION

The maxillary sinus, or antrum of Highmore, so named because this antrum, meaning a cavity or hollow space especially found in bone, was first described by Nathaniel Highmore, an English anatomist of the seventeenth century, is generally larger than any of the other sinuses and lies chiefly in the body of the maxilla. It is actually present as a small cavity at birth, starting its development during the third fetal month and usually reaching its maximum development in early adult life about the eighteenth year. The capacity of the average adult antrum is from 10 to 15 ml., and its complete absence is quite rare. Often subcompartments, recesses, and crypts are present, being formed by osseous and membranous septa. Fig. 15-1 shows x-ray films that reveal this condition.

The maxillary sinus is pyramidal in shape with its base at the nasoantral wall and its apex in the root of the zygoma. The upper wall or roof in the adult is thin; it is situated under the orbit and is the orbital plate of the maxilla. This plate usually possesses a bony canal for the infraorbital nerve and vessels. The floor of the sinus is the alveolar process of the maxilla. In front the anterolateral or canine fossa wall is the facial part of the maxilla. The posterior or sphenomaxillary wall, which is of lesser importance, consists of a thin plate of bone separating the cavity from the infratemporal fossa. The nasal wall separates the sinus from the nasal cavity medially. The nasal cavity contains the outlet from the sinus, the ostium maxillae, which lies just beneath the roof of the antrum. The location of this opening precludes the possibility of good drainage when the individual is in a vertical position.

The sinus is lined with a thin mucosa, which is attached to the periosteum. The ciliated epithelium aids in the removal of excretions and secretions that form in the sinus cavity. The cilia hold foreign material at their tips much as twigs or leaves are held on the surface of many blades of grass. Waves of ciliary action carry the material from one ciliated region to another toward the ostium. These waves could be compared to gusts of wind indenting a wheat field from one side to the other. Only a pathological membrane that has deficient ciliary action or is devoid of cilia in whole or in part will allow foreign materials to rest on its surface.

238 Textbook of oral surgery

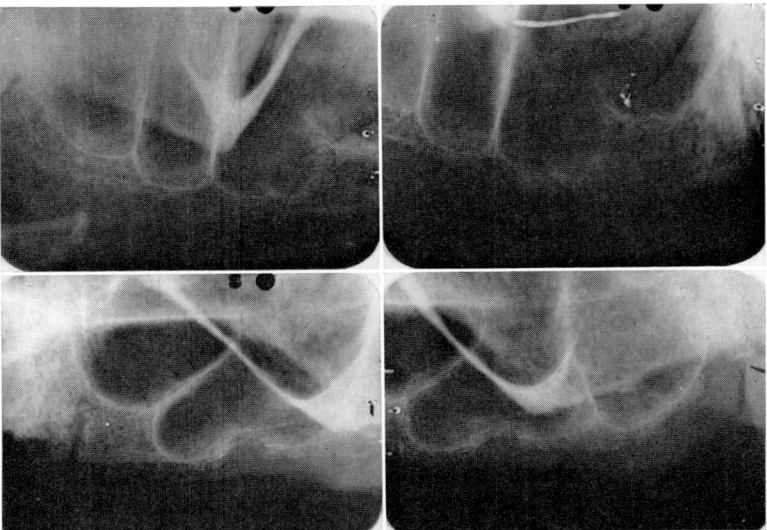

Fig. 15-1. Osseous septa in normal maxillary sinus. Left and right sides of same patient.

The thickness of the sinus walls is not constant, especially the roof and floor. The walls may vary in thickness from 2 to 5 mm. in the roof and from 2 to 3 mm. in the floor. Edentulous areas vary from 5 to 10 mm. In the event that the posterior wall is penetrated, causing entrance into the infratemporal fossa, care must be exercised in any operative procedure because of the presence of large vessels such as the maxillary artery and vein. Infraorbital and superior alveolar vessels are frequently ruptured in midfacial fractures, giving rise to the formation of hematomas in the antrum.

Below the floor are found the deciduous and permanent teeth, and quite often the roots of the permanent molar or premolar teeth may extend into the sinus itself. In children and infants, the floor of the sinus is always higher than the floor of the nose, so that better drainage is readily obtainable from window operations, which will be described later. In adults the reverse is true; the floor of the sinus is lower than the nasal floor.

The nerve supply is from the maxillary branch of the fifth cranial nerve, the posterosuperior alveolar branch of this nerve supplying the lining of the mucous membrane. Its blood supply is derived from the infraorbital artery, a branch of the maxillary artery. Some collateral supply is derived from the anterosuperior alveolar artery, a branch of the same vessel. The lymphatic supply is quite abundant and terminates into the submandibular nodes.

The functions or purposes of all the paranasal sinuses are as follows: (1) to give resonance to the voice (note the change in the sounds of words of persons with colds), (2) to act as reserve chambers to warm the respired air, (3) to reduce the weight of the skull. During inspiration the suction through the nasal cavity draws some warmed air from the sinuses. The sinuses are connected with the nasal cavities by openings or channels so that the mucous membrane of the sinuses is continuous with that of the nose. Because of this, ventilation and drainage of the sinuses are made possible.

Frequently radiographs reveal unusually large sinuses, with the root ends residing directly in the floor (Fig. 15-2). This may

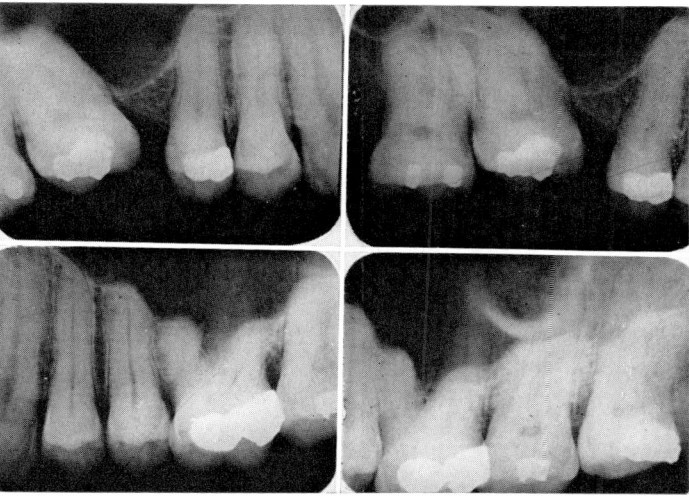

Fig. 15-2. Large sinus (left and right) with thin bony wall separating the floor from the apices of the teeth.

be confusing, resulting in an erroneous suspicion of pathology. Intraoral views are obtained of the opposite side and comparison is made; if the bony architecture is the same, then a diagnosis of no apparent pathology is readily made. The taking of skull pictures is to be encouraged because a study of them is most revealing and comparison of all the anatomical structures may be made readily. Of all the diagnostic aids used in the study of the maxillary sinus, the radiograph is the most dependable. Fig. 15-3 shows a skull film of normal, healthy sinuses.

In this connection, any time that the usual intraoral radiographs reveal the absence of a tooth in the arch and no history of previous extraction of that tooth is found, then extraoral views should be made. Many times the absent tooth will be shown to be aberrant and residing high in the superior part of the maxillary sinus. Figs. 15-4 and 15-5 show preoperative and postoperative views of this condition. Often these teeth will be the cause of headaches or neuralgias, and upon the removal of the displaced tooth and associated pathology these unpleasant conditions will disappear.

Toothache is frequently a symptom of maxillary sinus infection. The superior alveolar nerves run for a considerable distance in the walls of the antrum. They are contained with small blood and lymph vessels in narrow, sometimes anastomosing canals. Progressive expansion of the sinus in older persons invariably causes resorption of the inner walls of one or more of these canals, and thus the connective tissue covering the structures in the canals is brought into direct contact with the connective tissue of the mucoperiosteum of the sinus. This will cause involvement of dental nerves if sinus inflammation occurs. The quality of the pain sometimes resembles that of pulpitis. Examination of the teeth by cold stimulation will reveal, however, that not one but an entire group of teeth, sometimes all of the teeth in one maxilla, are hypersensitive.

DISEASES

Maxillary sinusitis occurs in the acute, subacute, and chronic forms. A careful diagnosis is important since the cure of the disease depends upon the removal of the cause. It is important to determine whether

240 Textbook of oral surgery

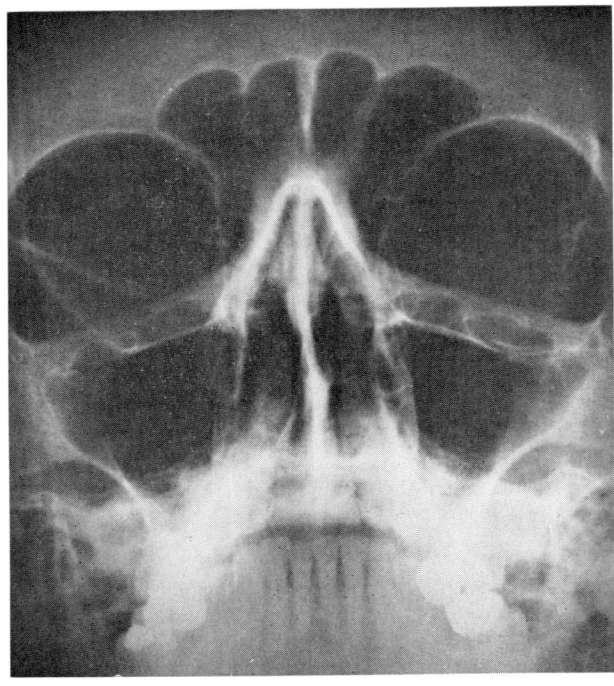

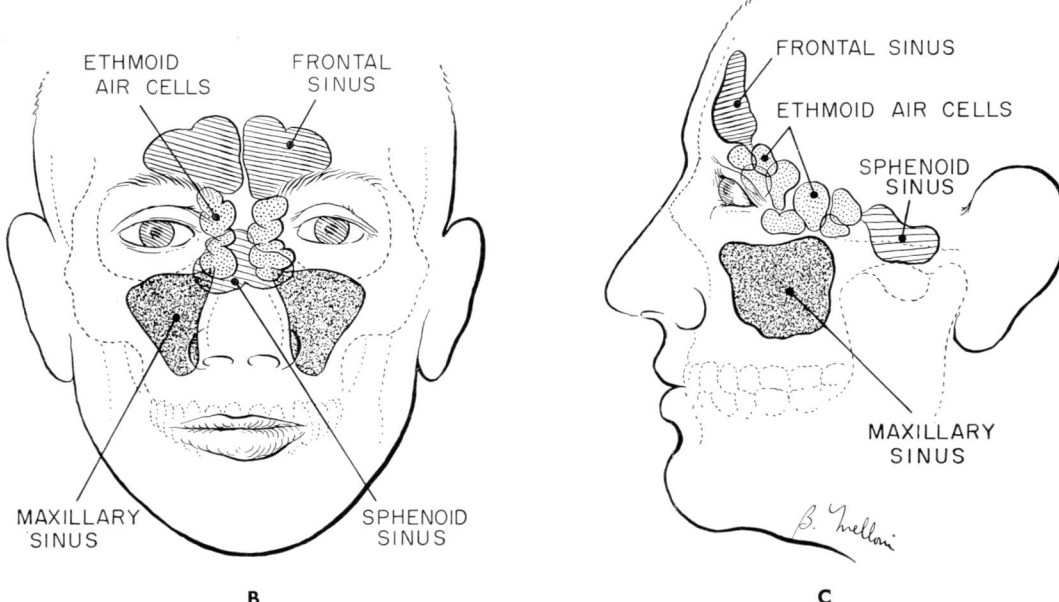

Fig. 15-3. **A**, Radiograph of normal healthy sinuses. **B**, Diagram of frontal view of paranasal sinuses. **C**, Diagram of lateral view.

Diseases of the maxillary sinus of dental origin 241

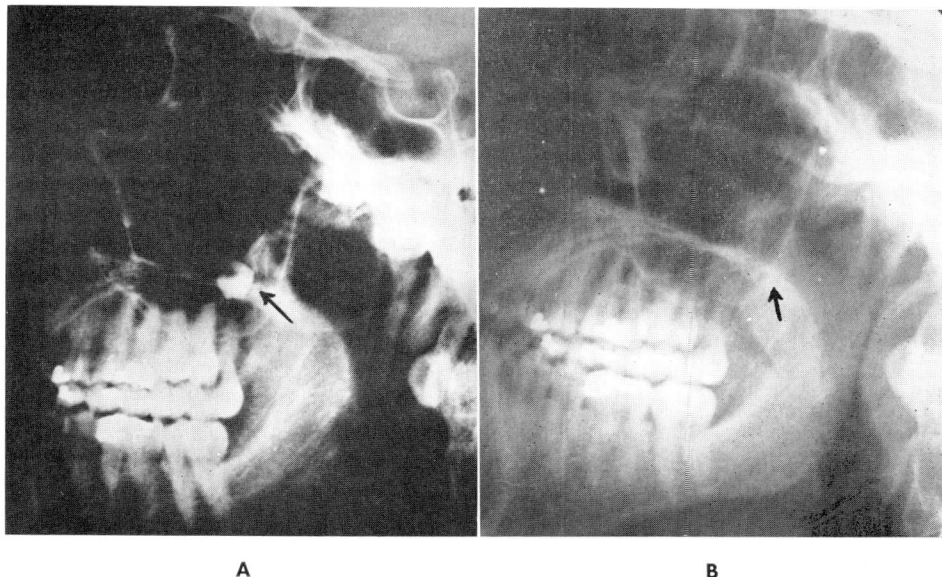

Fig. 15-4. **A**, Unerupted third molar residing half in and half out of the sinus. No apparent pathology of the antrum. **B**, Postoperative view. Removal of tooth was accomplished by exposure made through tuberosity approach so that the sinus was not involved.

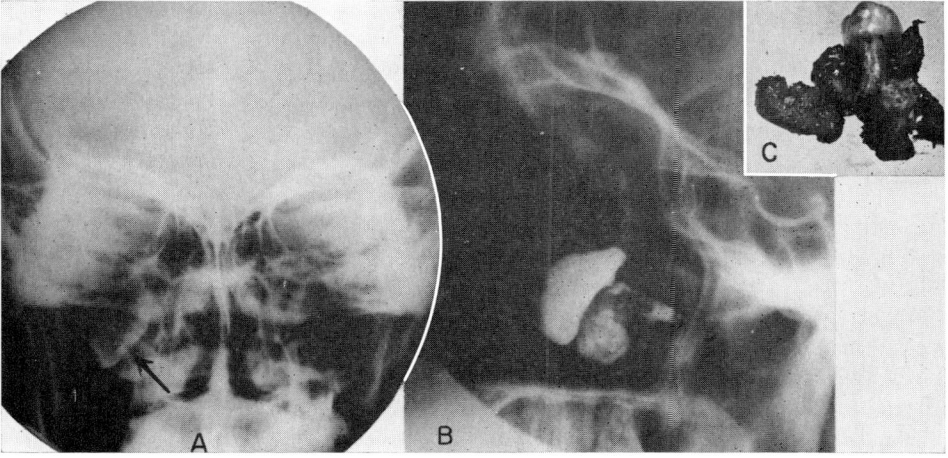

Fig. 15-5. **A**, Aberrant third molar located within maxillary sinus. **B**, Lipiodol in sinus disclosing presence of cyst. **C**, Surgical specimen showing tooth with cyst attached. The tooth and cyst were removed by means of a Caldwell-Luc approach.

or not any of the other nasal sinuses are involved. In many instances the maxillary sinus remains infected from the ethmoids or from the nose itself.

The symptoms of *acute* maxillary sinusitis depend upon the activity or virulence of the infecting organism and the presence of an occluded ostium. The main symptom is severe pain, which is quite constant and localized. It may seem to affect the eyeball, the cheek, and the frontal region. The teeth in that area may become extremely sore and painful. Any unusual motion or jarring may accentuate the suffering. The nasal discharge may at first be thin and watery and serous in character, but soon it becomes mucopurulent in form, dripping into the nasopharynx and causing a constant irritation. This produces spitting, swallowing, and a constant clearing of the throat. In the type of sinusitis that develops from infected teeth the secretion has a very foul odor. General toxemia develops with the disease, producing chills, sweats, elevation of temperature, dizziness, and nausea. Difficult breathing is quite common.

Subacute sinusitis is devoid of the symptoms associated with acute congestion such as pain and generalized toxemia. Discharge is persistent and is associated with nasal voice and stuffiness. Throat soreness is quite common. The patient feels run down, tires easily, and often cannot sleep well because of an irritating cough that keeps him awake. The diagnosis is based on the symptoms, rhinoscopy, transillumination, x-ray, sinus lavage, and a history of a persistent head cold or sinus attack of a few weeks' or months' duration.

Subacute sinusitis may be the interim stage between acute and chronic sinusitis, and many cases continue on to a stage of chronic suppuration. Proper medical and surgical treatment is important to prevent the acute case from ultimately becoming a chronic one. The relief may come on slowly or suddenly, but it usually takes place soon after improvement of drainage from the sinus reaches the point that the secretions are able to leave the cavity as rapidly as they form.

Chronic maxillary sinusitis is produced by the following factors: (1) repeated attacks of acute antritis or a single attack that has persisted to a chronic state, (2) neglected or overlooked dental focus, (3) chronic infection in the frontal or ethmoid sinuses, (4) altered metabolism, (5) fatigue, (6) overindulgences, worries, dietary deficiencies, and lack of sleep, (7) allergies, (8) endocrine imbalances and debilitating diseases of all kinds.

The fundamental pathological change in chronic sinusitis is that of cellular proliferation. The lining is thick and irregular. Fig. 15-6 shows the characteristic appearance of chronic antritis radiographically. In some cases the lumen of the cavity may be almost occluded by the thickened membranes. This edematous process involves the ostium, causing a complete blockage, so that drainage ceases. Medical treatment is of little value in chronic sinus disease. Roentgen-ray therapy and short-wave diathermy are advocated, but are of questionable value without the establishment of proper sinus drainage. This can best be done by performing an intranasal antrostomy or antral window. Conditions conducive to early repair are supplied by the establishment of adequate drainage. The success obtained by this procedure along with other conservative measures properly carried out has practically eliminated the need of radical procedures on the maxillary sinus.

PATHOLOGY

It is generally estimated that from 10% to 15% of the pathology involving the maxillary sinus is of dental origin or relationship. This includes accidental openings in the floor of the antrum during the extraction of teeth, the displacement of roots and even entire teeth into the antrum during the attempted removal of teeth, and infections introduced

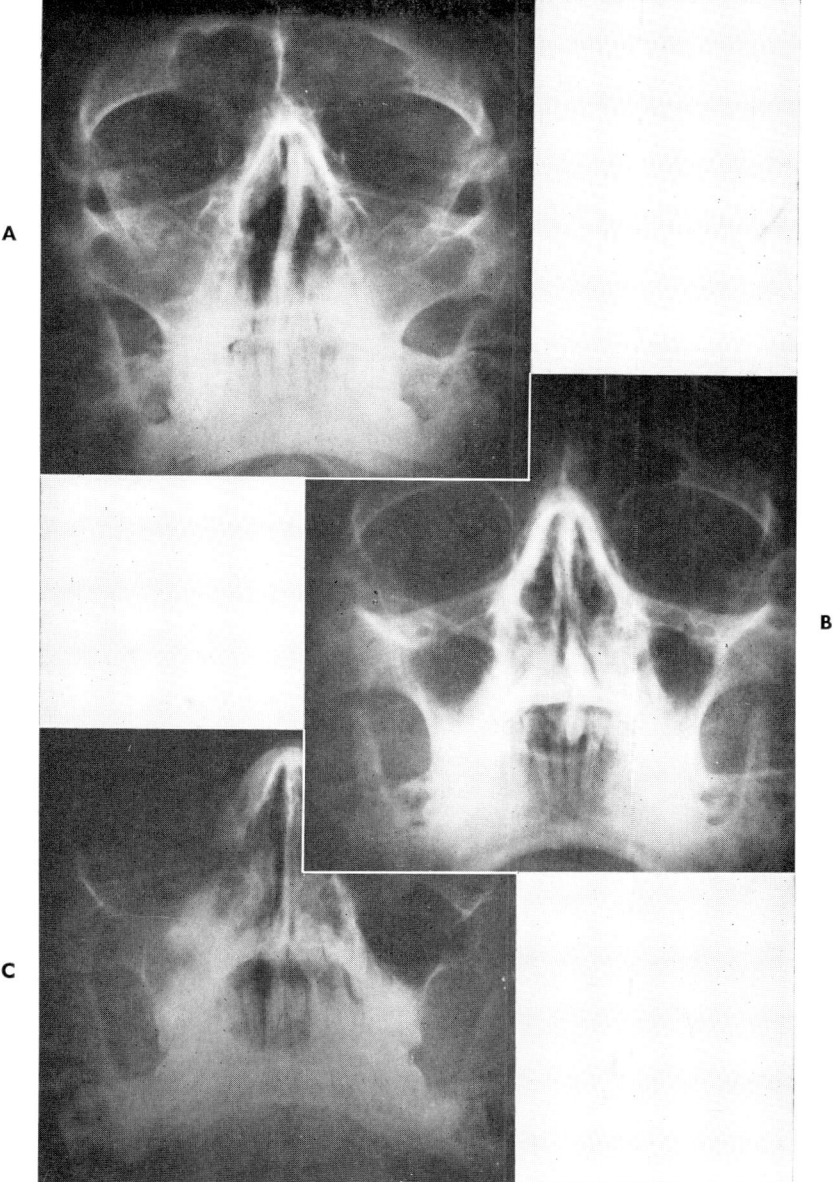

Fig. 15-6. **A,** Marked clouding of each maxillary sinus. **B,** Thickening of the mucosal lining associated with chronic maxillary sinusitis. **C,** Clouded right antrum produced by trauma that caused fracture of the right infraorbital rim.

through the antral floor from abscessed teeth, either of the apical or the parietal variety. Usually the infections are most likely to occur in those cases in which the roots of the teeth are separated from the floor of the antrum by a very thin lamella of bone, but many cases are reported in which this bone is quite thick and heavy.

Empyema of the sinus may occur as a result of too active currettage of root sockets following extractions. This procedure, of course, is frowned upon, and only light and gentle curettement, if any, should ever be employed. The blind and indiscriminate use of the curet is to be condemned since it is the means of spreading infection into bone and soft tissues in any part of the mouth. However, it is possible at times for the infection to involve the sinus for no apparent reason.

Dentigerous cysts are often found in the sinus. Other pathological entities include cysts of the mucosa of the sinus, benign and malignant neoplasms, osteomyelitis, antral rhinoliths, and polyps. Angiomas, myomas, fibromas, and central giant cell tumors seldom invade the sinus. Cystic odontomas may encroach on the sinus. They are usually incapsulated and can be shelled out readily without involving the antrum. The osteoma, a benign tumor, is often treated radically when it invades this area. If it obliterates the sinus, it often causes mechanical constriction to vital structures so that a hemimaxillectomy is necessary.

Ameloblastoma invading the sinus causes marked expansion of both facial and nasal walls. X-ray studies usually disclose the character of the lesion. Mixed tumors undergo malignant changes and result in rapid growth and invasion of this area. Connective tissue lesions such as fibrogenic and osteogenic sarcomas seldom involve the sinus. If they do occur, it is usually in childhood, and they offer a poor prognosis. Unfortunately, characteristic symptoms of malignant tumors develop in this region when the disease has reached an inoperable stage.

Epidermoid carcinoma of the antrum is more common than sarcoma. These conditions may be present for some time without producing clinical evidence. The teeth may become loose and pain develop. If extraction of the teeth is done, the sockets fail to heal. Metastases to vital organs may cause death before local extension occurs. Often swelling of the face is the chief reason for seeking medical advice. In the interest of early diagnosis, close attention should be given to persistent or recurrent pain in the teeth or face without clear-cut dental cause. Early diagnosis is pertinent whether the dentist assumes the responsibility of the treatment of the disease or not.

Trauma such as fractures of the maxilla with associated crushing of the sinus region sometimes occurs. Occasionally, following traumatic zygoma impactions, the zygoma is forced into the sinus. An acute sinus infection may follow because of the retention of an accumulation of blood in the sinus.

TREATMENT
Accidental openings

If information is obtained from the preoperative radiographs that the root ends of the teeth to be extracted penetrate the floor of the sinus, and if this condition is suspected after exodontia is completed, the patient is instructed to compress his nares with his fingers and blow his nose gently. If an opening has occurred through the membrane lining the sinus, the blood that is present in the tooth socket will bubble.

If this opening is quite small and great care is exercised, such as the avoidance of the use of irrigations, vigorous mouth washing, and frequent and lusty blowing of the nose, then in the majority of the cases a good clot will form and organize and normal healing will occur. At no time should these sockets be packed with gauze, cotton, etc. because in most instances these procedures will perpetuate the opening rather than serve as a means of causing it to close. Probing of the sockets with instruments

Diseases of the maxillary sinus of dental origin **245**

must be avoided as much as possible so that infection will not be introduced into uncontaminated areas.

If the floor of the antrum is completely disrupted and portions of the bone remain on the roots of the teeth after their removal and inspection reveals a large patent opening, then immediate closure should be done. Primary closure reduces the possibility of contamination of the sinus by oral infections and diseases. Such immediate closure circumvents pathological changes of the sinus, which may persist for some time and require considerably more effort to manage and cure. It often prevents the formation of an oral-antral fistula, which would require subsequent surgery of a more difficult and extensive nature.

A simple procedure that yields good results for the closure of large accidental sinus openings is described as follows. The mucoperiosteum is raised both buccally and lingually, and the height of the alveolar ridge is reduced at the site of the opening quite substantially. The edges of the soft tissue that is to be approximated are freshened so that raw surfaces will be in contact with each other. Relaxing incisions are made as illustrated in Fig. 15-7. Suturing may then be done without tension. These edges are drawn together with mattress sutures and reinforced with multiple, interrupted black silk sutures, No. 3-0 (Fig. 15-8). This type of material is preferred to the absorbable type (for example, catgut) because it obviates the possibility of the sutures coming out too soon, which could possibly limit the success of the closure. These are left in place from 5 to 7 days. Nose drops are prescribed to shrink the nasal mucosa and promote drainage.

The anatomical proximity of the roots of the molar and bicuspid teeth to the floor of the sinus leads to potential infection of the sinus either by direct extension of an apical abscess or through the accidental perforation of the sinus floor during exodontia. A fractured root apex that is separated from the floor of the sinus by a paper-thin lamina of bone can easily be pushed into the sinus and inoculate it with virulent bacteria. Unless the operator is skillful in the removal of such an accidentally displaced root tip, manipulation and trauma will usually be

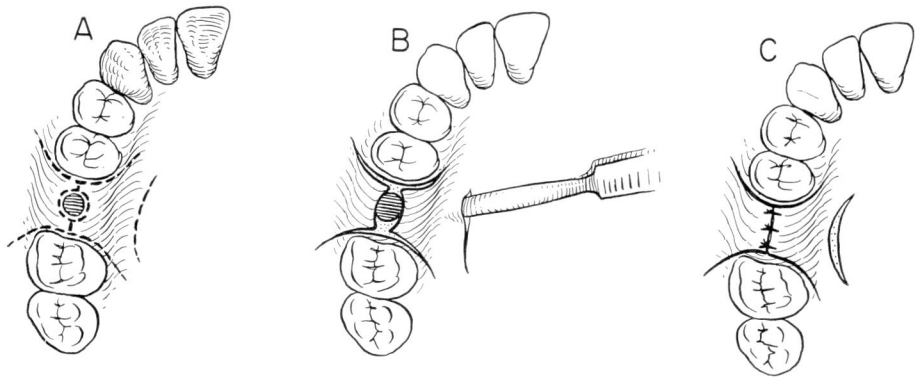

Fig. 15-7. Closure of large accidental sinus opening in the dentulous arch. **A,** Incisions are made around teeth and across opening. A relaxing incision is made on the palate, avoiding the palatine artery. The buccal and lingual alveolar walls are reduced with a rongeur. **B,** Mucosal edges on the ridge are freshened and flaps are raised. A periosteal elevator raises the palatal mucoperiosteum so that approximation of mucosal edges is made possible. **C,** Flaps are sutured. Healing should take place by primary intention. The palatal wound is left open.

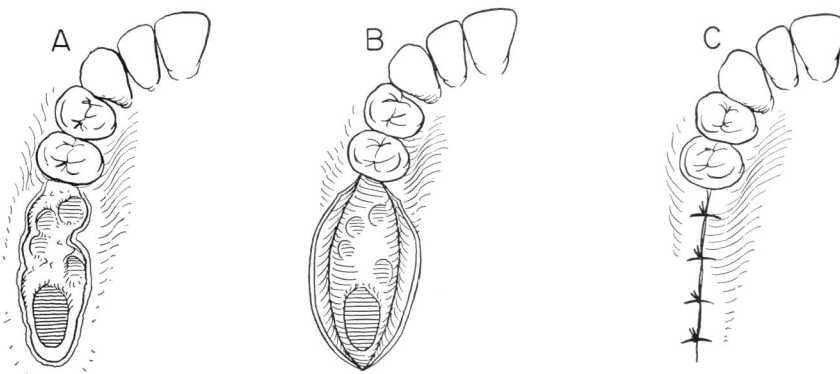

Fig. 15-8. Closure of large accidental sinus opening in edentulous areas (loss of maxillary tuberosity). **A**, Sinus opening immediately after extraction. **B**, Reduction of buccal and lingual walls to allow coaptation of buccal and lingual soft tissue flaps. The soft tissue flaps are trimmed conservatively to form a somewhat even line. **C**, Flaps sutured.

followed by an acute infection. If a short, precise primary endeavor to remove the root tip is unsuccessful, it should be abandoned and the wound encouraged to heal. If the wound is large, the buccal and palatal mucoperiosteum should be approximated.

The patient should be informed of the existence of the displaced root fragment. The surgical approach for removal of a root in the maxillary sinus should not be made through the alveolus after the primary attempt to recover the root has been done. It should be made through a Caldwell-Luc incision, which will permit adequate visualization of the entire sinus.

Preoperative considerations

Anesthesia for operation on the maxillary sinus may be either local or general, depending upon the operator's choice and the type especially indicated for the case concerned. If general anesthesia is to be employed in the hospital, then of course that becomes the responsibility of the anesthesiologist.

In the event that local anesthesia is to be employed, this may be obtained quite satisfactorily in the following manner. The patient is premedicated with 100 mg. of pentobarbital sodium and 0.4 mg. of atropine about 30 minutes prior to operation. Then a pledget of cotton saturated with cocaine (5% to 10% solution) or pontocaine (2% in ephedrine) is carefully applied just above and below the inferior turbinate. This is left in place 10 to 15 minutes. An anterior infraorbital nerve block or a second division block then is administered, using any local anesthetic agent of choice.

It should be stressed strongly that any patient who receives the application of cocaine to the oral or nasal mucosa should not be left alone, but should be constantly observed by someone trained to recognize the symptoms of sensitivity and shock that may occur in those individuals who are sensitive to the drug. When an idiosyncrasy is present, positive and immediate steps must be instituted, including the intravenous injection of agents such as Pentothal sodium and the employment of oxygen therapy. This may be lifesaving, and delay or failure to recognize symptoms may precipitate a crisis that may lead to a fatality. These conditions are quite rare, and if such is suspected, tests for sensitivity may be made. The ophthal-

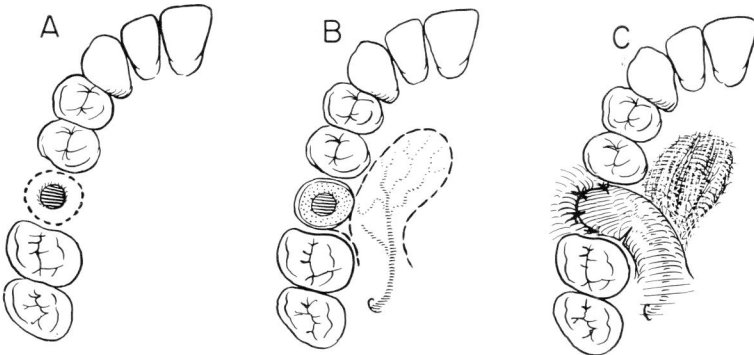

Fig. 15-9. Palatal flap to close chronic oroantral fistula. **A**, The hard and soft tissues surrounding the fistula are freshened. The buccal tissue is undermined. **B**, A mucoperiosteal flap is designed and raised. It must contain the artery. **C**, The flap is swung over the defect, tucked under the buccal flap, and sutured to place. Note V of tissue removed on lesser curvature to minimize folding. The donor area is packed with gauze or surgical cement.

mic test is easy to do and consists of dropping some of the substance that is to be used into one of the patient's eyes. This will produce a conjunctivitis within 5 minutes if the patient is sensitive to the drug; no harm will occur to the eye otherwise.

The skin test may be used in the patient suspected of an idiosyncrasy. It is done by making a wheal or bleb with the drug between the dermis and epidermis; if a marked erythema develops within 5 minutes, that particular drug should not be used. These tests require only the expenditure of a few minutes of time, but may be the means of saving hours of worry, confusion, or even the individual's life. Definitive tests are made by an allergist.

Closure of the oroantral fistula

Closure of the oroantral fistula, especially in the case of a large opening, may be accomplished very well by employing the palatal flap method (Fig. 15-9). A pedicle flap raised from the palate is thick and has good blood supply, so the chances of success are definitely enhanced. The design of the flap can be determined by a trial or practice procedure prior to surgery. A cast of the maxilla showing the defect or opening is made, and a soft acrylic palate is formed on this cast. The flap is outlined on the acrylic, the incision made, and the flap turned, covering the defect. This provides a preview of the results that should be obtained. The material may be sterilized and placed in the mouth for use at the time that the incisions are made through the mucoperiosteum of the palate. This procedure will show that the flap that is to be raised will be adequate to cover the opening.

With a No. 15 blade, the tissue is incised, and the flap is raised. A V-shaped section of the tissue may be excised at the region of greatest bend to prevent folding and wrinkling. The pedicle is raised with the periosteum and of course should contain a branch of the palatal artery. The margins of the fistular defect are freshened and the edges undermined. The flap is then tucked under the undermined edge of the buccal flap. This procedure permits two raw or fresh bleeding surfaces to be in contact. Using mattress sutures the tissues are drawn in good contact, and the margins are sutured with multiple interrupted sutures. Catgut is not used because it may not hold for a sufficient length of time for healing to occur. The silk or Dermalon sutures

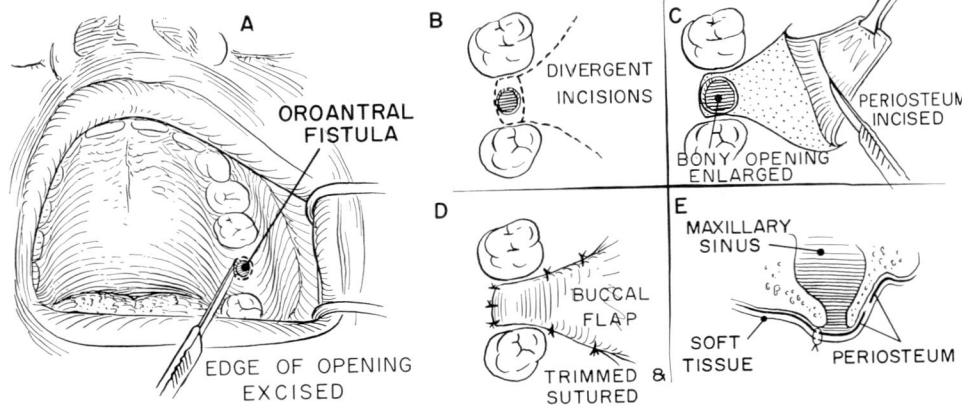

Fig. 15-10. Berger's sliding flap technique for oroantral closure. **A**, Edge of opening excised. **B**, Two divergent incisions carried from the opening into the mucobuccal fold. **C**, Flap elevated and bony opening made large enough for inspection and cleansing of sinus. Several horizontal incisions are made through the periosteum on the underside of the flap, which allows the flap to be extended. **D**, Flap trimmed to meet palatal tissue and closed with mattress sutures followed by interrupted sutures. **E**, Cross-sectional view of closure, showing stretching of flap allowed by incised periosteum.

should be left in position for from 5 to 7 days. The exposed bone at the donor site on the palate may be covered with surgical cement or a gauze strip saturated with compound tincture of benzoin.

Berger, a dentist, described in 1939 a very satisfactory method of closing oroantral openings by obtaining tissue from the buccal or cheek area (Fig. 15-10). The tissues that form the rim of the fistula are incised. From the extreme edges diagonal incisions are made through the mucoperiosteum to the bone. The incisions are carried upward into the mucobuccal fold. The flap is elevated, exposing the bone defect. In the undersurface of the flap the periosteum is incised horizontally at different points, care being taken to incise the periosteum only, so that there will be no interference with the blood supply. The incision in the periosteum lengthens the flap so that it may slide down over the opening. Mattress sutures are then introduced over the area, and definite coaptation is secured. The edges are sutured with multiple black silk sutures, which are allowed to remain in place for from 5 to 7 days.

The Berger technique can be combined with the Caldwell-Luc operation. Chronic antral infection, so often present in the patient with a persistent fistula, must be eradicated and antral polyps removed before healing can occur. To obtain good access to the antrum in the combined technique, the anterior limb of the flap used in the Berger technique is extended forward in the sulcus from its upper end, making a separate Caldwell-Luc incision unnecessary.

Another method of closure that seems quite simple and has been successful was described by Proctor. He places a cone-shaped piece of preserved cartilage into the defect. The tooth socket is prepared by curettement, and the cartilage is wedged into place. It is important to have the cartilage of sufficient size so that it can be definitely wedged into place. If loose fitting, it may become dislodged and drop out before the membrane grows over it, or it may pass upward into the sinus and become a foreign body.

Gold disks, or 24-karat, 36-gauge gold plate, have been used most successfully by many oral surgeons over the country.[1] The procedure is practical, effective, and uncomplicated. The involved sinus is thoroughly cleaned and adequately exposed. It is imperative that the sinus be as free from infection as possible. The bone is prepared for the reception of the metal, and then the metal is placed over the opening and maintained there by suturing the soft tissue flaps over it. The patient is placed on an antibiotic to reduce the possibility of an antral or soft tissue infection. A nasal spray is advised to maintain good nasoantral drainage and avoid stasis over the gold implant.

The possible closure of oroantral fistulas by means of free, full-thickness transplants obtained from the opposite side of the palate or from the mucobuccal fold is an approach that should not be overlooked. It is feasible and uses tissue that is not foreign to the mouth since it is a transfer of tissue from one part of the mouth to another. The donor site heals readily, being protected initially by the application of compound tincture of benzoin or sedative dressings.

Causes of failure in the closing of an oroantral fistula may be listed as follows:

1. Complete elimination of all infection within the antral cavity prior to closure not accomplished. This may be done by lavage and/or antibiotics that have been proved effective against the bacteria present.

2. The patient's general physical condition not adequately explored and treated. Such diseases as diabetes, syphilis, and tuberculosis can influence adversely the normal healing of wounds.

3. Flaps placed over the opening with too much tension, and failure to provide a fresh or raw surface at the recipient site of the flap.

The best insurance for a successful closure is the obtaining of good drainage from the sinus to the nose by the establishment of an intranasal antrostomy prior to making any attempt to close the chronic fistula. This may be performed in the following manner. A cotton pledget with 2% pontocaine (in ephedrine 1% solution) is applied to the inferior meatal wall and the inferior turbinate. After anesthesia is established the wall is penetrated with a punch or trocar, which will make a sufficiently large opening to admit cutting forceps. The window is enlarged in all directions until a diameter of at least 2 cm. is obtained at its narrowest point. It is important to lower the nasoantral ridge to the floor of the nasal cavity. If any of the ridge is left standing, it might defeat the entire purpose of the new opening, which is to permit a free flow of secretions from the sinus into the nose.

Caldwell-Luc operation

The indications for this radical sinus operation are many, including the following:

1. Removal of teeth and root fragments in the sinus. The Caldwell-Luc operation eliminates blind procedures and facilitates the recovery of the foreign body.

2. Trauma of the maxilla when the walls of the maxillary sinus are crushed or when the floor of the orbit has dropped. This type of injury is best corrected by the approach furnished by this operation.

3. Management of hematomas of the antrum with active bleeding through the nose. The blood may be evacuated and the bleeders located. Hemorrhage is arrested with epinephrine packs or hemostatic packs.

4. Chronic maxillary sinusitis with polypoid degeneration of the mucosa.

5. Cysts in the maxillary sinus.

6. Neoplasms of the maxillary sinus, which are best removed by this technique.

The surgical procedure employed is described as follows. With the use of the anesthetic best suited for the patient, the mouth and face are prepared in the usual manner. If the patient is asleep, he will be intubated and his throat packed along the anterior

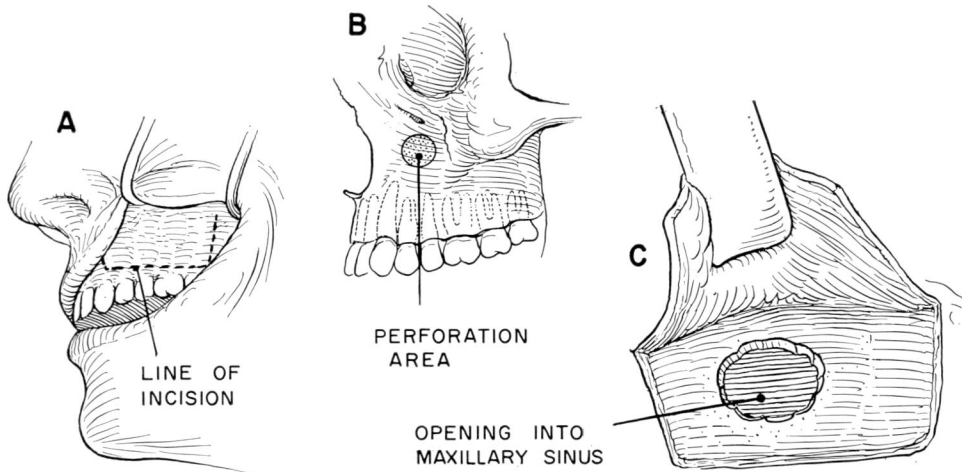

Fig. 15-11. Caldwell-Luc operation.

border of the soft palate and tonsillar pillars. The upper lip is elevated with retractors. A U-shaped incision is made through the mucoperiosteum to the bone. Vertical incisions are made in the cuspid and second molar areas from points just above the gingival attachment up to and above the mucobuccal fold. A horizontal line connecting the two vertical incisions is made in the alveolar mucosa several millimeters above the gingival attachments of the teeth. The tissue is elevated from the bone with periosteal elevators, going superiorly as high as the infraorbital canal. Care is exercised here to prevent injury to the nerve. An opening is made into the facial wall of the antrum above the bicuspid roots by means of chisels, gouges, or dental drills, and this is enlarged by means of bone-cutting forceps to a size that permits inspection of the cavity. The size ultimately obtained is about the size of the end of an average index finger.

The opening should be made high enough to avoid the roots of the teeth in that area. The purpose of the operation (for example the removal of root ends or foreign bodies) is readily accomplished. Seldom is the radical removal of the entire sinus mucosa required, but if it is deemed advisable, this is readily done by means of periosteal elevators and curets. The cavity is cleansed, and the soft tissue flap is replaced and sutured over the bone with multiple, interrupted black silk sutures. These are allowed to remain for a period of from 5 to 7 days. Fig. 15-11 illustrates the approach in the Caldwell-Luc operation.

Anesthesia of the cheek and teeth may follow injury to the infraorbital nerve or nerves of the teeth during chiseling of the bony wall. Swelling of the cheek is common, but usually disappears in a few days. The prognosis is good, and the development of severe conditions is quite rare.

SUMMARY

Intimate juxtaposition of the antrum and the roots of the teeth with their surrounding alveolar bone is complicated by occasional maxillary sinusitis of dental origin. Teeth and roots that are to be removed from the alveolus sometimes slip above the thin bony plate separating the alveolus from the sinus. Sometimes they lodge between the bone and the antrum membrane.

Frequently they enter the antrum, in which case the problem of the opening in the antrum cavity is complicated by an opening into the mouth as well as residual dental infection in the alveolus. The operator is then faced with the problem of deciding how far to probe through the alveolus for a lost root or tooth, whether the buccal plate of the alveolus should be opened at that site, or whether a Caldwell-Luc operation is indicated.

The oroantral fistula is a problem that requires detailed attention to the management of a flap in the mouth. However, in all these conditions the problem of antral infection is potential or real. For the sake of obtaining the best results and to give the patient the benefit of mutual or specialized knowledge, a close liaison between the otolaryngologist and the oral surgeon and the unhesitating call for consultation, if needed and available, are certainly to be encouraged.

REFERENCE

1. Fredrics, H. S., Scopp, I. W., Gerstman, E., and Morgan, F. H.: Closure of oroantral fistula with gold plate: report of case, J. Oral Surg. 23:650, 1965.

Chapter 16

TISSUE TRANSPLANTATION

Philip J. Boyne

The rapid advancements made by research in areas of tissue and organ transplantation during the past two decades have led to marked changes in clinical and surgical treatment procedures in many specialties of the health sciences. It was fully anticipated that a renewed interest in transplantation techniques in oral surgery would evolve in such a dynamic environment.

Although cartilage and, more rarely, skin grafts have been used occasionally in the treatment of acquired and developmental defects involving the oral cavity and facial bones, the most commonly utilized tissue in oral surgical transplantation procedures has been bone.

In bone implantation procedures, as in the grafting of any organ or tissue, transplant substances are of three types:
1. *Autogenous* grafts, composed of tissue taken from the same individual
2. *Homogenous* (allogeneic) grafts, made up of tissues removed from a genetically unrelated individual of the same species
3. *Heterogenous* (xenogeneic) grafts, composed of tissue from a donor of another species

---

The assertions and opinions contained herein are those of the author and are not to be construed as reflecting the views of the Navy Department or the Naval service at large.

Historically, attempts have been made for centuries to employ bone graft materials in surgical procedures. In 1668 Van Meekren is recorded as having successfully transplanted heterogenous bone from a dog to man in restoring a cranial defect.[1] Hunter conducted experiments in the eighteenth century on the host response to bone grafts, noting the phenomena of resorption and remodeling of the graft matrix. The first successful autogenous bone graft was reported by Merrem[2] in 1809. Macewen reportedly transplanted homogenous bone successfully in clinical patients in 1878.[1,2]

Various forms of devitalized bone from an animal source have been used clinically during the past half century. Orell in 1938 produced a graft material from bovine bone by the use of strong alkalis.[3] Boiling and defatting procedures have been employed in the treatment of animal bone prior to its use in heterogenous grafting.[3,4] Bovine osseous tissue grafts treated with chemicals such as ethylenediamine,[5] hydrogen peroxide,[6] and strong detergents[7] have also been used clinically.

Attempts have been made to preserve homogenous bone by the use of chemical agents. Merthiolate coagulation was employed for some time as a method of storing bone taken at autopsy.[8] The drastic treatment of human bone by physical or chemical agents, however, is now generally thought to be an inferior method of tissue preservation. Cryobiological methods of storage were first employed by Inclan,[9] who is credited with developing the first modern bone bank in 1942. Following the use of refrigeration (above freezing temperatures) for the preservation of bone, Wilson[10] developed a bone bank using freezing techniques. Methods of storage currently used in bone banks are generally cryobiological in nature, employing various procedures of cooling, freezing, or freeze-drying.

CRITERIA USED IN BONE GRAFT EVALUATION

In evaluating the clinical and histological effectiveness of various bone graft materials the following criteria are usually employed:
1. The graft must be biologically acceptable to the host.
2. The graft must actively or passively assist osteogenic processes of the host.
3. The graft material should withstand mechanical forces operating at the surgical site and contribute to internal support of the area.
4. Ideally, the graft should become completely resorbed and replaced by host bone.

Of primary importance is the first of these requisites, that of biological acceptability. This highly essential criterion refers to the existence of tissue immunological compatibility.

IMMUNOLOGICAL CONCEPTS APPLIED TO ORAL SURGICAL TRANSPLANTATION PROCEDURES

The various methods of transplanting living autogenous tissues, while frequently presenting surgical and technical problems, do not as a rule involve immunological complications. However, graft rejection phenomena must be given serious consideration when homogenous or heterogenous bone and cartilage implants are used in oral surgery. The basis for these rejection phenomena is reviewed in the following paragraphs to more fully identify the clinical response to various graft materials.

The immune response

The process by which the host rejects foreign graft material is a manifestation of an immunologically specific tissue reaction called the *immune response*. In the past it has been customary to explain the immune process within the context of disease susceptibility. The human body does not possess a natural immunity to many types of invading organisms. The immune process is initiated by exposure of the human host to invading bacteria, viruses, or parasites. The initial invasion of the host by these agents results in the production in the tissues and body fluids of specific substances that are capable of reacting with and destroying the invading agents.[11] The invading agent causing the initiation of the immune response is called an *antigen*. The specific protein developed in the body in response to the antigen is called an antibody or an *immune body*. This specific protein antibody is available to combine with the initiating antigen should it again invade the host organism. It is this reaction between the antigen and the antibody that occurs on subsequent exposure or invasion by the antigenic substance that is called the *immune response*.

Tissue immunity and humoral immunity. Two types of immunity are described in relationship to the mechanism of antibody release in the host. The cell most often implicated in antibody production is the plasma cell. Large lymphocytes and reticulum cells are also known to produce moderate amounts of antibody. These cells are capable of releasing their formed antibody into the circulatory body fluids, hence the name *humoral immunity*.

Other cells of the invaded host may also respond to foreign antigens. These cells, however, do not release antibody into the intercellular fluids of the host, but do react, often violently, with foreign material containing the antigens, giving rise to the so-called *tissue immunity*, which as the name implies operates at the cellular level.[11,12] Humoral immunity lasts only as long as specific antibody persists in the body fluids. Tissue immunity may last indefinitely. Antibodies operating in tissue immunity are produced by tissue cells that generally do not renew themselves as rapidly as those of the lymphoid series. The development of immunity in these cells therefore may persist for many years.

Immune response applied to tissue transplantation. Because we tend to think of the immune response in terms of infectious disease processes, it is not always appreciated that organic material taken from one person as part of a tissue graft may be foreign to another individual. The rejection of tissue grafts made between members of the same species is called a *homograft response*. This rejection of the living homogenous graft is the result of the cellular reaction of the host to the transplanted antigens. Such rejection is not immediate, however, and a homograft transplanted into a normal animal enjoys an immunological latent period during which its healing is indistinguishable from an autograft.[11,12]

The length of this latent period depends upon the disparity between donor and host (that is, the genetic relationship of the two). Genetic similarity between the donor and recipient of a transplanted tissue appears to be the major factor responsible for the success of the graft[13] (for example, skin homografts transplanted between closely related mice (inbred strain) may remain in place for over a month; skin homografts between different lines of mice may on the other hand be destroyed in an acute inflammatory reaction within a few days).

The second set response. The destruction of a tissue homograft leaves the recipient host in a specifically immune state (a condition of heightened resistance that may last for months). A second homograft from the same donor transplanted within this period is destroyed much more rapidly than its predecessor; indeed, these second transplants (the so-called "white grafts") are even rejected with little or no evidence of beginning revascularization. This is called a "second set" reaction and has been demonstrated in most tissue transplants, including bone and teeth.[12,30,31]

All available evidence at present indicates that humoral or circulating antibodies do not play a significant part in solid tissue homograft rejection.[14]

Methods used to attenuate the immune response in grafting. In attempting to solve the problems of incompatability in grafting from one individual to another, two approaches have been used.[11,15] One approach attempts to modify the *host* immune mechanisms to block the rejection of the graft. Various methods have been used to effect this modification in experimental animals, including thymectomy, the use of high and low dosage of antigen, the use of irradiation, and the employment of immunosuppressive drugs. The second method attempts to alter the inherent *graft* antigenic properties so that the normal immune defenses of the host will not be stimulated.[15] (Irradiation, freezing, and freeze-drying all tend to diminish graft antigenicity.[15-17])

The first of these approaches is highly experimental, and except for the use of the immunosuppressive drugs in major organ transplants (for example, kidney and heart), this type of treatment has not been extensively used clinically. The second method has, however, been used in the successful storage and preservation of homogenous bone and cartilage[15] for use in oral surgery.

STORAGE AND PRESERVATION OF HOMOGENOUS BONE FOR GRAFTING

The most successful tissue storage methods used in the banking of homogenous bone have been cryobiological in nature; that is, the use of cooling, freezing, or freeze-drying environments.[15-17] Bone grafts preserved by cryogenic methods are more rapidly and completely revascularized, resorbed, and remodeled than are homografts that have been deproteinized, boiled, or otherwise drastically treated.

The application of cryobiological techniques to bone preservation is predicated upon the unique histological nature of osseous tissue. Unlike many soft tissue and organ systems having large cell populations, bone and cartilage are composed of relatively small numbers of living cells with large amounts of calcified and noncalcified intercellular matrix, which is considered to be nonviable. Since the survival of the cells of a homogenous bone graft is not necessary, nor even desirable because of the previously discussed immunological factors, a method of storage that will bring about this cellular death without deleteriously altering the remaining osseous structure of the graft material is considered to be essential for the development of an effective graft substance. This is accomplished by freeze-drying[17] and by most controlled methods of freezing to low temperatures. Since the cells of a cryobiologically preserved bone graft do not survive, the assistance on the part of the graft to osteogenic processes of the host is purely passive. No active osteogenic stimulation is expected of these grafts. Such grafts offer their extracellular matrix as a system of absorbable surfaces over which new bone of the host may grow to reconstruct the grafted defect.

While clinical evaluation of freeze-dried homogenous bone has indicated that implants preserved in this manner are highly acceptable homografts, disadvantages associated with freeze-drying techniques have interfered with a more generalized use of this osseous material. These disadvantages relate to equipment costs, to the relatively large personnel requirements necessary for the performance of the aseptic autopsies, and for the processing and storing of the bone product. Efforts to minimize these disadvantages have been directed toward the elimination of the need for aseptic autopsies by sterilization of the bone following its procurement by less time-consuming, nonsterile procedures. The sterilization methods employed have been in the form of irradiation from a cathode and cobalt source, and chemical sterilization through such agents as ethylene oxide and beta propiolactone.[18]

FORMS OF HOMOGENOUS BANKED BONE AVAILABLE

Freeze-dried and frozen homogenous bone can be produced in various anatomical forms to conform to the needs of different oral surgical procedures.

Cancellous iliac crest bone can be ground into particles having a diameter of approximately 2 to 10 mm. for use in confined intrabony defects following cyst enucleation (Fig. 16-1). Smaller cancellous particles may be used in periapical areas following curettage, and larger cancellous chips may be used in recontouring procedures of the alveolar ridge. Shira has also utilized cancellous homogenous freeze-dried chips in the treatment of nonunion of fractures of the mandible.[22]

Frozen or freeze-dried split rib grafts may be used as onlays to improve width and contour of deficient edentulous ridges[19] (Fig. 16-2) and to cosmetically restore other facial bone deficiencies (Fig. 16-3).

It may appear paradoxical that homogenous bone preserved in this manner will at times produce a better recontouring onlay implant than will an autogenous graft. The slow remodeling rate of the homogenous bone in comparison to the fresh cancellous autograft permits the onlay graft to maintain the desired contour for longer periods of time postoperatively. Fresh autogenous bone grafts not infrequently are resorbed rapidly with no accompanying replacement of the graft by host osseous tissue to maintain the correct contour.

Although considered to be second-rate graft materials, cryobiologically preserved

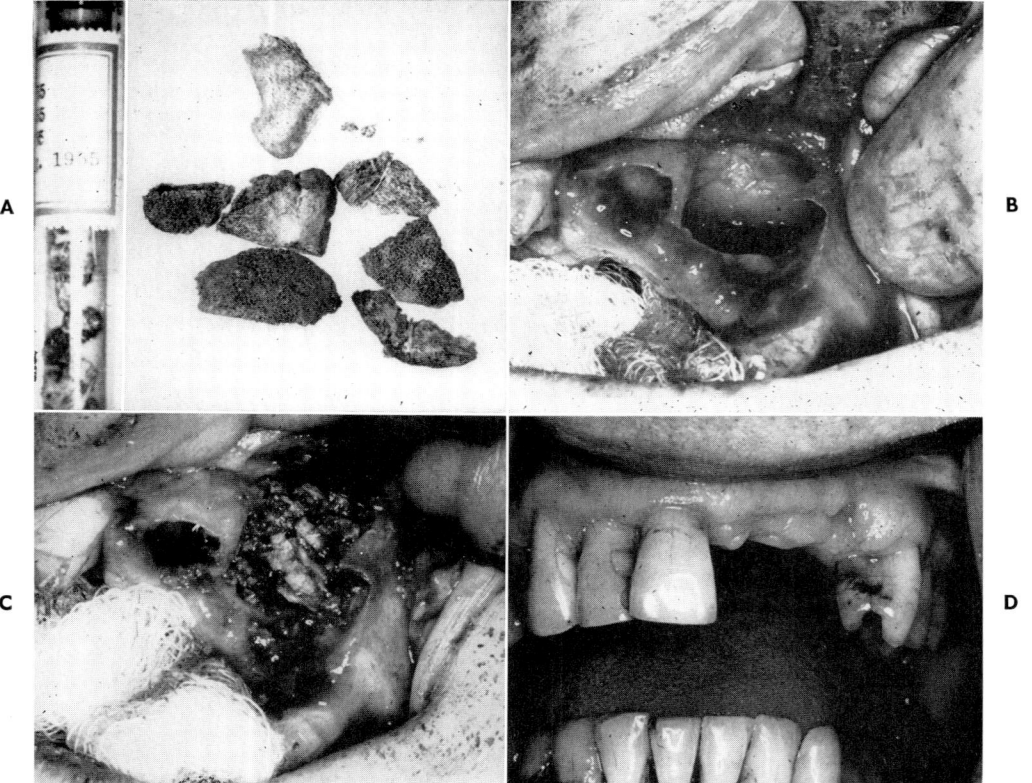

Fig. 16-1. **A,** Freeze-dried homogenous cancellous bone prior to implantation in an intrabony cystic defect. **B,** Osseous defect following enucleation of a radicular cyst involving maxillary anterior teeth. **C,** Intrabony defect is filled with freeze-dried homogenous bone particles. **D,** Three weeks postoperatively the alveolar ridge is well healed with acceptable width and contour having been restored.

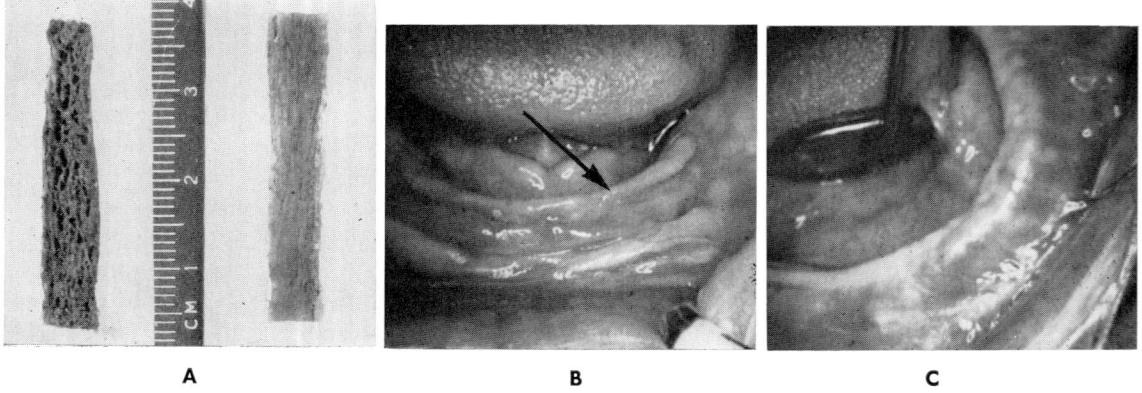

Fig. 16-2. **A,** Freeze-dried split rib grafts prior to implantation to restore deficient edentulous ridges. **B,** Preoperative view of a severely atrophied mandibular ridge (arrow) with redundant soft tissue alveolar folds and epulis fissuratum. **C,** One year after restoration of the deficient edentulous alveolar ridge by the use of onlays of freeze-dried split rib homografts.

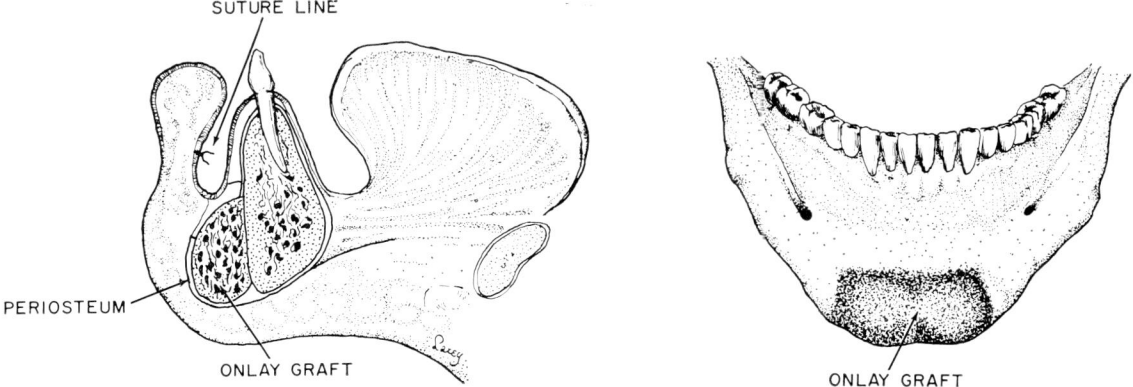

Fig. 16-3. Restoration of deficient mentum with onlays of freeze-dried homografts of split rib.

bone homografts are used in the surgical treatment of the indicated minor defects and can be used in selected cases as substitutes for larger autogenous bone transplants in patients in whom the operation necessary to obtain an autogenous graft is contraindicated.

Cryobiologically preserved homogenous cartilage has been extensively utilized in restoring contour defects of the facial bones. Recently, freeze-dried homografts of cartilage have been used to restore deficient edentulous alveolar ridges.[19] This material is as acceptable to the human host as would be a similarly treated bone graft. Freeze-dried or frozen cartilage can be easily reconstituted and shaped with a scalpel to fit the host defect.

If the cartilage homograft is placed within a soft tissue pocket, fibrous encapsulation and a prolonged resorption of the implant occurs. This host reaction in certain soft tissue implant areas restoring facial defects is considered to be advantageous since the cartilage graft will remain in place for longer periods of time, maintaining the desired postsurgical contour.

Cartilage placed subperiosteally and well immobilized will unite with the underlying bone by the formation of reactive osseous tissue.[19] The cartilage implant in such a recipient site will gradually be replaced with host bone.[19] The bone replacement rate of cartilage onlays placed subperiosteally on edentulous alveolar ridges is generally slower than that of similarly implanted bone grafts. Thus in the selection of the graft material to be used in these areas, any disadvantage of the slow remodeling and replacement of subperiosteally placed implants of homogenous cartilage must be weighed against the advantage of ease of manipulation of the cartilagenous tissue as opposed to the more rigid bone graft material.

PREPARATION OF HETEROGENOUS BONE FOR GRAFTING

While properly preserved hard tissue homografts have a place in oral surgical procedures, the expense of preparing bone in an acceptable manner has not been conducive to the widespread establishment of tissue banks in hospital centers. For this reason a continuing effort has been made through the years to develop an acceptable heterogenous bone graft material.

Cross species bone and cartilage transplants stimulate an immune response on the part of the host. Studies have shown that while in the case of bone homografts the main antigens are associated with nucleated marrow and bone cells contained in the transplant, in the case of heterografts the osseous matrix and the serum proteins are also potentially highly antigenic.[15] As a result the problem of rendering animal bone acceptable to the human host becomes increasingly difficult. Since the major antigenic component of animal bone is contained within the organic fraction of the tissue, this portion of the bone must either be altered or removed to render the product acceptable to the human host.

The problem of cross-species antigenicity in bone heterografting procedures has been approached for the most part by treating animal bone material by vigorous chemical measures to remove, alter, or destroy the organic portion of the osseous tissue. Consequently, while many chemical techniques have been described in the literature for the processing of heterografts, relatively few reports have appeared of the use of freezing and freeze-drying in heterogenous bone preservation and storage.[20]

As previously mentioned, the treatment of bovine bone by boiling in water,[4] boiling in alkalies (such as potassium hydroxide),[3] macerating in hydrogen peroxide,[6] and extracting with ethylenediamine[5] has been used in the past to render potentially antigenic heterografts acceptable to the host (Fig. 16-4). The preservation of beef bone by storage in alcohol and in ether also has been described. However, extensive clinical and histological evaluations of most of these methods have indicated serious disadvantages that preclude the clinical use of these materials.

Recent attempts to produce an acceptable heterograft from calf bone by the use of a process that included treatment with chemical detergents and freeze-drying resulted in a product which, while acceptable as a space-occupying implant in certain minor osseous defects, has not developed into an effective substitute for autogenous, or even preserved homogenous, bone.[21]

Animal cartilagenous tissue treated by various means has also been investigated as a heterogenous implant material. Such materials have not enjoyed significant clinical acceptance.

Various organic extracts of animal bone have been used in the past in an effort to produce an inductor substance that would stimulate bone formation. The most recent

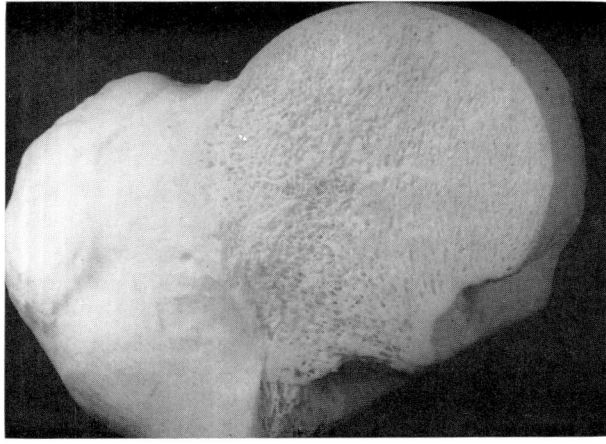

Fig. 16-4. View of a specimen of ethylenediamine-treated bovine bone demonstrating the effect of removal of all organic material from osseous tissue. The cancellous spaces are exposed and cleared of all organic material.

studies of such materials have involved evaluation of the properties of the mucopolysaccharide fraction of bone and the effects of chondroitin sulfates on bone repair.[23] The result of the use of these extracts has been at best equivocal, and to date no clinical application is apparent.

Thus research efforts have not at the present time produced a clinically acceptable heterogenous bone graft material.

AUTOGENOUS BONE GRAFTS

Cancellous autogenous bone grafts continue to be the material of choice in dealing with oral surgical defects that involve the bridging of discontinuity defects (for example, fracture nonunions), the surgical treatment of malocclusions (Fig. 23-42), the management of large intrabony cavities, and the treatment of defects in which previous homografts have failed (Fig. 16-5). Autogenous bone is usually taken from the iliac crest, the rib, or more rarely the tibia. In young children the rib is the preferred donor site. After puberty the iliac crest may be used.

Autogenous bone chips obtained at operation from the oral cavity are usually qualitatively and quantitatively poor. Very little cancellous bone is present at the operative sites of the usual oral surgical procedures. Most of the osseous specimens obtained from alveolectomies, ostectomies, and osteotomies are composed of cortical bone. Such cortical chips are of little osteogenic value. They may, however, be used as an acceptably banked homograft is employed, to fill well-demarcated intrabony defects and to restore contour to deficient osseous areas.

CURRENT EXPERIMENTAL STUDIES ON BONE GRAFT PROCEDURES

Some of the most promising studies relating to bone grafting procedures in oral surgery have been those involved in the evolution of new grafting techniques from investigations of normal osseous healing mechanisms.

Through appropriate intravital labeling with tetracycline, it has been possible to delineate areas of enhanced osteogenic activity following injury or surgical trauma to the facial bones.[24] These areas of osteo-

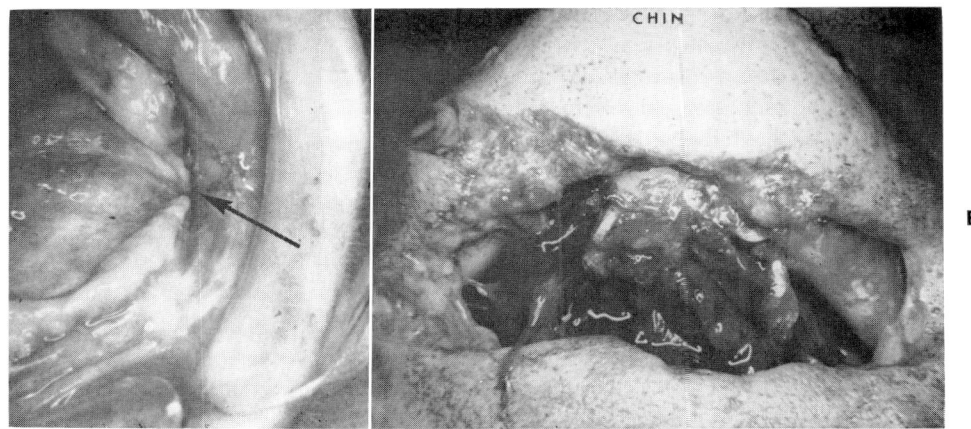

Fig. 16-5. Two examples of the application of autogenous bone grafts to oral surgical defects. **A**, Autografts are used to bridge large gaps of missing osseous tissue as in this fracture nonunion occurring in the molar area of a mandible (arrow). **B**, Autografts are used in restoring discontinuity defects produced by trauma as in this lacerated wound of the submental area with extensive loss of mandibular bone.

genic potential have been intensively investigated to determine the feasibility of utilizing these regions as sites for developing new oral surgical procedures and new bone grafting techniques. It has been demonstrated that it is possible to predict anatomical loci of osseous reparative response following surgical trauma.[24,25]

One area of enhanced osseous reparative response was found to occur along the lingual aspect of the mandible following buccal bone removal in alveolectomy procedures in dogs and monkeys. This subperiosteal lingual area has been found to be an excellent site for onlay implantation of graft materials (Plate 1).

It has been found that in experimental fractures of the body of the mandible in Rhesus monkeys, callus formation in endosteal areas predominates over subperiosteal callus proliferation in effecting bony union. These observations have led to renewed investigation of the use of autogenous cancellous bone chips containing viable marrow as inlayed grafts in discontinuity defects. Experimental comparisons are currently being carried out of gap-spanning grafts placed in various positions in an effort to obtain the most optimal anatomical placement of grafts at surgery.

Another aspect of the relationship of osseous repair to grafting procedures involves the optimal time for bone implantation. Important studies have been made of the histological effect of delayed grafting procedures in which bone implants were placed several days after an initial surgical trauma.[26]

The effect on graft acceptance of altering the recipient site by surgical procedures such as fenestration of the host bone walls is also being investigated.

Recently, experimental studies have demonstrated the marked osteogenic potential of hemopoietic marrow. Marrow taken from the iliac crest or sternum can be transplanted autogenously to alveolar ridge sites to effect new bone formation in intraosseous defects. By the use of special implant devices employing cellulose acetate filters to contain the marrow transplants it has been possible to produce new bone growth on the superior supracortical surfaces of edentulous ridges.[27] Autogenous hemopoietic marrow and autogenous cancellous bone containing marrow appear to be the only types of bone graft material that are capable of actively inducing osteogenesis. (As mentioned previously, properly preserved homogenous bone in certain graft sites can passively assist the osteogenic process of the host, but this type of graft material is not actively osteogenic.)

Through both experimental laboratory procedures and clinical experience it is possible to offer an overall evaluation of the surgical use of most types of bone graft materials at the present time. The relative effectiveness of the most common types of graft materials is given in the following outline. This evaluation was based on repeated experiments with laboratory animals, using various test systems.

First-rate grafts
  1. Viable autogenous marrow
  2. Viable autogenous cancellous bone, fracture callus
  3. Viable autogenous osteoperiosteal grafts
  4. Autogenous cortical cancellous bone with intact blood supply
Second-rate grafts
  1. Autogenous cortical bone
  2. Homogenous freeze-dried bone
  3. Homogenous frozen bone
Third-rate grafts
  1. Detergent-treated freeze-dried heterogenous bone
  2. Ethylenediamine-treated heterogenous bone
  3. Urea-treated fat-extracted heterogenous bone
  4. Improperly preserved homogenous bone
  5. Fresh homogenous bone
Fourth-rate grafts
  1. Boiled fat-extracted heterogenous bone
  2. Fresh heterogenous bone

Current research studies indicate that the most promising graft material for intraoral

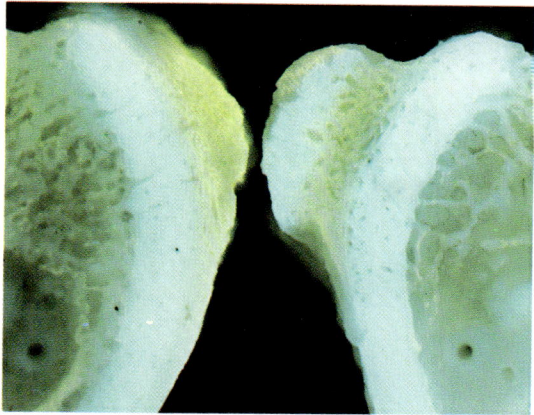 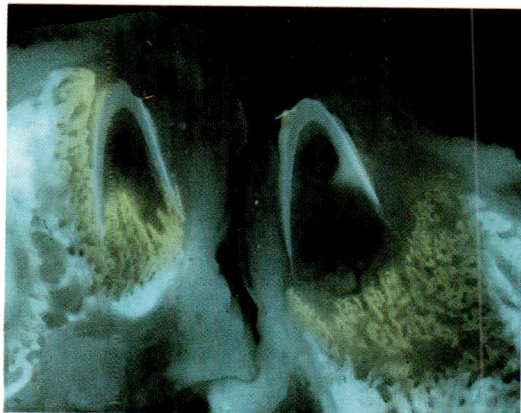

Plate 1. Photomicrograph taken with ultraviolet illumination of ground, unstained cross sections of dog alveolar ridges. The edentulous lingual areas had been implanted with onlays of freeze-dried homogenous bone. The specimen on the right taken at 6 weeks is exhibiting tetracycline-induced fluorescence in an area of reactive bone formation bonding the graft to the host wall. The specimen on the left taken at 12 weeks is demonstrating remodeling and replacement of the entire graft with fluorescing new bone.

Plate 2. Photomicrograph taken with ultraviolet illumination following intravital labeling with tetracycline demonstrating homogenously transplanted incisor teeth in a dog. Yellow-fluorescing new bone formation can be seen entering the pulp chamber and replacing the normal pulpal tissue of the transplanted tooth bud on the left. The transplant on the right is not as yet exhibiting pulpal metaplasia.

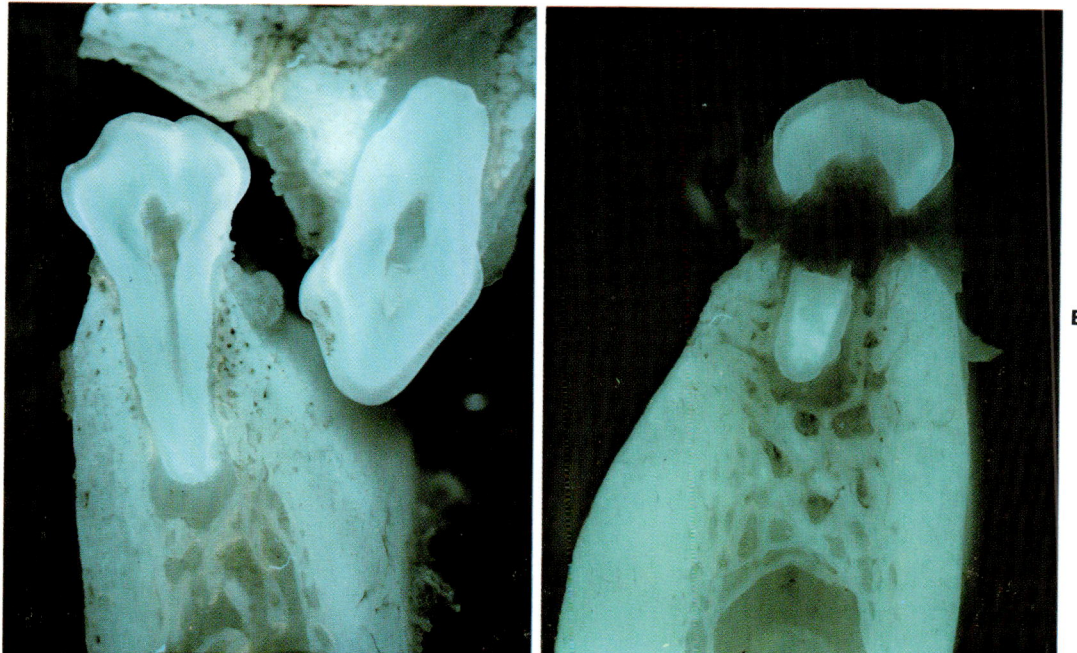

Plate 3. A, Transplanted, fully formed homogenous teeth in a dog after intravital labeling with tetracycline at 6 weeks postoperatively, demonstrating beginning resorption of the root of the transplant. Ultraviolet illumination reveals areas of tetracycline-induced yellow fluorescence indicating new bone formation surrounding the tooth. **B,** A similarly transplanted tooth 12 weeks postoperatively with tetracycline labeling demonstrating marked resorption leading to a complete separation of the crown from the radicular portion. New bone formation indicated by yellow fluorescence is occurring around the root.

use may be some combination of an acceptably preserved homograft and autogenous marrow. Marked osteogenic properties have been observed with the use of this combination of tissues in experimental animals.[28,29]

The possibilities of combining recently acquired knowledge of graft materials with the results of present studies on osseous repair phenomena offer exciting areas for the more effective adaptation of future surgical techniques.

TOOTH TRANSPLANTATION

During the past quarter of a century research investigation of homogenous tooth transplantation procedures has greatly increased. This renewal of interest in the centuries-old surgical exercise of dental transplantation was occasioned by the advent of antibiotic therapy and the almost simultaneous development of tissue banking and storage procedures.

Good evidence supports the view that teeth are capable of being antigenic.[30-33] The failure of tooth transplants to elicit overt immune responses may be the result of several factors. One interesting theory proposes to explain this lack of detectable immune response on the basis of the alveolus being a site of immunological privilege not subject to the usual laws of transplantation.[34] Recent work has tended to disprove this reasoning, however.[31,32] The rejection phenomenon following tooth transplantation, although not of the same magnitude as that elicited by other types of tissues, may be evidenced by the following:

1. A chronic inflammatory infiltration of cells surrounding the transplant and infiltrating the pulpal tissue[31]
2. Failure of the pulp to function as a dentin-forming agent and to assist in the completion of the structure of the tooth root
3. Fibrous encapsulation and root resorption with replacement by osseous tissue

It has been suggested that two phases are present in the immune response of the host to allogeneic homografts of teeth:

1. An early phase as part of a reaction to the soft tissue portion of the transplant
2. A later, weaker phase in reaction to the less antigenic hard structure of the tooth[33]

Homogenous tooth transplantation

Many attempts have been made to preserve tooth buds by refrigeration, by various freezing techniques, and by tissue culturing. In the final evaluation these attempts have been in general unsuccessful. Clinical acceptance without immediate rejection has been recorded following the transplantation of homogenous teeth previously stored under these various conditions. However, no tissue culture or cryobiological method has been able to preserve the pulp so that it has assumed a functional state subsequent to transplantation.[31] Necrosis of transplanted pulpal tissue invariably occurs following the storage of developing teeth by freezing and tissue culturing. Such necrosis results, of course, in a failure of further root development, and the pulp is gradually replaced by host fibrous and osseous tissue (Plate 2).

In the transplantation of pulpless fully matured teeth from a homogenous source, initial apparent acceptance has been obtained. However, ankylosis and progressive root resorption are the almost universal sequelae of such surgical procedures (Plate 3).

Although experimental work continues in evaluating the effects of tissue culturing and cryobiological storage techniques on tooth banking, the present level of investigation does not support the extensive clinical use of homogenous tooth transplantation.

Autogenous tooth transplantation

Although experimentation with tooth homografts has not been productive clinically, autogenous transplantation of teeth has during the past several years enjoyed a measure of success. A resurgence of clinical research in this area has occurred, with new surgical techniques developed in an effort to improve the transplantation success rate. A detailed surgical procedure has been described by Hale[35] and others[36,37] for the transplantation of developing third molars to the first molar position in the younger age groups. Proper patient selection is considered to be most important. Adequate mesiodistal width of the host implant site, absence of acute periapical or periodontal inflammatory states, and general oral health of the patient are emphasized.[35] The optimal root development of the tooth to be transplanted is approximately 3 to 5 mm. of root growth apical to the crown.[35] The recipient site is prepared surgically by removing the interseptal bone with bur or rongeurs and by removing bone at the crest of the ridge to produce the proper size of alveolus to receive the transplant (Fig. 16-6, A). The transplant is removed from the donor site by elevator and forceps. In one technique the portion of the dental follicle surrounding the transplant may be removed.[35] Damage to the soft tissue of the root sac, however, must be avoided (Fig. 16-6, B). The tooth is placed in the recipient site just below the level of occlusion and stabilized with stainless steel

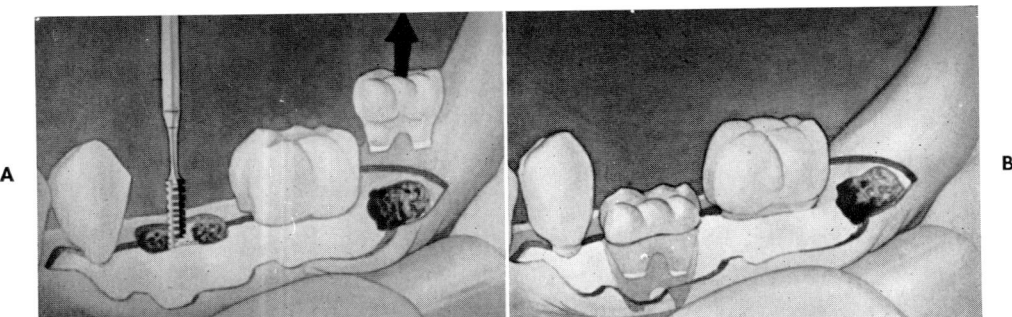

Fig. 16-6. A, The host site is prepared by removal of interseptal bone following the elevation of a mucoperiosteal flap from the retromolar to premolar area and following extraction of the first molar tooth. B, The third molar transplant is positioned below the level of occlusion in the recipient alveolus. (Courtesy Dr. Merle L. Hale.)

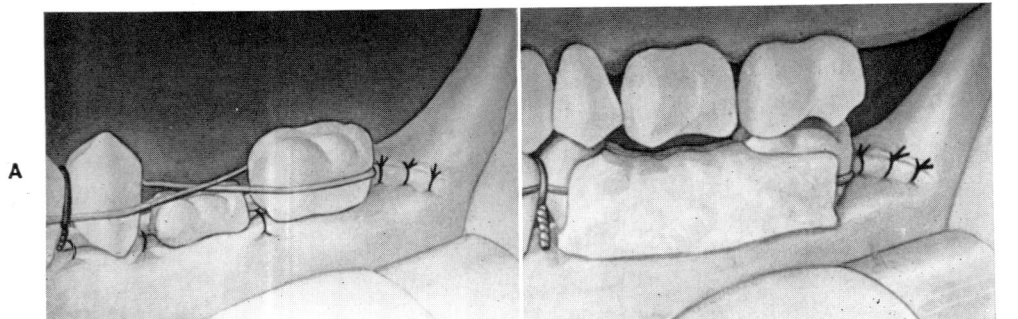

Fig. 16-7. A figure-of-eight stainless steel wire ligature is placed around the adjacent teeth to stabilize the transplant. B, A surgical cement pack is placed over the wire ligature and transplant. (Courtesy Dr. Merle L. Hale.)

wire ligatures crossed over the occlusal surface of the transplanted crown (Fig. 16-7, A). Surgical cement is packed around the transplant and the crossed wire ligatures (Fig. 16-7, B). Some surgeons prefer to use an acrylic splint for stabilization. The surgical cement splint is usually allowed to remain in place for 14 days; acrylic splints may be employed for longer periods.

In another technique[37] the developing third molar tooth is removed with the operculum, gubernaculum, and follicle intact and transplanted to a first or second molar recipient site beneath a mucogingival flap.[37] An acrylic splint is also constructed in this procedure to maintain the intercoronal space and prevent occlusal drift of the teeth mesial and distal to the transplant. As the transplant erupts into position the splint is trimmed to permit proper tooth movement.

Various success rates using this procedure have been reported in the literature with 5-year successes observed in 50% of the cases in some instances.[36,37] Failure of complete root formation frequently occurs, and root resorption is not uncommon. The cause of such resorption has often been attributed empirically to damage to the surrounding periodontal structures in the surgical transplantation procedure. Root resorption phenomena in autogenous tooth transplants have been studied by various techniques. Some investigators have found that the absence of periodontal ligament surrounding a transplanted tooth has not induced root resorption if a portion of the accompanying alveolar bone could be implanted along with the grafted tooth.[38] Others have shown that the transplantation of teeth together with surrounding periodontal ligament and bone has resulted in an extensive root resorptive process.[39]

The autotransplantation of fully developed teeth has been attempted using various surgical techniques. The transplantation of fully matured impacted maxillary cuspid teeth has been effected in a one-stage procedure. Initial attachment of the periodontal ligament following surgery can be demonstrated, and the transplanted tooth may be retained as a member of the dental arch for varying periods of time.[40] Root resorption eventually occurs, however, and rarely do these transplants remain in place for longer than 5 years postoperatively.

Reimplantation

Reimplantation refers to a dental procedure that is in reality a form of autogenous transplantation in which the avulsed or extracted tooth is returned to its original alveolus. Reimplantation of avulsed or partially avulsed teeth with incompletely formed roots and with or without a concomitant fracture of the surrounding alveolar bone may be undertaken in many cases. Proper splinting is usually essential in retaining the reimplanted tooth in the dental arch, although in some cases the reimplanted tooth can be digitally repositioned in such a manner as to make further mechanical splinting unnecessary.

Referral to the endodontist for root canal therapy may become necessary if revascularization of the pulpal tissue does not occur postoperatively.

Immediate endodontic therapy is necessary in reimplantation surgery involving completely avulsed teeth with fully formed roots and in all cases in which a considerable time has elapsed between the accidental avulsion of the teeth and the institution of treatment.

Of the dental transplantation procedures used at the present time, the autogenous grafting of the developing third molar appears to be the most successful. Good evidence supports the autogenous transplantation of the third molar tooth as a practical procedure in selected cases.

SUMMARY

Current and projected investigations of bone and tooth transplantation are directed toward solving clinical oral surgical problems that are immunological, anatomical, and physiological in nature. Research in these problem areas must of necessity bring to bear the work of other disciplines in evolving new and effective clinical procedures. Root resorption following both homogenous and autogenous tooth transplantation, rejection of chemically treated osseous heterografts, the adaptation of grafted areas to alterations in function, the determination of the optimal time and anatomical location for grafting, all these are problems that must be solved to evolve more efficacious oral surgical transplantation procedures of the future.

REFERENCES

1. Carnesale, P. G.: The bone bank, Bull. Hosp. Spec. Surg. 5:76, 1962.
2. Merrem: Adnimadversiones quaedam chirurgicae experimentes in animalibus factur illustratae. Giessae, 1810. Cited by Peer, L. A.: Transplantation of tissues, Baltimore, 1955, The Williams & Wilkins Co., p. 152.
3. Orell, Svante: Surgical bone grafting with "os purum", "os novum" and "boiled bone", J. Bone Joint Surg. 19:873, 1937.
4. Beube, F. E.: Periodontology, diagnosis and treatment, New York, 1953, The Macmillan Co., p. 571.
5. Losee, F. L., and Hurley, L. A.: Successful cross-species grafting accomplished by removal of donor organic matrix, NM004006.-09.01, Report, Naval Med. Res. Inst. 14:911, 1956.
6. Maatz, R.: Clinical tests with protein-free heterogenous bone chips, Bull. Soc. Int. Chir. 19:607, 1960.
7. Bassett, C. A. L., and Creighton, D. K.: A comparison of host response to cortical autografts and processed calf heterografts, J. Bone Joint Surg. 44A:842, 1962.
8. Reynolds, F. C., Oliver, D. R., and Ramsey, R.: Clinical evaluation of the merthiolate bone bank and homogenous bone crafts, J. Bone Joint Surg. 33A:873, 1951.
9. Inclan, A.: The use of preserved bone grafts in orthopaedic surgery, J. Bone Joint Surg. 24:81, 1942.
10. Wilson, P. D.: Experiences with a bone bank, Ann. Surg. 126:932, 1947.
11. Guyton, A. C.: Textbook of medical physiology, ed. 2, Philadelphia, 1961, W. B. Saunders Co., p. 174.
12. Peer, L. A.: Transplantation of tissue, vol. II, Baltimore, 1959, The Williams & Wilkins Co., p. 41.
13. Bach, F., and Hirschhorn, K.: Lymphocyte interaction: a potential histocompatibility test in vitro, Science 143:813, 1964.
14. Silverstein, A. M., and Kraner, K. L.: The role of circulating antibody in the rejection of homografts, Transplantation 3:535, 1965.
15. Bassett, C. A. L., and Rüedi-Lindecker, A.: Bibliography of bone transplantation, Addendum No. VI, Transplantation 2:668, 1964.
16. Chalmers, J.: Transplantation immunity in bone homografting, J. Bone Joint Surg. 41B:160, 1959.
17. Hyatt, G. W.: The bone homograft—experimental and clinical applications, Symposium on Bone Graft Surgery, Am. Acad. of Orth., Surgeons Instructional Course Lectures 17:133, 1960.
18. Boyne, P. J.: The cryopreservation of bone, Cryobiology (in press).
19. Boyne, P. J., and Cooksey, D. E.: The use of cartilage and bone implants in restoration of edentulous ridges, J.A.D.A. 71:1426, 1965.
20. Guilleminet, M., Stagnara, P., and Perret, T. D.: Preparation and use of heterogenous bone grafts, J. Bone Joint Surg. 35B:561, 1953.
21. Boyne, P. J., and Luke, A. B.: Host response to repetitive grafting of alveolar ridges with processed freeze-dried heterogenous bone, Int. Assn. for Dental Research., Abstracts of 45th General Meeting, Abs. No. 51, March, 1967.
22. Shira, R. B., and Frank, O. M.: Treatment of nonunion of mandibular fractures by intraoral insertion of homogenous bone chips, J. Oral Surg. 13:306, 1955.
23. Moss, M., Kruger, G. O., and Reynolds, D. C.: The effect of chondroitin sulfate in bone healing, Oral Surg. 20:795, 1965.
24. Boyne, P. J., and Kruger, G. O.: Fluorescence microscopy of alveolar bone repair, Oral Surg. 15:265, 1962.
25. Boyne, P. J.: Osseous repair of the postextraction alveolus in man, Oral Surg. 21:805, 1966.
26. Siffert, R. S.: Delayed bone transplantation, J. Bone Joint Surg. 43A:407, 1961.
27. Richter, H. E., Sugg, W. E., and Boyne, P. J.: Stimulation of osteogenesis on dog mandible by autogenous bone marrow transplants, J. Oral Surg. (in press).
28. Burwell, R. G.: Studies in the transplantation of bone, VII. The fresh composite homograft—autograft of cancellous bone, J. Bone Joint Surg. 46B:110, 1964.
29. Boyne, P. J.: Unpublished data.

30. Ivanyi, D.: Immunologic studies on tooth germ transplantation, Transplantation 3:572, 1965.
31. Coburn, R. J., and Henriques, B. L.: The development of an experimental tooth bank using deep freeze and tissue culture techniques, J. Oral Ther. 2:445, 1966.
32. Coburn, R. J., and Henriques, B. L.: Studies on the antigenicity of experimental intraoral tooth grafts, Int. Assn. for Dental Res., Abstracts of 44th General Meeting, Abs. No. 103, March, 1966.
33. Valente, L. J., and Shulman, L. B.: Transplantation immunity to a single subcutaneously implanted tooth in mice, Int. Assn. for Dental Res., Abstracts of 44th General Meeting, Abs. No. 107, March, 1966.
34. Shulman, L. B.: The transplantation antigenicity of tooth homografts, Oral Surg. 17:389, 1964.
35. Hale, M. L.: Autogenous transplants, Oral Surg. 9:76, 1956.
36. Fong, C. C.: Autologous and homologous tooth transplantation, seminar of Dental Tissue Transplantation, School of Dent., Univ. of Calif. at San Francisco, Nov., 1965, p. 2-8.
37. Apfel, H.: Autoplasty of enucleated prefunctional third molars, J. Oral Surg. 8:289, 1950.
38. Weinreb, M. M., Sharav, Y., and Ickowicz, M.: Behavior and fate of transplanted tooth buds. I. Influence of bone from different sites on tooth bud autografts, Transplantation 5:379, 1967.
39. Luke, A. B., and Boyne, P. J.: Study of histologic repair responses following osseousdental transplantation, Int. Assn. for Dental Res., Abstracts of 45th General Meeting, Abs. No. 144, March, 1967.
40. Boyne, P. J.: Tooth transplantation procedures utilizing bone graft materials, J. Oral Surg. 19:47, 1961.

Chapter 17

WOUNDS AND INJURIES OF THE SOFT TISSUES OF THE FACIAL AREA

Robert B. Shira

GENERAL CONSIDERATIONS

Trauma to the facial area produces a variety of injuries. These injuries may be simple and limited to the soft tissues, or they may be complex and involve the underlying skeletal structures. Of all injuries, none perhaps is of more concern to the patient than those involving the facial region. All efforts, therefore, should be directed toward restoration of the injured parts to normal or as near normal as possible. Regardless of the type of wound encountered, early care is of the utmost importance to ensure restoration of normal function and prevent facial disfigurement.

Wounds involving the soft tissues of the facial area are commonplace. In the past the more severe wounds were encountered as the result of gunshot fire and implements of war. With the advent of the modern automobile, however, a devastating instrument has been placed in the hands of the public, and transportation accidents are occurring with increasing frequency. Injuries resulting from these accidents are severe and complex, and, with the exception of the loss of tissue, they often approximate the type of injury seen in war.

Care of soft tissue injuries of the face is usually performed in the emergency rooms of hospitals by the assigned personnel. The oral surgeon, however, should be capable of rendering treatment for this type of injury. If he should be the only one available, he should certainly accept the responsibility for the early correct management of the facial wound. In times of war or civilian catastrophe his training in this field would prove of great value. In this age of thermonuclear warfare, with attack upon large population centers an ever-present possibility, casualties would undoubtedly be produced in such catastrophic numbers that care of the facial injuries might well be the responsibility of the oral surgeon. While it is realized that in normal circumstances care of the facial soft tissue injuries might not be delegated to the oral surgeon, he should nonetheless be capable of proper management of these wounds should the occasion arise.

Unless the soft tissue injuries are associated with intracranial injuries, fractures of the skull, or other serious injuries, even severe facial wounds are usually not destructive to life. Therefore, initial attention should be directed to any concomitant condition that, if uncorrected, would have serious consequences. It has frequently been said, "It is better to have an asymmetrical body than a symmetrical corpse." First priority should therefore be given, when indicated, to such lifesaving procedures as establishment and maintenance of a patent airway, arrest of hemorrhage, recognition and treatment of shock, recognition of associated head injuries, and treatment of intra-abdominal or thoracic wounds. These injuries are frequently of such severity that unless corrected early, the patient may die. While the facial wounds are important and should be treated as soon as possible, their management cannot take precedence over these lifesaving procedures.

When the general condition of the patient has stabilized and his life is no longer endangered, attention should be directed to the soft tissue wounds of the face. Open wounds in this area should be cleansed and closed as soon as possible, since conclusive evidence shows that early closure of these wounds is desirable. Wounds that are debrided and closed within the first 24 hours do much better, and the results from an esthetic, functional, and psychological standpoint far exceed any result possible when treatment is delayed. Early closure seals off the pathways of infection and promotes rapid healing, which keeps scar tissue and contracture at a minimum. It also reduces the need for nursing care, improves the patient's morale, and permits an early return to a satisfactory method of feeding.

CLASSIFICATION OF WOUNDS

Various types of soft tissue wounds are encountered, and a classification is indicated because of the individual management problems associated with the various wounds.

Contusion

A contusion is a bruise, usually produced by an impact from a blunt object without breaking the skin (Fig. 17-1). It affects the skin and subcutaneous tissue and usually causes a subcutaneous hemorrhage that is self-limiting in nature. Ecchymosis usually becomes evident in approximately 48 hours.

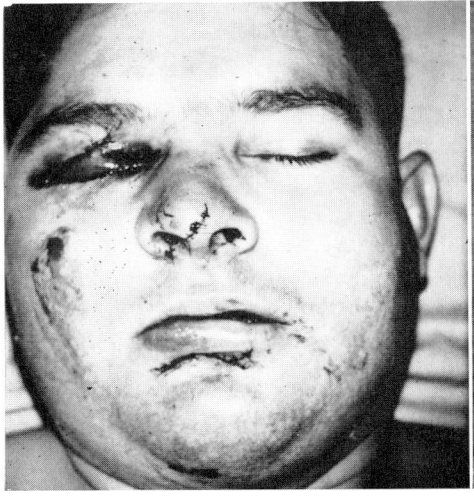
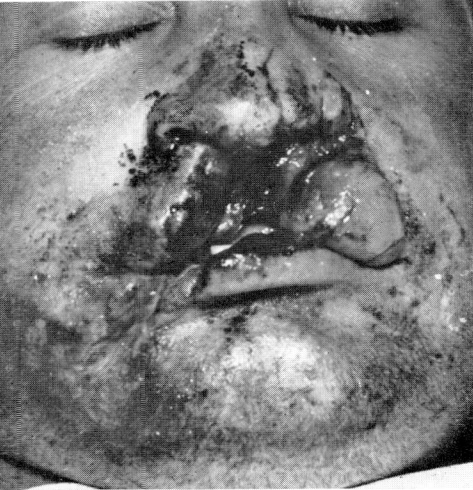

Fig. 17-1. Facial injuries that include a contusion of the right eye, an abrasion of the right cheek, and lacerations of the eyelid, nose, and lower lip. (Walter Reed Army Hospital.)
Fig. 17-2. Gunshot wound involving the lips, nose, and oral cavity. (Letterman Army Hospital.)

Abrasion

An abrasion is a wound produced by the rubbing or scraping off of the covering surface (Fig. 17-1). It results from friction, is usually superficial, and presents a raw, bleeding surface.

Laceration

A laceration is a wound resulting from a tear. It is the soft tissue wound most frequently encountered and is usually produced by some sharp object such as metal or glass (Fig. 17-1). It may be shallow or deep and may involve underlying vessels and nerves. When caused by a sharp object, leaving a clean-cut wound with sharp margins, this type of wound is referred to as an "incised" wound.

Penetrating wound

Penetrating wounds are usually puncture-type wounds produced by a sharp object such as a knife, ice pick, nail, etc. They are usually deep and frequently involve other structures such as the mouth, nose, or maxillary sinus. They may be small or large, depending upon the object producing the wound.

Gunshot, missile, and war wounds

These wounds are in reality penetrating wounds, but are usually classified separately because of the extensiveness of the wounds and the specialized problems encountered in their management. They are frequently further classified as penetrating wounds when the missile is retained in the wound, perforating wounds when the missile produces a wound of exit, and avulsive wounds when large portions of the soft or osseous structures are carried away or destroyed. These wounds are produced by gunshot, shrapnel, or other projectiles (Fig. 17-2). They vary greatly in character, depending upon the speed, shape, and striking angle of the projectile. High-velocity bullets usually cause small wounds of entrance and large, ragged wounds of exit.

Upon striking bone or teeth, fragmentation of these structures frequently occurs, producing secondary missiles that cause extensive internal trauma. Low-velocity projectiles often become distorted upon meeting resistance and cause marked comminution and internal destruction of the wound. Great tissue disorganization with associated fractures of the underlying skeleton and involvement of other facial structures, such as the eyes, nose, oral cavity, and maxillary sinus, is characteristic of these wounds. Shrapnel and blasts produce multiple penetrating wounds with the projectile frequently becoming distorted and scattered throughout the wound. While marked comminution of bone is seen in this type of wound, much less traumatic loss of the soft and osseous tissue is experienced. Multiple metallic foreign bodies are retained in the wound. Gross contamination is present in all these wounds. Fragments of clothing, dirt, metal, and other debris are often carried deep into the wounds and frequently result in infections of serious proportions.

Burns

Burns frequently involve the soft tissues of the face. They are caused by contact with flames, hot liquids, hot metals, steam, acids, alkalies, roentgen rays, electricity, sunlight, ultraviolet light, and irritant gases. Burns are classified as *first degree*, which produces an erythema of the skin; *second degree*, which produces vesicle formation; and *third degree*, which causes complete destruction of the epidermis and dermis, extending into or beyond the subcutaneous tissue.

TREATMENT OF WOUNDS
General considerations

When trauma and wounding are inflicted, at least four major phenomena develop that may threaten life unless measures are instituted to control and finally correct the conditions. First, blood is lost, not only to the exterior, but also into the damaged tissue. Second, tissue is damaged, with derangement of the physiology of the tissue and production of a suitable medium for bacterial growth. Third, the defense against bacteria is broken, which allows the wounds to become contaminated by bacterial invasion of the tissues. Fourth, mechanical defects may develop. These defects may be of major proportion such as blockage of the airway, hemothorax, pneumothorax, cardiac tamponade, or increased intracranial pressure, or they may be minor problems such as defects of the soft tissues. These four factors frequently are not limited to the traumatized area alone, but may provoke a response in every system of the body. The more severe the injury, the more pronounced will be the systemic response.

Nature has provided the body with an efficient and effective healing response to these major phenomena. Immediately after injury, vasoconstriction, coagulation of the blood, and retraction of blood vessels tend to arrest the local hemorrhage. Damaged, nonvital tissue becomes necrotic and produces a slough that tends to rid the wound of damaged tissue. Wound contamination produces an antibody and leukocytic response that combats the invasion of infectious organisms. Finally, tissue defects may be corrected by proliferation of capillaries, fibroblasts, and epithelium. These natural reparative processes are often sufficient to bring about healing of minor wounds, but in the larger and more complicated wounds, surgical procedures are indicated to complement and assist these natural healing processes. The surgeon's aim should be to aid the body's healing response, and this chapter will deal with the surgical procedures involved in treatment of the specific types of wounds encountered in the facial areas.

Treatment of contusions

Contusions are minor injuries and treatment should be conservative. It consists for the most part of observation, and seldom are definitive measures necessary. Hemorrhage is usually self-limiting as pressure of the extravasated blood builds up within the tissues. The tissue usually remains viable, so necrosis and sloughing are absent. Since the trauma is produced by a blunt force, the skin is usually not broken, and contamination and infection of the wound are seldom seen. No tissue defect results from this type of injury, and as the hematoma resorbs, normal contour and function are restored. Because of the hemorrhage in the deeper structures, the contused area first turns blue and later yellow. In this type of wound nature's reparative processes are usually sufficient to produce complete resolution without surgical intervention. Surgical intervention is indicated only to control hemorrhage that does not stop spontaneously, to evacuate a hematoma that does not resolve, or to suture a superimposed laceration. These complications are rarely encountered.

Treatment of abrasions

Abrasions, being caused by friction, are superficial wounds involving varying amounts of the surface. They are usually painful since removal of the covering epithelium leaves nerve endings in the subcutaneous tissues exposed. Hemorrhage is no problem because major vessels are not involved and the involved capillaries retract and are occluded by thrombi. The tissue damage is superficial, and necrosis and sloughing usually do not occur. These wounds occasionally become infected, but are so superficial that local therapy is usually sufficient to control the infectious process. If the wound does not extend below the level of the rete pegs of the epithelium, healing without mechanical defect or scarring can be anticipated.

Minimal treatment is indicated for the abraded wound. It should be thoroughly cleansed by mechanical scrubbing with one of the surgical detergent soaps and followed by an antiseptic solution such as

Zephiran. A dressing is usually not required since an eschar that serves to protect the wound forms rapidly. Epithelization rapidly occurs beneath the eschar, and healing without scar formation is the rule. Occasionally an infection develops under the eschar. When this occurs, the eschar must be removed to permit access to the infected area. Local application of one of the analine dyes or antibiotic preparations, together with continued mechanical cleansing, is usually sufficient to control the infection. Systemic or parenteral antibiotic therapy is seldom necessary for this type of wound.

Prevention of traumatic tattoo. Abrasions are frequently produced by traumatic episodes that cause dirt, cinders, or other debris to be ground into the tissue. It is extremely important that these foreign bodies be removed, particularly if they are pigmented. If allowed to remain in the wound, a traumatic tattoo would result that produces an unsightly defect (Fig. 17-3). These particles should be removed by mechanical cleansing. The surrounding area should be cleansed with one of the detergent soaps and then isolated by sterile towels. A local anesthetic solution is then injected and the involved area meticulously scrubbed with a detergent soap or sterile gauze. Frequent irrigation of the field with sterile saline solution aids in washing the particles from the wound. If the particles are firmly imbedded, it may be necessary to substitute a stiff brush for the gauze, and frequently a sharp-pointed instrument must be utilized to remove the particles from the tissue. A dental spoon excavator is ideal for this procedure. The procedure is tedious and time-consuming, but the importance of the removal of these particles cannot be overemphasized. The golden opportunity is at the time of original treatment, for if allowed to heal in the wound, their removal at a subsequent time poses a difficult problem.

Following this mechanical cleansing a wound resembling a second degree burn is produced. This may be left open, but it frequently requires the application of a dressing. Thin mesh gauze applied to the wound and then covered with tincture of benzoin forms a good protective dressing, although petrolatum or scarlet red gauze may also be used.

Treatment of lacerations

Early primary closure. Lacerations constitute the most common of the facial injuries and vary from superficial cuts to deep, complex wounds involving underlying body cavities. Whenever possible, these wounds should be treated within a few hours of the injury, and seldom is a patient so severely injured that early closure of the facial lacerations cannot be accomplished. Even though these wounds may be grossly contaminated, primary closure early within the first 24 hours is preferred to the radical excision of suspected tissue and the open treatment of the resultant wound as recommended for wounds of other parts of the body (Fig. 17-4). Successful closure of facial lacerations requires meticulous attention to detail and depends upon complete cleansing of the wound, adequate debride-

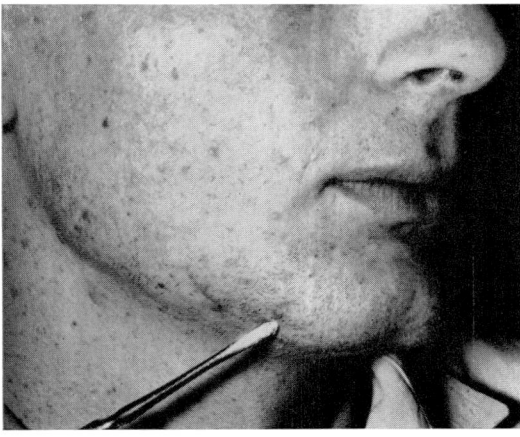

Fig. 17-3. Traumatic tattoo resulting from impregnation of the skin with multiple metallic foreign bodies. (Letterman Army Hospital.)

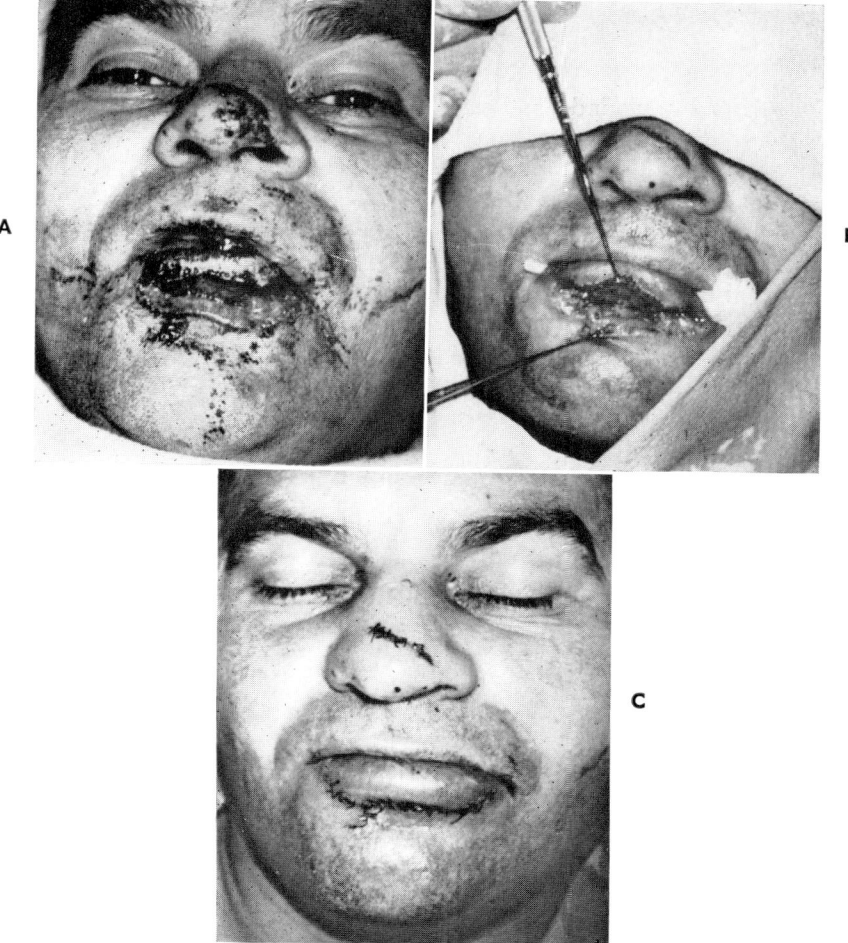

Fig. 17-4. **A,** Laceration of the lower lip 6 hours after injury. This is an ideal situation for early primary closure. **B,** Wound after cleansing and conservative debridement. **C,** Laceration closed by early primary suture. (Walter Reed Army Hospital.)

ment, complete hemostasis, proper closure of the wound, and adequate supportive therapy.

Cleansing of the wound. After local or general anesthesia has been obtained, mechanical cleansing of the wound is necessary. The skin about the wound should be scrubbed with a surgical detergent soap, and occasionally ether or one of the other solvents may be needed to remove grease or other foreign substances. The wound is then isolated with sterile towels and scrubbed vigorously. A constant stream of water applied by an Asepto or similar syringe assists in washing the debris from the wound. All areas should be investigated and cleansed, and any foreign bodies encountered should be removed. Great care in the removal of superficial pigmented foreign bodies to prevent a traumatic tattoo is again emphasized. If hematomas are found, they should be removed, for an ideal culture media for infectious organisms would be produced if they were allowed to remain. Hydrogen peroxide flushed through the wound is of value in eliminating the hematomas (Fig. 17-4, B).

Debridement. After the wound has been thoroughly cleansed the area is redraped and a conservative debridement is performed. The facial structures are richly supplied with blood and appear to possess a resistance to infection seen in few other tissues. Radical debridement is therefore not indicated. Only the necrotic, obviously nonviable tissue need be removed. It is occasionally difficult to differentiate between viable and nonviable tissue. Bleeding from a cut surface or contracture of a muscle when stimulated is evidence of viability, but when in doubt about viability, conservatism is recommended. Rough, irregular, ragged, or macerated margins should be excised to diminish the ultimate amount of scar formation. Lacerations that have been cut on the oblique require excision of the edges of the skin so that the margins will be perpendicular to the skin surface (Fig. 17-4, B).

Hemostasis. Control of hemorrhage in lacerated wounds is essential. Nature provides a degree of hemostasis by vasoconstriction and thrombi formation, but hemorrhage from larger vessels or from the debrided surfaces of the wound must be controlled. Vessels that persist in bleeding are clamped and tied with ligatures. No. 2-0 or 3-0 absorbable or silk ligatures may be used for the ties. Care in grasping the cut ends of vessels to avoid inclusion of excessive amounts of subcutaneous tissue will limit the amount of scar formation. An alternate procedure for smaller bleeding points is to clamp the bleeding point with a hemostat and touch the instrument with the high-frequency coagulation current. Hemostasis must be complete, and the wound should be carefully inspected for frank hemorrhage or seepage of blood. No primary suturing is indicated until complete hemostasis has been secured.

Closure of the wound. After the wound has been cleansed and debrided and hemostasis is complete, the wound is ready for closure. The object of closure is the accurate coaptation of the layers of tissue with elimination of all dead spaces. The tissues should be handled gently, utilizing tissue hooks rather than forceps whenever possible. If the wound involves the mucosa, this structure should be accurately reapproximated as the first step in closure. An

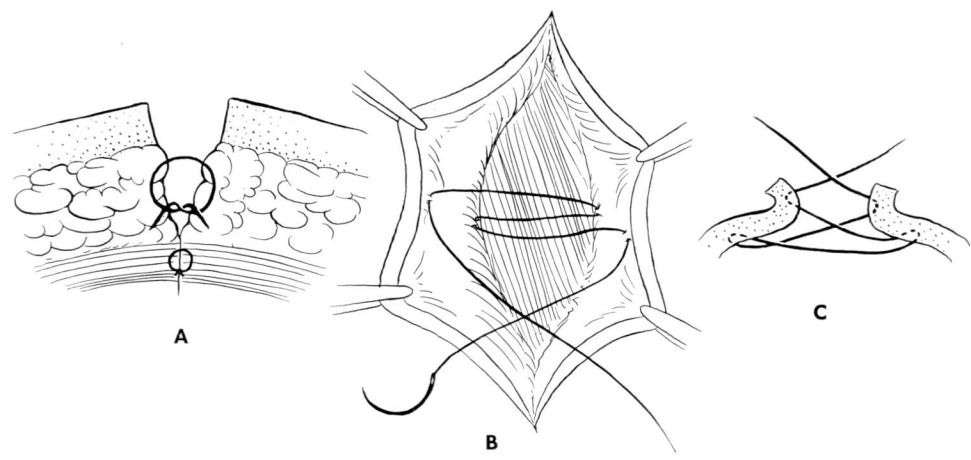

Fig. 17-5. **A**, Inverted buried sutures for closure of the deeper structures. **B** and **C**, Gillies' near-far far-near relaxing suture, which is valuable in relieving tension on the skin margins.

attempt to form a watertight seal of the mucosa by interrupted No. 4-0 or 5-0 nonabsorbable sutures is made. If at all possible, any fractures of the facial bones that may be present should be reduced at this time before completing the closure of the soft tissue. If the soft tissue wounds are closed first, the subsequent manipulative procedures necessary for reduction of the fractures frequently cause a disruption of the soft tissue wound. After the fractures are reduced, the deeper muscle and subcutaneous layers are closed by inverted buried interrupted sutures, with care being taken to eliminate all dead spaces (Fig. 17-5). If tension appears to be affecting the wound, the employment of the Gillies near-far far-near relaxing suture will aid in approximating the subcutaneous tissue and in relieving the tension on the skin (Fig. 17-5). Catgut or No. 3-0 silk sutures are utilized for the closure of the deeper layers.

The final step in closure of the subcutaneous tissues is the placement of fine subcuticular sutures just beneath the cutaneous surface (Fig. 17-6). These sutures should accurately reapproximate the subcutaneous tissues and relieve all tension of the skin margins. If any undue tension is encountered, undermining of the skin may be necessary prior to placement of the subcuticular sutures. The skin is approximated by No. 4-0 or 5-0 silk or Dermalon interrupted sutures placed in adequate numbers to ensure apposition. The sutures should be placed at equal distance and equal depth on either side of the wound. They should be placed in such a manner that a slight eversion of the skin margins is produced (Fig. 17-7). The interrupted sutures will

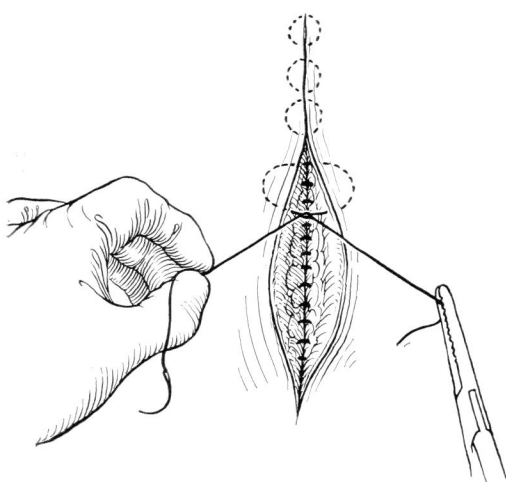

Fig. 17-6. Fine subcuticular sutures beneath the skin, which accurately reapproximate the subcutaneous tissues.

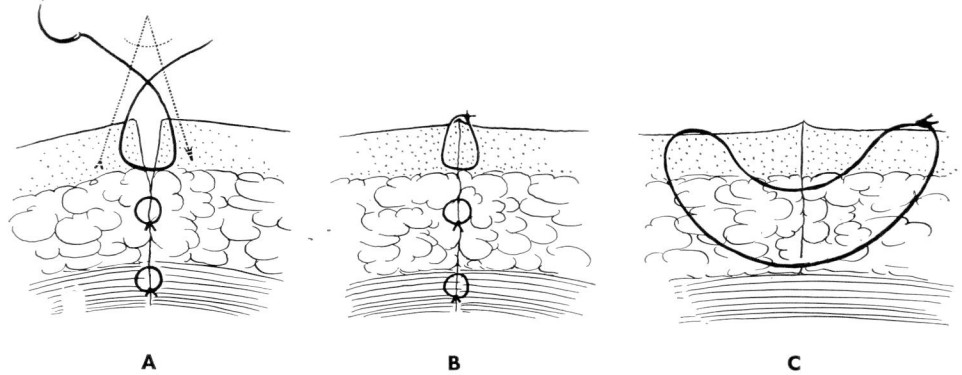

Fig. 17-7. A, Interrupted skin sutures are placed after deep layers have been closed. **B,** Eversion of the skin margins should be produced with interrupted skin sutures. **C,** Vertical mattress suture is a useful adjunct in obtaining the proper eversion of the skin margins.

produce this eversion if properly placed. An occasional vertical mattress suture, however, may be necessary as supplementary support (Fig. 17-7).

Little difficulty is encountered in closing the small or moderately large wounds by this method, particularly if no tissue has been lost. In suturing extensive, complicated lacerations, it may be difficult to determine the proper position of the tissues. In these instances a start should be made at a known point, such as the corner of the mouth, ala of the nose, or the corner of the eye (Fig. 17-8). Each remaining segment is then bisected with a suture until closure is complete. Key surface sutures at these points may be necessary. These may be placed deep into the tissue, but should never be placed far from the wound margins since wide placement is conducive to unsightly scar formation. Fine subcuticular sutures placed between the key sutures will approximate the subcutaneous structures before insertion of the skin sutures. Larger wounds in which no key points are involved may also present difficulties in realignment. Such wounds should be managed by placing a key suture in the center, dividing the wound in half. Each half is then bisected until final closure is accomplished.

Delayed primary closure. For various reasons all lacerated wounds cannot be treated within the initial safe period for primary closure. Such wounds become edematous, indurated, and infected, and early primary closure should not be attempted (Fig. 17-9, A). A program of wound preparation should be instigated and followed by a delayed primary closure when conditions are suitable. Chipps and associates have outlined an excellent regime for the preparation of wounds for secondary closure, and their observations stem from a vast experience gained at Tokyo Army Hospital during the Korean conflict. The regime they recommend includes an initial examination and debridement, at which time all obvious devitalized and infected tissues are removed. Concomitant fractures of the facial bones, if present, should then be immobilized. Adequate drainage should be maintained, and an effective and specific antibiotic regime employed to combat any infection that may be present. Continuous moist dressings applied to the injured tissues assist greatly in preparing the tissues

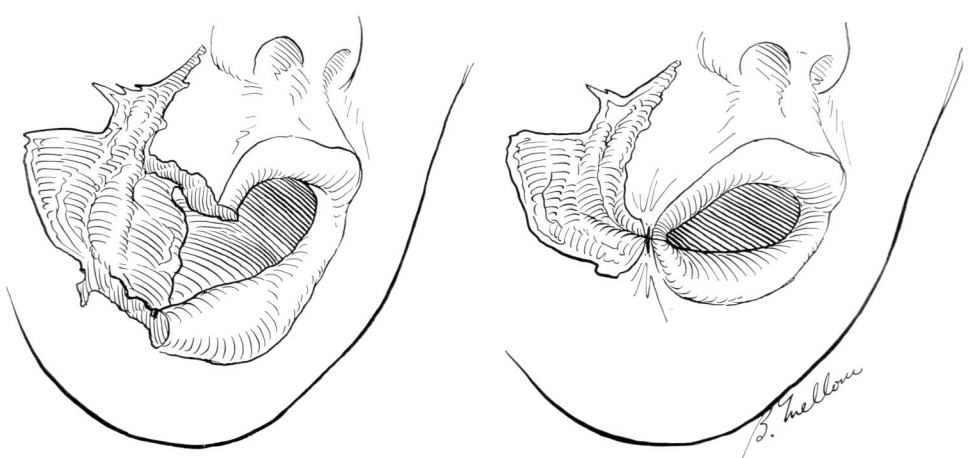

Fig. 17-8. Diagrams that illustrate the principle of starting at a known point, in this instance the corner of the mouth, in suturing large lacerations.

for closure. The wounds should be observed daily, and when necrotic areas are discovered, they should be removed by tissue forceps. Wounds involving the oral cavity should be isolated and oral feeding prohibited to eliminate contamination and fermenting food debris from entering the wound. To accomplish this, feeding by a Levin tube is usually employed. This regime rapidly controls infection, reduces edema and induration, and renders the wound amenable to delayed primary suture in from 5 to 10 days. The wounds are then closed as described under initial primary closure. Success depends upon how well the surgeon adheres to the surgical procedures previously described (Fig. 17-9, *B*).

Supportive therapy. The successful treatment of wounds requires consideration of several other factors such as the need for drains, the type of dressing, and the prevention or treatment of various infections.

Drains. Superficial lacerations do not require drainage. Deeper wounds, however, particularly those involving the oral cavity, should have a Penrose or rubber dam drain inserted. This allows the escape of serum and tissue fluids and prevents the collection of these substances in the deeper structures. Drains may be placed between the sutures or through a stab incision approximating the original wound. Drains should be removed in from 2 to 4 days.

Dressings. After suturing, some type of protective dressing is indicated. Small wounds may be covered by fine-mesh gauze, which is then painted with collodion and allowed to dry. Larger wounds require a secure pressure dressing. This dressing should offer tissue support and exert sufficient pressure on the tissue to prevent additional bleeding or the collection of fluid in the subcutaneous areas. A strip of fine-mesh gauze or nylon is usually placed over the sutured wound, and then gauze fluffs, reinforced by elastoplast, are added. Ace bandages, followed by adhesive tape, are applied to exert moderate pressure on the wound. The dressings should be changed in 48 hours. Sutures are removed on the fourth or fifth day, and a collodion dressing is placed over the wound for another 3 or 4 days.

Prevention of infection. All lacerated wounds are contaminated and infected by the time they are seen for treatment. While this infection is frequently subclinical, efforts should be made to keep the infection

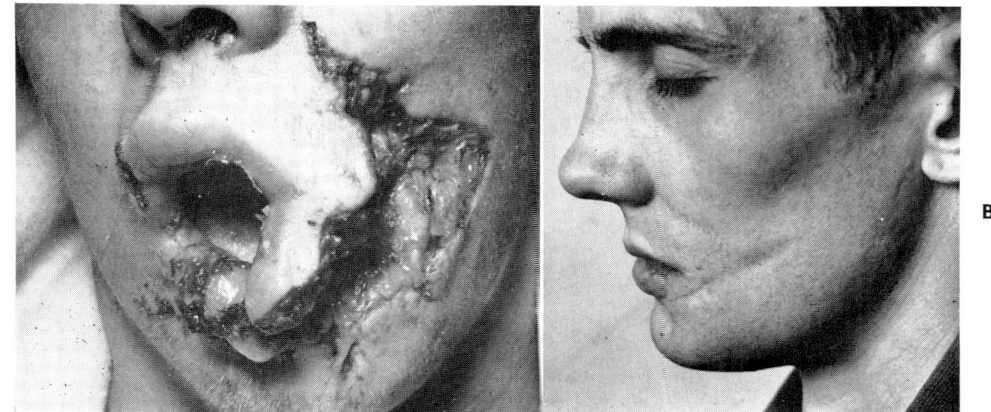

Fig. 17-9. **A**, Facial laceration as it appeared 11 days after injury. Note the sloughing, edema, and induration. This wound was treated by delayed primary closure. **B**, Six months after delayed primary closure. (Letterman Army Hospital.)

at a minimum and to eliminate it as soon as possible. This is accomplished by strict adherence to sterile techniques, thorough cleansing of the tissue, complete hemostasis, conservative but adequate debridement, wound closure that eliminates all dead spaces, and adequate supportive care. This supportive care includes the intelligent utilization of antibiotics and/or chemotherapy. Prophylactic utilization of these substances is indicated in all major wounds as a safeguard against infection.

Prophylaxis against tetanus. Because all wounds of the face are contaminated and are frequently produced by accidents that force dirt and debris into the wound, protection against infection by the *Clostridium tetani* organism must be provided. This is particularly true of laceration, puncture, and gunshot wounds. Tetanus infections are so catastrophic and have such a high mortality rate that if any possibility exists of a wound being contaminated by this organism, active prophylaxis must be provided. In a large segment of the population an active immunity against tetanus has been developed as the result of inoculation with the tetanus toxoid. An injured person who has been so immunized should receive a "booster" dose of 1 ml. of tetanus toxoid as soon after injury as possible. Tetanus toxoid alone is of little value to the injured patient in whom no active immunity has developed, for the development of antibodies within the body would probably be too small and too late to prevent tetanus.

Patients who have not been vaccinated with tetanus toxoid or who have been incompletely vaccinated should receive a dose of tetanus toxoid followed by the intramuscular administration of 250 units (1 ml.) of tetanus immune globulin of human origin. In children the dosage is 2.3 units per pound of body weight. The human tetanus immune globulin must not be administered intravenously and should not be given at the same site as the tetanus toxoid. The recommended dosages will provide protection for approximately 28 days, and the period of protection may be extended by subsequent injections. Antibiotics such as penicillin and tetracycline are effective against vegetative tetanus bacilli; however, they have no effect against toxin. The effectiveness of antibiotics for prophylaxis remains unproved, and if used, they should be given for at least 5 days.

Failures in primary closure. Whereas the majority of lacerated wounds heal without complications by primary intention, some do break down. Chipps and co-workers report that 30% of the facial wounds observed at Tokyo Army Hospital during the Korean conflict failed to heal by primary intention. In an analysis of these cases they found that six major factors were responsible for this wound breakdown. These were (1) tight closure of the wound without provision for deep tissue drainage, (2) inadequate use of pressure dressings, (3) failure to close the mucosa on the oral surface of the wound, (4) secondary hemorrhage, (5) secondary manipulation of the repaired wound, and (6) inadequate antibiotic therapy. It is obvious that these problems in wound disruption stem, primarily, from failure to meticulously apply the standard surgical principles of wound treatment. If these principles are strictly adhered to, failure will be kept to a minimum.

Treatment of puncture type of penetrating wounds

Most objects producing wounds to the facial areas also produce lacerations, so the isolated puncture wound is rarely seen in this region. When it does occur, the wound of entrance is usually small, but may penetrate deeply into the underlying tissue and involve the mouth, nose, or maxillary sinus. This type of wound is dangerous in that it may carry infection deep into the tissue, and the possibility of tetanus infection is always present.

Treatment should be conservative and directed primarily at the control of infection. The wound should be thoroughly irrigated and cleansed under sterile conditions. Hemostasis usually presents no problem because the bleeding stops spontaneously unless larger vessels are involved. Excision of the wound is not usually indicated since it would require a wide incision to expose and explore the depths of the wound, and the resultant scarring would be objectionable. Debridement is not indicated with most wounds of this type, and unless an infection complicates the wound, necrosis and sloughing are rare. Measures to control infection are of primary interest, with particular emphasis being given to prophylaxis against tetanus. The wound should not be closed by primary suture, but should be allowed to remain open to heal by granulation. Because of the small wound of entrance, healing usually occurs with little deformity. If an unsightly scar or depression results, it should be managed as a secondary procedure after complete healing and revascularization have taken place.

Treatment of gunshot, missile, and war wounds

Injuries produced by gunshot and other missiles traveling at varying speeds will be considered together since the resulting wounds present the same problems. These wounds are only occasionally seen in civilian practice, but they become an immediate and major problem in time of war. With the changing pattern of warfare and the possibility of mass casualties resulting from thermonuclear attacks, wounds resulting from missiles and other flying projectiles assume new importance. As seen with lacerations, these wounds vary considerably in extent and character. Many appear hopeless at first sight, but surprising results are usually obtainable by careful surgical technique.

In no other type of facial wound is attention to emergency lifesaving procedures so important. Since these wounds are usually extensive, first attention must be given to the general condition of the patient, and measures to ensure an adequate airway, arrest of hemorrhage, and control of shock must be instigated. The very nature of these wounds produces conditions that tend to interfere with the upper respiratory passages, and if not corrected early, they may lead to disastrous consequences. If any doubt exists as to the ability to maintain a patent airway by conservative methods, no hesitancy should delay the performing of a tracheostomy. Control of hemorrhage is usually not a major problem. Although the facial areas are well supplied with blood vessels, they are mostly small in caliber and well supplied with elastic fibers, and when severed, they retract into bony canals and are occluded by thrombi. The searing action of the missile itself occludes many of the vessels. If hemorrhage becomes a problem, pressure to the bleeding area is usually sufficient to control the bleeding; however, on occasion it may be necessary to clamp and ligate larger vessels. Shock is not a constant finding, but is observed in the more severe injuries. When encountered, hemorrhage must be arrested and the blood volume restored as soon as possible to prevent the condition of shock from progressing to its irreversible stage. Surgery can usually be performed as soon as the blood pressure and pulse become stabilized at the desired levels. Neurological disorders must be recognized and carefully evaluated before instigation of treatment. As a rule, treatment of the soft tissue may be started when the vital signs have stabilized.

The method of treatment depends upon the problems encountered in each individual case. Gunshot wounds in civilian practice usually receive definitive treatment within a matter of hours, whereas definitive treatment of war wounds may be early or markedly delayed. Regardless of which situation exists, when certain fundamental principles are followed, satisfactory results may be obtained.

Whenever possible, this type of wound

should be managed by early primary closure. A general policy of working from the inside out should be followed. Wounds involving the maxillary sinus, palate, and tongue should be sutured first, followed by suturing of the oral mucosa. Associated fractures should then be reduced and immobilized, followed by closure of the soft tissue wound (Fig. 17-10).

Unfortunately not all gunshot and missile wounds can be treated early, and many are seen after edema, necrosis, and gross infection are present. Perhaps in no other group of wounds is the delayed primary suturing after a period of wound preparation more effective. By adequate wound cleansing, debridement, utilization of continuous moist dressings, and control of infections, these wounds may be prepared for closure in from 5 to 10 days. The wound is ready for suturing when the edema and inflammation have subsided, when the suppuration has ceased, and when healthy granulation tissue is present. The wound edges containing the granulation tissue are excised and the tissues sutured in layers as described earlier in this chapter (Fig. 17-11).

Not all gunshot and missile wounds can

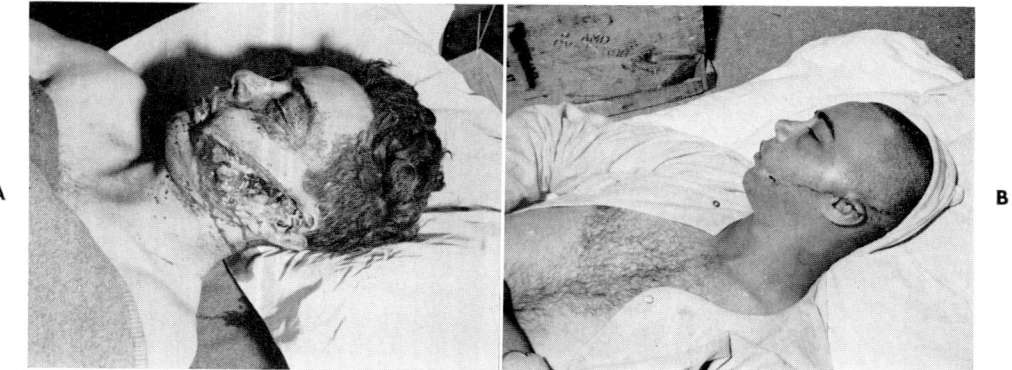

Fig. 17-10. Gunshot wound treated by early primary closure. **A,** Preoperative condition. **B,** Appearance 10 days after operation. (AFIP 55-321-641-47.)

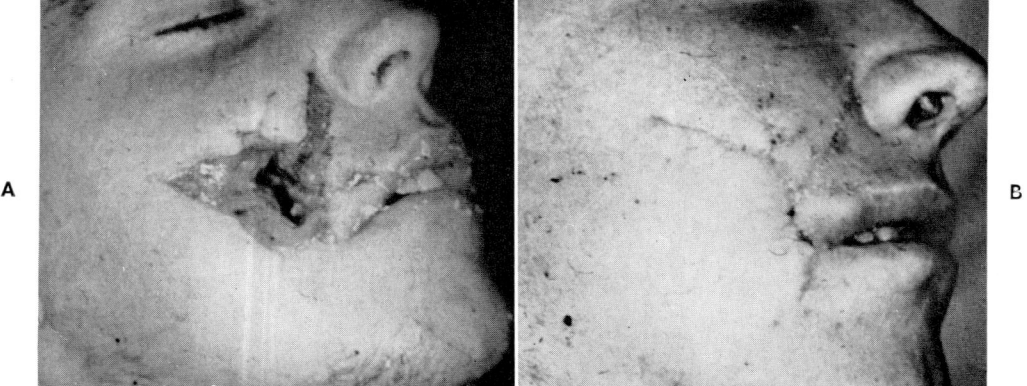

Fig. 17-11. Gunshot wound treated by delayed primary closure. **A,** Condition on admission. **B,** Ten days after operation. (Courtesy Colonel James E. Chipps.)

be closed by primary or delayed primary suture. The large avulsive-type wounds, particularly in which considerable loss of osseous structures has occurred, are not amenable to this procedure. If closed primarily, such wounds may show marked distortion of the remaining tissue and produce unsightly cosmetic defects. However, if the bony fragments can be immobilized in proper position, or if an intraoral splint can be utilized to restore normal facial contour, either primary suturing or delayed primary suturing should be utilized if sufficient soft tissue is present. This practice will often

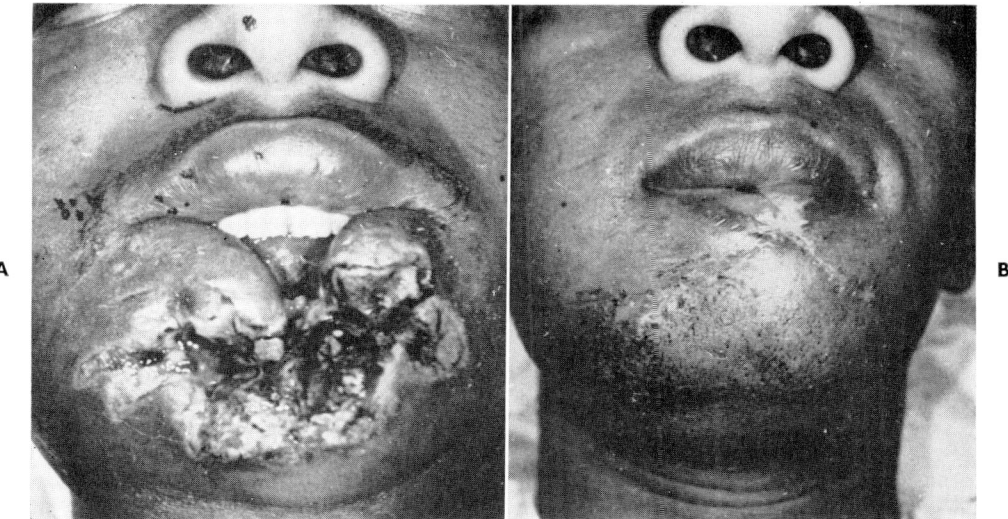

Fig. 17-12. Avulsive wound with moderate loss of soft tissue and bone. An acrylic splint was utilized to stabilize the bony fragments and restore facial contour before the soft tissue was sutured over the defect. **A**, Condition on admission. **B**, Restoration of an acceptable facial contour. (Courtesy Colonel James E. Chipps.)

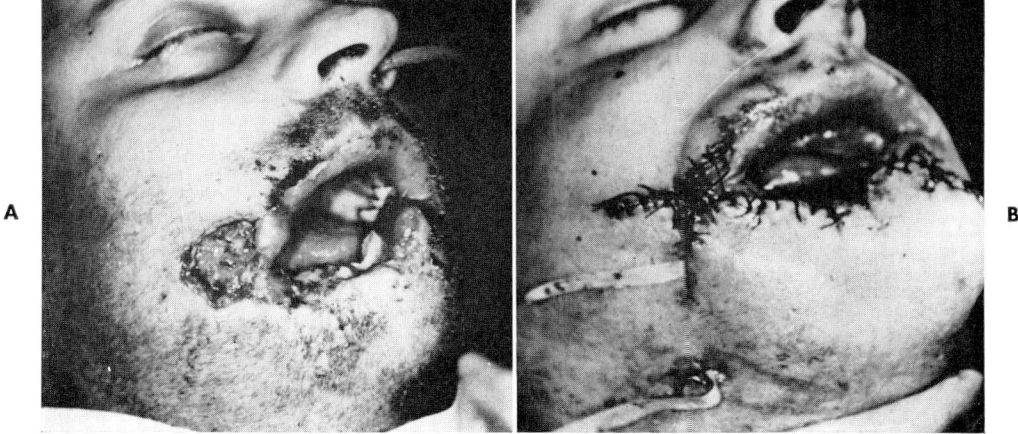

Fig. 17-13. **A**, Wound with loss of substance at lower lip and corner of mouth. **B**, Suture of mucous membrane to skin. (Courtesy Colonel James E. Chipps.)

produce an acceptable cosmetic result and reduce the number of reconstructive procedures needed later (Fig. 17-12). Avulsive wounds in which it is impossible to restore the normal facial contour by immobilization of fractures or utilization of intraoral splints, or wounds with extensive loss of soft tissue, must be handled differently. In such instances suturing the skin margins to the oral mucosa (Fig. 17-13) is an acceptable procedure. Reconstructive surgery to restore facial contour can be performed later.

Foreign bodies

Gunshot and missile-type injuries are often complicated by foreign bodies carried into the wound. These foreign bodies range from the superficially located debris resulting from explosions and powder blasts to the deeply penetrating bullets or metallic fragments of gunfire. They include such objects as pigmented debris, clothing, bullets, splinters of metal, wood, glass, and stone. Fractured teeth and detached segments of bone may also act as foreign bodies. The question often arises as to the advisability of the removal of these objects. No rule applicable to all conditions can be set forth, but several fundamental principles are worthy of mention. The superficial blast-type of multiple foreign bodies should be removed within the first 24 hours to prevent the development of a traumatic tattoo (Fig. 17-14). Any foreign bodies encountered during the cleansing and debridement of the wound should, of course, be removed. This is particularly true of glass, gravel, wood, teeth, or unattached bone segments, for if allowed to remain, infection and delayed healing may result. Metallic bodies present a different problem. Many of these become fragmented and are often so widely scattered throughout the tissue that complete removal is virtually impossible. In evaluating metallic fragments in a wound the possible deleterious effects of these objects must be weighed against the effect of

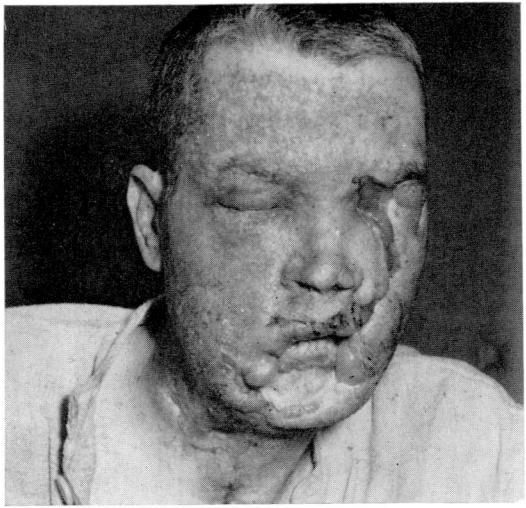

Fig. 17-14. Extensive traumatic tattoo resulting from a shrapnel blast. The metallic fragments are so deeply embedded in the tissue that a permanent tattoo will result. (AFIP B-688-D.)

the surgical procedure necessary for their removal. Many metallic fragments are sterile and will remain in the tissue indefinitely without injurious effect. An old adage often quoted is, "When a bullet ceases to move, it ceases to do damage." While this is not literally true, it is worth remembering. It is considered unwise to perform an extensive surgical procedure to remove these fragments if they are not readily accessible at the time of debridement. It is better to allow them to remain in the tissue, and if any complications develop, removal can be accomplished as a secondary procedure.

Gunshot, blast, and missile wounds are notoriously contaminated, and special precautions are indicated to prevent infection. Antibiotic therapy should be instituted as soon after injury as possible and continued until primary healing is complete. War wounds inflicted in the Korean conflict were for the most part badly contaminated, yet infection was rarely seen by the time the casualties arrived at definitive treatment centers in the United States. This is attributed to the fact that the patients were given antibiotic therapy soon after injury and maintained on this therapy until healing had occurred. If infection did develop, definitive bacteriology and antibiotic sensitivity tests were available to ensure that the proper antibiotic was being used. Tetanus is also an ever-present possibility, and prophylaxis against this infection must be provided. It must also be remembered that tetanus may be a late development in these wounds. Once the organisms are established, they are capable of forming spores that are highly resistant and may remain viable for years. They may lie dormant in the tissues and be activated by some secondary surgical procedure and produce typical tetanus infections. When secondary procedures are necessary on these previously contaminated wounds, it is wise to provide additional protection against this infection.

TREATMENT OF BURNS

The treatment of burns is usually not included in textbooks on oral surgery and rightly so since the specialist in this field is seldom called upon to treat this type of injury. Because of the current emphasis on mass casualty care, however, and the need for all members of the healing arts to have basic knowledge of the problems that will be encountered in the event of a thermonuclear attack, brief coverage of burns of the facial region is included, with particular emphasis on initial treatment measures.

Burns are perhaps the most severe injuries to which man is exposed, and like so many of the injuries discussed previously, they may vary greatly in extent and severity. Their classification as first, second, and third degree burns depends upon the depth of tissue involved. The severity of a burn wound can be estimated from the depth of the wound and the amount of the body surface involved. The deeper the wound and the greater the surface involved, the more severe the burn. Burns, like other wounds, invoke a systemic response that is proportional to the extent of the wound. It has been estimated that a burn of the entire face involves only approximately 3% of the body surface. Thus, isolated burns of the face seldom produce a serious systemic reaction. The isolated facial burn, however, is the exception since facial burns are usually associated with burns on other portions of the body. Collectively these wounds may produce systemic problems of major proportion; therefore, brief consideration of these problems must be given.

The major systemic problem is shock. Immediately after a burn injury a diminution of blood volume occurs as a result of the loss of fluid from the wound and into the interstitial spaces. This results in a hemoconcentration and a loss of colloids and electrolytes. Oligemic (hypovolemic) shock will occur unless the loss of blood volume is corrected. Consequently, therapy to prevent shock is of primary importance and consists of restoration of the normal blood volume, including colloids and electrolytes. The amount of fluid to be replaced is sometimes difficult to determine, and the exact ratio of colloids to electrolytes has not been determined. Use of the hemoglobin determination and hematocrit are of value in replacement therapy, and a workable estimate of replacement needs can usually be determined by knowing the patient's weight and the extent of the burned surface. The estimated need for replacement in the first twenty-four hours can be derived from the following formula:

Colloid (blood, plasma, or plasma expander) = Percentage of body burned × Body weight × 0.25

Electrolyte = Percentage of body burned × Body weight × 0.50

Glucose in water = 2,000 ml.

Requirements for the second 24 hours are half the amount of colloids and electrolytes estimated for the first 24 hours plus 2,000 ml. of glucose in water. By the third day the moderately burned patient can usually be maintained on oral intake of fluids, whereas the severely burned patient will continue to require intravenous therapy, which should consist primarily of electrolyte-free water.

In addition to the loss of fluids and electrolytes, other systemic responses are frequently seen. Destruction of red blood cells, certain endocrine abnormalities, as well as aberrations in protein and carbohydrate metabolism are encountered. It is obvious that the systemic involvement is of major concern in the overall treatment of the burned patient.

The burn wound varies with the depth of the injury. First degree burns first become blanched and then an edema and erythema appear. Small intra-epithelial blisters may form. In a few days the surface epithelium may slough, leaving a healthy granulating epithelium. Second degree burns rapidly produce vesicles and blisters that separate the epidermis into layers. Sloughing is more prominent than in first degree burns. Third degree burns produce complete destruction of all layers of the skin. Necrosis deep in the wound is seen, and suppuration is common. Sloughing occurs in approximately 2 weeks, leaving healthy red granulation tissue in the base of the wound.

Therapy

Treatment of the burned patient may be divided into two categories—supportive care and local care of the wound. Only the initial therapeutic measures and first-aid procedures will be considered.

In supportive care the prevention and treatment of shock are of primary importance. With minor burns this problem is not encountered, but it is of major importance in extensive burns. Control of infection is important, and the aggressive use of prophylactic antibiotics is efficacious in prevention and control of infections. Grossly contaminated burn wounds also call for prophylaxis against tetanus.

Pain is a problem in the burned patient. This is usually controlled within a few days by the local treatment of the wound, but in the early periods systemic sedation is indicated. This sedation should be administered with caution, particularly to the patient in shock, and doses should be kept to the minimum.

Thorough cleansing of the burned surface is the first consideration in the initial care of first and second degree burns. Bland soap and sterile water gently applied are usually sufficient to cleanse the wound, but occasionally some solvent is necessary to remove oil or grease. The wound is then debrided of all devitalized epithelium, and any vesicles or blisters are removed. Hemorrhage is not a problem in the burn wound, and infection at this initial stage is seldom encountered. Treatment from this point may utilize either the open or closed method. In the former the wound is left open without covering, and within 48 hours a dry, firm, brownish eschar will form. This eschar protects the underlying wound, and unless infection develops, epithelization will proceed under this protective covering. If cracks in the eschar develop, it should be debrided for a short distance on either side and moistened fine-mesh gauze should be packed into the defects as a precaution against infection. The eschar will eventually fall off, leaving healthy healing tissue exposed.

In the closed method of burn therapy, after the wound has been cleansed and debrided, fine-mesh plain or petrolatum gauze is applied directly to the burned area. A large, occlusive-type dressing is then applied and supported by an elastic bandage reinforced with adhesive tape. This dressing affords protection to the open wound, prevents infection, and relieves pain. It is not necessary to redress the burned areas, except to change the outside bandages, until the wound is healed. If infection becomes a complication, the dressings must be changed, but if the wound has been thoroughly cleansed and the primary dressing is adequate, infection seldom occurs.

Local treatment of third degree burns that involve the full thickness of the skin is essentially the same as for second degree burns. After early cleansing and debridement a dressing is applied, which is allowed to remain for 10 to 14 days. When the dressing is changed the necrotic, destroyed tissue can be removed with tissue forceps. If the wound becomes suppurative, the dressing will require changing before this time, and local as well as parenteral antibiotic therapy should be employed. Third degree wounds should be treated as soon as possible by skin grafting. If no infection is present, grafting is possible when the necrotic tissue is removed. If this wound is allowed to heal by granulation, marked scarring with contracture and deformity will result.

Burns of the face do equally well with either the open or closed method of treatment. The open method is usually employed, but this has the disadvantage of pain during the first 48 hours while the eschar is forming. This pain can be controlled by sedation. Utilization of the closed method is sometimes difficult to apply to facial wounds because of the difficulty in maintaining pressure dressings on the face. If dressing changes become necessary, pain becomes a factor.

First-aid treatment depends a great deal on the extent and seriousness of the wound. For minor burns, which include most of the isolated burns of the face, local care of the wound and relief of pain are usually all that is necessary. Close observation of the patient is essential, and any signs of shock or other systemic reactions call for aggressive therapy. Prophylaxis against infection should be administered as indicated. Patients with severe burns should be hospitalized and replacement therapy started immediately. The burned surfaces may be treated by either the open or closed method, depending upon the conditions encountered in each individual case.

One type of burn that presents a serious emergency is the flash or flame burn that involves the upper respiratory passages. Such burns often damage the mucosa of the respiratory tract, and the resultant edema may progress so rapidly that respiratory embarrassment and asphyxia may occur. In such an emergency, tracheostomy may be lifesaving (Fig. 17-15).

Burns in mass casualty care

In the case of mass casualties resulting from thermonuclear attack, burn injuries will undoubtedly constitute a major problem. They will result primarily from exposure to the flash of the explosion or from fires ignited by the explosion. In planning for the types of burn casualties from such an explosion it has been convenient to divide them into four categories, depending upon the magnitude and severity of the injury: self-care burns, moderate burns, severe burns, and overwhelming burns.

Because of the great number of casualties

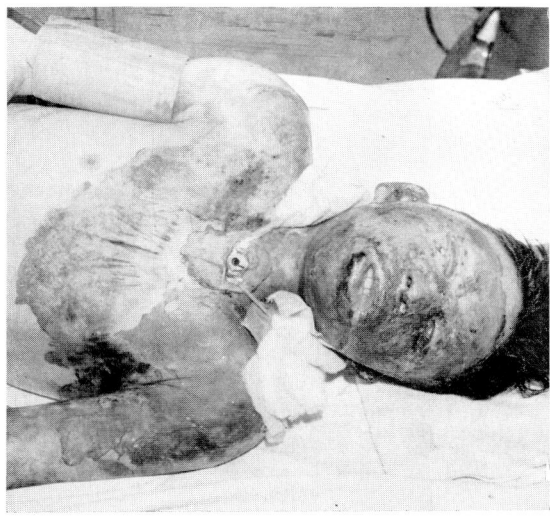

Fig. 17-15. Extensive burn of face that involves the oral cavity and upper respiratory passages. Tracheostomy was necessary to maintain a patent airway. (AFIP 56-8078.)

that may occur simultaneously, undoubtedly insufficient personnel will be available to provide complete medical care, and many patients will of necessity have to depend upon self-care for survival. It is expected that this group will represent the largest number of burn casualties. Most of these burns will be of the flash variety, which are primarily second degree burns on the exposed surfaces of the body.

Flash burns do well without covering, and the open method of treatment may be the only treatment available. The chief deterrent to this method is pain, and most patients would undoubtedly attempt to cover their wounds. Since sterile dressings may be a critical item, a bland nonirritating ointment applied to the burned surface would afford considerable relief. Fluids should be taken by mouth, and if electrolytes are necessary, the oral fluids can be fortified with the following substances: 3 Gm. of salt (NaCl) and 1.5 Gm. of soda ($NaHCO_3$) added to a liter of water; this makes a satisfactory electrolyte solution for oral use. Prophylaxis against infection should also be provided.

Persons with moderate burns would require more extensive therapy. They would undoubtedly need some intravenous colloids and electrolytes. During the early period when definitive care is not available, however, they could be managed with oral electrolytes, oral antibiotics, and sedation to control pain. Wounds should be covered by anything available to prevent further contamination.

Severe burns would require aggressive therapy. Patients with severe burns would be unable to tolerate large quantities of fluid by mouth and would be dependent upon intravenous therapy. Antibiotics to control infection and sedation for pain should be administered, and, if available, some occlusive type of dressing should be applied to the wound. This type of casualty should be given a high priority for definitive care.

Overwhelming burns would carry a poor prognosis. Even under ideal situations with optimum care administered by trained personnel, the mortality in these cases would be at least 50%. In event of mass casualties, treatment under such adverse conditions would be anything but ideal, and few of the patients with overwhelming burns would be expected to survive. Patients with this type of injury should be made as comfortable as possible and given the lowest priority for definitive treatment.

MISCELLANEOUS WOUNDS
Intraoral wounds

Because of the isolated position of the oral cavity and the protection afforded by the lips and cheeks, wounds of the intraoral soft tissues are relatively rare. The majority of these injuries are part of the complex wounds involving other facial structures and have been considered under other sections of this chapter. Isolated wounds, however, do occur, and they warrant separate attention.

Any type of wound may occur in the oral cavity. Direct blows to the oral mucosa are virtually impossible, so primary contusions seldom occur. Secondary contusions of the oral mucosa, however, are frequently seen as a part of extensive contusions involving the lips or cheeks. In these wounds the mucosa becomes swollen as blood extravasates into the submucosal tissue, and with time the entire area takes on a purplish hue. Treatment of intraoral contusions is not necessary. Infection is no problem, and as normal reparative processes take place the blood clot is gradually resorbed, the discoloration fades, and the tissues return to normal in approximately 10 days.

Abrasions are common in the oral cavity. They may result from any type of trauma that produces a frictional or scraping effect on the mucosa. Characteristic abraded wounds are produced by the irritation of a dental prosthesis, a malposed tooth, or a rough filling. Abraded mucosal surfaces are also caused by habitual lip or cheek chewers or by the occasional accidental self-inflicted bite. These wounds are superficial and require little therapy other than removal of the traumatizing force. Once the irritation has been corrected, the wounds heal rapidly without scar formation. If pain is a factor, the local wound may be covered with tincture of benzoin, which will seal off the nerve endings and afford relief for varying periods of time.

Lacerations are the most common of the isolated intraoral wounds and, for the most part, present little difficulty in management. Lacerations of the oral mucosa are frequent findings in traumatic injuries of the face. This is particularly true of lip lacerations since the external trauma forces the lip against the sharp incisal edges of the anterior teeth. Accidents caused by the slipping of dental burs or disks during dental procedures or the injudicious use of exodontia instruments are added causative factors for lacerations of the mucosa. If treated early, most of these lacerated wounds can be closed by primary suture without debridement. Hemorrhage can usually be controlled by pressure, although it may occasionally be necessary to clamp and tie larger bleeding vessels or active bleeding points. Lacerations limited to the oral mucosa are seldom of sufficient depth to warrant closure of the submucosal tissues as a separate layer, and suturing of the mucosa with No. 4-0 or 5-0 interrupted, nonabsorbable sutures is usually all that is necessary. Deep wounds of the tongue, lip, or floor of the mouth that are occasionally of sufficient magnitude to warrant closure in layers are the exceptions. Mucoperiosteum that has been stripped from the bone should be repositioned and sutured at the earliest opportunity.

A lacerated wound that deserves special mention is the one resulting from tears of the palatal mucosa secondary to injuries of the maxilla, which include vertical fractures of the hard palate. These maxillary fragments are occasionally displaced laterally, which may result in a tear of the covering mucosa and produce a communication with the nasal fossa. If these mucosal tears are not sutured early, a nasal-oral fistula may develop that requires a difficult secondary plastic procedure to obtain a closure. If treatment is possible within a few hours after the injury, the maxillary fragments are usually sufficiently mobile to permit the manual molding of the fragments into their proper position, where they can be stabilized with an arch bar. The tears of the palatal mucosa may then be sutured without difficulty. It is obvious that these palatal lacerations must be sutured before intermaxillary immobilization of the fractures. This early primary suturing of the palatal mucosa is a gratifying procedure and, if properly carried out, will prevent the formation of a troublesome fistula.

Intraoral puncture wounds are usually the result of falls or accidents while some hard, pointed object is being held in the mouth. This is a common accident of young children, who frequently run and play with lollipop sticks or similar objects in their mouths. A puncture-type wound results when the sharp object is forcibly driven into the soft tissue. When the soft palate is involved, an actual perforating wound may be produced. Similar puncture wounds of the cheek, tongue, floor of the mouth, or palate are seen as the result of accidental slipping of an elevator during exodontia procedures. The wounds resulting from these injuries are more alarming than dangerous. The puncture wound seldom bleeds profusely, and the tissues usually collapse and obliterate the defect when the penetrating object is withdrawn. The perforations of the soft palate are eliminated by contracture of the muscles around the perforation. Examination to ensure that no part of the perforating object is left in the wound as well as measures to prevent infection are usually the only therapy indicated. Suturing is not necessary. In fact this is contraindicated since the wounds should be allowed to heal by granulation. Any accompanying lacerations should, of course, be sutured.

Most burns of the mouth are minor problems and closely simulate first or second degree burns of the skin. They result most frequently from heated instruments or from drugs used during dental procedures that accidently come in contact with the mucosal surfaces. Treatment is almost entirely directed to the local wound since systemic reaction to such limited burned surfaces is highly improbable. The mucosal surface sloughs early, leaving a raw, denuded submucosal surface. These exposed surfaces are painful, and treatment is directed toward relief of pain and prevention of secondary infection. Systemic sedation is frequently necessary, but considerable relief can be obtained if the burned areas are dried and coated with tincture of benzoin. When large areas of the mucosa are involved, such treatment is not feasible. These patients should be given one of the topical anesthetic solution such as the viscous type of lidocaine or a 0.25% solution of pontocaine to apply to the burned surfaces. A bland, nonirritating diet should be prescribed since any tart or acid food will aggravate the pain. Secondary infection of the wounds should be prevented. Local application of one of the aniline dyes is helpful, and occasionally systemic antibiotic therapy is indicated. These burns heal rapidly without scarring, and the mucosa returns to normal in approximately 10 days.

Serious burns do occur in the oral cavity. The flash or flame type of burn of the upper respiratory tract may also involve the oral cavity, and the rapidly developing edema of the mucosa may create a real emergency. In such instances tracheostomy is indicated as a lifesaving procedure, and general supportive therapy should be instigated immediately. The oral burn is usually superficial, and treatment of the local wound should be delayed until the patient's general condition has stabilized. Treatment of the oral wound is essentially the same as previously outlined.

Burns from accidental contact with strong acids and alkalies may be serious. As a rule these substances are swallowed rather than retained in the mouth, and damage to the esophagus and stomach are more common and dangerous than the injuries of the oral cavity. When these substances are retained in the mouth for any appreciable time, however, full-thickness mucosal burns resembling third degree burns of the skin may result. They produce deep necrosis of the tissue that sloughs in from 10 to 14 days, leaving a red, granulating bed. These wounds usually heal by granulation with marked scarring and contracture (Fig. 17-16). When feasible, split-thickness skin grafts should be placed on the granulating surfaces when the slough is removed. This, however, is frequently impossible, and the skin grafting must be done as a secondary procedure. The seriousness of these chemical burns may occasionally be minimized by prompt first-aid measures. If they are

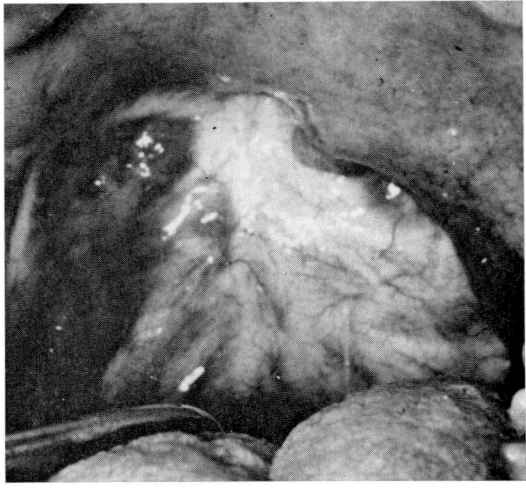

Fig. 17-16. Scar tissue of soft palate and pharynx following accidental swabbing of the throat with phenol. (Walter Reed Army Hospital.)

neutralized with an agent that in itself is not destructive to tissue and then followed by repeated irrigations of the mouth, the depth of the burn may be limited and the resultant scar contraction minimized.

Another oral burn that causes serious consequences is the electric burn. This is seen most frequently in babies who place electric cords in their mouth and chew the cord until a direct short is established. Flash burns occur from the arcing of the electricity, and deeper tissue burns result from the electricity surging through the tissues. Changes ranging from erythema to actual charring may result. In severe electric burns the systemic response is severe and immediate and must be treated vigorously if the child is to survive. Treatment of the local wound depends upon the extent of the injury. Superficial burns heal spontaneously without incident, but deeper burns that destroy considerable tissue heal by granulation with marked distortion of the tissues, which usually requires secondary procedures for correction. In all instances control of infection is essential.

Severed parotid ducts

Facial lacerations in the region of the parotid gland occasionally sever the parotid duct. This should receive attention at the time of original wound closure to prevent the formation of an external salivary fistula. If both ends of the duct are visible, direct anastomosis of the severed ends is possible. A metal probe or polyethylene catheter is placed into the lumen of the duct, bridging across the severed portion. The duct is then repaired by suture over this probe or catheter, followed by closure of the remaining portions of the external wound. The probe or catheter is removed in approximately 3 days and the flow of saliva stimulated. Once salivary flow has started through the repaired duct, danger of stricture or stoppage of salivary flow is minimal.

Repair of the parotid duct is not always feasible, but a very simple alternate procedure produces excellent results. It consists of placing a rubber drain from the mouth into the lacerated region of the cheek through a stab wound in the oral mucosa adjacent to the severed duct. The external wound is then tightly closed, and the saliva is forced to flow along the rubber drain, thus creating a fistulous opening into the mouth. The rubber drain is maintained in position with sutures for 5 or 6 days, and a permanent fistula that functions as a new opening for the parotid secretions is established.

REFERENCES

1. Artz, C. P.: Treatment of burns in atomic disaster, Publication No. 553, Management of Mass Casualties, AMSGS, WRAMC, Washington, D. C.
2. Bethea, H.: The treatment of disfiguring injuries to the exposed part of the face, Surg. Clin. N. Amer 33:109, 1953.
3. Blair, V. P., and Ivy, R. H.: Essentials of oral surgery, ed. 4, St. Louis, 1951, The C. V. Mosby Co.
4. Bradley, J. L.: Primary treatment of maxillofacial injuries, Oral Surg. 9:371, 1956.
5. Brown, J. B.: The management of compound injuries of the face and jaws, South. M. J. 32:136, 1939.
6. Brown, J. W.: Characteristics of war wounds of the face and jaws, Army Dent. Bull. 12:292, 1941.
7. Chipps, J. E., Canham, R. G., and Makel, H. P.: Intermediate treatment of maxillofacial injuries, U. S. Armed Forces M. J. 4:951, 1953.
8. Department of Army Technical Bulletin: Management of battle casualties, Tech. Bull. Med., p. 147, 1951.
9. Department of Army Technical Bulletin: Early medical management of mass casualties in nuclear warfare, Tech. Bull. Med., p. 246, 1955.
10. Erich, J. B., and Austin, L. T.: Traumatic injuries of facial bones, Philadelphia, 1944, W. B. Saunders Co.
11. Erich, J. B.: Management of fractures of soft tissue injuries about the face, Arch. Otolaryng. 65:20, 1957.
12. Ferguson, L. K.: Surgery of the ambulatory patient, ed. 2, Philadelphia, 1947, J. B. Lippincott Co.
13. Fry, W. K., Shepherd, P. R., McLeod, A. C.,

and Parfitt, G. J.: The dental treatment of maxillo facial injuries, Philadelphia, 1945, J. B. Lippincott Co.
14. Gants, R. T.: Shock in management of mass casualties, Publication No. 569, Management of Mass Casualties, Walter Reed Army Institute of Research, WRAMC, Washington, D. C.
15. Gillies, H. D.: Plastic surgery of the face, London, 1920, Oxford University Press.
16. Harding, R. L.: The early management of facial injuries, Mil. Surgeon 112:434, 1953.
17. Hartgering, J. B., and Hughes, C. W.: Field resuscitation, Publication No. 573, Management of Mass Casualties, Walter Reed Army Institute of Research, WRAMC, Washington, D. C.
18. Hughes, C. W.: Debridement, Publication No. 557, Management of Mass Casualties in Nuclear Warfare, Walter Reed Army Institute of Research, WRAMC, Washington, D. C.
19. Ivy, R. H.: Manual of standard practice of plastic and maxillo facial surgery, Philadelphia, 1942, W. B. Saunders Co.
20. Karsner, H. T.: Human pathology, ed. 8, Philadelphia, 1955, J. B. Lippincott Co.
21. Kazanjian, V. H.: Early suturing of wounds of the face, J. Amer. Dent. Ass. 6:628, 1919.
22. Kazanjian, V. H.: An analysis of gunshot injuries to the face, Int. J. Orthodont. 6:96, 1920.
23. Kazanjian, V. H., and Converse, J. M.: The surgical treatment of facial injuries, Baltimore, 1949, The Williams & Wilkins Co.
24. Kwapis, B. W.: Early management of maxillofacial war injuries, J. Oral Surg. 12:293, 1954.
25. McIndoe, A. H.: Surgical and dental treatment of fractures of the upper and lower jaws in wartime, Proc. Roy. Soc. Med. 34:267, 1941.
26. Ochsner, A., and DeBakey, M. E., editors: Christopher's Minor surgery, ed. 7, Philadelphia, 1955, W. B. Saunders Co.
27. Ordman, L. J., and Gillman, T.: Studies in healing of cutaneous wounds, Arch. Surg. 93:857, 1966.
28. Parfitt, J. G.: The dental treatment of maxillofacial injuries, Philadelphia, 1945, J. B. Lippincott Co.
29. Parker, D. B.: Synopsis of traumatic injuries of the face and jaws, St. Louis, 1942, The C. V. Mosby Co.
30. Robinson, I. B., and Laskin, D. M.: Tetanus of the oral regions, Oral Surg. 10:831, 1957.
31. Rowe, N. L., and Killey, H. C.: Fractures of the facial skeleton, Baltimore, 1955, The Williams & Wilkins Co.
32. Rush, J. T., and Quarantillo, E. P.: Maxillofacial injuries, Ann. Surg. 135:205, 1952.
33. Schultz, L. W.: Burns of the mouth, Amer. J. Surg. 83:619, 1952.
34. Smith, Ferris: Plastic and reconstructive surgery, Philadelphia, 1950, W. B. Saunders Co.
35. Soberberg, B. N.: Facial wounds in Korean casualties, U. S. Armed Forces M. J. 2:171, 1951.
36. Sparkman, R. S.: Lacerations of parotid duct, Ann. Surg. 131:743, 1950.
37. Sturgis, S. H., and Holland, D. J., Jr.: Observations on 200 fracture cases admitted to the 6th general hospital, Am. J. Orthodont. (Oral Surg. Sect.) 32:605, 1946.
38. Thoma, K. H.: Oral surgery, ed. 4, St. Louis, 1963, The C. V. Mosby Co.
39. Thoma, K. H.: Traumatic surgery of the jaws, St. Louis, 1942, The C. V. Mosby Co.
40. Department of Army Circular 40-47, Tetanus prophylaxis, Washington, D. C., 25 March, 1968.
41. Stewart, F. W.: The consultant, J. Oral Surg. 26:297, 1968.

Chapter 18

TRAUMATIC INJURIES OF THE TEETH AND ALVEOLAR PROCESS

Merle L. Hale

TRAUMATIC INJURIES

Traumatic injuries to the teeth and the alveolar process are an all too frequent childhood and teenage accident and a not uncommon adult injury. A traumatically injured tooth is a distressing accident for the patient, and often the final dental restoration leaves much to be desired in appearance as well as in function (Figs. 18-1 and 18-2).

Review of a long series of such accident cases established that, on the basis of frequency, the patient's age must be considered as one of the predisposing causes. The greatest incidence appears to be from 7 to 11 years of age (Fig. 18-3). At this period in the development of the anterior teeth the crowns are especially vulnerable because of the large pulp chambers. Also, at this "toothy age" these teeth frequently erupt in positions of isolated prominence in the arch, and they are inevitably exposed to accidents.

Clinical evaluation of the injury

Accidents that produce traumatic injuries to the teeth often are accompanied by hemorrhage, swelling, and laceration of tissue. Such injuries tend to frighten people, and this may complicate the examination procedures. When a small child has been hurt, considerable emotional tension is usually exhibited on the part of both the patient and the parents. By the time the unhappy twosome or threesome reaches the dentist the situation may easily have developed into a very difficult problem. To cope with such accidents properly the dentist must conduct himself in a calm and reassuring

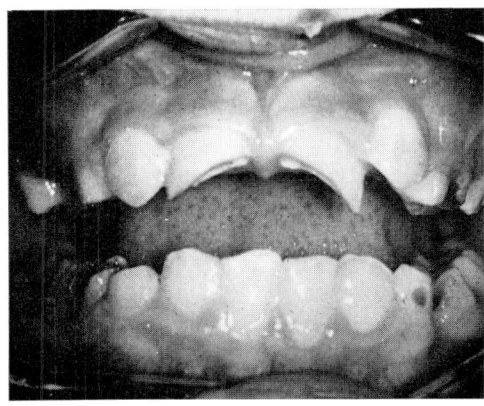

Fig. 18-1. The functional, esthetic, and psychological effects of a dental accident such as illustrated are distressing and often leave a lifetime mark on the patient.

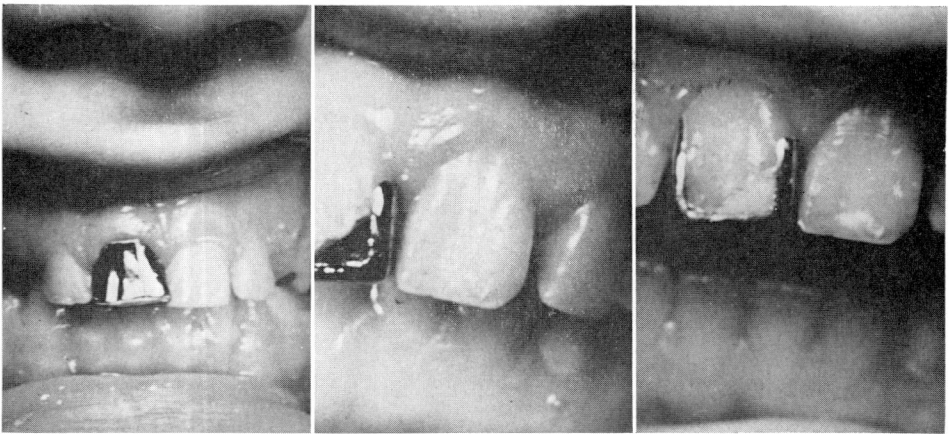

Fig. 18-2. Three case photographs representing dental restorations frequently used in the treatment of traumatic injuries. Permanent disfigurement often follows.

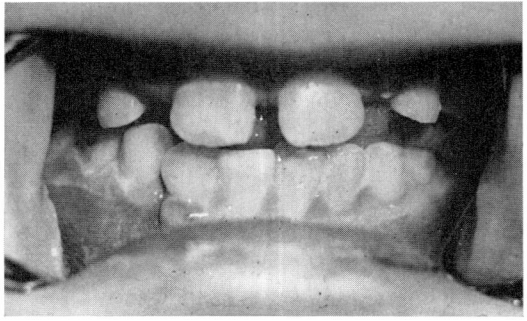

Fig. 18-3. The "toothy age," between 7 and 11 years of age.

manner, and in spite of the adverse conditions he must be able to make an accurate diagnosis and decide immediately how to proceed with treatment. It is often expedient to have one of the parents hold the child while the clinical and radiographic examinations are made. To try to reason with a small child at such times is futile. Gentleness, understanding, and a direct approach to the problem are imperative. In accomplishing the clinical examination it is necessary to inspect the teeth and alveolar process carefully with a mouth mirror and by digital examination.

The extent of these dental accidents can be evaluated as follows:

First, the injury to the tooth should be classified (Fig. 18-4).

- Class I fracture: A fracture of only the enamel cap of the crown of the tooth
- Class II fracture: An injury extending into the dentine, but with no exposure of the pulp
- Class III fracture: An extensive injury to the coronal portion of the tooth with a pulp exposure
- Class IV fracture: A fracture occurring at or below the cementoenamel junction of the tooth

Second, one should determine clinically if the tooth has been merely loosened or completely displaced from the socket, or if it has been forced deeper into the supporting structures. Thus the injured tooth can be classified as *luxated, avulsed,* or *impacted* (Fig. 18-5).

Finally, by digital manipulation, any suspected alveolar fracture should be evaluated. Frequently during such a procedure minor displacements of the alveolar process, or even slight displacement of teeth, can be detected and sometimes advantageously reduced at once.

Since many of these accident patients have mixed dentitions, it is all the more

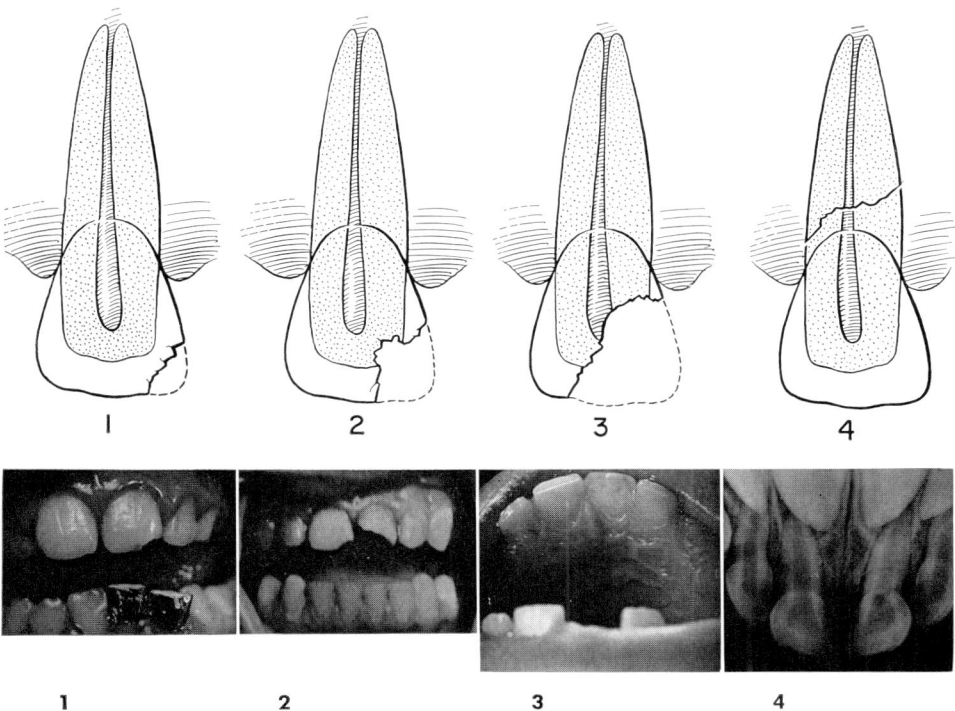

Fig. 18-4. Four cases have been selected, one to typify each of the classifications of injuries to the teeth. 1, Class I fracture: fracture of the enamel cap only. 2, Class II fracture: fracture line includes dentine, but no pulp exposure. 3, Class III fracture: fracture of crown with exposed pulp. 4, Class IV fracture: fracture of root below the cervical line of the crown.

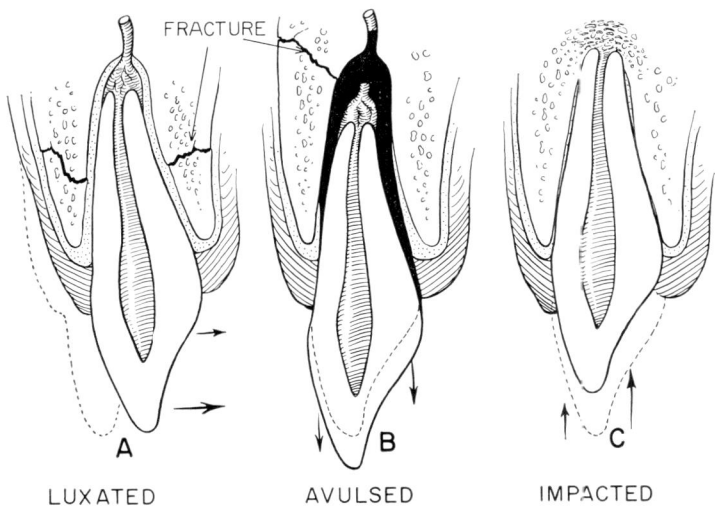

Fig. 18-5. Types of traumatic displacement of a tooth from the socket. A, The tooth has been loosened and moved. B, The tooth has been displaced from the socket, as represented by the dotted and solid lines. C, The tooth has been impacted into the alveolus, as represented by the dotted and solid lines.

important that the mouth be charted so that this information will be readily available to aid in later interpreting the radiographs and in planning the necessary supporting treatment.

Radiographic evaluation of the injury

In completing the radiographic examination it is usually necessary to secure more than one angle or line of exposure to demonstrate fractures. Therefore periapical and occlusal films should be used intraorally. Occasionally, extraoral exposures will be required, with both lateral and posteroanterior views. Satisfactory radiographs may help verify clinical impressions and often provide additional findings that are not revealed by the clinical examination alone.

It is necessary to study radiographically the odontogenesis of the apical ends of the teeth receiving the trauma. If the x-ray films reveal a large, funnel-shaped root canal with an incompletely developed apex, it is logical to assume that the vascular supply to the embryonal tissues in the developing apex will assist repair more speedily than if the root canal and apex are those of a fully developed tooth (Fig. 18-6).

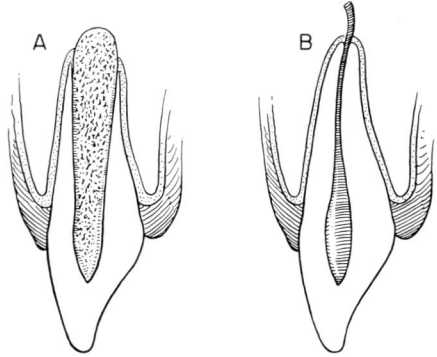

Fig. 18-6. A, Incompletely developed tooth, with embryonal tissues present over the open apical area. B, A fully developed tooth. Note the narrowing of the apical end of the root canal and the absence of embryonal tissues.

Completing the diagnosis and treatment plan

When the clinical and radiographic examinations have been accomplished, sufficient information should be available to permit completion of the diagnosis. At this point, it must be decided whether the injured tooth should be treated as a vital or a nonvital tooth. This diagnostic opinion should be based upon knowledge of the following conditions:

1. The stage of development of the root end of the tooth
2. The extent of injury to the tooth itself
3. The condition of the supporting alveolus

Therefore, if the injured tooth is not fully developed and has an immature apex, if the coronal injury does not involve the pulp, and if the supporting alveolar fracture will retain itself after reduction or can be readily retained by splinting, then all evidence points toward treating the injured tooth as a vital tooth.

Fully developed teeth with mature apices present a much more difficult diagnostic problem. If a fully developed tooth has only been loosened, but not avulsed or impacted, then it should be considered for treatment as a vital tooth, provided nothing more severe than a Class I or II coronal fracture is involved.

If the treatment of the injured tooth as a vital tooth should prove unsuccessful, or if it seems to be contraindicated at the time of the examination, it will be necessary to treat it as a nonvital tooth. At the time of this decision a root canal treatment plan may be formulated.

Splinting is usually necessary to retain all displaced teeth in a satisfactory arch position until the supporting structures have healed adequately to retain them. The time factor of the healing period is best evaluated by direct clinical testing of the mobility of the tooth in question.

The basic principle to consider in the treatment of the traumatically loosened or displaced vital tooth is the prognosis for the repositioned tooth. Vascular nourishment of the pulp must be reestablished if possible. If the blood supply to the pulp is lost, the pulp will become necrotic or gangrenous, and this will necessitate early recognition and appropriate treatment. In fully developed teeth the root canal, as revealed by x-ray films, has become narrowed or constricted. It is very unlikely that such a tooth, if displaced or impacted, can become revascularized as a vital tooth. If the injured tooth appears not to be fully developed in the radiographic studies, or if by direct examination of such a displaced tooth the mesenchymal tissue is found to be present and intact in the cupped-out apex, then repositioning the tooth and retaining it by splinting is justified until sufficient time has lapsed to permit it to prove itself.

Early coronal discoloration alone, especially in teeth having incompletely developed apices, is not sufficient indication for an immediate root canal treatment or extraction. The accumulated extravasated blood in the pulp normally releases hemoglobin, which causes discoloration of the tooth. If, however, the pulp becomes revascularized through the embryonal tissues in the apical area, the injured tooth may recover and continue to be a vital tooth.

In the treatment of a Class I fracture of the coronal portion of the tooth it is usually necessary to reduce irregularities along the fracture line of the crown by the use of abrasive disks or stones (Fig. 18-7). This procedure tends to reduce irritations to the tongue and lips and minimizes the chance of other fracture lines developing under stress along the unprotected enamel rods. This can usually be accomplished at the time of the preliminary examination and often requires no anesthesia.

For the treatment of other than a Class I fracture of the coronal portion of the tooth the patient will require additional supportive treatment from his dentist. Extended treatment of injuries to a fractured tooth other than emergency treatment as previously discussed will not be included here since this subject is covered in excellent detail in numerous operative and pedodontia texts.

Splinting procedures

Injuries to a tooth alone, without displacement from the socket or a fracture of the alveolus, do not require splinting procedures. However, to stabilize a repositioned tooth, with or without an alveolar fracture, and to protect the organizing clot at the apex to enhance revascularization of the tooth, it is necessary to splint this type of injury.

Numerous techniques for this type of stabilization or support have been advocated. As a general rule the simple, easily managed procedures such as the application of Erich arch bars or an Essig-type splint are adequate measures (Fig. 18-8). The primary purpose is to stabilize the repositioned tooth, or teeth, to minimize traumatic stress on the organizing clot. Sometimes a heavier arch bar or sectional bar is indicated if an impacted alveolar fracture requires slow, elastic traction to secure a functional position.

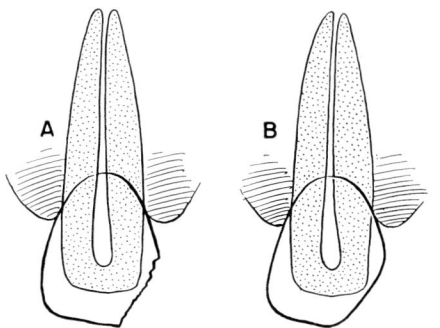

Fig. 18-7. **A**, An irregular fracture of the crown of a maxillary central incisor tooth. **B**, After treatment with fine abrasives such as sandpaper disks and fine mounted dental stones to remove sharp and irregular enamel rods.

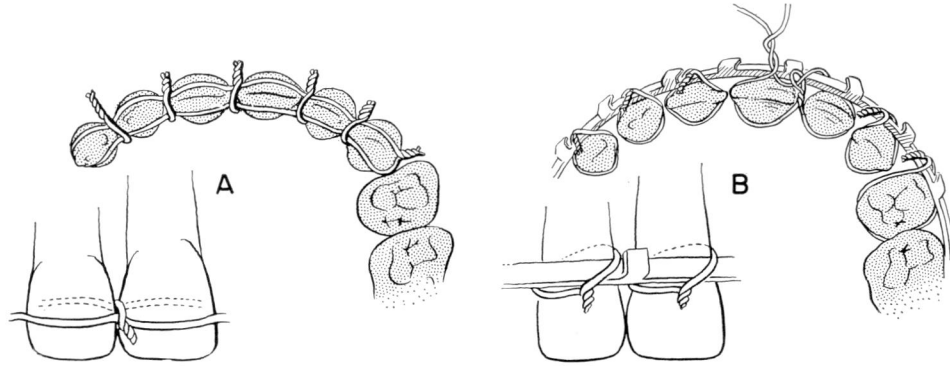

Fig. 18-8. Two techniques that may be used advantageously to stabilize and reposition teeth that have been injured. **A,** Essig type of splinting with 0.018-inch stainless steel fracture wire. **B,** Erich arch bar. This bar is readily contoured and ligated to the arch, and yet by its design it affords good support for intermaxillary traction when needed.

Anesthesia

The patient's need dictates the type of anesthesia necessary for the accomplishment of any surgical procedure.

Occasionally, if the patient is seen soon after an injury, minor manipulations and repositioning procedures may be tolerated without any anesthetic. However, most of these procedures are painful, and to effectively control the pain and allay the apprehension of the patient some type of anesthesia is indicated together with preoperative and postoperative sedation.

For the uncooperative and fearful child, or adult, it is usually desirable to complete the examination insofar as possible and then to schedule the surgical procedure under general anesthesia. The reassurance to the patient that he will be asleep and not be hurt during the necessary surgery often will aid in quieting him, and this fact alone may permit a more complete preliminary clinical and radiographic evaluation of his injuries.

Postoperative considerations and care

The concept of stages of healing in the repair of bone fractures can be applied in principle to the repair of the displaced tooth, with or without an alveolar fracture.

To the period immediately after the traumatic insult, and continuing for approximately 24 to 72 hours, the term *hematoma phase* has been aptly applied. During this period the blood clot is forming and beginning to undergo its earliest organization.

From approximately the third day through the first 3 weeks the healing progresses and may be described as the *fibrous repair phase*. During this period every precaution should be taken to prevent additional injury to the organizing blood clot by any traumatic movement of the tooth in the socket. During this period, however, gentle, slow repositioning stresses are usually tolerated without impediment to the healing of the supporting tissues.

The fourth through the sixth week usually is considered to be the *final bone-forming phase* in the repair of the supporting tissues. During this period the bone formation is completed, and any undesirable movement or traumatic stress at this time may result in a nonunion or malunion and a surgical failure.

It should be remembered that most traumatic wounds of the oral cavity are open, and because of the bacteria normally present in the mouth, all such injuries should be treated as infected wounds. The same basic principles in surgical care should be applied here as to any other contaminated wound. Special attention to oral hygiene should be stressed, and systemic antibiotic coverage should be administered as indicated.

An understanding of surgical principles, coupled with the proper use of antibiotics, should encourage conservative treatment of teeth in the line of an alveolar fracture. Such teeth as are determined on the basis of clinical and radiographic findings to have a favorable prognosis should be carefully retained until they have had ample time to prove their status.

REFERENCES

1. Arwill, T.: Histopathologic studies of traumatized teeth, Odont. T. **70:**91, 1962.
2. Baume, L. J.: Physiologic tooth migration and its significance for the development of occlusion, J. Dent. Res. **29:**330, 1950.
3. Penick, E. C.: The endodontic management of root resorption, Oral Surg. **16:**344, 1963.
4. Skieller, V.: The prognosis for young teeth loosened after mechanical injuries, Acta Odont. Scand. **18:**171, 1960.
5. Korns, R. D.: Incidence of accidental injury to primary anterior teeth, J. Dent. Child. **27:**244, 1960 (abst.).
6. Ellis, R. G.: The classification and treatment of injuries to the teeth of children, ed. 4, Chicago, 1960, The Year Book Medical Publishers, Inc.
7. Hale, M. L. Pediatric exodontia, Dent. Clin. N. Amer., pp. 405-419, July, 1966.
8. Clark, Henry B., Jr.: Practical oral surgery, ed. 3, Philadelphia, 1965, Lea & Febiger, pp. 350-404.

Chapter 19

FRACTURES OF THE JAWS

Gustav O. Kruger

GENERAL DISCUSSION
Etiology

Fractures of the jaws occur most often because of automobile collisions, industrial or other accidents, and fights. Since the mandible is a hoop of bone articulating with the skull at its proximal ends by two joints, and since the chin is a prominent feature of the face, the mandible is prone to fracture. The mandible has been compared to an archery bow, which is strongest at its center and weakest at its ends, where it breaks often.

The chin is a convenient feature at which an adversary can aim. It is interesting to note that often the patient will not identify his adversary to the oral surgeon or to the police after a fight. He prefers to gain revenge in like manner later. This philosophy increases the number of jaw fractures, and if the patient has not had 6 months of good healing before the second altercation, he himself may be a candidate for a bone graft to the original site of injury.

A recent survey of 540 fractured jaw cases at District of Columbia General Hospital revealed that physical violence was responsible for 69% of the fractures, accidents for 27% (including automobile accidents, 12%, and sports, 2%), and pathology for 4%. Males experienced 73% of the fractures, whereas females experienced only 27%. Private hospitals in the same area report a preponderance of automobile accidents as the main cause of jaw fractures. Hospitals in industrial cities report a high incidence of industrial accidents.

The automobile has made serious injury to the face and jaws commonplace. Violent forward deceleration causes injury to the head, face, and jaws. When the car stops quickly the head hits the dashboard, steering wheel, rearview mirror, or the windshield. A middle face fracture can result in which the maxilla, nose, zygoma, and perhaps the mandible are fractured. The National Safety Council, automobile manufacturers, and other groups are suggesting various safety features, including seat belts, dashboard padding, rearview mirror of different design, telescoping steering wheel, push-away windshield, and dashboard with recessed or absent knobs. It seems sensible to insist that children always ride in the back seat since fewer major facial fractures occur to back-seat riders. The most dangerous seat in the automobile is the front seat next to the driver.

A fracture can occur more easily in a jaw that has been weakened by predisposing factors. Diseases that weaken all bones can be factors. Examples include endocrine disorders such as hyperparathyroidism and postmenopausal osteoporosis, developmental disorders such as osteopetrosis, and systemic disorders such as the reticuloendothelial diseases, Paget's disease, osteomalacia, and Mediterranean anemia. Local disorders such as fibrous dysplasia, tumors, and cysts can be predisposing factors. A patient turning over in bed can experience a pathological fracture if the jaw is weak enough.

Classification

Fractures are classified into various types, depending upon the severity of the fracture and whether or not the fracture is simple, compound, or comminuted (Fig. 19-1).

A simple fracture is one in which the overlying integument is intact. The bone has been broken completely, but it is not exposed to air. It may or may not be displaced.

A greenstick fracture is one in which one side of a bone is broken, the other being bent. It is difficult to diagnose sometimes, and it must be differentiated on the roentgenogram from normal anatomical marks and suture lines. It requires treatment since resorption of the bone ends will occur during the healing process. Functioning of the member and muscular pull can result in a nonunion during healing if the bone ends are not held rigidly in place. However, the time required for healing usually is minimal. This type of fracture is seen often in children, in whom the bone will bend rather than break through.

A compound fracture is one in which an external wound is associated with the break in the bone. Any fracture that is open to the outside air through the skin or mucous membrane is assumed to be infected by outside contaminants. Unfortunately, almost all jaw fractures that occur in the region of the teeth are compounded. The jaw will respond to stress by fracturing through its weakest part. Rather than fracture through the full thickness of the bone at an interdental space, it will separate through a tooth socket and then extend from the apex of the socket to the inferior border. The periodontal membrane and the thin alveolar

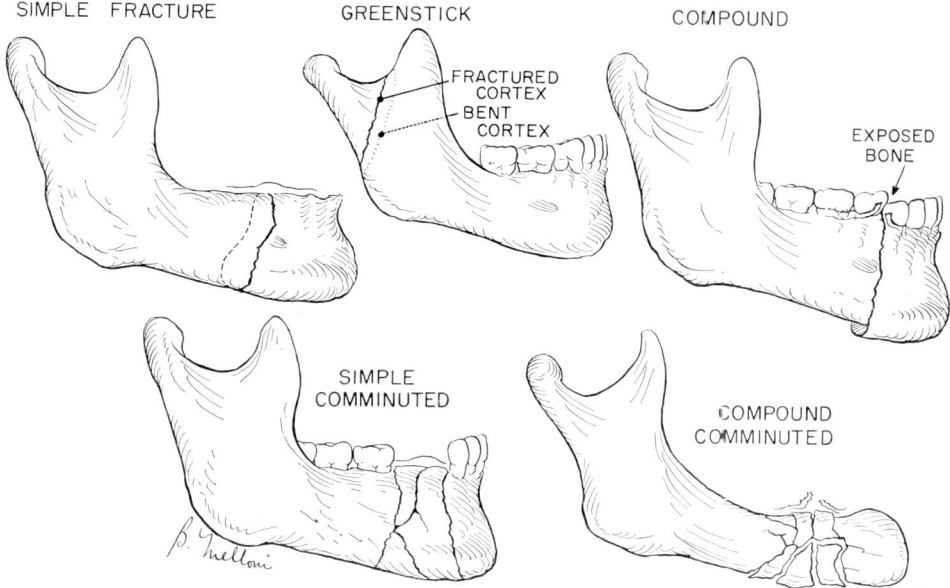

Fig. 19-1. Fracture types.

mucosa are broken at a point adjacent to the tooth. The edentulous mandible will harbor a simple fracture more frequently. Even though the fracture may be displaced so that a "hump" appears on the ridge, the periosteum and overlying tissues can "give" a little since the tissues have no close attachment to the teeth.

The oral surgeon is accustomed to dealing with fractures that are compounded into the mouth. The antibiotics have aided in controlling the potential infection. The bones of the jaws appear to have a degree of natural resistance to oral infection. A fracture that is compounded through the outside skin is more difficult to manage, and an osteomyelitis may develop more readily. The orthopedic surgeon finds that compounded fractures of the long bones are much more difficult to manage than simple fractures. This is partly the result of the introduction of plain dirt as well as outside organisms and partly of the fact that the fractured bone ends are more distracted so that one end of the bone can penetrate the skin.

A comminuted fracture is one in which the bone is splintered or crushed. It may be simple (that is, not open to outside contaminants) or compounded. Fractures of the vertical ramus of the mandible are composed sometimes of ten or more fragments, and yet because of the splinting action of the masticatory muscles no displacement occurs, nor is compounding present. If comminution occurs in the body of the mandible, the treatment is sometimes revised. Although an open reduction might be done normally (in which the bone is exposed surgically, holes are drilled, and wires are placed to hold the fragments in place), such a procedure would force stripping of the periosteum from the many small bone fragments, and healing would be delayed. A closed procedure may be substituted to ensure viability of the fragments.

Gunshot wounds are usually compound comminuted fractures, and usually bony substance is lost where the missile has traversed.

The District of Columbia General Hospital survey found the following incidence of jaw fractures: simple fractures 23%, compound fractures 74%, and comminuted fractures 3%.

Examination

Every patient who has suffered a head or face injury should be examined for the possibility of a jaw fracture. Not infrequently a leg fracture is treated and facial wounds are sutured only to discover several days or weeks later that a jaw fracture exists. Fractures are more difficult and in some cases impossible to treat satisfactorily at the later date. In most large hospitals every head injury is examined routinely by the oral surgery service while the patient is still in the accident room.

The general condition of the patient and the presence or absence of more serious injuries are of prime concern. Asphyxia, shock, and hemorrhage are conditions that demand immediate attention. Extensive soft tissue wounds of the face are cared for before or concomitantly with the reduction of bony fractures except in the few cases in which the fractures can be treated by direct wiring before soft tissue closure is accomplished.

A history should be written as soon as feasible. If the patient cannot give a good history, the relative, friend, or police officer should be asked for a statement. Relevant details of the accident should be placed in the record. The events that took place between the time of the accident and the time of arrival at the hospital should be recorded. The patient should be questioned regarding loss of consciousness, length of unconscious period if known, vomiting, hemorrhage, and subjective symptoms. Medications given before arrival at the hospital are recorded.

Questions regarding past illnesses, current medical treatment immediately preceding the accident, drugs being taken, and known drug sensitivity should be asked now. If the patient is uncomfortable, the detailed medical history can be deferred until later. Routine medical examination can be done now or later, according to the judgment of the internist.

Upon examining the patient to determine if jaw fracture is present and its location, it is well to look for areas of contusion. This will provide information about the type, direction, and force of the trauma. The contusion sometimes can hide severely depressed fractures by tissue edema.

The teeth should be examined. Displaced fractures in dentulous areas are demonstrated by a depressed or raised fragment and the associated break in the continuity of the occlusal plane, particularly in the mandible (Fig. 19-2). Usually a tear in the mucosa and concomitant bleeding are noted. A characteristic odor is associated with a fractured jaw, which perhaps results from a mixture of blood and stagnant saliva. If no obvious displacement is present, manual examination should be done (Fig. 19-3). The forefingers of each hand are placed on the mandibular teeth with the thumbs below the jaw. Starting with the right forefinger in the retromolar area of the left side and with the left forefinger on the left premolar teeth, an alternate up-and-down motion is made with each hand. The fingers are moved around the arch, keeping them four teeth apart, and the same movement is practiced. Fracture will allow movement between the fingers, and a peculiar grating sound (crepitus) will be heard. Such movement should be kept to a minimum since it traumatizes the injured site further and allows outside infection to enter.

The anterior border of the vertical ramus and the coronoid process should be palpated within the mouth.

The mandibular condyles should be palpated on the side of the face. The forefingers can be placed in the external auditory meatus with the balls of the fingers turned forward. If the condyles are situated in the glenoid fossae, they can be palpated. The unfractured condyles will leave the fossae when the jaw is opened. This maneu-

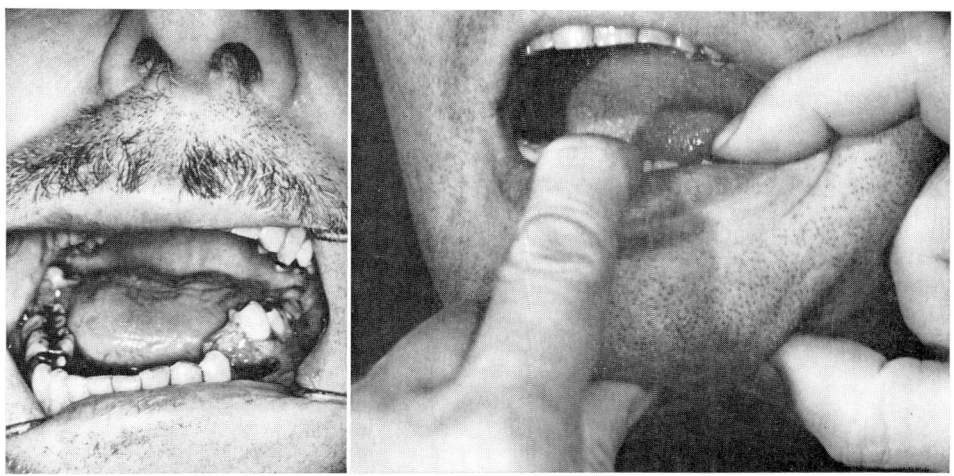

Fig. 19-2. Fig. 19-3.

Fig. 19-2. The continuity of the occlusal plane disrupted by a fracture.
Fig. 19-3. Clinical examination for fracture of mandible.

ver should be done carefully and sparingly. The patient will experience pain on opening and inability to open properly if a fracture is present. The unilateral condylar fracture is suspected following a shift of the midline toward the affected side upon opening. A step sometimes is noted on the posterior or lateral borders of the vertical ramus of the jaw in a low condylar neck fracture if edema has not obscured it.

The maxilla is examined by placing the thumb and forefinger of one hand on the left posterior quadrant and rocking gently from side to side, following with the same procedure on the right posterior quadrant and then on the anterior teeth (Fig. 19-4). If a complete fracture is present, the entire maxilla might move. An old fracture or one that has been impacted posteriorly will not move. The latter will be reflected in a malocclusion.

In a unilateral fracture one half of the maxilla will move. This must be differentiated from an alveolar fracture. The unilateral maxillary fracture usually will have a line of ecchymosis on the palate somewhere near the midline, whereas the alveolar fracture will be confined to the alveolar ridge.

If a maxillary fracture is demonstrated, the facial aspect of the maxilla and the nose should be observed. A pyramidal fracture extending upward in the nasal area may be present. Besides loose bones the patient usually will have a nosebleed (epistaxis) and black eyes.

All patients with facial injury should be examined for a transverse facial fracture. These fractures are overlooked sometimes because of facial edema and soreness. The examining finger should palpate the infraorbital ridge (Fig. 19-5, A). A step in this

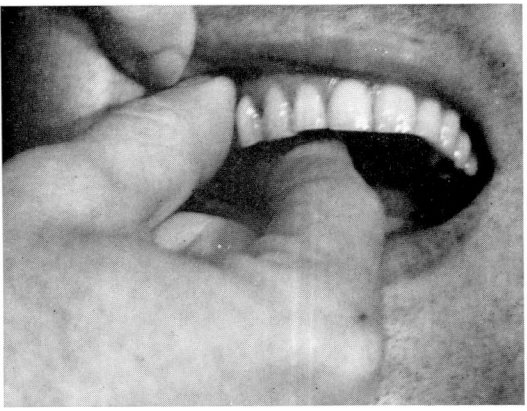

Fig. 19-4. Clinical examination for fracture of maxilla.

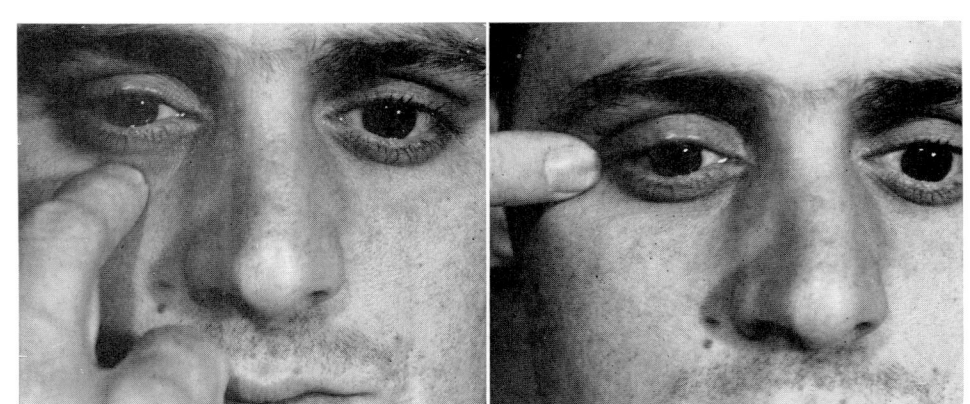

Fig. 19-5. A, Palpation of infraorbital ridge. B, Palpation of lateral rim of the orbit for separation of the frontozygomatic suture.

area indicates a fracture. The normal ridge has a roughened area here, which should not be mistaken for a fracture. The lateral aspect of the bony orbit should be palpated next (Fig. 19-5, *B*). Careful examination may reveal a separation of the frontozygomatic suture line. It is found usually if the infraorbital ridge is fractured.

The arch of the zygoma should be palpated. A fracture may be found here even if no other facial or jaw fracture is present. If the infraorbital and lateral orbital areas reveal fractures, the body of the zygoma is detached from the maxilla, and frequently one or more posterior fractures are present in the zygomatic arch. Careful palpation may reveal the fracture. A dimple over the course of the zygomatic arch is pathognomonic of a fracture (Fig. 19-6). Overlying edema may make the clinical diagnosis difficult. By standing in front of the patient and pressing a tongue blade from the center of the zygoma to the lateral aspect of the temporal bone on each side, the oral surgeon will note a difference in angulation between the blades, which will aid in the diagnosis of a depressed zygomatic arch (Fig. 19-7). A depressed body of the zygoma may allow a gravitational depression of the orbital contents. The edge of a tongue blade held in front of the pupils of the eyes will incline away from a horizontal plane if one eye is lower than the other.

When a maxillary fracture is suspected, several signs should be looked for before proceeding with manual examination as described above.

1. Bleeding from the ears. This requires differentiation between a middle cranial fossa fracture, a fracture of the mandibular condyle, and even a primary wound in the external auditory canal. Other neurological signs are present with the cranial fracture. A neurosurgical consultation is necessary to help differentiate the above conditions. However, the experienced oral surgeon can diagnose the condylar fracture and thereby

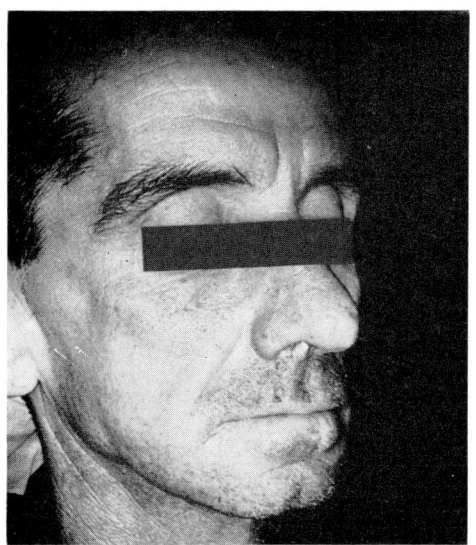

Fig. 19-6. A dimple over the zygomatic arch indicates a depressed fracture.

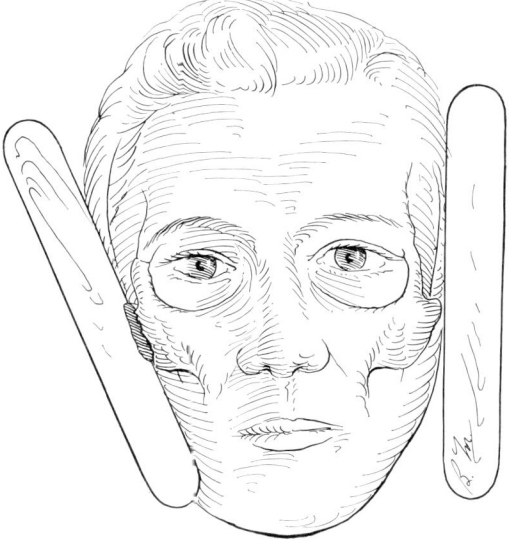

Fig. 19-7. A tongue blade pressed on the zygoma and the temporal bone will incline medially in the presence of a fractured zygomatic arch.

facilitate the neurological examination. The patient with a suspected or diagnosed cranial fracture is the responsibility of the neurologist or neurosurgeon. Fractures or other wounds are treated only when he considers the patient to be out of danger, which in some cases may be a week or two later.

2. Cerebrospinal rhinorrhea. If the cribriform plate of the ethmoid bone is fractured in a complicated maxillary fracture, cerebrospinal fluid will leak out the external nares. Quick diagnosis can be made by placing a handkerchief under the nose for a moment and then allowing the material to dry. Mucus associated with a head cold will starch the handkerchief, whereas cerebrospinal fluid will dry without starching. If doubt exists, test the collected material for glucose.

Movement of the maxilla of any type in the presence of cerebrospinal rhinorrhea is dangerous. Infectious organisms can be pushed up into the dura and a meningitis may result. A few years ago the neurologist insisted that time be allowed for a granulation tissue covering to form over the distracted bone ends so that infection could not enter the meninges when maxillary fracture reduction was attempted. Complete reduction often was not possible by that time. With the antibiotics the reduction is now allowed earlier. Properly reduced bones allow earlier and better soft tissue healing over them, with less bridging of voids between distracted bone ends.

3. Neurological signs and symptoms. Lethargy, severe headache, vomiting, positive Babinski reflex, and a dilated and widely fixed pupil or pupils are signposts that point to possible neurological trauma. Neurological consultation should be sought.

Radiographic examination. A patient should be radiographed if indications suggest that a fracture exists. Three extraoral films are routinely made: posteroanterior jaw and right and left lateral oblique jaws. The films should be examined in the wet, paying particular attention to the bone borders, where most of the fractures appear.

If a fracture is suspected in the vertical ramus or in the condyle, the oblique lateral view on that side can be remade to concentrate on the suspected area. A lateral temporomandibular radiograph can also be made. If necessary, the x-ray beam can be directed posteriorly through the orbit to a cassette held to one side of the back of the head to obtain a proximolateral view of the condyle head.

In suspected maxillary fractures a Waters view (nose-chin position taken from a posteroanterior exposure) should be made. If a zygomatic fracture is suspected, a "jughandle" view is made with the tube near the patient's umbilicus and the cassette at the top of the head. Maxillary fractures are difficult to diagnose on the radiograph even by the trained oral surgeon or the radiologist. When a definite conclusion cannot be reached, a lateral skull radiograph should be made. If the frontonasal suture line is opened on the radiograph, the possibility is strong that a maxillary fracture exists. The absence of this sign, however, does not eliminate the possibility of maxillary fracture.[1]

In cases in which a fracture is demonstrated, intraoral radiographs should be made at the fracture sites before definitive treatment is given. Extreme trismus or a severely injured patient would preclude this. Intraoral views generally provide excellent definition because of the proximity of bone to the film. They sometimes show fractures that are not seen on the standard views, notably alveolar process, midline maxilla, and symphyseal fractures. The condition of the adjacent teeth and detailed information about the fracture can be obtained by this procedure.

The diagnosis of a double fracture at one site, particularly in the mandible, should be made guardedly. A lateral jaw radiograph is not often so made that the fractures of the lateral cortex and the medial cortex

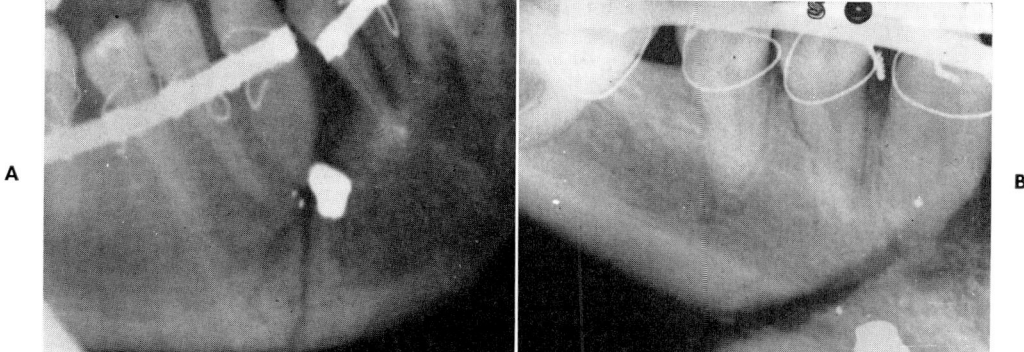

Fig. 19-8. **A,** Lateral jaw radiograph showing an apparent double fracture. Note that the two radiolucent lines converge at the inferior border. **B,** Intraoral radiograph of the same case, showing that only a single fracture exists. Note metal fragment.

superimpose exactly. The two fractured cortical plates may be interpreted mistakenly as two fractures through the body of the bone. (See Fig. 19-8.)

From a medicolegal point of view a permanent record in the form of radiographs is necessary. In any case in which a fracture might be suspected it is better to err on the safe side and make the minimum extraoral radiographs, namely, the posteroanterior jaw and right and left lateral oblique jaw films. In children or young adults in whom consideration of the total amount of radiation is a factor, a leaded rubber sheet can be used to cover the gonads and neck.

First aid

The primary consideration is to have a live patient. Accordingly, immediate measures should be taken to assure that his general condition is satisfactory. Specific treatment of fractures in the severely injured patient is given anytime from hours to weeks later.

If the airway is not patent, the fingers should be placed at the base of the tongue and the tongue pulled forward. Dentures, broken-off teeth, and foreign objects should be removed carefully if the finger can reach them. Suction should be employed for secretions and blood. A rubber airway can maintain a patent airway temporarily, or a suture can be placed through the midline of the tongue and tied to the clothing or affixed to the chest wall with adhesive tape. Mandibular fractures may involve the muscular attachment of the tongue with attendant posterior displacement and resultant asphyxia. If serious consideration is given to performing a tracheostomy, it should be done. An emergency tracheostomy may be needed, or, if time and facilities are available, an elective tracheostomy can be done.

Shock is treated by placing the patient in shock position with the head slightly below the level of the feet. Warm blankets are placed over him. Excessive heat in the form of hot-water bottles is as dangerous as cold. Whole blood is given for definitive treatment of major shock.

Hemorrhage is rarely a complication of jaw fractures unless deep vessels in the soft tissue (for example, maxillary artery, facial vessels, lingual vessels) are involved. Even if the inferior alveolar vessels are severed in the bony canal, the hemorrhage is not severe. Hemorrhage from other wounds, however, demands immediate attention. In most cases the proper pressure point can be held with finger pressure until the vessel can be clamped and tied.

Patients with head injury should not receive morphine except possibly in case of severe pain. Morphine may complicate further the function of the respiratory center. Tetanus antitoxin is given after a sensitivity test if the skin is broken, provided the patient has not been immunized. If the patient has been previously immunized, then a 1 ml. booster dose of tetanus toxoid is given. This is done in the accident room.

The best treatment for jaw fractures is immediate intermaxillary fixation. Ideally, the permanent fixation that will be used to treat the fracture should be placed within hours after the injury. In a good many large hospitals the intern is instructed to place intermaxillary fixation immediately following clinical and radiographic examination regardless of the time of day or night. The patient then is sedated further, given antibiotics and other necessary supportive measures, and ice packs are placed on the face. If these procedures are done soon after admission, the patient is more comfortable. The broken ends of bone are not moving or in malposition, and therefore the nerve is not traumatized. The organization of the blood clot, which takes place in the first few hours, will not be disrupted by further manipulation in the majority of instances. Intraoral wiring is more difficult to apply the next morning when edema and the trismus associated with reflex spasms of the muscles have occurred. If further treatment is necessary, it is discussed after the immediate measures have been instituted and adequate postoperative radiographs are available for interpretation.

Temporary fixation should be placed if definitive fixation is not feasible. Some sort of fixation should always be placed, to keep the patient comfortable and to keep the fragments in as good position as possible. A head bandage is the most simple form of fixation. The four-tailed bandage (Fig. 19-9) is one method that can be used. Ivy loops can be placed as temporary measures (see p. 320). A method that has been

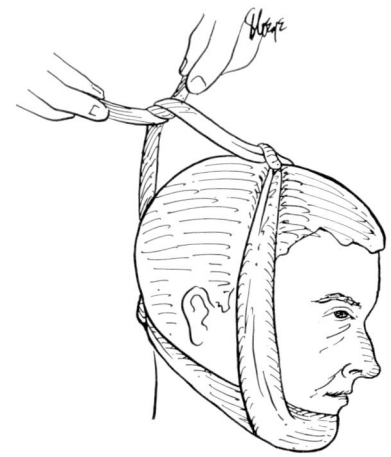

Fig. 19-9. The four-tailed bandage.

valuable is to string No. 4-0 dress clamps on thin, 28-gauge stainless steel wire. Four of these can be placed in as many minutes, and elastics are stretched between them.

Treatment

The treatment of fractures is directed toward placing the ends of the bone in the proper relation so that they touch and maintaining this position until healing occurs. The term used for positioning the bone is *reduction* of the fracture. The term used for maintaining the position is *fixation*.

Closed reduction. Several methods of reduction are available. The simplest method is closed reduction, that is, manipulation without surgically exposing the bone to view. In long bones the orthopedic surgeon pulls or manipulates the bone under the intact skin until the fracture is in proper position. The story is told of an old Scottish physician who had a bucket of sand in the corner of his office. A patient suffering a wrist fracture would be directed against his will to pick up the bucket. In so doing, the fractured parts would align themselves perfectly, and a plaster cast was applied.

Most early jaw fractures can be reduced manually. In older fractures in which the bony segments are not freely movable, traction supplied by rubber bands between the jaws exert a powerful, continuous force, which will reduce an obstinate fracture in 15 minutes to 24 hours. The elastic traction overcomes three factors: the active muscular pull that distracts the fragments (the main cause for malposition), the organized connective tissue at the fracture site, and the malposition caused by the direction and force of the trauma. A maxillary fracture often is pushed back by force, and it must be brought forward by manual manipulation or elastic traction. Rarely do the bones require surgical separation except in the case of delayed treatment when a fracture has healed in malposition (malunion).

Open reduction. It is not feasible to reduce all fractures satisfactorily by closed procedures. The often-encountered fracture at the angle of the mandible is difficult to reduce because it is difficult to counter the powerful pull of the masticatory muscles in that area. In the case of the angle fracture, however, open reduction is done more for fixation than for reduction. When the bone is surgically exposed, holes are drilled on either side of the fracture, wire is crossed over the fracture, and the bone ends are brought into good approximation. Besides good fixation, the fracture can be reduced exactly by direct vision. Perfect approximation is not always present following closed procedures. It might be stated in passing, however, that jaw fractures that occur within the dental arch are reduced to a fraction of a millimeter by the action of the dental facets of one arch guiding the other arch into the preexistent occlusion. This is not so likely to be true in fractures in other parts of the body, where manipulation is necessarily done through large muscle masses. Reduction in these latter instances need not be as critical as in jaw fractures, which must present an exact occlusion.

Another advantage of open reduction, particularly in a late fracture, is the opportunity for the surgeon to clean out the organizing connective tissue and debris between bone ends that would delay healing in the new position if left interposed.

Disadvantages of open reduction are: (1) the surgical procedure removes the natural protective clot at the site, and the limiting periosteum is incised; (2) infection is possible even with extreme aseptic procedures and antibiotics; (3) a surgical procedure is necessary, which increases time in the hospital and other hospital costs; and (4) a skin scar is present.

Fixation. The orthopedic surgeon reduces a simple fracture of the long bones by a closed procedure and then employs a plaster cast for fixation. The oral surgeon frequently combines the two procedures by the use of one apparatus. When the bones of the jaws contain teeth, the occlusion of the teeth can be used to guide the reduction. By placing wires, arch bars, or splints on the teeth and then extending elastic bands or wires from the mandibular to the maxillary arch, the bones are held in proper position through proper and harmonious interdigitation of the teeth. Plaster casts are not necessary or feasible.

The fixation of jaw fractures is approached in graduating steps. Usually intermaxillary fixation by means of wires, arch bars, or splints is the first step. In many cases that is all that is needed. If this is insufficient, however, direct wiring through holes in the bone is done by an open procedure. This is done in addition to the intermaxillary fixation.

Methods other than open reduction and direct bone wiring have been employed to manage the angle fracture. Distal extensions from intraoral splints and external extensions from plaster headcaps to a hole in the distal fragments have been discarded by and large. Fixation by medullary pins is used sometimes. The parts are reduced, and a long, sharp, stainless steel pin is drilled into the length of the bone, crossing the fracture line. The pin is used more often in

306 Textbook of oral surgery

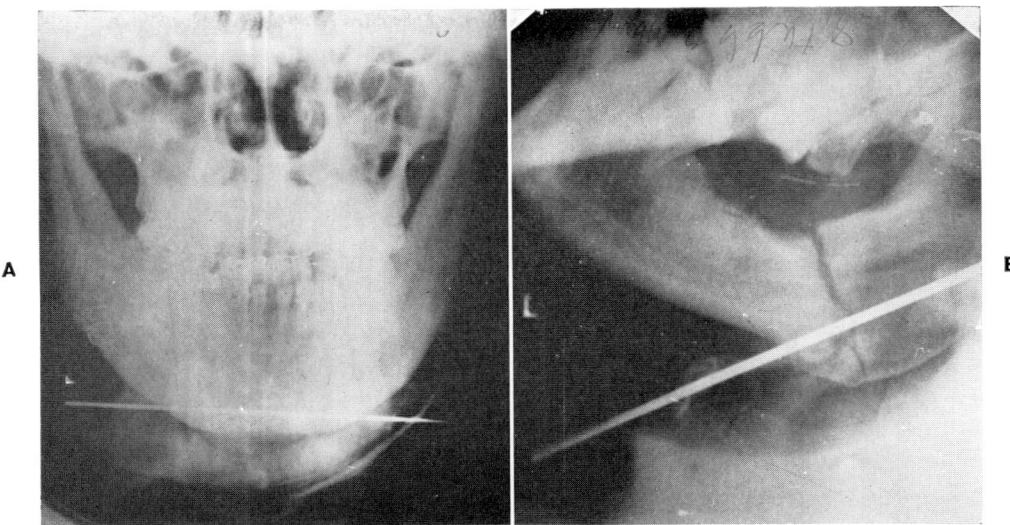

Fig. 19-10. **A,** Kirschner wire placed across symphysis fracture. **B,** Steinmann pin placed through angle fracture.

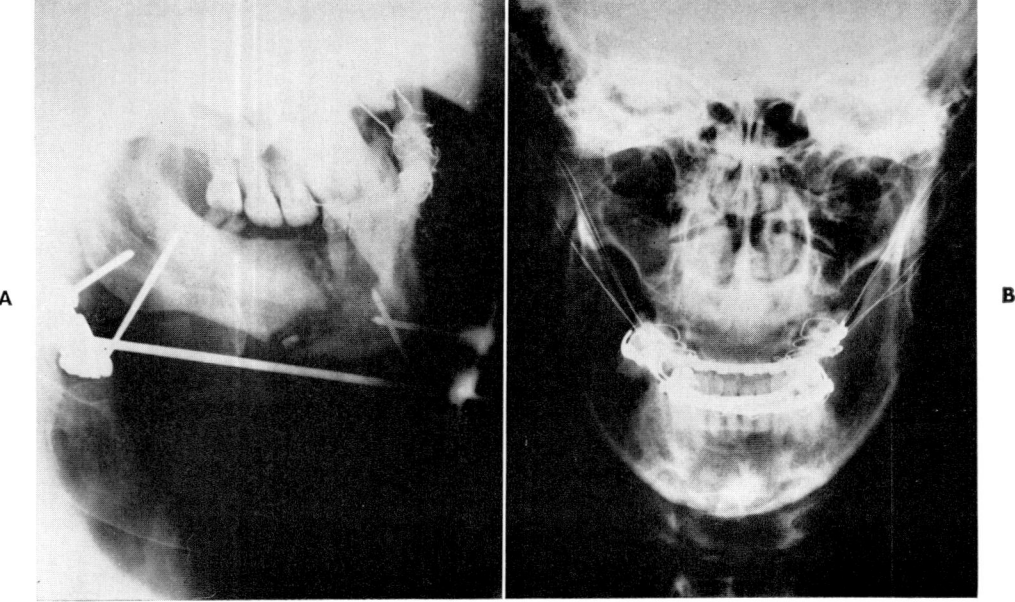

Fig. 19-11. **A,** Skeletal pin fixation. **B,** Circumzygomatic wire suspension of maxilla.

mandibular symphysis fractures and rather infrequently in mandibular angle fracture. (See Fig. 19-10.)

Skeletal pin fixation is used often (Fig. 19-11, *A*). In simplest form a screw pin, 8 cm. long with a diameter of 2 mm., is drilled into the lateral aspect of the jaw through the skin and subcutaneous tissues, through the outer bone cortex, the spongiosa, and just through the inner bone cortex. Another pin is drilled on the same side of the fracture. Two pins are drilled on the other side of the fracture. The pins are attached to each other by a connecting apparatus, and the two connecting units are united across the fracture by a stout metal rod. This is a closed procedure that is simple, but many failures are associated with it. If it is performed by an inexperienced person, the pin will not engage the inner cortex, and the entire assembly will become loose at an inopportune time.

Maxillary fractures must be maintained against the base of the skull. A plaster headcap with extensions has been used for years. Recently, internal wiring has been used more often. Wires are suspended over the intact zygomatic arches or holes are drilled into an unfractured bone superior to the fracture such as the infraorbital ridge or the bone just above the zygomaticofrontal suture line (Fig. 19-11, *B*). Wires are passed then beneath the skin and the maxilla is thereby suspended. Since this suspension is not visible the patient can go about his business during recovery. Less chance exists for movement of the fracture during healing than with the plaster headcap.

It is interesting to note changes in the thinking of the profession over the years regarding open reduction. In the years before World War II open operations on bones frequently resulted in osteomyelitis. Complicated jaw fractures were treated by all manner of gadgets. Bicycle spokes, fancy castings, and man-from-Mars outfits were used. In the years since the beginning of World War II the popular procedure has been the open reduction. The antibiotics, the introduction of metals tolerated by the tissues, and the more predictable results were largely responsible. The gadgets had been uncomfortable to the patient, sometimes inefficient in approximating the bony segments, and the surgeon never knew when one would slip at a crucial moment.

The trend is beginning to regress a bit at present. Largely responsible are the occasional infection of the open wound that is resistant to many antibiotics and the fact that the results are not always that much better despite the increased amount of surgery. A tremendous backlog of experience with open procedures can be compared now with conservative procedures. The fractured mandibular condyle is an example. A few years ago almost every fractured condyle was considered for open reduction. Now only a selected few are done. However, many indications exist for open procedures if no other method will give a comparable satisfactory result. Open reduction is still preferable to most of the modern gadgets.

HEALING OF BONE

Healing of bone can be divided into three overlapping phases. *Hemorrhage* occurs first, associated with clot organization and proliferation of blood vessels. This nonspecific phase occurs during the first 10 days. *Callus formation* occurs secondly. A rough "woven bone" or primary callus that looks like burlap is formed in the next 10 to 20 days. A secondary callus in which the Haversian systems form "in every which way"[2] forms in 20 to 60 days. *Functional reconstruction* of the bone is the third phase. Mechanical forces are important here. The Haversian systems are lined up according to stress lines. Excess bone is removed. The shape of the bone is molded to conform with functional usage so that bone may be added to one surface and removed on another side. It takes 2 to 3 years, for example, to completely reform a fracture of the human femur.

Weinmann and Sicher[3] divide the healing of fractures into six stages:

1. Clotting of blood of the hematoma. When a fracture occurs, the blood vessels of the bone marrow, the cortex, the periosteum, the surrounding muscles, and adjacent soft tissues rupture. The resultant hematoma completely surrounds the fractured ends and extends into the bone marrow as well as into the soft tissues. It coagulates in 6 to 8 hours after the accident.

2. Organization of blood of the hematoma. A meshwork of fibrin is formed in the organizing hematoma. The hematoma contains fragments of periosteum, muscle, fascia, bone, and bone marrow. Most of these fragments are digested and removed from the scene. Inflammatory cells, which are so necessary for the hemorrhagic phase of bone healing, are called forth by this diseased tissue rather than by bacterial organisms. Capillaries invade the clot in 24 to 48 hours. Fibroblasts invade the clot at about the same time.

The proliferation of blood vessels is a characteristic of the early organizing hematoma. A good blood supply is important. The capillary beds in the marrow, cortex, and periosteum become small arteries to supply the area of fracture. As they become more tortuous a slower flow results in a richer blood supply. At this stage proliferation of capillaries occurs throughout the hematoma. The hyperemia associated with the slow flow of blood through tortuous vessels is responsible for mesenchymal proliferation. Protein building blocks created by the richer blood supply form the basis for mesenchymal proliferation.

Resorption of bone is a characteristic of an older hematoma. The torrents of blood running through the area of active hyperemia, and not disuse atrophy, cause resorption of bone. When the blood gets into the actual site of fracture where the capillary bed lies (which Johnson likens to a "swamp"), the flow is slowed. This area of passive hyperemia is associated with proliferation of bone. Calcium ion level is increased in this swamp area by the capillary bed.

3. Formation of fibrous callus. The organized hematoma is replaced by granulation tissue ordinarily in 10 days. The granulation tissue removes necrotic tissue primarily by phagocytic activity. As soon as this function is completed the granulation tissue develops into a loose connective tissue. The end of the hyperemic phase is characterized by a decrease in the number of white cells and partial obliteration of the capillaries. The fibroblasts are now most important. They produce numerous collagenous fibers, which are termed fibrous callus.

4. Formation of primary bony callus. Primary callus forms between 10 and 30 days after fracture. Structurally it has been compared to a crudely woven burlap. The calcium content is so low that primary callus can be cut with a knife. It is for this reason that primary callus cannot be detected on the roentgenogram. It is an early stage that serves only as a mechanical prop for the formation of secondary callus.

Primary callus has been considered in different categories, depending upon location and function (Fig. 19-12).

Anchoring callus develops on the outside surface of the bone near the periosteum. It extends some distance away from the fracture. Young connective tissue cells of the fibrous callus differentiate into osteoblasts, which produce this spongy bone.

Sealing callus develops on the inside surface of the bone across the fractured end. It fills the marrow spaces and goes out into the fracture site. It forms from endosteal proliferation.

Bridging callus develops on the outside surface between the anchoring callus on the two fractured ends. This callus is the only one that is primarily cartilaginous. Some question remains on this point in the heal-

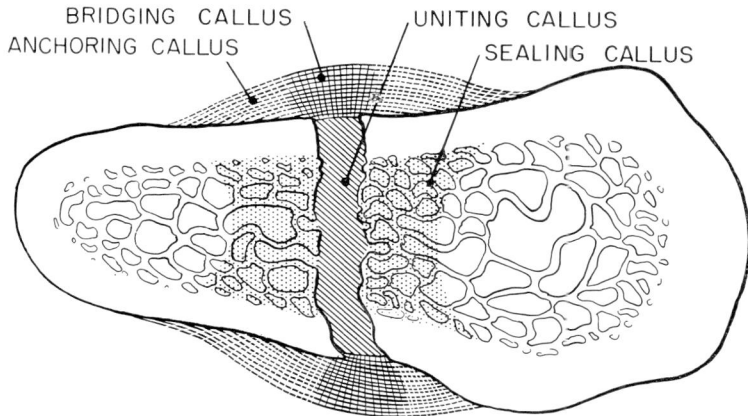

Fig. 19-12. Types of primary callus forming in a healing fracture.

ing of the mandible since it is one of the bones formed originally in membrane rather than by replacement of cartilage. The question has been raised whether true bridging callus forms in mandibular fractures. However, cartilage cells have been identified in such areas of healing in the mandible.

Uniting callus forms between the ends of bones and between areas of other primary calluses that have formed on the two fractured parts. It does not form until the other types of callus are well developed. It forms by direct ossification. Extensive resorption of the bone ends has occurred by this time. Therefore, rather than mere ossification of the interposed connective tissue at the fracture site, the uniting callus forms in the area of resorption as well. A well-united fracture is the result.

5. Formation of secondary bony callus. Secondary bony callus is mature bone that replaces the immature bone of the primary callus. It is more heavily calcified, and therefore it can be seen on the roentgenogram. It differs from other skeletal bone, however, by the fact that the pseudo-Haversian systems are not formed in any uniform pattern. It is composed of laminated bone that can withstand active use. Therefore fixation can be removed when secondary callus is seen on the roentgenogram. Formation of secondary callus is a slow process, requiring from 20 to 60 days.

6. Functional reconstruction of the fractured bone. Reconstruction proceeds over months or years to the point where the location of the fracture usually cannot be detected histologically or anatomically. Mechanics is the major factor in this stage. As a matter of fact, if a bone is not subjected to functional stress, true mature bone will not form. True Haversian systems that are oriented by stress factors replace the nonoriented pseudo-Haversian systems of secondary callus. The secondary callus that is formed in abundance is sculptured to conform with the size of the remainder of the bone. The entire bone is molded by mechanical factors if the healing has not taken place in exact alignment. Steps are reduced on the one side and deficiencies are filled in on the other side. This process seems to take place in alternative waves of osteoclastic activity and osteoblastic activity.

FRACTURES OF THE MANDIBLE
Causes

Two principal components are involved in fractures: the dynamic factor (blow) and the stationary factor (jaw). The common causes for setting in motion the dynamic factors have been discussed at the beginning of the chapter. Physical violence and automobile accidents lead the list in a municipal hospital administering to a preponderance of indigent patients. However, in studies conducted in private hospitals, industrial accidents rate as a close second to automobile accidents. In these hospitals the incidence of physical violence is extremely low, usually about 10%.

The dynamic factor is characterized by the intensity of the blow and its direction. A light blow may cause a greenstick or simple unilateral fracture, whereas a heavy blow with "follow through" may cause a compounded, comminuted fracture with traumatic displacement of the parts. The direction of the blow largely determines the location of the fracture or fractures. A blow to the right of the chin may result in a fracture of the mental foramen region on that side and a fracture of the angle of the mandible on the other side. Force applied to the point of the chin might result in symphysis and bilateral condyle fractures. Severe force may push the condylar fragments out of the glenoid fossa.

The stationary component has to do with the jaw itself. Physiological age is important. A child, with his growing bones, can fall out of a window to experience a greenstick fracture or no fracture at all, whereas an elderly person, whose heavily calcified skull can be compared to a flower pot, can trip over a rug and suffer a complicated fracture.

Mental and physical relaxation prevents fractures associated with muscular tension. A bone that has severe tensions placed upon it by all-out contractions of its attached muscles requires only a slight blow to fracture it. Intoxicated persons have fallen from rapidly moving vehicles only to suffer bruises. The muscle masses serve as tissue cushions when relaxed, but the same muscles under tension form strain patterns in the bones.

Vulnerability of the jaw itself varies from one individual to another and from time to time in the same individual. A deeply impacted tooth will make the angle of the jaw vulnerable, as will physiological and pathological conditions such as osteoporosis or a large cyst. Heavier deposition of calcium in the trained athlete will reduce jaw fractures. Jaw fractures in boxers are almost nonexistent because of increased calcification, the use of padded boxing gloves and rubber mouthguards, and a training factor.

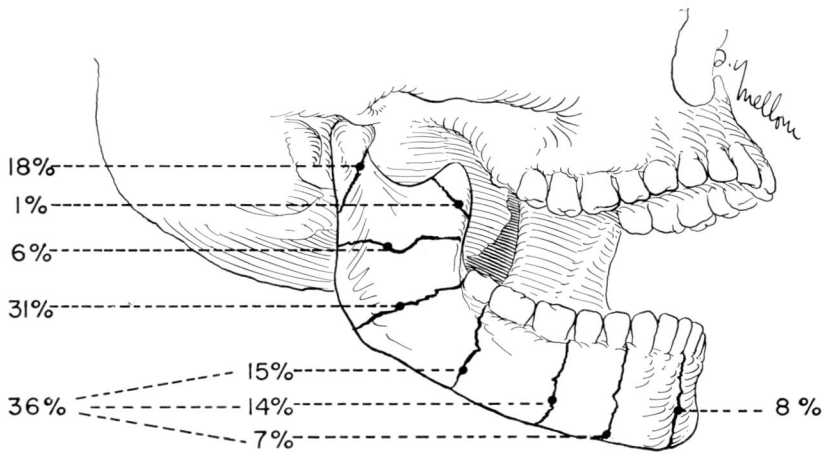

Fig. 19-13. Sites of mandibular fractures.

Location[4]

In the series quoted previously (p. 296) the following incidence of fracture, by sites, occurred in the mandible (Fig. 19-13).

Angle	31%	Symphysis	8%
Condyle	18%	Cuspid	7%
Molar region	15%	Ramus	6%
Mental region	14%	Coronoid process	1%

The most common bilateral fracture was in the angle-mental regions.

Displacement

The displacement of a fracture of the mandible is a result of the following factors.

Muscle pull. The intricate musculature attached to the mandible for functional movement distracts the fragments when the continuity of the bone is lost (Figs. 19-14 to 19-18). The action of balances between

Text continued on p. 316.

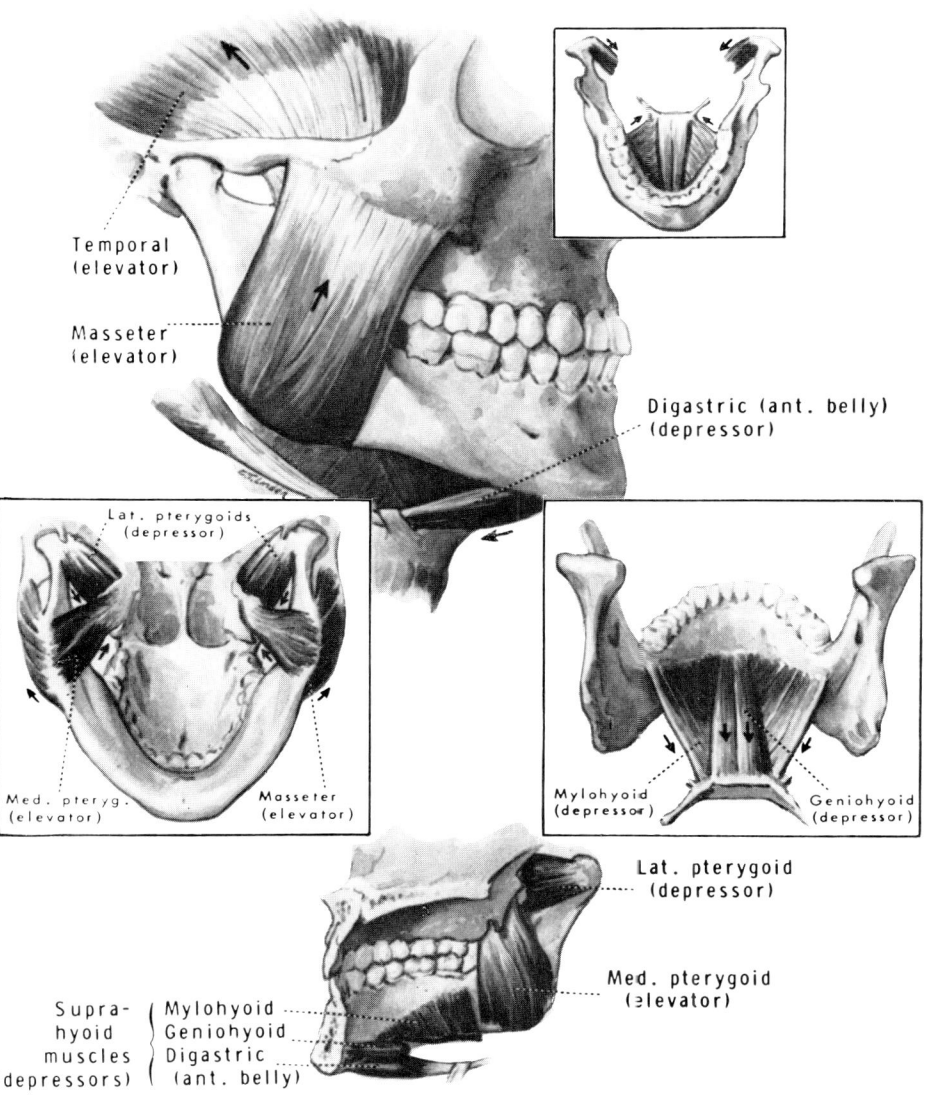

Fig. 19-14. Muscles of the mandible. (From Massler, M., and Schour, I.: Atlas of the mouth; courtesy American Dental Association.)

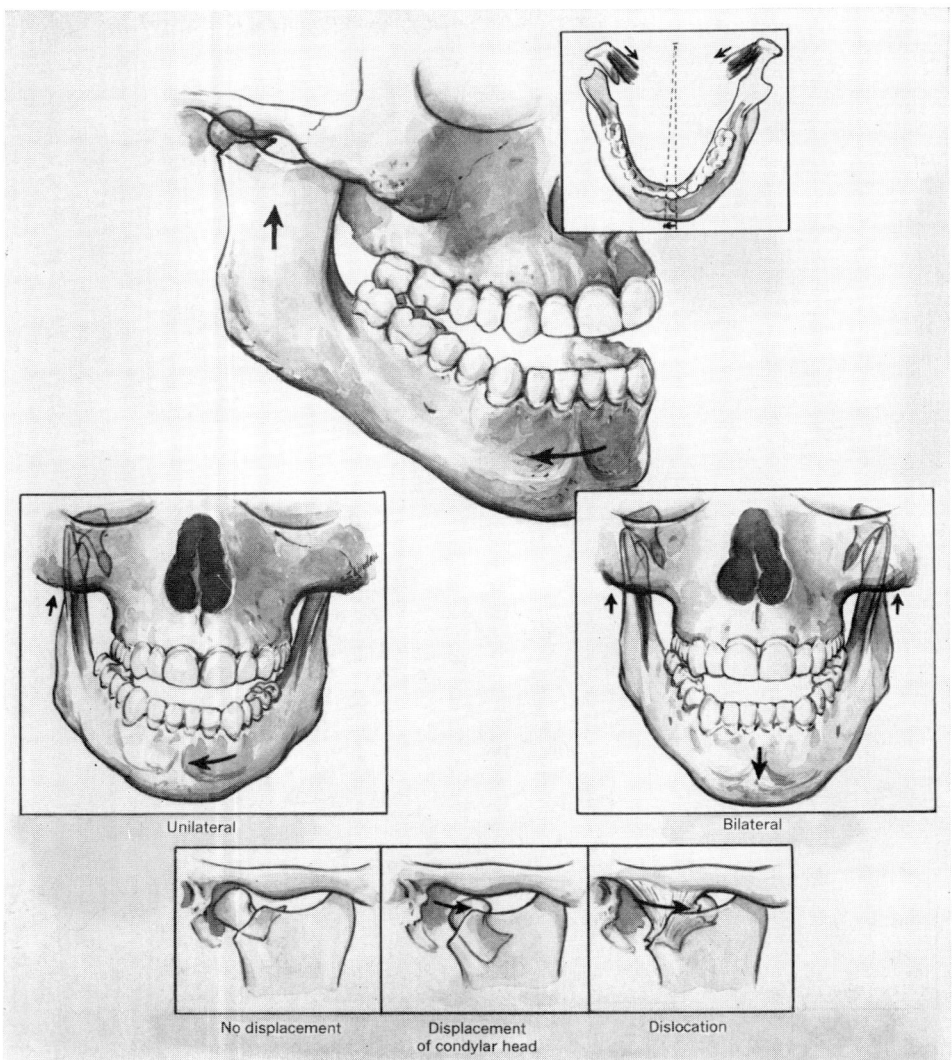

Fig. 19-15. Fractures of the neck of the condyle. (From Massler, M., and Schour, I.: Atlas of the mouth; courtesy American Dental Association.)

Fractures of the jaws **313**

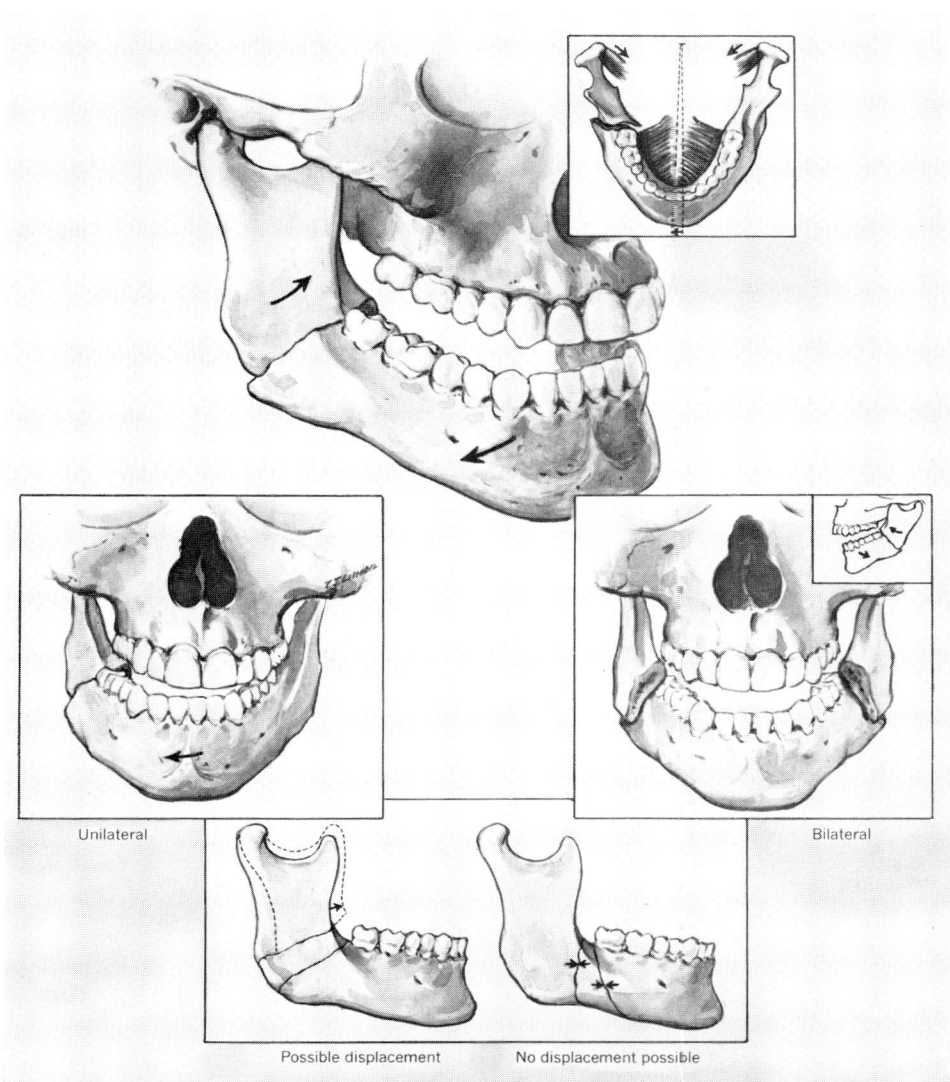

Fig. 19-16. Fractures of the angle of the mandible. (From Massler, M., and Schour, I.: Atlas of the mouth; courtesy American Dental Association.)

314 Textbook of oral surgery

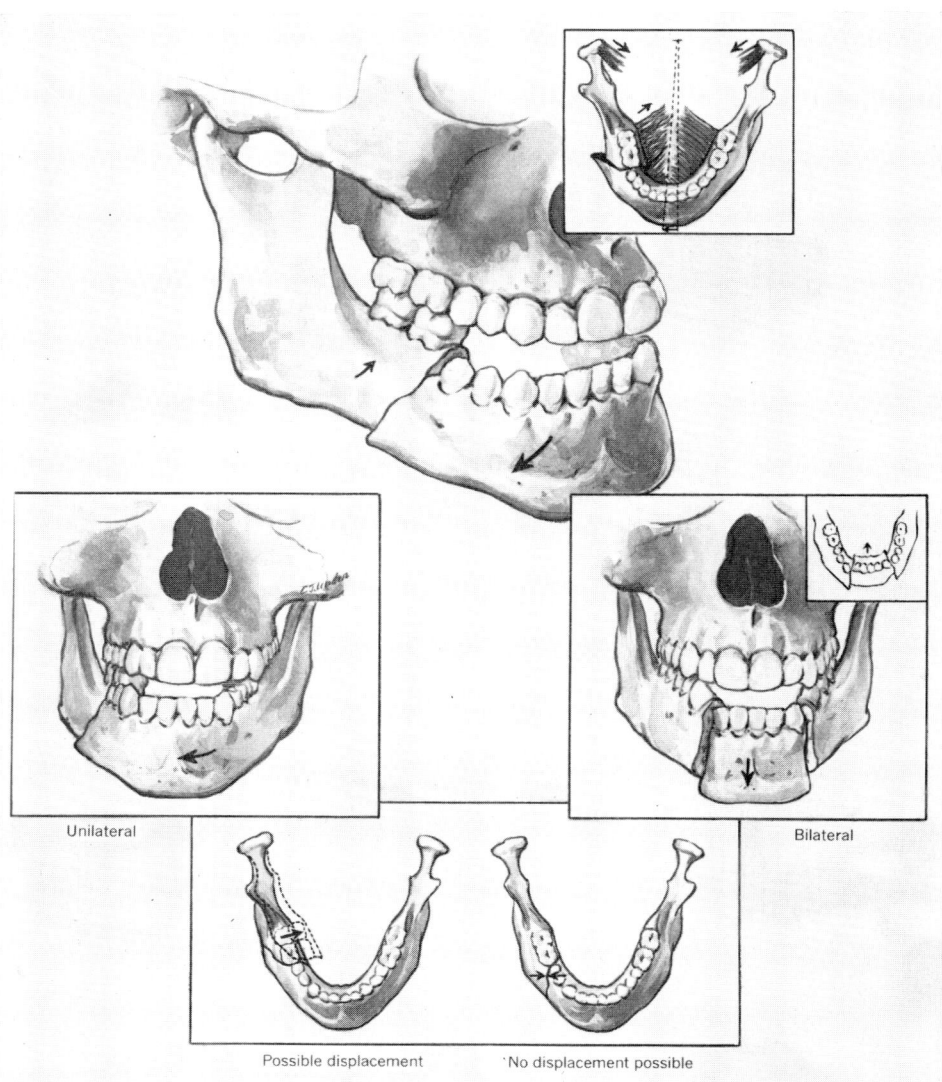

Fig. 19-17. Fractures of the body of the mandible. (From Massler, M., and Schour, I.: Atlas of the mouth; courtesy American Dental Association.)

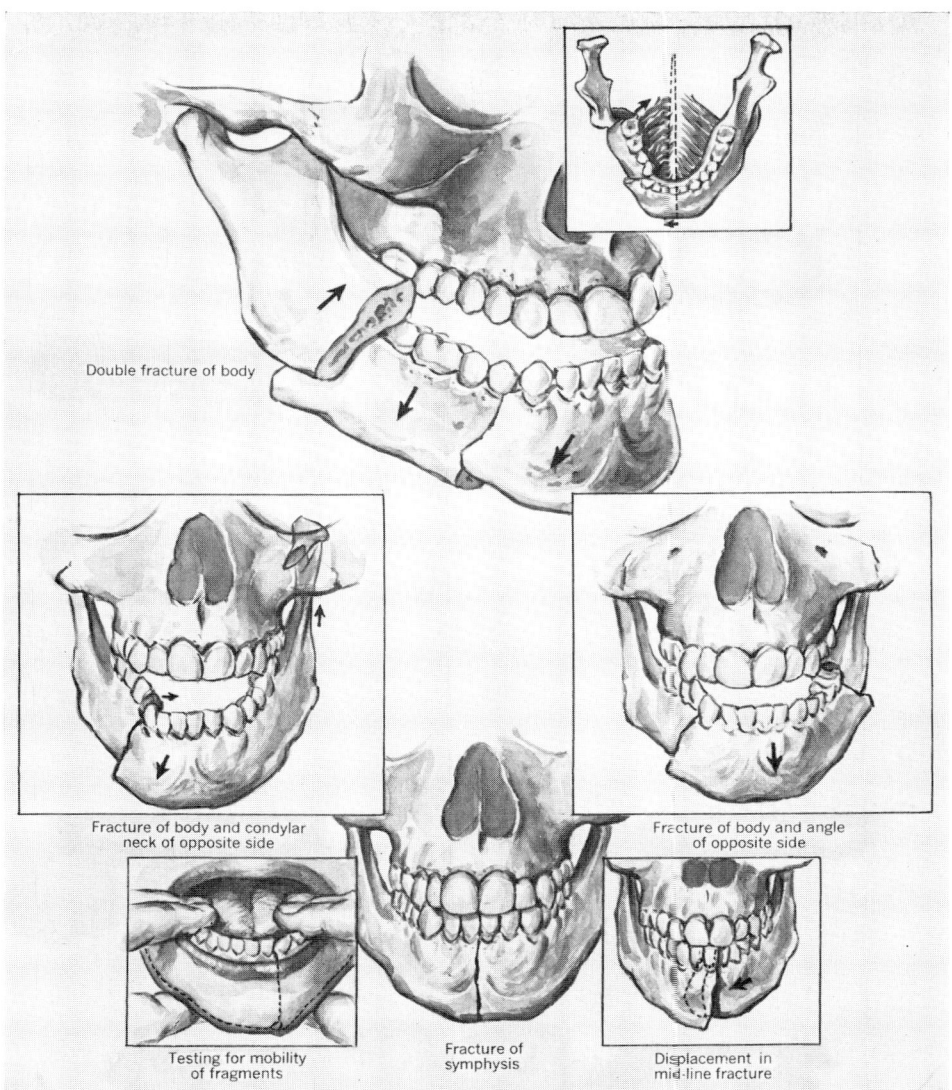

Fig. 19-18. Multiple fractures of the mandible. (From Massler, M., and Schour, I.: Atlas of the mouth; courtesy American Dental Association.)

sets of muscles is lost, and each muscle group exerts its own force unopposed by another muscle group. The "sling of the mandible," namely, the masseter and medial pterygoid muscles, displaces the posterior jaw fragment upward, aided by the temporalis muscle. The opposing force, namely, the suprahyoid muscles, displaces the anterior fragment downward. These forces would balance themselves if attached to an intact bone.

The posterior fragment usually is displaced medially, not because of lack of muscular balance as much as because the functional direction of pull is medial. The medial pterygoid muscle is largely responsible. The superior constrictor of the pharynx exerts medial pull from its multicentric origin on the mylohyoid ridge, pterygomandibular raphe, and hamular process to its insertion on the occipital bone. The lateral pterygoid muscle attached to the condyle will help, and in the case of the condylar fracture it will tend to displace the condyle medially.

Fragments situated in the anterior portion of the jaw can be displaced medially by the mylohyoid muscle. Symphysis fractures are difficult to fixate because of the bilateral posterior and slight lateral pull exerted by the suprahyoid and digastric muscles.

Direction of line of fracture. Fry and associates[5] classified fractures of the mandible as "favorable" and "unfavorable," depending upon whether or not the line of fracture was in such direction as to allow muscular distraction. In the mandibular angle fracture the posterior fragment will be pulled upward if the fracture extends forward toward the alveolar ridge from a posterior point on the inferior border. This is termed an unfavorable fracture (Fig. 19-19, *A*). However, if the inferior border fracture occurs further anteriorly and the line of fracture extends in a distal direction toward the ridge, a favorable fracture is present (Fig. 19-19, *B*). The long angle of the anteroinferior portion will lock the posterior fragment mechanically to withstand upward muscular pull.

These distractions are in a horizontal plane, and so the terms horizontal unfavorable and horizontal favorable are used. Most angle fractures are horizontal unfavorable.

Medial displacement can be considered in similar fashion. Oblique fracture lines

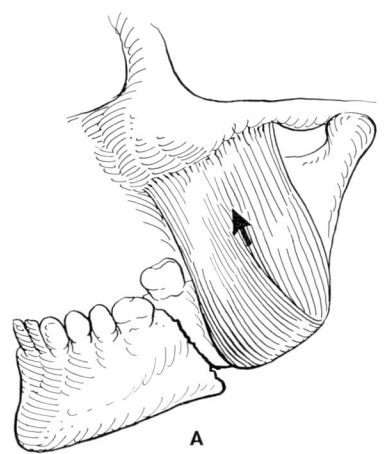 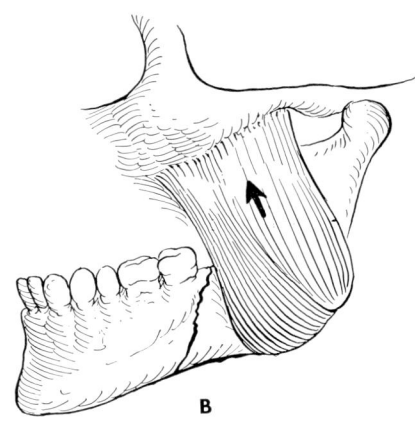

Fig. 19-19. **A,** Horizontal unfavorable fracture. **B,** Horizontal favorable fracture.

can form a large buccal cortical fragment, which will prevent medial displacement. If the mandible could be viewed directly downward from the upper jaw so that the occlusal surfaces of the teeth are seen in button fashion, a vertical unfavorable fracture line extends from a posterolateral point to an anteromedial point (Fig. 19-20, *A*). No obstruction to medial muscular pull is present. A vertical favorable fracture extends from an anterolateral to a posteromedial point (Fig. 19-20, *B*). Medial muscular displacement is prevented by the large buccal cortical fragment.

Force. Factors such as the direction of the blow, the amount of force, the number and location of fractures, and the loss of substance as in gunshot wounds are not as important in displacing mandibular fractures as they are in maxillary fractures except insofar as they form the basis for later muscular distraction. Force in itself can displace fractures by forcing the bone ends away, impacting the bone ends, or pushing the condyles out of their sockets, but secondary displacement by muscular pull is stronger and more significant in mandibular fractures.

Force that compounds a fracture or comminutes it serves to complicate the treatment. Events that follow the initial fracture can also complicate it. An initially undisplaced fracture may be displaced by trauma, such as rolling, in the same accident. Placing the patient face down on a stretcher or injudicious and unskilled examination may displace bone segments. Lack of temporary support of the jaw, particularly in the case of a fractured skull, often leads to functional and muscular displacement, which is painful and difficult to treat later.

Signs and symptoms[6]

1. *History of injury* is invariably present, a possible exception being a pathological fracture.
2. *Occlusion* indirectly offers the best index of recently acquired bony deformity.
3. *Abnormal mobility* with bimanual palpation of the mandible is a reliable sign of fracture. By this procedure separation between mandibular fragments is differentiated from mobility of teeth.
4. *Pain* with movements of the mandible or upon palpation of the face often is a significant symptom. When condylar movements are restricted and painful, a condylar fracture should be suspected.
5. *Crepitus* with manipulation or mandibular function is pathognomonic of a fracture. However, this is elicited with considerable pain to the patient in many cases.
6. *Disability* is manifested by the pa-

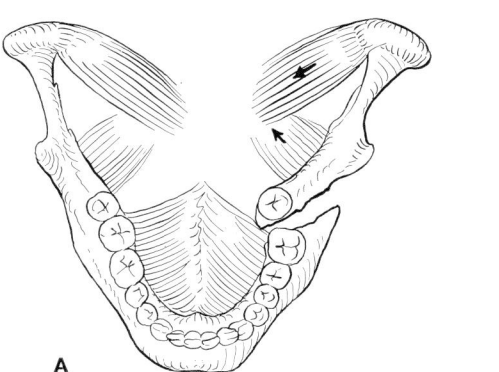 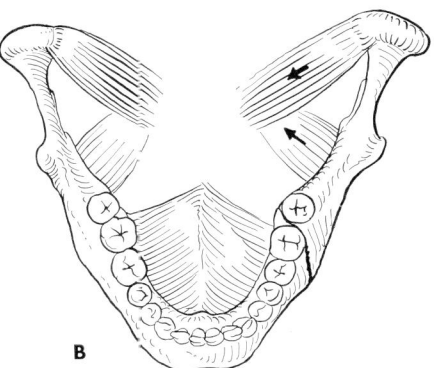

Fig. 19-20. **A,** Vertical unfavorable fracture. **B,** Vertical favorable fracture.

tient's inability to masticate because of pain or abnormal motility.

7. *Trismus* is seen frequently, especially in fractures through the angle or in the ramus region. This is a reflex spasm mediated through the sensory pathways of the disrupted bone segments.

8. *Laceration* of the gingiva may be seen in the region of the fracture.

9. *Anesthesia* may be noted, especially in the gingiva and lip up to the midline, when the inferior alveolar nerve is injured.

10. *Ecchymosis* of the gingiva or mucosa on the lingual or buccal surfaces may be suggestive of a fracture site.

11. *Salivation and fetor of breath.*

Treatment methods

Treatment of the fracture consists of reduction and fixation. In the case of long bones this is often done in two stages, particularly if much manipulation is necessary for reduction. In simple mandibular fractures reduction and fixation are accomplished together. The apparatus that is used to keep the jaws together during healing will often reduce the fracture as well. If multiple-loop wiring is placed, no attempt is made to reduce the fracture until the wiring on each jaw is complete. When the jaws are brought together and intermaxillary elastic traction is placed, the occlusion of the teeth will help to orient the fractured parts into good position. Exceptions occur, of course. Fractures that occur beyond the tooth-bearing portion of the mandible, such as the angle, will not be reduced if initially displaced. Other examples are edentulous jaws and old fractures that are partially healed, which require continuous elastic traction for reduction.

Intermaxillary fixation, that is, fixation obtained by applying wires or elastic bands between the upper and lower jaws to which suitable anchoring devices have been attached, will successfully treat most fractures of the mandible. The main methods for such fixation are wiring, arch bars, and splints.

Wiring

Multiple-loop wiring. The Armed Services and many civilian institutions use this method almost exclusively. The four posterior quadrants are wired.

Preparation. Local anesthesia with sedation, or sedation alone, is used. General anesthesia is used occasionally when further treatment is necessary after the wiring. Even then it is better to have the interdental wiring completed the day or night before the operation so that the time of the operating room personnel and prolonged general anesthesia are not needlessly required. The wiring is done in a dental chair if possible.

A local anesthetic can be given by two pterygomandibular blocks in the mandible and simple infiltration in the maxilla. Bilateral block anesthesia combined with sedation in a patient who later will be put on his back in bed can be dangerous because of lingual anesthesia. The patient should sit in a chair until the anesthesia has disappeared.

If the contact points of the teeth are not too tight and broad, and if the interdental gingival tissue is not too close to the contact points, no anesthesia is necessary. Sedation alone is adequate if care is taken that the fracture zone is not traumatized by undue movement. Premedication with either Demerol hydrochloride (50 to 100 mg.) or pentobarbital sodium (100 to 200 mg.) parenterally is adequate generally. For severe pain or to render the patient almost completely insensible to manipulative pain for 20 minutes, 75 to 100 mg. of Demerol hydrochloride can be given intravenously to an average adult. This must be administered slowly over a 2-minute interval.

Armamentarium. The materials used for multiple-loop wiring are as follows:

Wire, 26-gauge stainless steel, cut into lengths of 20 cm. and placed in a cold-sterilizing

solution 20 minutes before use; wire cut on a bevel so that the bevel can act like a needle point if it must go through tissue
Solder, soft No. 20 resin core
Hegar needle holders (two)
Wire cutters
Blunt-nosed crown and bridge pliers
Discoid dental instrument

Technique. One end of the wire is placed on the buccal side of the teeth, starting at the midline (stationary wire). The other end goes around the last tooth in the arch (for example, the second molar) and into the mesial interproximal space and emerges under the stationary wire. Then it is bent back above the stationary wire into the same interproximal space. It is delivered to the lingual side and bent around the next tooth (first molar) and into the interproximal space between the molar and the premolar. The wire that goes around each tooth and over and under the stationary wire is called the working wire (Fig. 19-21, A).

To make uniform loops on the buccal side, a piece of solder is placed on the buccal surfaces of the teeth over the stationary wire. It can be pressed against the teeth with the finger. The working wire therefore emerges under the stationary wire as well as under the solder, and then it is turned back and passed over the wire and solder to reenter the same interproximal space.

Each time the wire emerges on the buccal side it should be grasped with the needle holder and pulled firmly to reduce slack. The left hand should provide counterpressure on the buccal surfaces of the teeth. The discoid instrument is used to move the wire under the height of contour of the teeth on the lingual side.

When the arch segment has been wired, the working wire and the stationary wire are crossed at the mesial side of the canine or first premolar. They are crossed 1 cm. away from the tooth; the needle holder is placed over the cross and twisted clockwise until the wire almost touches the tooth. With the discoid instrument the wire is pushed beneath the cingulum of the cuspid. The wire is then grasped with the needle holder at the turn nearest the tooth and turned until the tooth surface is contacted. Backward pressure always is placed on the needle holder when wires are tightened.

The solder is cut midway between the last two buccal loops, bent outward, and twisted gently out of the last loop. The

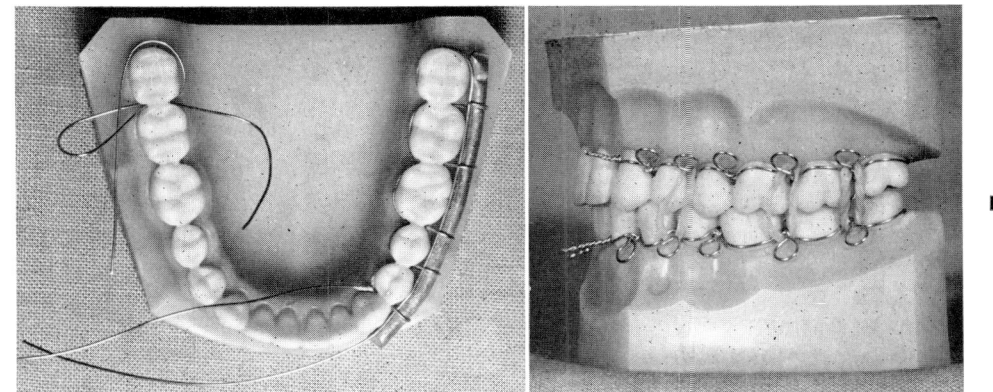

Fig. 19-21. A, Multiple-loop wiring. Note the buccal stationary wire and the lingual working wire that is threaded back and forth through interproximal spaces. B, Completed multiple-loop wiring.

wire loop then is given a three-quarter turn in a clockwise direction with the needle holder or pliers. Another cut is made in the solder between the next two loops and the small distal piece is withdrawn. The loop is tightened with a three-quarter turn. This is continued until all of the solder has been removed. Then, starting in the back, each loop is given another half turn. The multiple-loop wiring should be firm by this time (Fig. 19-21, B).

The same procedure is followed in the other three quadrants of the mouth. If elastic traction will be used, the loops should be bent away from the occlusal plane so that hooks are formed. If wire will be used between the jaws, the loops are bent toward the occlusal plane.

It is desirable to use elastic traction routinely. This overcomes muscular distraction so that reduction is accomplished more easily, and it serves as a positive force to overcome muscular spasm when the jaw first tires of its forced closed position. If the mouth should have to be entered in the immediate postoperative period for relief of vomiting or the placement of an endotracheal tube for subsequent operation, the removal of the elastic bands is a simple matter. As an emergency procedure, particularly if the patient will be transported later, a wire can be placed on the buccal side under the elastics, bent back on itself over the elastics, and the two ends tied to clothing over the chest. If actual vomiting (not retching) occurs, the patient can jerk the wire and remove the elastic fixation immediately. This procedure is used rarely in civilian hospitals.

Elastic traction is obtained by stretching small or large Angle orthodontic elastics from an upper to a lower wire loop. A 14- or 16-gauge rubber catheter can be cut into bands that provide stronger traction. If the fracture does not position itself properly, elastics can be placed in different directions rather than straight up and down. If the chin fragment is too far forward, several strong elastics can be placed from the lower cuspid region to the upper second bicuspid region. Often the angled elastics can be replaced by straight elastics in one day, thereby eliminating a possibility of overreduction.

Ivy loop wiring. The Ivy loop embraces only two adjacent teeth, and it provides two hooks for elastics. An individual Ivy loop is applied more quickly than multiple-loop wiring, although several Ivy loops are necessary in a dentulous arch. If many teeth are missing, adjacent teeth can be used satisfactorily by this method. If a wire should break, it is simpler to replace a single Ivy loop than it is a multiple-loop wire.

The armamentarium is the same. The wire is 26 gauge cut in 15 cm. lengths. A loop is formed in the center of the wire around the beak of a towel clip and twisted once. These wires can be stored in an accident room in cold-sterilizing solution.

The two tails of the wire are placed in the embrasure from the buccal to the lingual side (Fig. 19-22, A). If difficulty occurs, a piece of dental floss can be doubled through the loop. The floss then is carried past the contact point and the wire pulled through the embrasure from the lingual to the buccal side. The floss is removed. One wire tail is carried around the lingual surface of the distal tooth, pushed through the embrasure on the distal side of that tooth, and bent around the buccal surface. It is threaded through the previously formed loop or just under the loop. The other wire tail is carried around the lingual surface of the mesial tooth, passed through the embrasure on the mesial side of that tooth, and meets the first wire. The two wires are crossed and twisted together with the needle holder. The loop is then tightened and bent toward the gingiva. The crossed wires are cut, and a small rosette is made to serve as an additional hook. The rosette is wound clockwise below the greatest circumference of the tooth for two turns and then flattened toward the

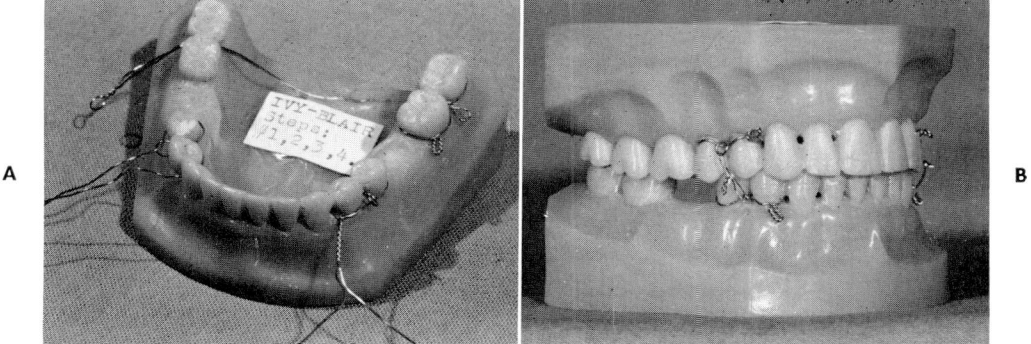

Fig. 19-22. **A,** Ivy loop wiring. **B,** Completed Ivy loop wiring. Intermaxillary fixation can be obtained by the use of wire or elastics simply by bending the loops down or up.

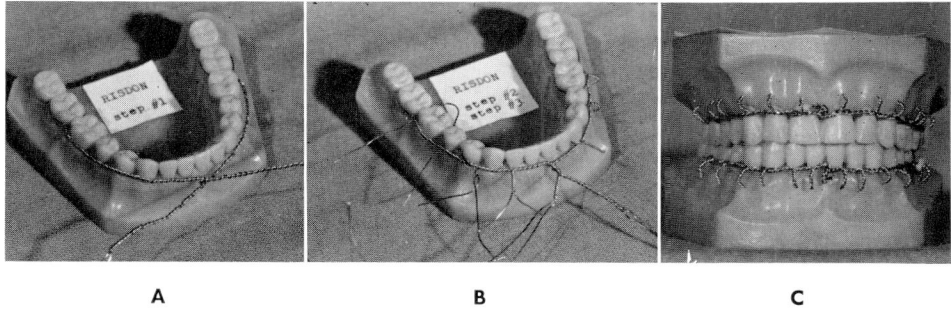

Fig. 19-23. Risdon wiring. **A,** Formation of wire arch bar. **B,** Ligation of separate teeth to wire arch bar. **C,** Completed wiring ready for elastic bands.

tooth (Fig. 19-22, *B*). One or two of these Ivy loops are placed in each quadrant. Elastic traction then is placed between the jaws.

Risdon wiring. A wire arch bar tied in the midline is especially indicated for symphysis fractures. A 26-gauge stainless steel wire 25 cm. long is passed around the most distal strong tooth so that both arms of the wire extend to the buccal side. The two wires, which are of equal length, then are twisted on each other for their entire length. The same procedure is followed for the other side of the arch. The two twisted strands are crossed in the midline and twisted around each other (Fig. 19-23, *A*).

A rosette is formed. Each tooth in the arch then is ligated individually to the wire arch (Fig. 19-23, *B*). One wire is passed over the arch wire and the other is passed under the arch wire. After tightening, a small hook is formed with each twisted strand (Fig. 19-23, *C*). Intermaxillary traction is obtained by stretching elastic bands between the hooks in each arch.

Arch bars

Arch bars are perhaps the ideal method for intermaxillary fixation. Several types of ready-made arch bars are used. The rigid type requires either an impression and a stone cast to which the bar can be adapted

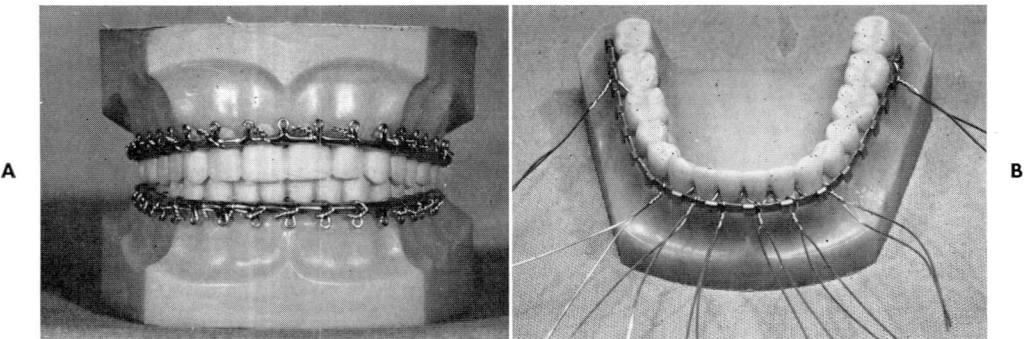

Fig. 19-24. **A**, Rigid arch bars. **B**, Soft type arch bar. Note that the incisor and canine teeth are wired before the bar is placed, and the bar is then wired to the anterior teeth fixation. The posterior teeth are ligated directly to the bar.

carefully by a two-plier technique or a person skilled in the bending of prosthetic bars who has sufficient time to adapt it in the mouth (Fig. 19-24, *A*). A soft type is available that can be bent with the fingers. It must be remembered that teeth lashed to any type of bar can be moved orthodontically if the bar has not been fitted skillfully.

The soft bar can be fitted using two large needle holders, although wire-bending pliers are better (Fig. 19-24, *B*). In an unfractured maxilla the bending should be started at the buccal side of the last tooth. The bar is adapted accurately to each tooth. The pliers or needle holder should be kept close together so that previously adapted portions are not bent again. By starting at one end of the bar, progressing past the midline, and finishing at the other end, the bar can be adapted readily and quickly without producing bulges. The bar should be shortened properly and the end filed smooth with a gold file. An overextended bar will cause soft tissue necrosis and severe pain. The midline of the jaw should be marked on the bar during bending so that it will be reseated accurately. As a general rule the bar should not cross a fracture line except in a greenstick fracture. The bar is cut and adapted to each segment of a fractured jaw.

Wiring the bar to the teeth is relatively simple. Thin 30-gauge wire is used. Before seating the bar, wires are placed on the anterior teeth to seat tightly under the cingulum to resist displacement of the bar to the incisal level. A small loop of wire is placed by "jumping" the contact point or by threading through the two embrasures. The wires are crossed and grasped with a needle holder close to the labial enamel surface. Three fourths of a turn is given to the wire after the wire has been pushed below the cingulum. This is done to each anterior tooth.

The bar then is placed between the open ends of the wires. The midline mark is adjusted, and care is taken that the hooks on the arch bar project upward in the maxilla and downward in the mandible. The individual anterior wire ends are crossed over the bar, grasped, and twisted. The posterior teeth are then ligated individually to the bar. One end of a 7 cm. length of wire is passed from the buccal side under the bar through one embrasure, circled around the lingual side of the tooth, and then pushed back from the lingual side through the next embrasure to pass over the bar.

The crossed wires are grasped 2 mm. away from the bar, and backward pressure is placed on the needle holder before a turn is made. This pressure is maintained during any tightening operation. When the turns approach the bar, the wire is again grasped with the needle holder further away from the bar and turns are made until the previous turns are reached. The turned strand is cut 7 mm. away from the bar while the holder still has the wire in its beaks so that the cut strand will not be lost in the mouth. The strand is grasped close to the bar and given a final turn. The end is turned under the bar so that the lips and cheeks will not be traumatized.

All teeth should be ligated to the bar. This rule has few exceptions.

Perhaps the main failings of the bar technique are improper adaptation of the bar, ligation of an insufficient number of the teeth, and inefficient tightening of the wires. Advantages associated with arch bars include less trauma, because of the thin wire, and greater stability in an arch that has many missing teeth, because the edentulous gaps can be spanned by a rigid appliance. If one wire should break during healing, the fixation will not suffer. The hooks on the bar also seem to be less irritating to the soft tissues.

Splints

Splints are used when wiring of the teeth will not provide adequate fixation or when horizontal splinting across a fracture zone is necessary, as well as in some cases in which immobilization of the fractured parts is indicated without closing the mouth by intermaxillary fixation. At one time splints with distal metal extensions were used to control the posterior fragment in angle fractures, but pain and unsatisfactory results have made it necessary to generally discontinue this procedure.

The acrylic splint is made from an impression so that it covers a minimum of the occlusal surfaces of the teeth and as much of the labial and lingual surfaces of the teeth as do not form an undercut. The gingival margins are not encroached. The lingual surface is continuous. The buccal surface is attached to the lingual portion behind the last molar either by continuous acrylic material or by a wire connector. A vertical cut is made in the midline of the labial flange through a large acrylic button. The splint is placed over the reduced fractured mandible, and the acrylic button is drawn together and held by wire. (See Fig. 19-25, A.)

The cast cap silver splint requires impressions of the opposing arches. The lower cast is sawed through the line of fracture. The cast is reassembled in proper occlusion and fixed in this position by pouring a base for the cast. The splint is formed to the gingival margins in 28-gauge sheet wax. Occlusal relations are established in the wax-up by bringing it into proper centric relation with the opposing casts while the

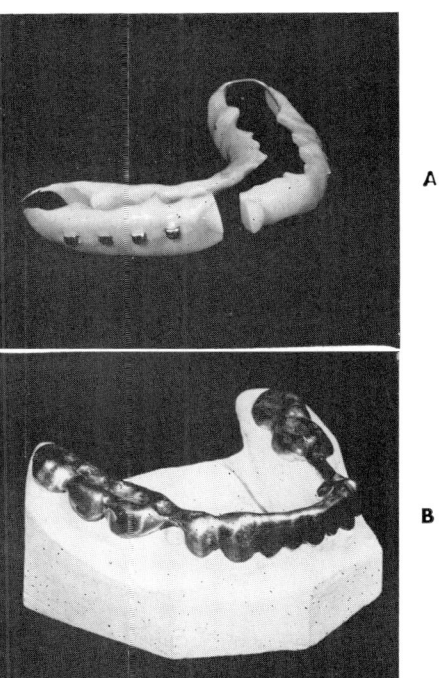

Fig. 19-25. A, Acrylic splint. B, Cast cap silver splint.

wax is soft. The cast is sprued with inlay wax. When the sprues are in place the wax-up is drawn from the stone cast in an occlusal direction while the wax is warm, to eliminate undercuts. The wax-up is mounted in a large crucible former in a single investment technique, with an asbestos liner in the ring. It is cast in coin silver at 1000° to 1500° F. and finished (Fig. 19-25, B).

The splint is cemented to the reduced fractured jaw. If the splint will be needed for weeks rather than months it is sometimes better to use zinc oxide and eugenol for cementation rather than crown and bridge cement, since the splints are often difficult to remove. The splints can be made of gold, and projections or hooks for intermaxillary fixation can be formed on them. Some gold splints are made in sections for specific purposes.

The splint is generally indicated for the very simple or the very complex case. If an oral surgeon suffered a simple mandibular fracture within the area of dentition he probably would prefer a cast cap silver splint so that his jaws would not be wired shut. In bone graft cases or in delayed union cases the splints are indicated since they provide long-term fixation in the presence of function.

Except for these general indications the use of splints is not great. The acrylic splint has fallen largely into disuse except for children with deciduous teeth, which are difficult to wire sometimes. The average fracture with good teeth is well on the way to good healing if wired immediately. The splinted patient requires impressions, temporary immobilization, delay of various degrees during construction of the appliance, and then later reduction and cementation. If a tooth should become acutely infected under a splint, a real problem is presented.

Orthodontic fixation is used oftener for elective surgery and long-term procedures rather than for traumatic surgery. It is especially indicated for alveolar fractures.

Circumferential wiring

Circumferential wiring ("wiring around") usually refers to the procedure of placing

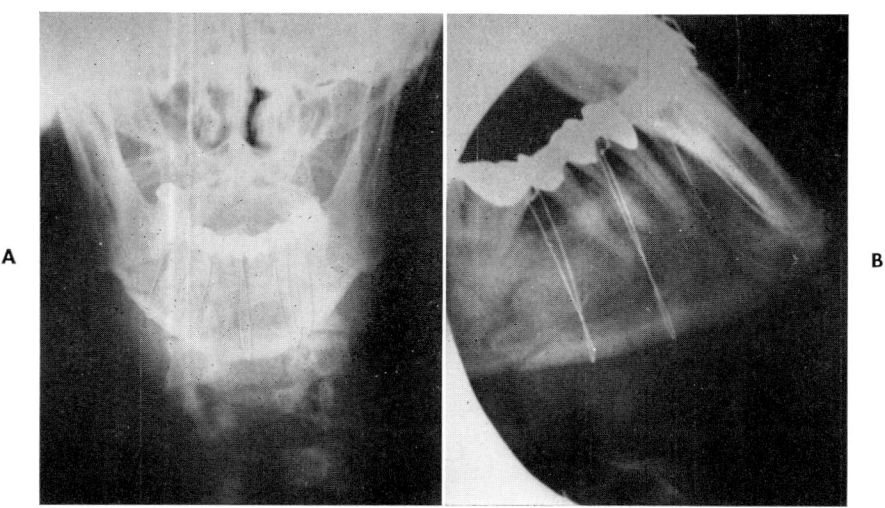

Fig. 19-26. **A,** Circumferential wiring around cast cap silver splint. The splint was cemented to the teeth. Circumferential wiring pulled the inferior border fragment upward. **B,** Lateral view.

wires around a mandibular denture and around the mandible so that the fractured mandible is held firmly into the denture, which serves as a splint. The fracture must be situated within the area covered by the denture base unless secondary procedures for the control of the other segment are contemplated. If the denture is fractured at the time of the accident, it can be repaired satisfactorily, sometimes with quick-cure acrylic (Fig. 19-26).

The mouth is rinsed with an antiseptic solution such as Metaphen 1:10,000 or Zephiran 1:10,000 to reduce the bacterial count. The skin is prepared in the usual manner. General or local anesthesia is satisfactory, although skin infiltration is necessary to supplement a local block procedure.

The simplest procedure consists of threading a long, straight skin needle with thin 28-gauge steel wire, which has been sterilized previously. The needle is bent into a slightly concave form with the fingers. It is passed through the floor of the mouth close to the mandible to emerge through the skin directly beneath the mandible. The needle is brought out of the skin, turned, and redirected into the same skin puncture hole. It is passed upward on the buccal side of the mandible close to the bone to emerge in the mucobuccal fold. The wires are cut near the needle. The two lingual and the two buccal wires are twisted over the denture, cut short, and formed into a rosette on the buccal side. At least three circumferential wires are placed, one near the distal end of the denture on each side and one at the midline. Occasionally two wires are placed in the anterior region. One side of the denture may have a wire placed anterior and another posterior to the fracture line. (See Fig. 19-27.)

The wires are sawed back and forth several times before tightening, to move them through the tissues to the inferior border of the mandible. Care is taken that a dimple does not persist at the skin wound. The skin around the wound should be released from the subdermal structures after the wires are tightened around the denture. A No. 11 surgical blade is used to release the skin, and a single skin suture is placed.

Several variations in technique are possible. A long, No. 17 hypodermic needle

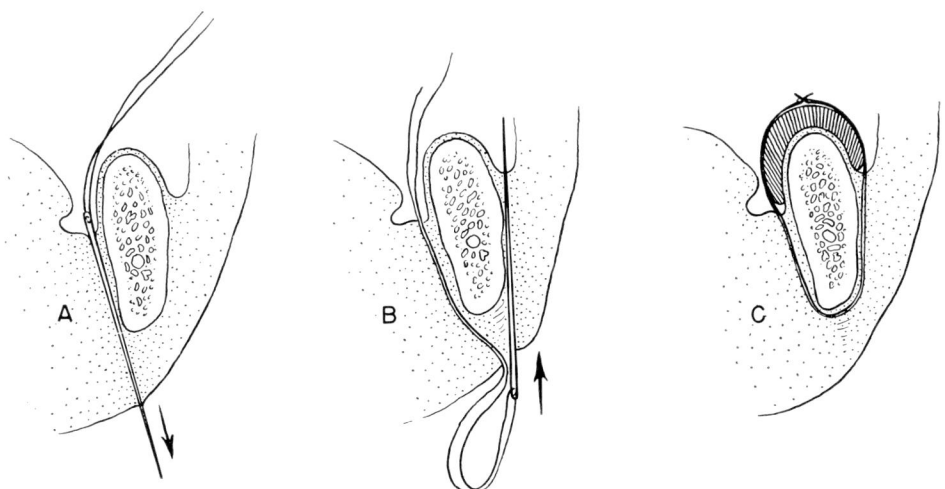

Fig. 19-27. Circumferential wiring technique with straight skin needle. **A**, Penetration of floor of mouth. **B**, Penetration of buccal sulcus. **C**, Wire around denture or splint.

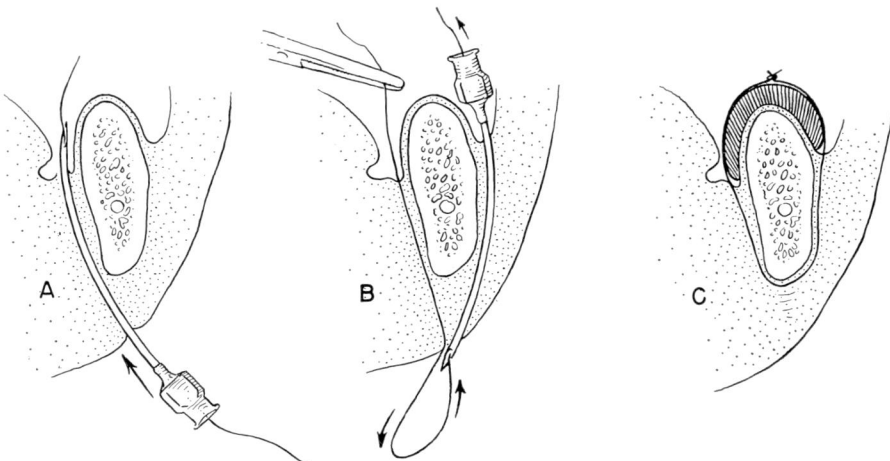

Fig. 19-28. Circumferential wiring technique with hypodermic needle. **A,** Penetration of floor of mouth from skin surface. **B,** Penetration of buccal sulcus from mucosal surface. **C,** Finished wiring.

can be used (Fig. 19-28). It is bent to a concave form and passed on the lingual side from the skin through the floor of the mouth. A single 26-gauge wire is introduced into the lumen from the skin side and grasped in the mouth with a hemostat. The needle then is removed. The same needle is introduced intraorally through the buccal fold to emerge through the same skin hole, and the other arm of the wire is threaded through the lumen from the skin side into the mouth.

If the hub of a second needle is cut off so that it can be removed from the wound, it can be introduced from the skin side into the buccal vestibule. The advantage of this method is the introduction of the two needles and the two arms of the wire from the skin surface into the more septic oral cavity, which will enhance the possibility of a noninfected skin wound.

Other variations have to do with the preparation of the denture. Holes for the wires can be drilled in the acrylic buccolingually between the teeth, just above the ridge. Danger of slipping is lessened, and the occlusal surfaces are not separated by the thickness of the wire. These holes also can be used for ligating the maxillary and mandibular dentures together for intermaxillary fixation following reduction, or hooks can be placed on the dentures for this purpose. The anterior teeth of the mandibular denture can be removed to provide better feeding and to eliminate the fulcrum created by the wire when it is tied over the teeth away from the ridge. Edentulous acrylic baseplate splints can be constructed if dentures are not available.

Skeletal pin fixation

Skeletal pin fixation is used in cases in which the management of a fractured bone segment is not satisfactorily accomplished by intermaxillary fixation. Fractures of the mandibular angle can be immobilized by skeletal pin fixation without surgically exposing the fracture. Fragments bridged by a bone graft are immobilized by skeletal pin fixation. Fractures in edentulous jaws can be treated in similar fashion.

At the time of World War II skeletal pin fixation became popular for several reasons. The Armed Services and the British treated simple as well as complicated fractures by this method, without supplement-

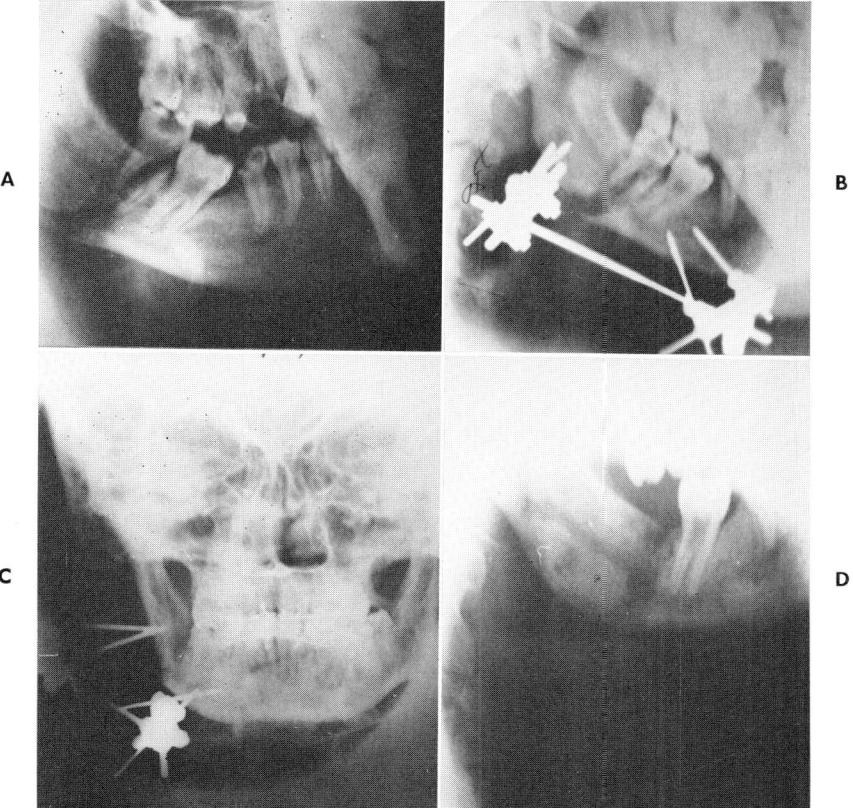

Fig. 19-29. **A**, Compound fracture extending through molar tooth, complicated by infection. The posterior fragment has been distracted upward by muscular pull. **B**, Skeletal pin fixation in position. **C**, Posteroanterior view. Note intermaxillary wiring. The fractured tooth was removed after this radiograph was made. **D**, Healing 3 months later.

ing it with intermaxillary fixation, so that the transported patient who suffered from motion sickness was not endangered by drowning in vomitus, and limited duty was made possible without liquid diet restrictions. Men practicing in, as well as out of, the Armed Services could treat complicated fractures without having training in open procedures.

Skeletal pins can be placed under general anesthesia or local block anesthesia supplemented by skin infiltration. It can be done in the dental chair or preferably in the operating room, where greater safety and convenience are possible. Strict asepsis is necessary. The skin must be prepared thoroughly, the field must be draped, and the operating team must be scrubbed and wear gloves and gowns.

Following skin preparation the inferior and superior borders of the mandible are palpated and marked on the skin with a dye such as gentian violet on an applicator stick. The line of fracture is marked, and the general location of the inferior alveolar canal is marked following reference to the radiograph. Intermaxillary fixation should be placed beforehand if used. (See Fig. 19-29.)

The pins are positioned usually by an

eggbeater-type drill. Two are placed at a 40-degree angle to each other on one side of the fracture, and two are placed similarly on the other side. If each pin is started 20 degrees from the vertical plane, a 40-degree divergence between them will result. The pins should not be placed closer to the fracture line than 1 cm. The skin is tensed directly over the bone. The pin in the drill is placed on the skin and pressed directly down to bone. The drill is rotated slowly under moderate pressure. The revolving point will be felt to penetrate the outer cortex, traverse the softer spongiosa, and then enter the inner cortex. It should penetrate the entire inner cortex, but it should not be lodged more than 1 or 2 mm. in the medial soft tissues. The drill then is removed carefully from the pin. The pin should be tested for stability. If not stable, it has not penetrated the medial cortex and should be rotated deeper with a hand attachment.

Two pins are placed in the anterior fragment parallel to the inferior border. The two pins in the posterior fragment can be placed parallel to the inferior border also, provided that the location of the fracture is not so far back that the most posterior pin will be located in the thin bone at the angle of the jaw. If the most posterior pin location is at the angle, it is better to locate the second pin further up on the vertical ramus at the posterior border or in the retromolar area near the anterior border. The pins should be located halfway between the mandibular canal and the inferior border, and care is taken that they do not traverse the facial artery or vein. (See Fig. 19-30.)

A bar assembly is attached to the two anterior pins. A similar assembly is placed on the two posterior pins. A large bar is selected and placed in the attachments on the short bars so that it crosses the fracture. The fracture is manually reduced so that the inferior border is continuous to palpation and the lateral border is continuous. All attachments are then tightened securely with a wrench. A drop of collodion is placed around the pin entrances into the skin. Roentgenograms made in the operating room or later will demonstrate the accuracy of the reduction.

Properly placed pins will remain tight for several months in the absence of infection.

Many variations exist in the design of skeletal pin apparatus. The Thoma bone clamp is useful in cases in which infection

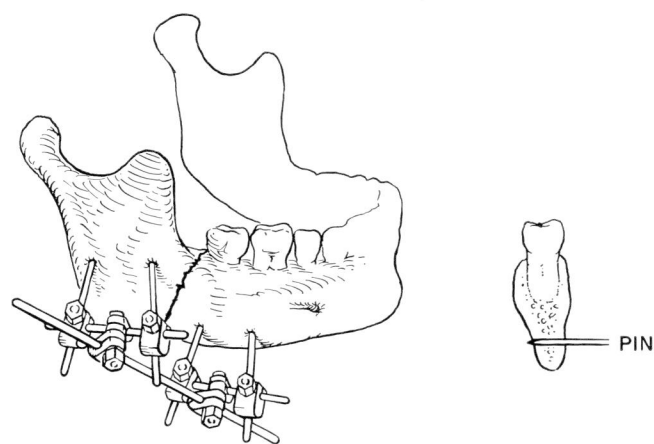

Fig. 19-30. Skeletal pin assembly. Note that the pin traverses both bony cortices.

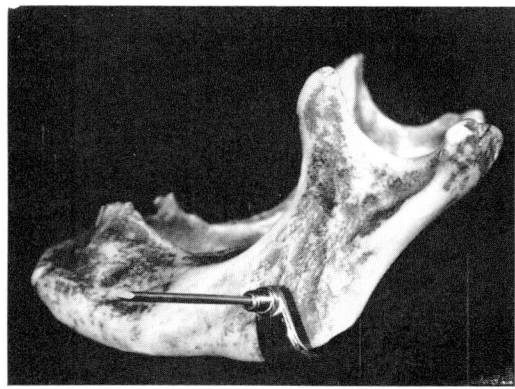

Fig. 19-31. Thoma bone clamp.

makes pins or transosseous wiring uncertain or in long-range treatment cases in which a bone graft is used (Fig. 19-31).

Some operators make use of an electrical drill to place pins rather than the manually operated eggbeater-type drill.

Open reduction

Open reduction with interosseous wiring is a definitive method for anchoring bone segments at the fracture site. Wire is placed through holes on either side of the fracture, reduction is accomplished under direct vision, and immobilization is obtained by tightening the wires. This procedure usually is reserved for fractures that cannot be reduced and immobilized adequately by closed methods. However, fractures that have soft tissue or debris interposed between the fragments and fractures that have healed in malposition are treated by open reduction.

One advantage to this method is direct visualization of the fractured parts, and consequently better reduction is possible. Oblique fractures, particularly those that present a short fracture on one cortical plate and a long one on the other plate (usually the lingual), are reduced with more precision. Complicated fractures are treated in this manner. It should be noted, on the other hand, that a severely comminuted fracture is not treated by open reduction if it can be avoided. The many small fragments may lose their vitality and be sloughed following an open procedure because the surrounding periosteal and soft tissue attachments and the traumatic hematoma and its binding, nutritive, and protective functions have been removed, and infection may be introduced.

Another advantage is firm fixation. Teeth can loosen, wires and appliances can slip, but the bone ends are still held close to each other. If teeth are present, open reduction should be supplemented by intermaxillary fixation for additional stabilization. Experience has shown that the direct interosseous wires cannot be relied on for complete immobilization of the fragments if unrestricted use of the jaws is permitted.

Open reduction is done almost always under general anesthesia in the operating room. Intermaxillary wiring should be in place. For that reason nasoendotracheal anesthesia is indicated. The most common site for open reduction is at the angle of the mandible, and the description will be for that procedure.

Preparation of the site of surgery, draping, and the surgical approach through the skin and soft tissues have been described in Chapter 2. The basic armamentarium is supplemented with the following instruments necessary for interosseous wiring:

2 Periosteotomes, dull and sharp
1 Bone rongeur
1 Mallet, metal, small
3 Chisels
1 Pliers, cutting, wire
4 Forceps, bone, Kocher
1 Retractor, malleable, narrow
1 Pistol drill, key, and drill points
  Wire, stainless steel, 24 and 30 gauge

Infiltration of the skin with a local anesthetic solution containing 1:50,000 epinephrine hydrochloride or other vasoconstrictor will eliminate clamping and tying the skin blood vessels, resulting in a smoother postoperative skin wound.

The bone is exposed and the fracture is visualized (see Chapter 2 for technique). The posterior fragment usually will be malplaced in a superior and medial position. Examination should be made of the cortical plates, particularly on the medial side. If the medial cortex is missing for some distance on one fragment, the location of the bur holes will have to be moved back until both cortical plates of that fragment can be traversed by one hole.

A flat ribbon retractor is placed under the medial side of the bone from the inferior border to protect the underlying soft tissue structures. The second assistant holds the superior soft tissue retractor across the face with his right hand and the ribbon retractor at the inferior border of the jaw with his left hand. The first assistant holds a syringe of normal saline solution in the right hand and the suction (if it is used) in the left hand. The operator holds the drill in both hands. Occasionally, secondary tissue retraction by the right hand of the first assistant is necessary near the drill bit.

An electrical drill is used more commonly than a mechanical eggbeater-type drill. The first hole should be started on the anterior fragment, near the inferior border, 0.5 cm. from the fracture site. The drill point should be sharp. Rotation is started at slow speed until the hole is started and then the speed may be increased, taking care that burning of the bone does not occur. The operator will feel the penetration of the outer cortex, the spongiosa, and the inner cortex. Saline solution is sprayed on the site during drilling. The drill is removed. Another hole is placed above the first one in the anterior fragment. It should not go through the inferior alveolar canal, being slightly below it. Usually it is well to place a 24-gauge wire in this hole immediately after the drill is removed and clamp the two ends with a hemostat outside the wound.

The ribbon retractor is repositioned under the posterior fragment. One hole is placed near the inferior border 0.5 cm. from the fracture site. Another hole is placed as high as possible above the first one and still just below the inferior alveolar canal. A wire is placed through this hole and clamped outside the wound.

The medial arm of the wire in the anterosuperior hole (Fig. 19-32, 2) crosses the fracture line and is threaded in the posteroinferior hole (3) from the medial to the lateral cortex (Fig. 19-32, A). It usually is difficult to locate the hole from beneath. Time can be saved by placing a thin 30-gauge wire in the second hole from a lateral to medial direction. This wire is doubled and the loop is introduced into the hole first. When recovered with a small curved hemostat from the medial aspect, the medial arm of the original wire is placed through the loop and bent back 3 cm. The thin double wire then is pulled upward (laterally) with care, to thread the original wire through the hole. The two arms of the original wire then are clamped outside the wound.

The medial arm of the wire in the posterosuperior hole (4) is threaded through the anteroinferior hole (1) from a medial to lateral direction, using a similar thin wire loop technique. It is clamped outside the wound.

The bone fragments are grasped with bone-holding or Kocher's forceps, although two No. 150 dental forceps may be employed, and the fracture is reduced by manipulating the fragments. If aberrant soft tissue and other debris are located between the bone fragments, it should be removed at this time. If necessary, major debridement should be done before the wires are placed. The wires are tightened while the assistant holds the bone ends in the reduced position. It is important to place upward traction on the needle holder while twisting the wires. After the wire has been tightened to within 3 mm. of the bone surface, a small periosteal elevator is placed on the underside (medial) of the bone and the

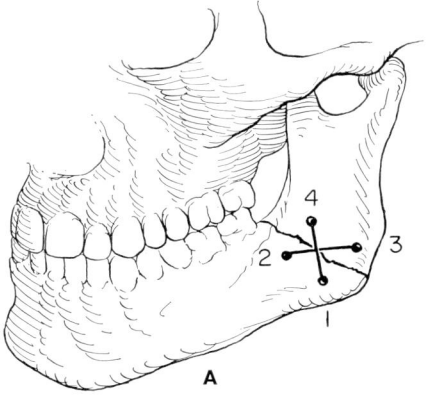 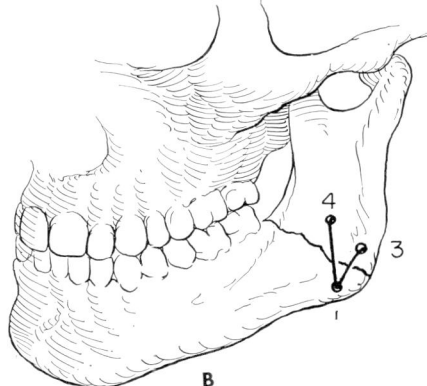

Fig. 19-32. Open reduction and interosseous wiring. **A,** Four-hole technique for mandibular angle fracture. **B,** Three-hole technique.

wire flattened against the bone. The needle holder grasps the strand of wire at the next to last turn, upward traction is made, and the wire is turned down to the bone surface.

The same procedure is followed for the other wire. The first wire is examined for tightness. The bone-holding instruments are removed, and the fracture reduction is inspected. Ordinarily no further manipulation will be necessary. The wire strands are cut off at a length of 0.7 cm., and the ends are turned carefully into the nearest bone holes.

Soft tissue closure is made by layers as described in Chapter 2. No drains are placed unless uncontrollable oozing of blood from deep areas is noted when the platysma muscle layer is being closed. After the skin sutures are placed, a small piece of sterile rayon is laid over them. Three 4 by 4 inch gauze sponges are placed over the rayon and held. The drapes are removed together with gloves and operating gowns. Blood and secretions are wiped from the face and neck. Skin areas adjacent to the bandages are painted with compound tincture of benzoin and allowed to dry. Many narrow strips (1 cm.) of adhesive tape 9 inches long are placed over the bandages and skin with a fair amount of tension since a pressure dressing is desired. An operating cap is placed on the head of the patient. A roll of elastic adhesive tape is wrapped around the chin, bandage, and head in modified Barton style. Last, a 1-inch strip of ordinary adhesive tape is placed on the cap over the forehead and the words "fractured jaw" are written upside down on it. This will remind recovery room personnel that the ordinary practice of holding the chin up to maintain a clear airway must be done with care, if at all.

It is possible to place too much bulk and pressure with the elastic adhesive dressing on the anterior throat instead of under the chin. Immediate respiratory embarrassment will result, necessitating revision.

The endotracheal tube should not be removed until the elastic adhesive dressing is in place. Anesthesia should be continued in sufficient depth until that time so that the patient will not "buck" on the tube. A carefully reduced fracture can be disturbed by "bucking" on the tube, particularly if it is not supported adequately by outside bandaging.

The postoperative orders should be written in the operating room. In most hospitals all preoperative orders are automatically cancelled by an operative procedure.

This basic technique has many variations.

Three bone holes are adequate usually (Fig. 19-32, B). This eliminates the need for the anterosuperior hole with the attendant threading of the wire immediately after drilling. All three holes are drilled. The posterosuperior hole (4) is drilled last, and a wire is placed through it. The medial arm of this wire in the posterosuperior hole is threaded into the anterior hole (1). Then one wire is placed from the anterior hole (1) to the posteroinferior hole (3). Two wires therefore are located in one anterior hole. The horizontal (1 to 3) wire is tightened first to impact the bone and then the oblique wire (1 to 4) is tightened to prevent upward muscle displacement. The first wire is examined for stability since it often requires another turn.

In the three-hole technique a figure-of-eight wire in two inferior holes offers advantages in providing downward traction as well as cross fracture traction. It is the technique used most today. A figure of eight is made on the inferior border, with the wires crossing near the fracture site. Both ends of the wire can be placed from the lateral side, eliminating the threading from the medial side.

Bone plates are used infrequently in new fractures of the jaws (Fig. 19-33). Healing seems to be delayed in comparison with wire techniques that pull the fractured ends together during convalescence. The screws in bone plates hold the bones rigidly. The technique of fastening the plates sometimes will allow a small distraction of the fragments, and the absence of minute functional stresses at the fracture site results in slower healing. Care must be taken that the screws and the plate are made of exactly the same alloy to prevent electrolytic currents from forming, which would cause dissolution of bone around the holes.[7] Even screws cast from the same alloy sometimes cause such currents. In the casting process the metals may have separated somewhat so that the head and point of the same screw are not a uniform alloy.

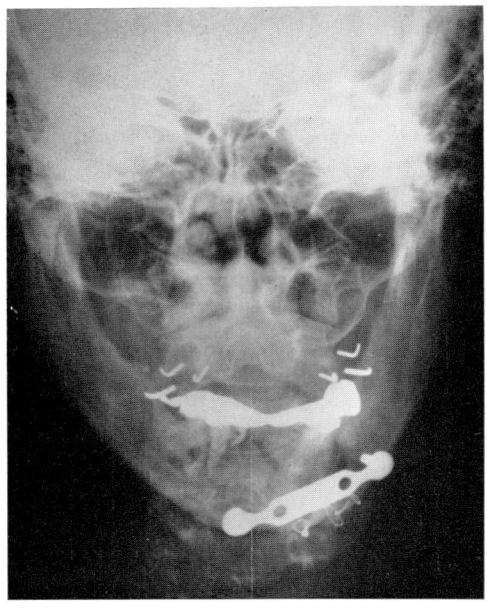

Fig. 19-33. Bone plate used to maintain telescoped comminuted symphyseal fracture. Cast cap splint on mandibular teeth; acrylic splint with metal lugs in edentulous maxilla.

In comminuted fractures that require open reduction, and occasionally in edentulous mandibular fractures that have a strong tendency to override, a metal gutter plate can be placed on the inferior border with screws or wires through bone holes. Ordinary wires without a bone plate will pull an overriding fracture together, but they will not hold an overriding fracture in proper distracted position unless other wires are placed in lateral directions. The principle of the slotted plate used by the orthopedic surgeon in fractures of the long bone is applicable here. Muscular pull across the fracture site is allowed to act to keep the fractured ends together during healing by the sliding of screws in a horizontal slot rather than in a hole in the plate.

The L splint has a right-angle bend across its top surface that is placed in a slot cut through the cortical plate across the frac-

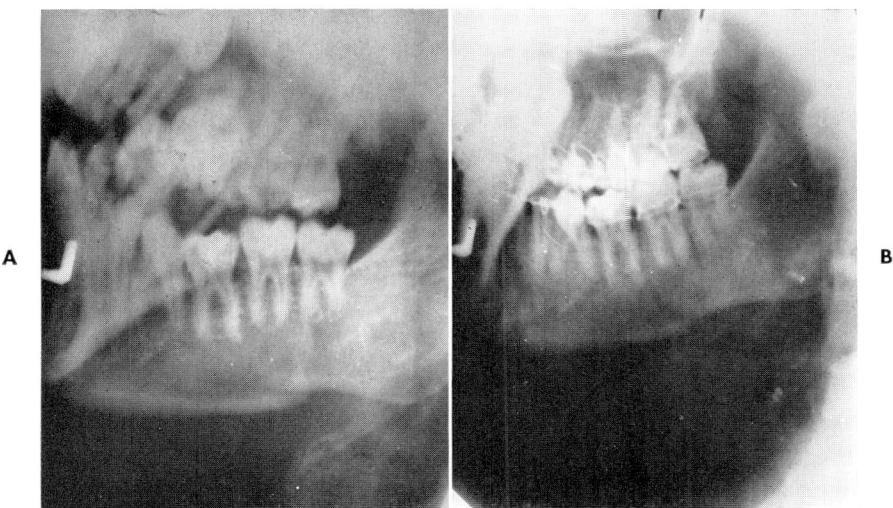

Fig. 19-34. **A**, Fracture in dentulous region distracted upward. **B**, Satisfactory reduction by simple interdental wiring and intermaxillary fixation.

ture zone. Because of its horizontal stability, only two screws are necessary. The L splint is less bulky and more stable than ordinary bone plates.[8]

Treatment of fractures of the mandible
Uncomplicated fractures

A large percentage of mandibular fractures can be treated by simple intermaxillary fixation. The fractures must be located within the dental arch, and at least one sound tooth should be present in the distal fragment. Although specific advantages are inherent in the use of one method over another in a specific fracture, by and large any method of intermaxillary fixation can be used. (See Fig. 19-34.) For example, multiple-loop wiring was used extensively and almost exclusively in the Armed Services during World War II. The beginning practitioner should be able to manage one method well. Variations can be considered with increased experience.

The question of the removal of a tooth in the line of fracture is managed often by the judgment of the operator. Before the sulfonamides and antibiotics it was always removed. Most experienced men still will remove this tooth. The following factors influence the decision: the absence of fracture or gross injury to the tooth; the absence of caries or large restorations; the absence of periodontitis; the location of the tooth, including esthetics and the possibility of arch collapse; the nature of the fracture; and the probability of adequate response to antibiotic therapy. If serious doubt exists whether or not to extract the tooth, it should be extracted. Persistent chronic infection or an acute abscess occurring later in treatment sometimes will require opening of the fixation to extract the tooth. Delayed union or nonunion can result.

As a matter of fact, infected and grossly carious teeth that are not in the line of fracture should be extracted before placing intermaxillary fixation. This can be done under the same anesthesia given for wiring.

Elastic traction is placed to overcome distraction and muscle spasm. With continued changing, elastic traction can be used throughout convalescence. If desired, the elastics can be replaced by intermaxillary wires after 1 week. The wires are easier to keep clean, and they seem to bother the patient less. Recalcitrant patients who desire a chicken dinner at the end of the third week sometimes require heavy intermaxillary wire fixation supplemented by elastic traction.

Antibiotics are useful for the first week as a prophylactic measure. It is advantageous usually to admit a fracture patient to the hospital. Many patients with simple fractures are treated in the outpatient clinic or office and then allowed to go home, where they are observed. However, a 24- or 48-hour admission will allow the patient to recuperate from his trauma and operation better, his new diet and drug therapy can be introduced to him, and he can be observed more closely.

Complicated fractures

Fractures that cannot be reduced and fixed properly by simple intermaxillary fixation require further measures. Usually the dentulous cases have intermaxillary fixation placed as a starting point.

Mandibular angle. Intermaxillary fixation is placed. The horizontal and vertical favorable fractures require no further treatment. A solid, unfractured tooth in the posterior fragment with an antagonist in the maxilla will preclude further treatment (Fig. 19-35). Conservatism is necessary in condemning such a tooth for extraction. Many experienced men on occasion have retained such a tooth when one root has been fractured, but as a rule the worry during the convalescent period does not make the procedure worthwhile. The oral surgeon who enjoys life treats the fracture in definitive fashion immediately.

Many methods for controlling the posterior fragment have been advocated. Some have been abandoned, and others are not generally accepted. Skeletal pin fixation and open reduction are the two main alternatives. Individual preference is a strong factor in choice. Skeletal pin fixation is satis-

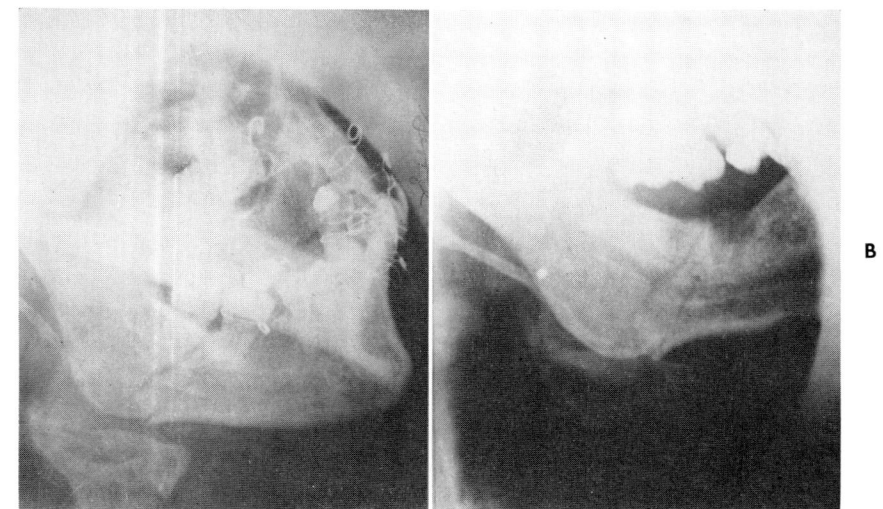

Fig. 19-35. **A,** Horizontal unfavorable angle fracture satisfactorily reduced by intermaxillary fixation, aided by the presence of an unfractured third molar in the line of fracture, preventing upward displacement. Note that this tooth is not wired. **B,** Healed fracture. The molar teeth were extracted after healing had occurred.

factory if it is placed properly. Pin fixation can be done in the office if necessary. The fact that much external hardware is in evidence during healing and the fact that open reduction takes only about 30 minutes longer to do influence many men toward open reduction. Open reduction, despite its drawbacks of the external scar, the loss of the original hematoma, the exposure of bone to possible infection, and the operating room procedure involved, still seems to provide more definitive treatment (Figs. 19-36 and 19-37).

Symphysis Simple wiring often provides satisfactory immobilization. Wiring of the teeth, particularly with the Risdon wiring across the fracture, will reduce the fracture adequately at the alveolar level, but separa-

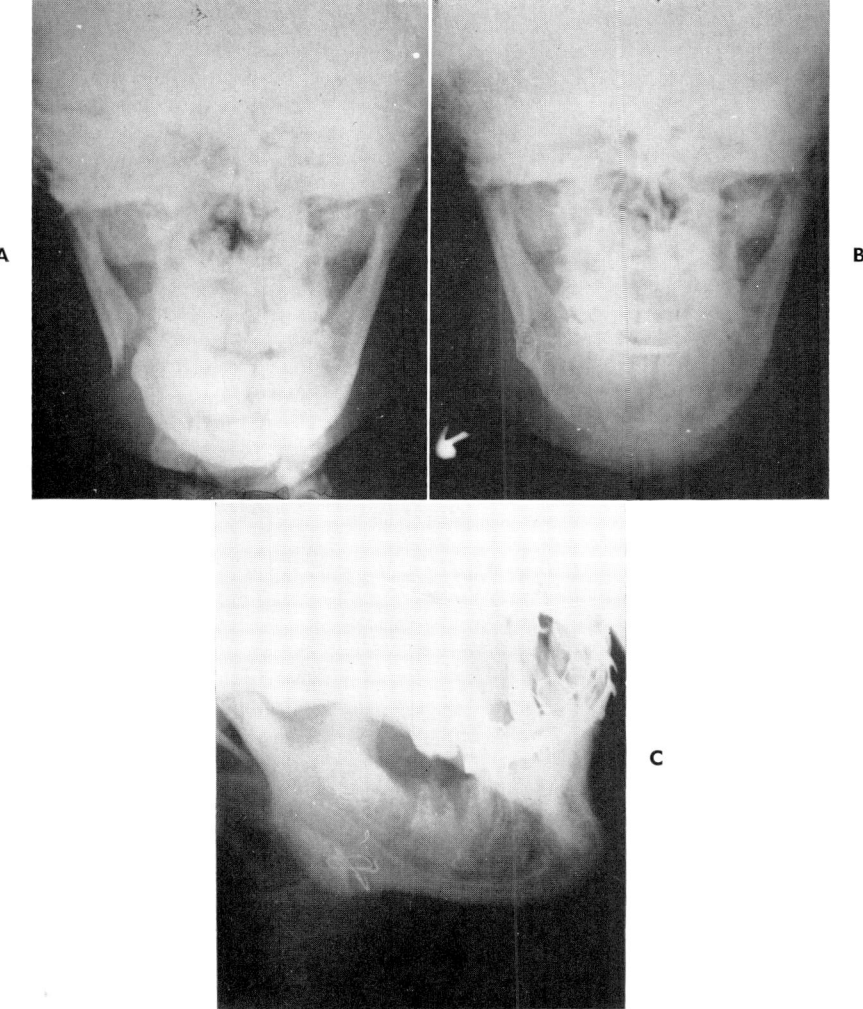

Fig. 19-36. Open reduction, four-hole technique. **A,** Preoperative radiograph. **B,** Postoperative radiograph. **C,** Lateral view showing details of interosseous wiring. The presence of the third molar in this case would not have aided reduction or fixation. The second molar was infected. Both molars were removed.

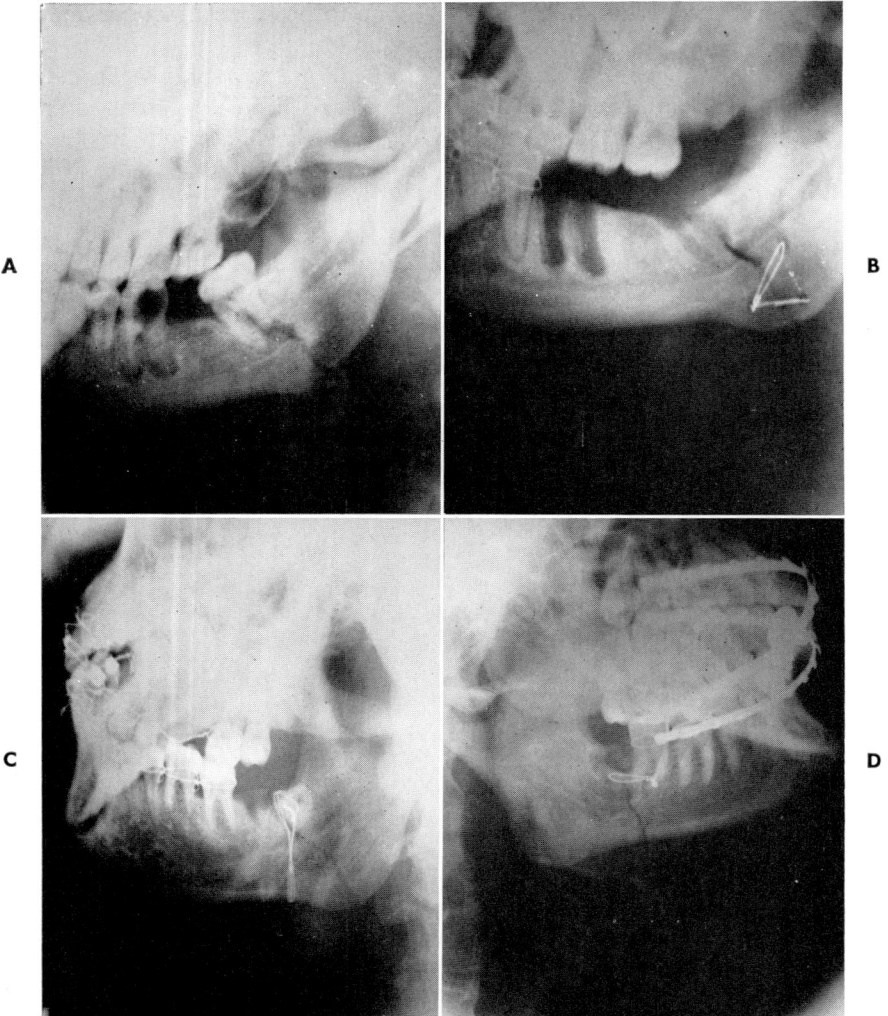

Fig. 19-37. Open reduction. **A,** Three-hole technique, preoperative radiograph. **B,** Postoperative radiograph. **C,** Similar case showing circummandibular wire placed from within the mouth, precluding an operating room procedure. A hole was drilled in the ascending ramus. **D,** Successful use of an intraoral wire through holes placed in the buccal osseous plates following fracture during odontectomy.

tion or telescoping may occur at the inferior border. If the wiring is tight and the inferior border separation is minimal, healing will be satisfactory (Fig. 19-38, *A*). However, the principal complication is collapse of the alveolar arch inward, which is difficult to prevent with dental wiring. A simple acrylic splint placed on the lingual aspect of the dental arch before wiring will prevent arch collapse.

Wide separation or other malposition requires further treatment. Skeletal pins can be used. A Kirschner wire or Steinmann pin (Fig. 19-38, *B*) can be driven across the chin by an electrical drill. This is done through the skin surfaces while the frac-

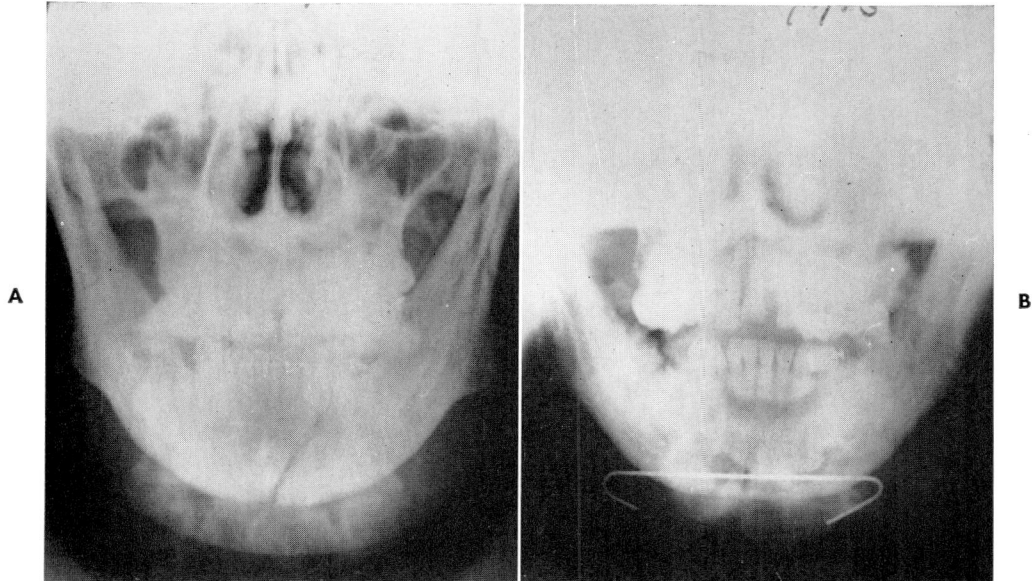

Fig. 19-38. **A**, Symphysis fracture reduced by multiple-loop intermaxillary wiring. **B**, Steinmann pin through symphysis.

tured ends are held in proper reduction. This is a relatively simple procedure that takes little time.

Open reduction in this region does not encounter large vessels, but the tissue attachments are difficult to raise. Care must be given to locating the linear scar beneath the chin within Langer's lines if practicable. More exact reduction and closer fixation are made possibly by open reduction. This method is valuable, especially in the grossly telescoped fracture (Fig. 19-39).

In symphysis fractures uncomplicated by condyle fracture, force of the blow has traumatized the temporomandibular joint, and ankylosis can occur if the jaw is not opened occasionally during the treatment period to free the joint. This maneuver is accomplished better if a lingual acrylic splint stabilizes the symphysis fracture.

Edentulous fracture. Circumferential wiring around a denture or acrylic splint is adequate in most cases (Fig. 19-40). All of the fragments must be covered by the denture base, and they must be held adequately to preclude auxiliary treatment. Fractures occurring distal to the posterior border of the denture, old telescoped fractures, and cases of severe trauma require skeletal pin fixation or open reduction. Some oral surgeons do not place dentures and intermaxillary fixation in edentulous jaws when skeletal pin fixation or open reduction is done, although others feel that all jaw fractures should have intraoral stabilization.

In the case of the angle-third molar region fracture that is not distal to the posterior border of the denture, the circummandibular wires should be placed around the anterior fragment. Muscular pull on the posterior fragment will elevate it so that further wires are not necessary in this area (Fig. 19-41).

Keeping the maxillary denture in is often a problem. If the maxillary denture fits well, and particularly if it has one or more minor undercuts, the two dentures con-

338 *Textbook of oral surgery*

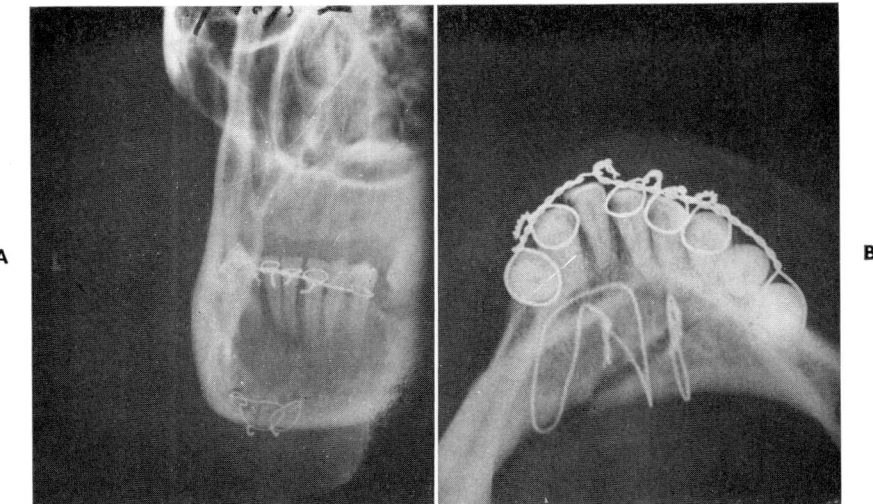

Fig. 19-39. **A,** Open reduction of symphysis fracture. **B,** Intraoral view to show figure-of-eight wiring to overcome characteristic tendency to telescope in symphysis fractures.

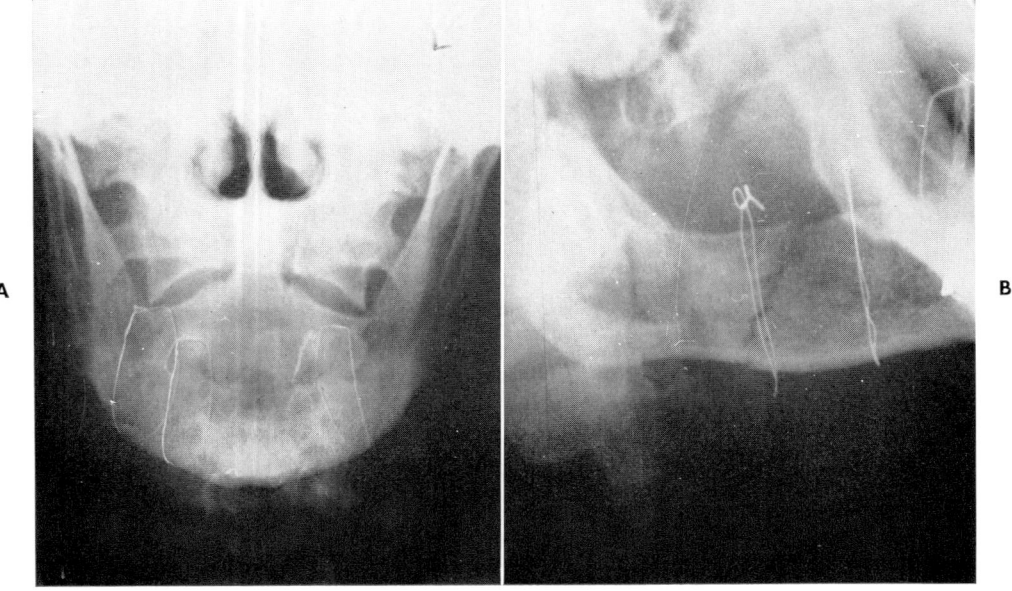

Fig. 19-40. **A,** Circumferential wiring around acrylic splint in edentulous patient. **B,** Lateral view.

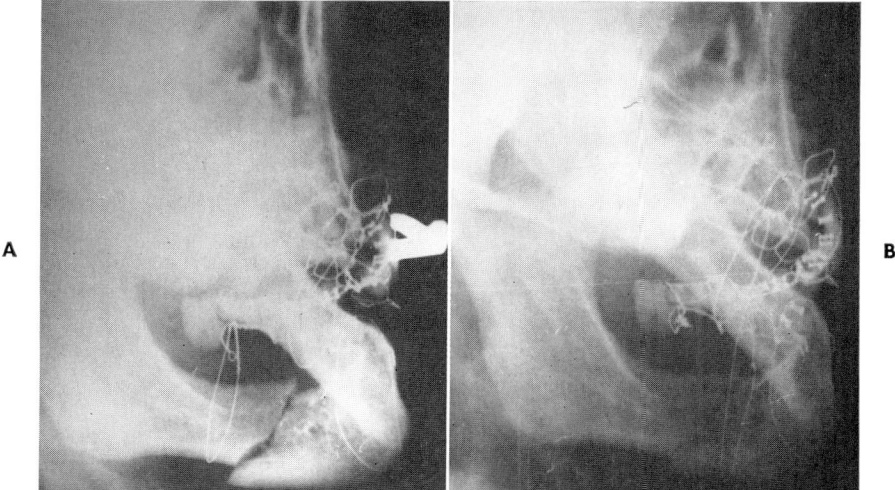

Fig. 19-41. **A**, Circumferential wire around denture, incorrectly placed. Tightening the wire distracted the posterior fragment upward. **B**, Same case after distal wire was replaced by a wire around the anterior fragment.

nected by intermaxillary fixation may stay in place. Older women with resorbed alveolar ridges will carefully slip the maxilla out of the assembled dentures when the surgeon has gone, turn to the next bed, and start to jabber incessantly. This is an eerie sight with the dentures closed and still moving in unison over fast speech. If the surgeon does not drop in unexpectedly he will find the jaws always fixed in position, and he will wonder why the fracture heals slowly, if at all.

A head bandage worn continuously is uncomfortable. The cooperative patient can wear an elastic support over the head and chin at night or even during the day. The uncooperative patient will require further stabilization. A simple method consists of direct wiring to the piriform fossa margins (Fig. 19-42).[9] Under local anesthesia, or general anesthesia supplemented by infiltration anesthesia, an incision is made high in the labial fold next to the midline of the maxilla. The bone is exposed by blunt dissection. The inferior border of the piriform fossa is followed laterally until the lateral border is reached, where a small hole is placed with a bur. Thirty-gauge wire is placed through the hole and brought out untwisted through the incision. The incision is closed with No. 3-0 catgut. The same procedure is carried out on the other side. The denture is removed from a cold-sterilizing solution and placed in the mouth. The wires are threaded through previously drilled holes in the labial flanges of the denture and tightened moderately. Dental compound is placed over the rosette, and a pressure bandage is placed over the lip.

Pernasal wiring is another method for fixing a denture to the maxilla.[10] A heavy awl is passed just inside the external nares directly through the mucosa and bone of the nasal floor and palate with simple pressure and rotation. A wire is looped through the eye of the awl at its point of emergence on the palatal side. The instrument is withdrawn upward through the palate, but only to a point just beneath the nasal epithelium. It is then guided anteriorly and inferiorly through the labial mucosa into the height of the vestibule. The wire is removed from the eye of the awl, the awl is withdrawn completely, and the two free wire ends

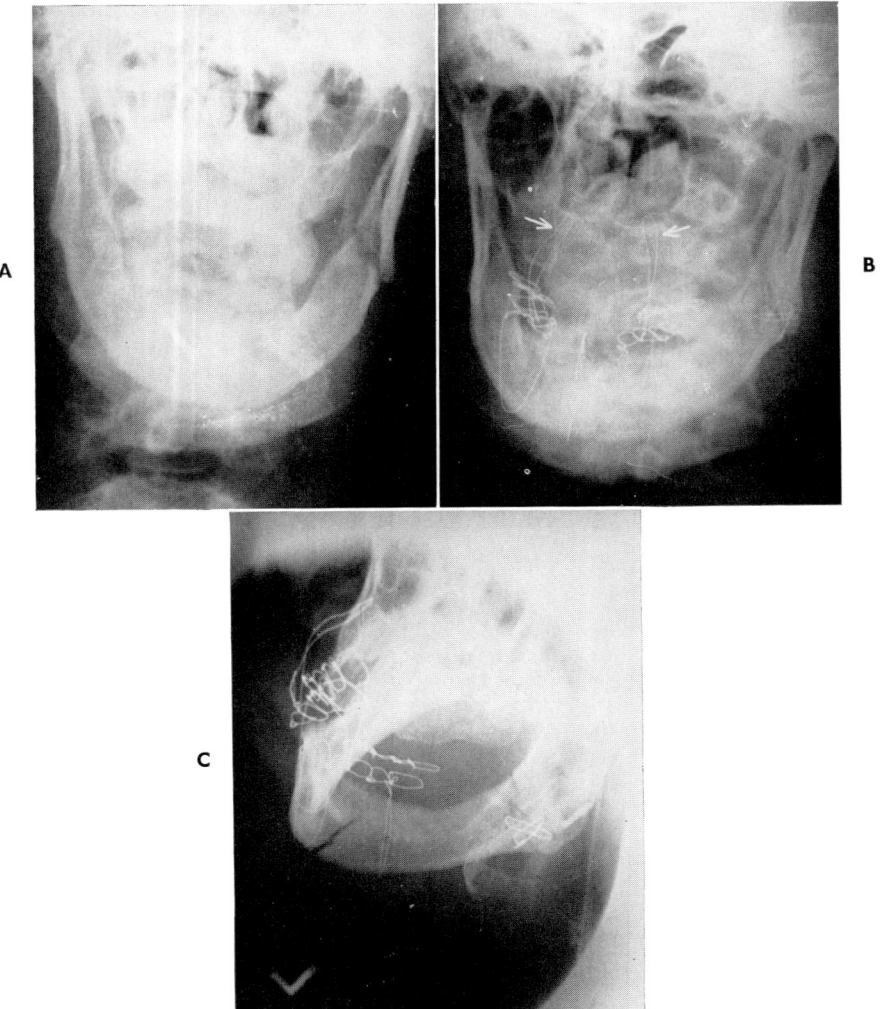

Fig. 19-42. Piriform rim wiring. **A,** Preoperative radiograph. **B,** Circumferential wiring. Piriform rim wiring extends to mandibular denture to aid in immobilizing dentures. **C,** Piriform rim wiring can be seen anteriorly. Note incidental interosseous wiring at angle.

(one palatal and the other vestibular) are drawn together around the prosthesis, through a palatal bur hole in the appliance, and tightened on the labial surface.

Circumzygomatic wires are useful also. A long, sharp instrument with a hole near the tip is introduced at the height of the buccal fold just distal to the maxillary first molar region and is pushed upward and posteriorly. A finger on the skin over the zygomatic arch guides the point medial to the arch to emerge on the skin. A wire is threaded into the eye of the instrument and the instrument is withdrawn into the mouth. The wire is disengaged. The instrument is introduced into the same oral wound and pushed in the same upward direction, this time to pass on the lateral side of the zygomatic arch and emerge through the same skin wound. The other arm of the

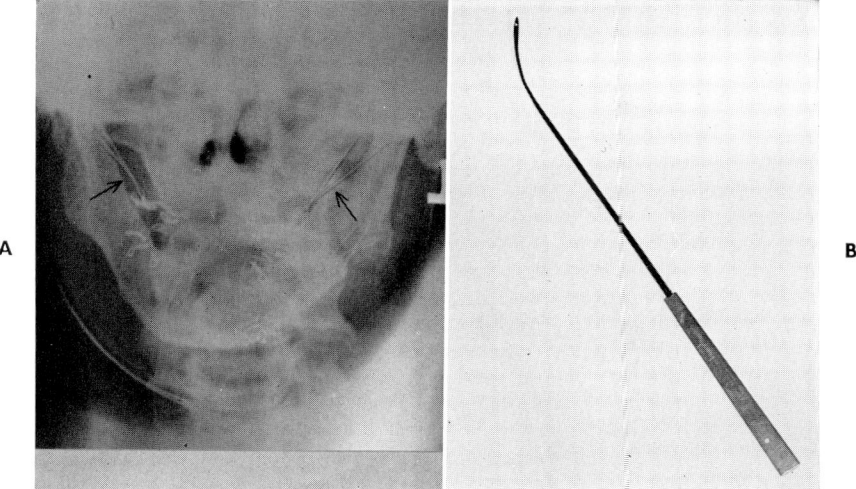

Fig. 19-43. A, Circumzygomatic and circummandibular wires used to stabilize splints for edentulous fracture fixation. B, Instrument for passing circumzygomatic wires (made by Dr. G. E. Morin).

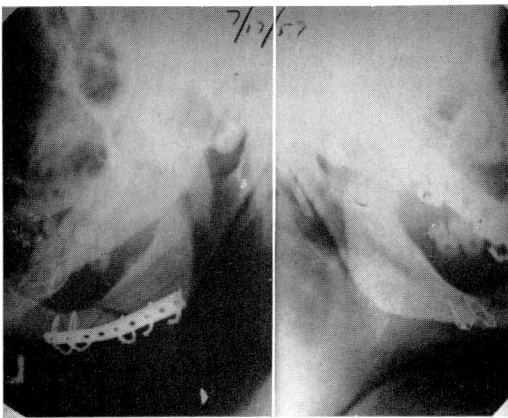

Fig. 19-44. Gutter bone plate used to stabilize triangular segment on inferior border. Note interosseous wiring on other side.

wire is threaded into the eye of the instrument and the instrument is withdrawn. The two arms of the wire are sawed back and forth until they contact bone, and they are attached to the maxillary denture flange in the molar region. A similar circumzygomatic wire is placed around the opposite zygomatic arch. The wires can be looped around the mandibular circumferential wires that secure the mandibular denture to the lower jaw (Fig. 19-43).

Open reduction of an edentulous fracture is done best with four holes, using heavy wire. If a triangular segment of bone is found on the inferior border (a not uncommon occurrence in edentulous fractures) and telescoping has occurred, a gutter bone plate on the inferior border will support the segment (Fig. 19-44).

Skeletal pin fixation is excellent. The thinness of the bone makes placement difficult at times. (See Fig. 19-45.)

Multiple fractures

Multiple fractures, in which four or more jaw fractures are present in the same person, occurred in 17% of the fractures in the District of Columbia General Hospital series. When multiple fractures occur in both jaws in the same patient, it is difficult sometimes to find a starting point for treatment. Many fragments at different occlusal levels require the establishment of a base-

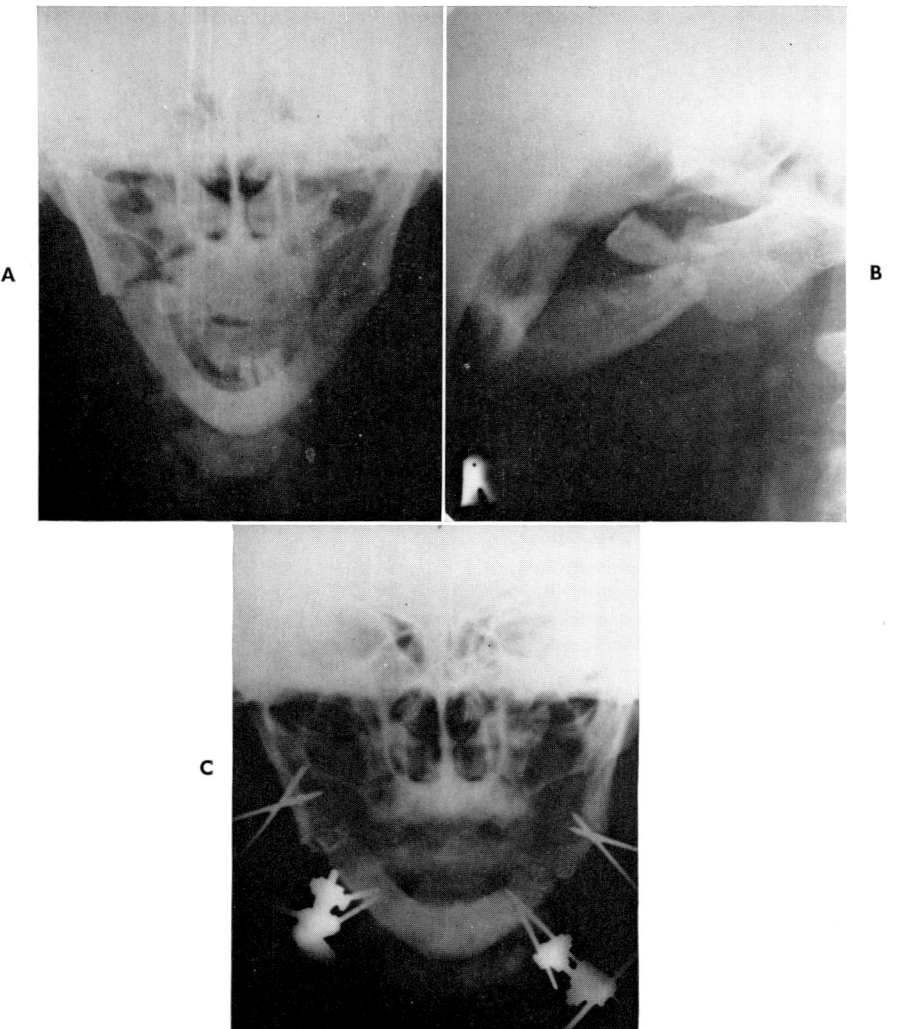

Fig. 19-45. **A,** Bilateral fracture in edentulous mandible. **B,** Lateral jaw radiograph showing collapse of fragments. **C,** Interosseous wiring supplemented by skeletal pin fixation.

line, which is usually the mandible. After the parts of the mandible have been reduced to a satisfactory plane of occlusion, other segments are fitted to it. If many mandibular segments are present, and if the maxilla is severely fractured so that it cannot be used to establish a plane of occlusion, impressions of the teeth are made and casts are poured. The casts are cut at the fracture lines and reassembled in normal occlusion, and a cast splint that has proper indentations on its superior surface to support the maxillary teeth is made for the mandible.

Multiple fractures that occur solely in the mandible often can be assembled by fixing the teeth of the individual segments to the intact maxillary arch. Wiring or divided arch bars are used. However, many teeth often are lost in this type of fracture. A

Fractures of the jaws 343

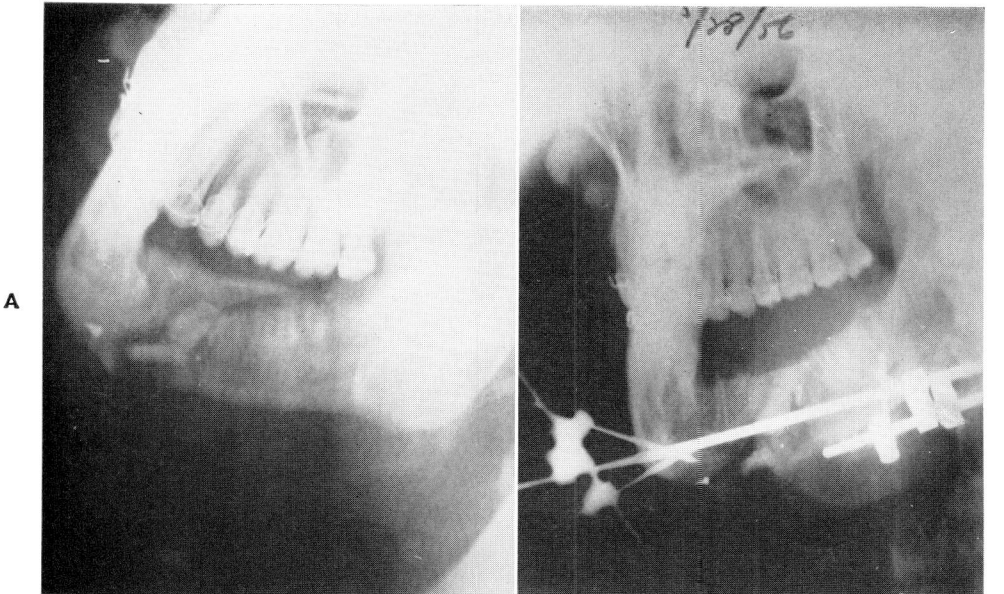

Fig. 19-46. **A**, Compound comminuted mandibular fracture. **B**, Treatment by skeletal pin fixation.

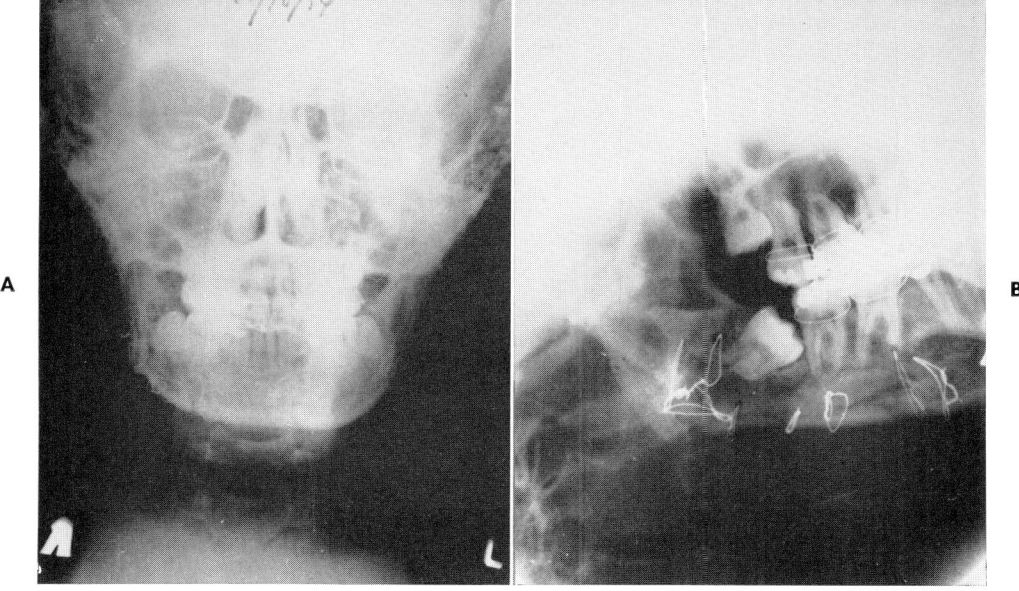

Fig. 19-47. **A**, Multiple fractures of right mandible treated by interosseous wiring. **B**, Impacted third molar successfully retained for stability.

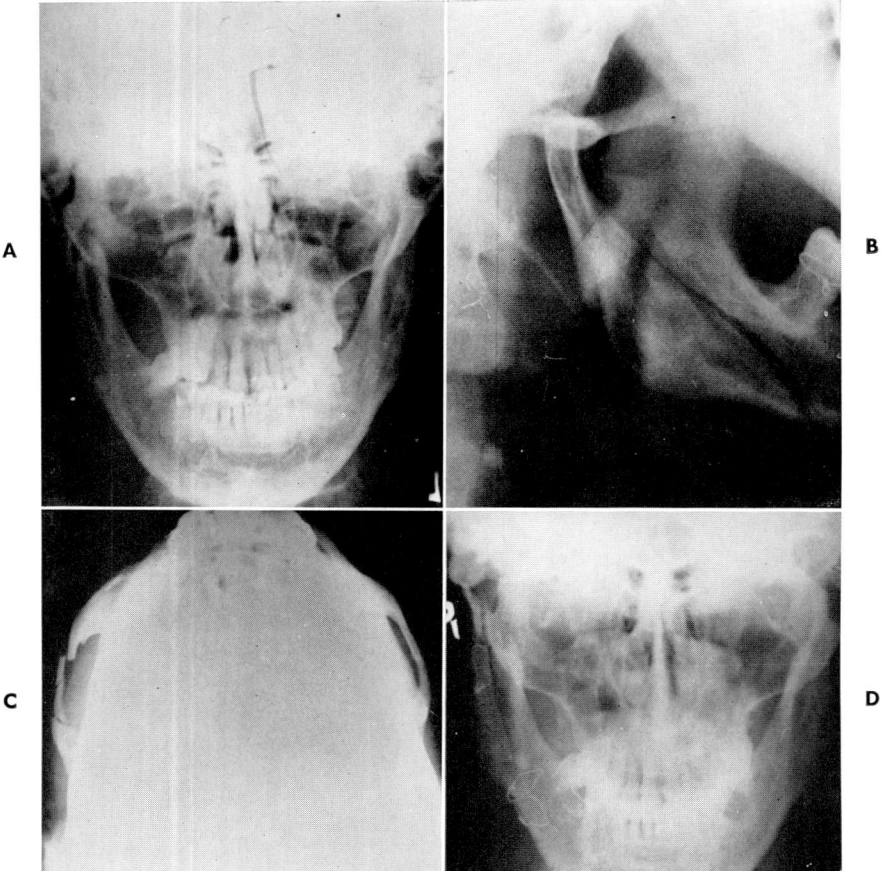

Fig. 19-48. Multiple fractures. **A,** Infraorbital rim, mandibular angle. **B,** Neck of condyle. **C,** Right zygomatic arch. **D,** Treatment by interosseous wiring through submandibular approach, followed by simple elevation of arch.

splint may be used for greater stability, but the splinted mandible in this case is wired to the maxilla to obtain and maintain good occlusion. Oblique fractures and horizontal fractures appearing on the inferior border are treated by circumferential wiring around the splint. Skeletal pins are difficult to place in many small fragments. Open reduction is a last resort. It is definitive treatment, but many small pieces are difficult to wire, and surgical exposure will deprive them of any last vestiges of mechanical and physiological support afforded by the surrounding soft tissues. (See Figs. 19-46 to 19-48.)

Fractures of the coronoid process (2% of the District of Columbia General Hospital series) often are not treated if no displacement has occurred (Fig. 19-49). The tendons of the temporalis muscle frequently are inserted low on the ramus, which will prevent displacement. If upward displacement does occur, open reduction can be done through an intraoral approach. An incision is made on the anterior border of the ramus, and direct wiring utilizing two holes

Fractures of the jaws 345

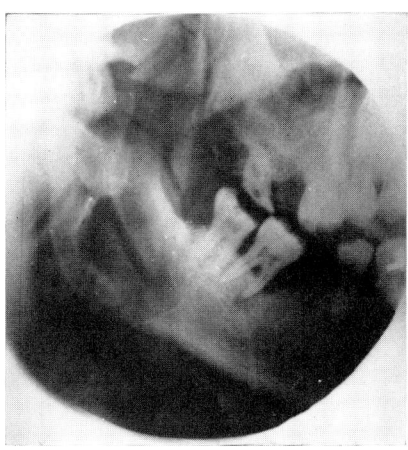

Fig. 19-49. Fracture of coronoid process with minimal displacement.

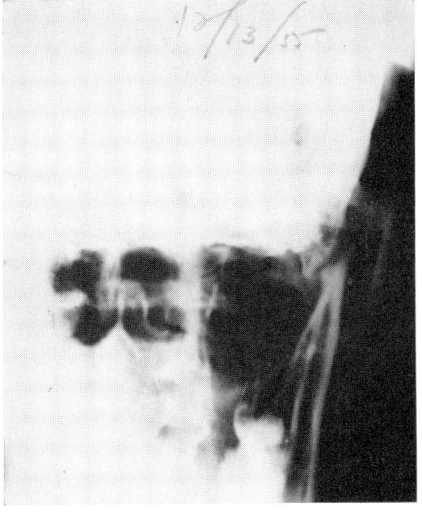

Fig. 19-50. Fracture of condyle with medial displacement.

is done. If reduction is not possible and impairment of function is present, the coronoid process is removed.

Condyle

The fractured mandibular condyle has been treated for many years by a closed procedure. Intermaxillary fixation is placed that immobilizes concomitant fractures and corrects the displacement of the jaws associated with the condyle fracture, that is, a shift of the midline toward the side of the fractured condyle and a slight premature posterior occlusion on that side. The fractured ends of the bone in the condylar region thereby are placed in a somewhat better relationship.

Because of muscular pulls and the stress of the blow, the condylar head often is dislocated forward or tipped medially out of the glenoid fossa (Fig. 19-50). Often the fractured neck of the condyle remains close to the fractured ramus portion. In a subcondylar fracture the fractured segment remains upright in a position lateral to the ramus. Attempts at intraoral as well as extraoral manipulation, the latter including lateral pressure by a sharp instrument through the skin ("ice-pick technique") and various pressure pads on the skin, are usually unsuccessful (Fig. 19-51).

Because of trauma to the joint structures, an ever-present danger exists of ankylosis of the condyle to the glenoid fossa. Healing in proper occlusion under intermaxillary immobilization is allowed to progress for 2½ weeks. At that time, with the patient in the dental chair, the jaw is opened carefully once, by the operator rather than the patient, care being taken that other fractures do not move, and fixation is again applied. This is done several times in the following weeks. The effect of this procedure is to disrupt the continuity of the fibrous callus in the condylar fracture area. Fibrous tissue rather than bone forms at the junction.

The fractured condylar head treated in this manner is nonfunctional. Because of this factor, together with a traumatic hematoma and the damaged synovial membranes, it ankyloses to the base of the skull. The ramus articulates on the edge of the condylar fragment by a fibrous joint. The functioning of the contralateral joint, together with the stability afforded by the fibrous joint, allows satisfactory function-

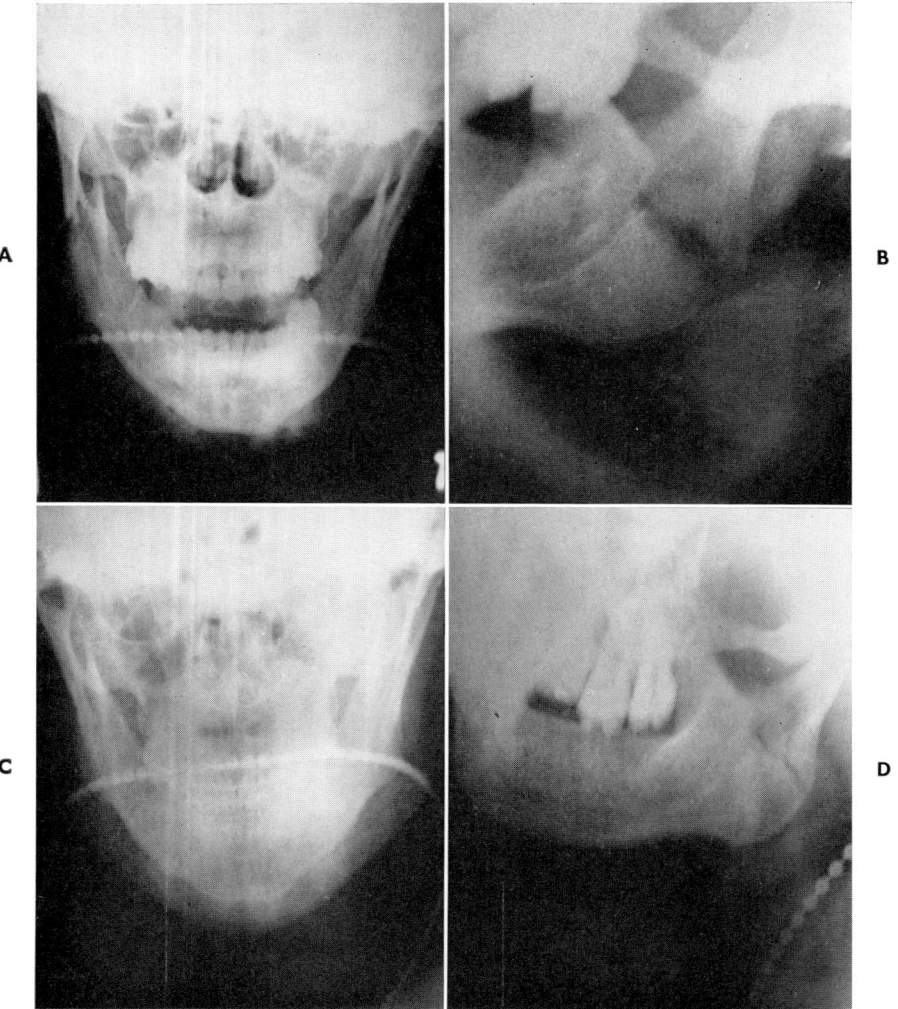

Fig. 19-51. **A** and **B**, Extracapsular fracture of condyle neck. Preoperative radiographs. **C** and **D**, Postoperative radiographs following "ice-pick" (closed) reduction. Note intermaxillary fixation.

ing in good occlusion. The patient can bite as hard on the side of injury as on the other side without experiencing pain.

Frequently, such manipulation during healing will create movement in the joint rather than in the fracture zone if it is done carefully, and primary healing of the fractured parts will occur with no ankylosis in the joint.

The head of the condyle that is displaced medially out of the glenoid fossa will ankylose if it touches bone. It is held in place by the soft tissues. Years later it seems to disappear. Fibrous tissue fills the joint cavity.

The occluding dental arches attached to a normal contralateral joint will not allow the ramus to move further upward to form an open bite, whether or not an ankylosed condylar fragment is present in the fossa.

Fractures of the jaws **347**

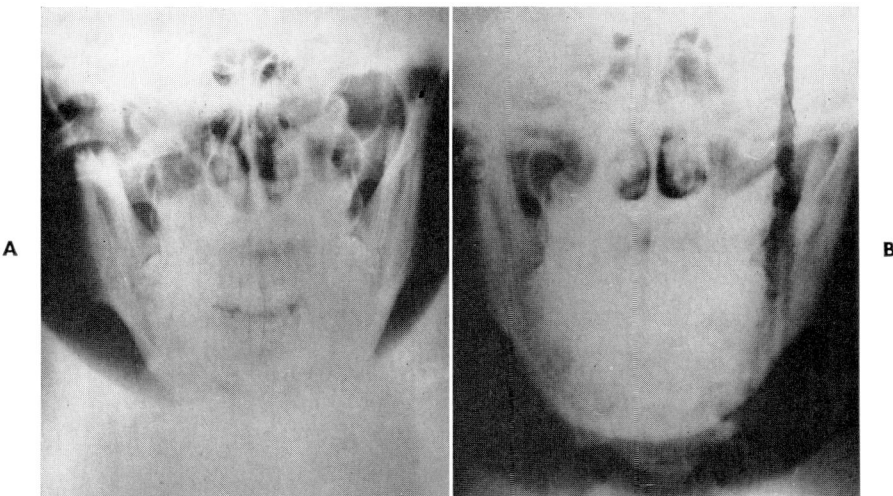

Fig. 19-52. **A,** Fracture of condyle with medial displacement. **B,** Interosseous fixation following reduction through preauricular exposure.

Evidence suggests that an attempt is made over the years to re-form the missing condyle from the remaining ramus portion.

Open reduction of condylar fractures has become popular since World War II. The condylar head is placed back in its original position in the glenoid fossa and wired to the ramus. Healing of the fracture takes place by direct bony union, and the healed member functions on the true joint rather than on an artificial fibrous joint.

The surgical procedure for the preauricular approach (Fig. 19-52) is made according to the description given in Chapter 2. Dissection is carried down to the articular capsule. Manual movement of the jaw at this time will demonstrate the joint structure. The capsule is incised horizontally if the fracture is intracapsular or if the condyle has been displaced medially out of the glenoid fossa. This is necessary for access. It is advantageous not to incise the capsule if possible since the lateral side of the capsule is stronger than the medial side, and the intact capsule stabilizes the condylar head.

A hole is placed in the fragment that lies most superficial. Special retractors such as those designed by Thoma are placed beneath the fragment to protect the maxillary artery. The ramus of the jaw may be pushed upward into the wound to visualize the inferior fragment better and distracted downward to gain access to the superior fragment. A hole is then placed in the other fragment.

The condylar fragment is repositioned carefully in the glenoid fossa. The management of this fragment is a delicate procedure. The fragment is difficult to find if it is displaced deeply to the medial side. It must be placed in its properly oriented position in the fossa with as little damage to the surrounding structures as possible. It must be held firmly while the hole is drilled. Any excessive pulling will bring the fragment completely out of the wound.

A wire is placed through the two holes, threading it from the lateral surface of the condylar fragment first and recovering it from the medial surface to the lateral surface of the inferior fragment by means of a thin wire loop. The wires are twisted over the reduced fracture. It is well to remove

348 *Textbook of oral surgery*

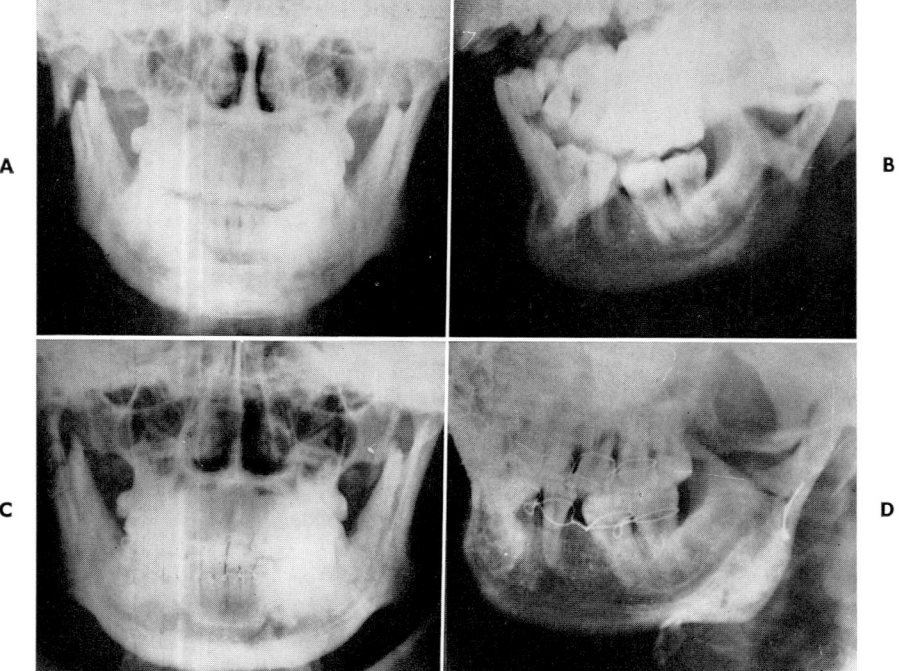

Fig. 19-53. **A,** Extracapsular condyle fracture with lateral displacement. **B,** Lateral jaw radiograph showing displacement. **C** and **D,** Postoperative radiographs following interosseous wiring.

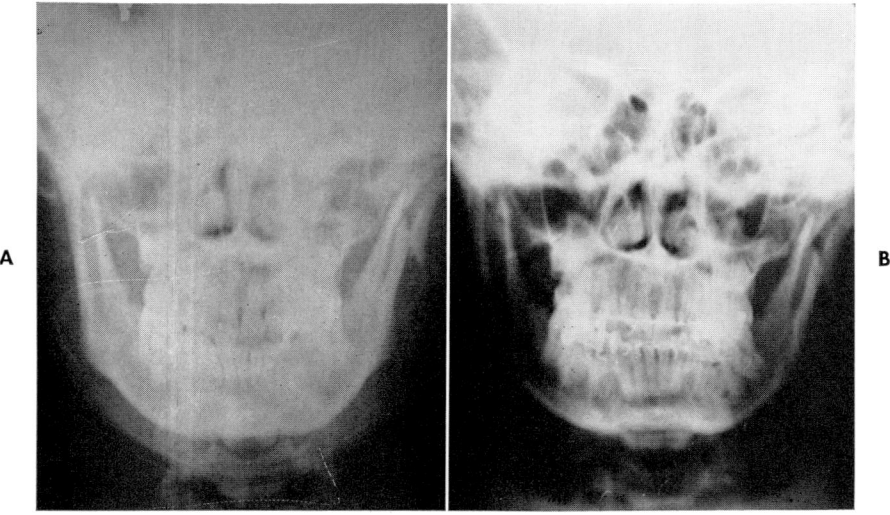

Fig. 19-54. Fracture similar to that shown in Fig. 19-53, with bone contact of fragments, which was successfully treated conservatively. **A,** Preoperative view. **B,** Postoperative view.

the attachment of the lateral pterygoid muscle to prevent redislocation of the condyle. Thoma immobilizes the severely displaced condyle that has few if any attachments by means of a catgut suture through holes to the glenoid fossa or by skeletal pin fixation between the condylar head and the eminentia articularis.

The wound is closed in layers, with particular attention to good closure of the articular capsule. A pressure bandage is placed over the wound, and a head bandage made with elastic adhesive tape is placed before the anesthesia is lightened. The endotracheal tube is removed before the patient "bucks" on it.

The submandibular approach is used if the fracture is situated outside of the capsule at the base of the condylar neck (Figs. 19-53 and 19-54). As a matter of fact, this approach is recommended for most cases of open reduction of the condyle. For a description of the surgical approach see Chapter 2. The fracture site can be exposed well by the use of long, narrow-angle Army-Navy retractors. It may be necessary at this stage to administer curare, 60 to 90 units, or succinylcholine hydrochloride, 20 mg., intravenously to provide muscular relaxation.

The same general technique of direct wiring, using two holes, can be employed as described previously. The thin fragments in the condylar neck are usually telescoped. Therefore the ordinary placement of wires will further telescope the fragments rather than hold them distracted in correct position. A small amount of telescoping of the fragments does not seem to affect correct function, particularly in the presence of poor dentition. Lateral contact of the bone ends is important to healing, although the healing is slower. Several methods to overcome telescoping are employed. A figure-of-eight wiring offers some advantage. If one cortex is longer than the other, one hole is drilled through both fragments and the fragments are wired together. A rounded gutter plate can be placed around the posterior border and wired into place, or a flat, three-pronged plate can be screwed into the lateral surface. The lateral pterygoid muscle attachment often is removed surgically to prevent subsequent dislocation through muscle spasm. Surgical closure of the wound and the immediate postoperative treatment are similar to the procedures described previously.

The Chalmers J. Lyons Club in 1947 reviewed the postoperative results of 120 cases of fractured condyles. They found that fractures treated by closed procedures healed satisfactorily without accurate alignment of the fragments, that ankylosis occurred infrequently, that disturbances to epiphyseal growth did not appear among the younger or skeletally immature patients, and that conservative methods of closed reduction and intermaxillary fixation were simple and effective.

In a 5-year survey of 540 jaw fractures at the District of Columbia General Hospital were found 115 cases of condylar fracture with a total of 123 condylar fractures (8 being bilateral). Of these, 16 were intracapsular, 64 were extracapsular, and 43 were subcondylar (a total of 107 extracapsular fractures). Thirteen cases were in children. Condyles were fractured in 21% of all cases of jaw fracture. Treatment was as follows: no treatment, 14 cases; conservative treatment, 96 cases; and open reduction, 12 cases. One case of postoperative ankylosis developed in a conservatively treated case.

The general consensus today in the management of the condyle fracture is toward conservative (that is, closed) treatment.[11-14] This is particularly true in the unilateral case. No figures are available to indicate the percentage of ankylosis following open reduction of the condyle, which would necessitate later resection of the condyle. This seems to be an infrequent complication. However, function following the open procedure does not seem to be better than that following the closed procedure, in spite of the rather time-consuming procedure in a hazardous location.

The bilateral case presents a different problem. If proper ramus height is afforded by a nondisplaced condylar fracture on at least one side, open bite may not result. If ramus height is collapsed on both sides, consideration should be given to an open procedure on at least one side. If a low extracapsular fracture occurs on one side, that side should be opened through a submandibular approach. True temporomandibular joint function then will be made possible through direct bone healing on the one side. Both sides can be wired directly if the fractures demand it.

Smith and Robinson[15] presented an interesting case of bilateral joint fracture. The fractures occurred several years apart. Re-

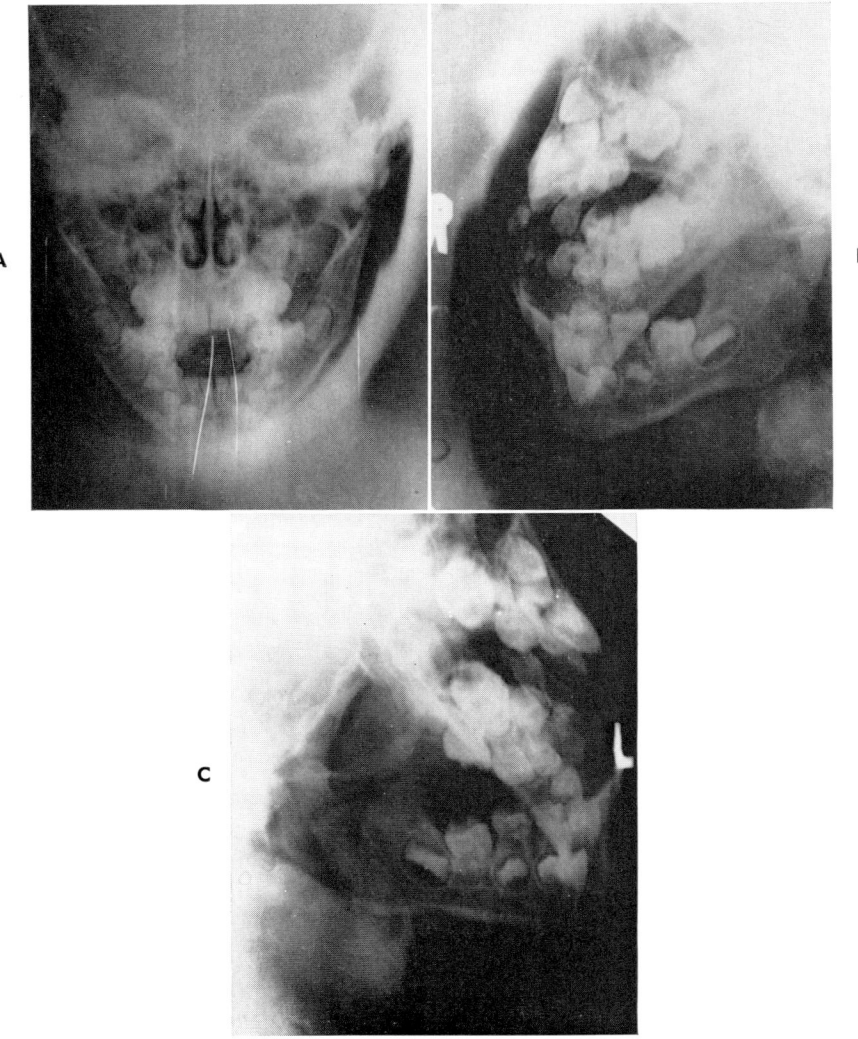

Fig. 19-55. Bilateral intracapsular condylar fractures with medial bowing in a child 6 years of age treated conservatively. A, Posteroanterior view. B, Right condylar fracture. C, Left condylar fracture.

peated intermaxillary wiring for a total of 3½ years was followed in each instance by open bite when the wires were removed. When the patient was presented to them, they performed a bilateral joint reconstruction by placing in each glenoid fossa a piece of bone that was designed to ankylose to the fossa and to the ramus. Later the two sides were resected at the graft-ramus junction and preformed metal guide plates were placed to form joint surfaces. Function was excellent.

Observation is continuing on condyle fractures in children (Fig. 19-55). The main growth center of the jaw is located in the condylar region. A study conducted elsewhere was said to show that portions of the growth center in rats extended some distance down the posterior border of the ramus. For this reason the separation of the growth center from the rest of the jaw is being studied.

The mandibular growth that is associated with the condylar growth center occurs between 1 and 5 years of age in the human being. A period of quiescence occurs from 5 to 10 years of age, followed by another period of active mandibular growth from 10 to 15 years of age. This latter growth is associated with muscular function more than with the growth center, which is not so important at this age. By this reasoning the most critical period for a condylar fracture would be from 1 to 5 years of age. Perhaps the most critical situation is a fracture-dislocation in a child 2½ years old or less.[16]

Numerous clinicians have presented radiographs showing re-formed rami following closed treatment of condylar fractures. Such reconstruction takes place in conformity with Wolff's law that the shape of the bone conforms to the stresses placed upon it during function. The process takes years to accomplish the end result.

Fractured jaws in children

Two considerations are primary in the management of fractured jaws in children. Deciduous teeth are difficult to wire, and growing jaws heal exceedingly fast.

Deciduous teeth have a bell shape. The

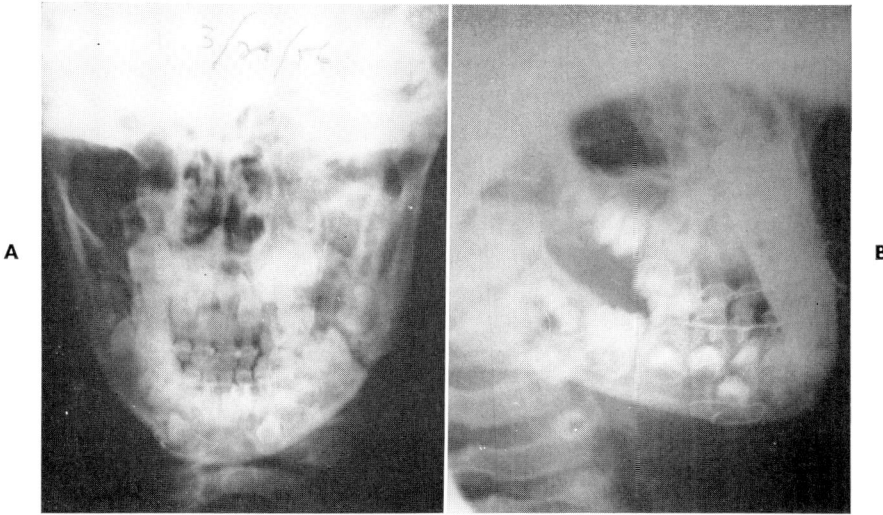

Fig. 19-56. **A**, Bilateral condylar fracture in a child treated by interdental wiring and intermaxillary fixation. **B**, Note interosseous wiring in canine area with retention of permanent tooth bud.

widest portion of the tooth is at the neck, where the wires are placed. For this reason many oral surgeons did not attempt to wire deciduous teeth in the past, turning to the use of acrylic splints instead. The splint has the advantages of stability and the elimination of time spent in wiring under general anesthesia. However, often it requires the use of circumferential wires. The main disadvantage is the time needed for construction, although if several sizes of preformed acrylic splints are available, one can be selected and adapted with dental compound for immediate insertion. Healing usually is complete in 3 or 4 weeks. If nearly a week is required for impressions and laboratory construction of the splint, the preliminary organization at the fracture site is broken up during reduction and placing of the splint.

The use of a finer wire (28 gauge) makes the wiring of deciduous teeth possible. If the permanent first molar and anterior teeth have erupted, retention is made easier. (See Fig. 19-56.)

Malpositioned angle fractures occurring in children are treated by open reduction. Condyle fractures are treated conservatively in most instances. Intermaxillary fixation is placed while the patient is under general anesthesia or heavy sedation. It is maintained for 2 weeks and the fracture then is examined. No fixation has been used in isolated instances, with apparently satisfactory results.

Feeding problems

The diet is a high protein, high caloric, high vitamin diet in liquid or semiliquid form. A successful sample diet* containing 2,100 calories is as follows:

Breakfast
    Fruit juice—½ cup
    Cereal—½ cup cooked, thinned with ½ cup milk, sugar to taste
    Milk—1 cup
    Coffee or tea as desired

*Courtesy Dietene Co., Minneapolis, Minn.

Midmorning
    Milk shake (4 level tbsp. of protein-vitamin-mineral supplement in 1 cup whole milk)

Lunch
    Meat—6 tbsp. thinned with ½ cup broth or bouillon
    Vegetable—¼ cup thinned with ¼ cup vegetable juice
    Potato—¼ cup mashed potato thinned with ¼ cup milk
    Fruit—¼ cup thinned with ¼ cup fruit juice
    Cocoa—1 cup
    Coffee or tea as desired

Midafternoon
    Milk shake (4 level tbsp. of protein-vitamin-mineral supplement in 1 cup whole milk)

Dinner
    Same as lunch, but substitute ½ cup strained cream soup for potato

Bedtime
    Milk shake (4 level tbsp. of protein-vitamin-mineral supplement in 1 cup whole milk)

Food selections

Beverages: Milk, cocoa, and milk shakes. Fruit and vegetable juices. Coffee, tea, etc. only if they do not interfere with schedule

Cereals: Coca Wheats, Cream-of-Wheat, Farina, Malt-o-Meal, Cream-of-Rice, corn meal—*thinned with milk*

Fruits: Applesauce, apricot, peach, pear—*strained and thinned with fruit juices*

Fruit juices: Apple, apricot, grape, grapefruit, orange, pineapple, tomato

Meat: Beef, lamb, pork, veal, liver—*strained and thinned with broth or bouillon*

Vegetables: Beets, carrots, wax beans, green beans, peas, asparagus, spinach, mashed squash—*strained and thinned with vegetable juice*

Vegetable juice: Can be the water used in cooking, or liquid from canned vegetables, or commercially prepared vegetable juices

Cream soup: Make with strained vegetable and milk or use commercial soup thinned with milk

Seasoning: Sugar may be added to tart juices or any seasonings used in any foods to suit your taste

Instructions to patient: Follow the feeding schedule above, selecting foods from the accompanying list. Larger amounts may be taken, but be certain to follow the basic meal plan. For the strained foods, you can use prepared baby foods or you can liquefy common table foods in a mechanical blender. Potatoes can be mashed or strained by hand. IMPORTANT: The three protein-vitamin-mineral nourishments ensure nutritional adequacy in this liquid diet and must be taken. Additional liquids and beverages may be taken, provided they do not interfere with above feeding schedule.

The patient should be fed six times a day. He is unable to obtain enough nourishment in the ordinary regime of three meals a day. Perhaps this is associated with the small particle size, which eliminates bulky pieces in the diet.

A calorie chart is important to the fracture patient. He should know how many calories are present in each ounce of the special mixture and how many are in supplementary foods and beverages. He should know also how many calories are necessary to maintain his weight at his present level of activity. The decision then is made whether he should maintain his present weight, gain, or lose weight. Some individuals will lose weight when loss is not indicated, and attention should be given to supplements that will make the diet as attractive as possible. Other persons will gain a tremendous amount of weight, especially with ice cream soda supplements. Some individuals who are overweight will use this situation to lose weight deliberately. This should be encouraged if the amount of loss each week is not too drastic and the patient receives adequate nourishment.

Many modern food advances have a place in this problem.[17] Milk and egg powders and protein supplements make nourishment possible without great quantity. The electric food blender makes possible a balanced diet of the same foods that the rest of the family eats rather than the monotonous dairy food diet. The meal is made more palatable by the electric blender because the individual vegetables and meat can be served as separate servings rather than as a nonspecific conglomeration. A soup preceding and a liquid dessert following the meal constitute a normal fare, except for particle size. The importance of meat in the diet is emphasized by faster healing, especially if the meat is not overcooked. Meats canned for babies are excellent if a food blender is unavailable, although they are expensive.

Intravenous feeding with a supplement of 5% protein hydrolysate and vitamins is the method of choice for the first 24 hours following the treatment of a fracture with intraoral complications or for a severely injured patient. This method keeps food out of the mouth until preliminary healing can take place, and it keeps food out of the stomach. A Levin tube placed into the stomach through the nose will allow feeding into the stomach and still keep food out of the mouth. It is a good method of feeding in the first few days following operation if oral wounds are present.

The patient who has an uncomplicated fractured jaw usually is better off to start with the diet for fractured jaw as soon as possible rather than to be fed intravenously. Ordinary spoon-feeding or a large-bore glass straw is satisfactory. Most persons have one or more teeth missing through which spaces the food material can be placed. If no teeth are missing the food material is brought, by means of a straw, into the oropharynx through the space existing behind the last molars. When the patient is recuperating well, usually he will want separate blenderized foods by spoon. The larger the entrance space the larger the particle size and the more bulk admissible, which avoids constipation.

An old adage states that as soon as the hospitalized fractured jaw patient complains about his food, he has recovered enough to go home.

Time for repair

Most mandibular fractures heal well enough to allow removal of fixation in 6 weeks. Occasionally the young adult will require only 4 or 4½ weeks. Children require 3 to 4 weeks.

Oral hygiene is difficult to maintain during immobilization. During hospitalization the mouth should be sprayed by means of a 10-pound pressure spray on a dental unit at least once each day. The patient must irrigate the mouth after every meal with saline solution, preferably with a water pik. The use of a soft brush is excellent. Failure to keep the mouth clean in a patient who is lying down will permit material to enter the eustachian tubes and allow a middle ear infection to start. The outpatient can have his mouth irrigated with a power spray once or twice each week. Elastics should be changed weekly.

Wires that irritate the lips and cheeks should be turned and the ends protected by dental compound, gutta percha, wax, or quick-cure acrylic.

Pain during healing is not common. For the first few days a satisfactory analgesia level is obtained by giving one 300 mg. tablet of aspirin each hour for four consecutive hours to obtain a satisfactory level, and one tablet every fourth hour to maintain the level. Each day that analgesia is needed the aspirin level should be built up by taking 1.2 gm. of aspirin in 4 hours and then maintained as outlined above. Some patients may not be able to tolerate this amount of salicylate. However, this method has been found by pharmacologists to be as equally effective as 30 mg. of codeine. Because of the possibilities of nausea and addiction, codeine should be used only if absolutely necessary. Then it is ordered in 60 mg. doses every 4 hours with salicylates.

At the optimum time for healing, callus formation should be seen on the radiograph. However, the surgeon should be guided by the clinical signs of union in determining the length of time immobilization is necessary since bone healing in the form of secondary callus takes place sometimes before it is demonstrable clearly on the radiograph. The intermaxillary elastics or wires are removed, and the fracture is tested gently with the fingers. If clinical movement occurs, the elastics should be replaced for another week. Reexamination is carried out at weekly intervals until healing has occurred. Even with the best of treatment some fractures will take several months to heal. In instances in which an unusual delay has occurred, a cast cap splint can be cemented over the fractured member so that the jaws can be opened. Function stimulates healing at this stage. If nonunion is inevitable, all fixation is removed, and the patient is allowed to rest for several months so that the bone ends may round off preparatory to a bone graft. It is not an isolated occurrence to find that the patient has bony union when he returns after moderate functional use of the jaw during the interim.

Following removal of the elastics the patient is seen daily for 3 days. If the occlusion and the fracture site remain satisfactory, the wiring or arch bars can be removed at that time. The patient should eat a soft diet for a week, until muscle and joint function have returned. Scaling and polishing of the teeth should be done, and minor occlusion disharmonies should be corrected by grinding.

Complications

Delayed healing in the properly reduced fracture occurs in the presence of inadequate or loosened fixation, infection, or a fault in the vital reparative effort.

Loosened fixation usually is associated with poorly placed wires. Wires that have not been placed under the cingulum in anterior teeth, or those that have not been tightened properly so that they stay under the cingulum, will not hold. The multiple-loop wiring technique fails if the strand of wire bridging an edentulous area is not twisted so that it fits the space exactly. For that reason the eyelet wire for double teeth or a thin wire wound twice around a single tooth is preferable in areas of missing teeth. Arch bars should be wired to every tooth in the arch.

The occasional patient who removes his elastics for a small chicken dinner should be strongly advised of the serious consequences. He should be warned that a bone graft is an interesting operation for the oral surgeon and that the patient himself will request such an operation when he tires of a flopping jaw.

Infection caused by bizarre and resistant organisms is becoming more frequent. A routine blood culture and organism sensitivity test should be done in all cases of postoperative infection. If pus forms, it should be cultured. Systemic and metabolic disease will cause delayed healing. In some instances the cause for delayed healing is not apparent even after a general medical survey, and healing takes months instead of weeks (Fig. 19-57).

Nonunion is an aftermath of delayed healing if the cause is not corrected. A bone graft is necessary. Sometimes freshening of the area through open reduction is sufficient. A technique for an intraoral approach, freshening, and the placing of homogenous bone chips has been successful.[18]

Malunion is healing in poor position. Poor treatment, an intercurrent accident, or a lack of treatment is responsible. The bone must be refractured and immobilized. However, there is a fine line in judging whether the degree of malposition requires treatment. If the clinical position is satisfactory and the radiograph reveals a small amount of malposition, no treatment may be necessary. Repositioning in this instance is called "treating the x-ray." If facial contours and esthetics are involved as a result of malunion, cartilage or bone onlays have been used successfully.

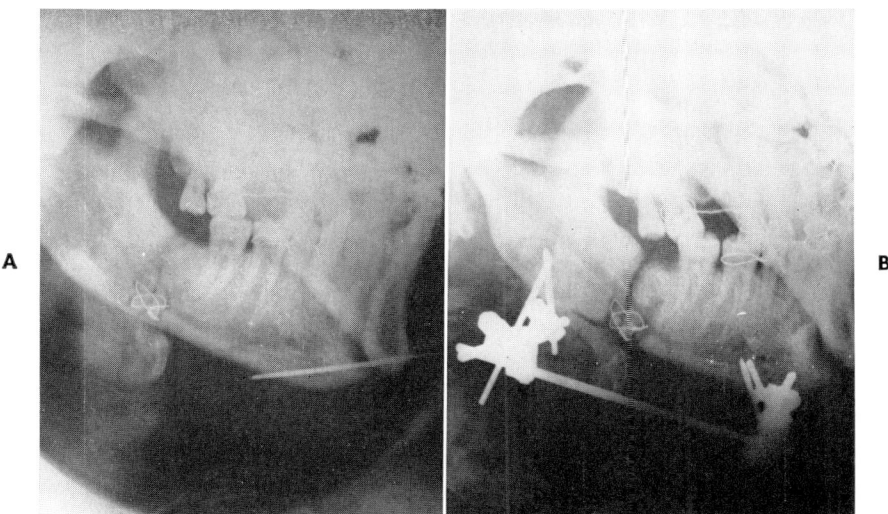

Fig. 19-57. **A**, Fractures at angle and symphysis treated by interosseous wiring and Kirschner pin. Patient had history of nonunion for earlier wrist fracture. Union occurred at symphysis, but nonunion complicated angle fracture. **B**, Three months later. *Proteus vulgaris* cultured and found resistant to antibiotics. Skeletal pin fixation. Interosseous wires later removed and area debrided before healing occurred.

FRACTURES OF THE MAXILLA

Maxillary fractures are serious injuries because they involve important adjacent structures. The nasal cavity, the maxillary antrum, the orbit, and the brain may be involved primarily by trauma or secondarily by infection. Cranial nerves, major blood vessels, abundantly vascular areas, thin bony walls, multiple muscular attachments, and specialized epithelia characterize this region in which injury can result in disastrous consequences.

Causes

Automobile injuries, blows, industrial accidents, and falls can cause such injuires. Rapid deceleration in a fast-moving vehicle can produce a typical middle face fracture known as a "dashboard injury." The force, direction, and location of the blow determine the extent of the fracture. In the District of Columbia General Hospital survey, maxillary fractures represented 6% of all jaw fractures.

Classification; signs and symptoms

Horizontal fracture

The horizontal fracture is one in which the body of the maxilla is separated from the base of the skull above the level of the palate and below the attachment of the zygomatic process. The horizontal fracture results in a freely movable upper jaw. It has been called a "floating jaw." An accessory fracture in the midline of the palate may be present, which is represented by a line of ecchymosis. The maxillary fracture can be unilateral, in which case it must be differentiated from an alveolar fracture. The alveolar fracture does not extend to the midline of the palate (Fig. 19-58).

Displacement is dependent upon several factors. The force of a severe head-on blow may push the maxilla backward. Muscular pull may do the same. In a low level fracture muscular displacement is not a factor. If the fracture is at a higher level, the pterygoid muscle attachments are included in the loose fragment, which is consequently retruded and depressed at the posterior end, resulting in an anterior open bite. Some fractures are depressed all along the line of separation. Many horizontal maxillary fractures are not displaced, and therefore the diagnosis is missed at first examination.

Evidences of trauma may be seen on the teeth, lips, and cheeks. Unless they are severely traumatized the anterior teeth should be grasped between thumb and forefinger and a forward-backward motion made. The molar teeth on first, one side and then the other should be similarly moved. A fractured jaw will move. The distally impacted jaw will not move, but diagnosis can be made from the malocclusion.

Radiographic examination will reveal the fracture on posteroanterior, lateral jaw, and Waters views. Fractures should not be confused with cervical vertebral shadows, nor must intervertebral shadows be diagnosed as fractures.

Pyramidal fracture

The pyramidal fracture is one that has vertical fractures through the facial aspects of the maxillae and extends upward to the nasal and ethmoid bones. It usually extends through the maxillary antra. One malar bone may be involved.

The entire middle of the face is swollen, including the nose, lips, and eyes. The patient may have a reddish injection of the eyes, associated with subconjunctival extravasation of blood, in addition to the black eyes. Hemorrhage is present in the nares. If a clear fluid is seen in the nose, cerebrospinal rhinorrhea must be differentiated from mucus associated with a head cold. An empirical test consists of collecting some of the fluid on a handkerchief or linen cloth. If it starches on drying, it is mucus; if it does not starch, it is cerebrospinal fluid that has escaped through the dura as a result of fracture of the cribriform plate of the ethmoid bone. It is for this reason that

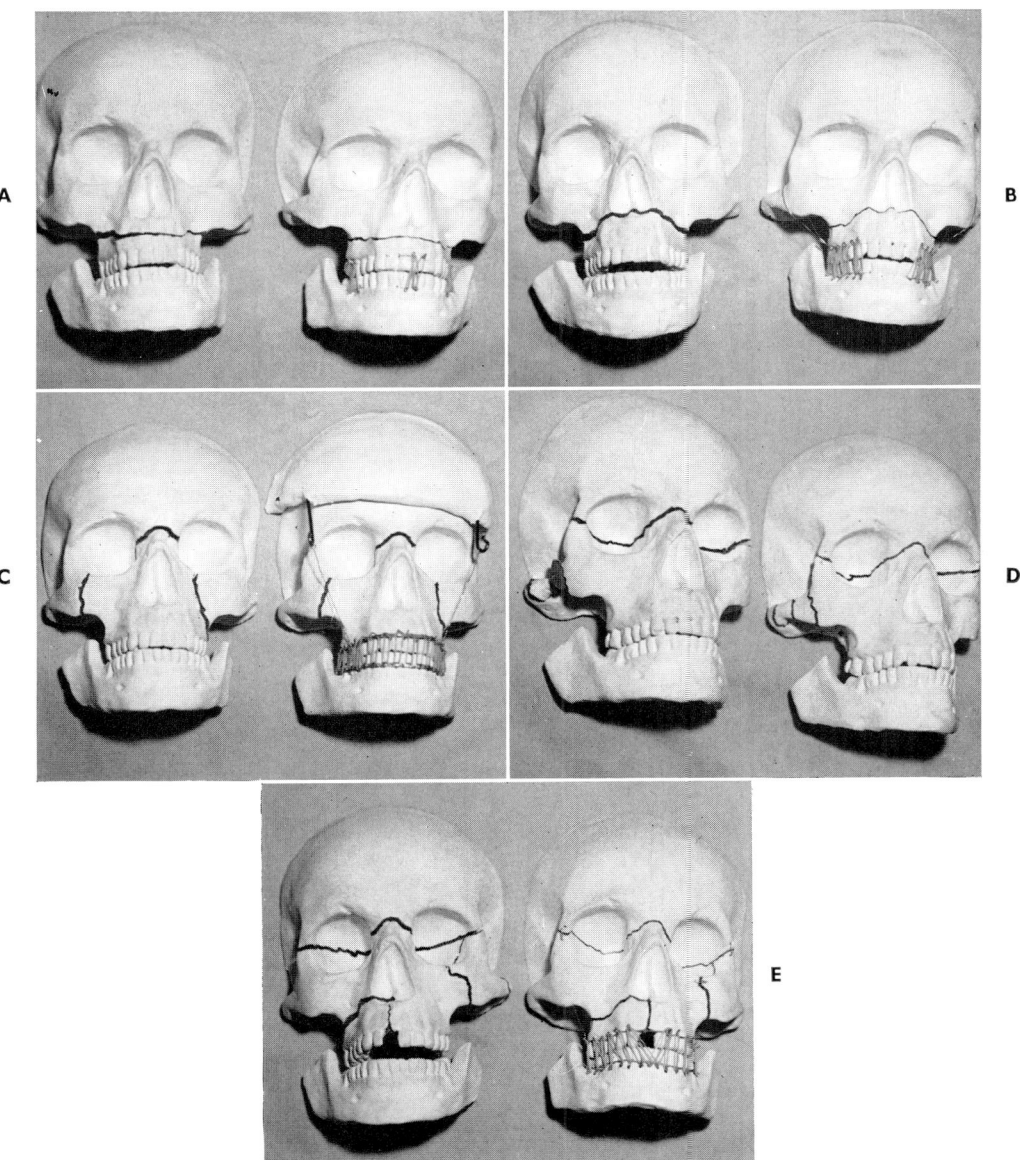

Fig. 19-58. **A**, Horizontal fracture, low level, treated by intermaxillary fixation. **B**, Horizontal fracture, high level. Note open bite. Treatment by intermaxillary fixation and circumzygomatic wiring. **C**, Pyramidal fracture treated by intermaxillary fixation and suspension from plaster headcap. **D**, Transverse fracture complicated by zygomatic arch collapse. Treatment by interosseous wiring at frontozygomatic sutures, simple elevation of zygomatic arch, and intermaxillary fixation. **E**, Multiple fractures. Note intermaxillary fixation, frontozygomatic wiring connected to maxillary arch bar, and infraorbital rim wiring.

clinical examination for suspected upper jaw fractures must be done gently with as little movement as possible. No palpation of the jaw is done in the presence of nasal fluid until cerebrospinal fluid is ruled out. Infected material can be pushed up into the dura if the cribriform plate has been fractured, and a meningitis can follow.

The neurosurgical service should be consulted if positive neurological signs are present or if a fractured skull is suspected. Discreet palpation over the vertex of the skull should be done following a head injury even if no evidences of skull fracture are noted. Edema masks skull depression that the examining finger often will find. The possibility of a basal skull fracture should not be overlooked in the severely injured patient. More than half of all cranial fractures are complicated by basal skull fractures. A history of unconsciousness is always present, and lesions of the cranial nerves (especially the abducens and facial) are characteristic signs. Battle's sign (ecchymosis in line of the posterior auricular artery in the mastoid area) becomes evident in 24 hours after fracture of the base of the skull. Increased temperature is associated with intracranial damage.

The patient with cerebrospinal rhinorrhea is the responsibility of the neurosurgical service until that service releases him. The neurosurgeon usually will permit temporary bandaging or wiring after a satisfactory antibiotic level is obtained, and definitive treatment is sanctioned often in anticipation of faster healing of the dura upon reduction of the bony walls. Previously no reduction was done until fibrous healing had taken place over the defect, at which time reduction of the fractures was difficult if not impossible to accomplish.

Diagnosis of all types of maxillary fractures is difficult at times. Palpation of bones through massive edema of the facial tissues is inexact. The radiographs are difficult to read. If fracture displacement is present, the radiograph will reveal steps and spaces at the cortical borders that can be corroborated clinically. The many structures, including the vertebrae, that are superimposed on the maxilla make radiographic diagnosis difficult in the absence of displacement. The statement has been made that a separation of the frontonasal suture line on the lateral head radiograph usually indicates a maxillary fracture elsewhere, although its absence does not exclude a fracture in the maxilla.[1]

The unconscious or dazed patient should have the facets of the teeth examined carefully to verify the correct occlusion if a suspected maxillary fracture is not confirmed clinically or radiographically.

Transverse fracture

A transverse fracture is a high level fracture that extends across the orbits through the base of the nose and the ethmoid region to the zygomatic arches. The lateral rim of the orbit is separated at the zygomaticofrontal suture line, the bony orbit is fractured, and the inferior orbital rim is fractured. The zygoma usually is involved either by a fracture of the arch or by a downward and backward displacement of the body of the zygoma.

Because the zygoma is involved, the transverse fracture usually is associated with other fractures. A pyramidal fracture often accompanies the transverse fracture. A unilateral transverse fracture is associated often with a unilateral pyramidal fracture on the other side. Combinations of the basic maxillary fractures are the rule rather than the exception. A severe middle face fracture includes transverse, pyramidal, and horizontal fractures, often in multiple form, zygomatic body and arch fractures, and fractures of associated structures such as the nasal and ethmoid bones.

Transverse fracture cases present a characteristic "dishface" facies because the central portion of the face is dished in. On profile the face appears spooned out in the nasal area because of fracture and posterior dislocation of the maxilla.

Orbital signs are important neurological signs. If one eye is widely dilated and fixed, a 50% probability of death from intracranial damage is present, and if both eyes are involved, the probability of death is 95%.[19] However, the neurosurgeon must differentiate this sign from other conditions such as alcoholism, morphinism, glaucoma, and previous eye operations. Cerebrospinal rhinorrhea, skull fractures, other neurological signs, and bleeding in the ears should be looked for. Bleeding from the ears usually means a middle cranial fossa fracture. However, trauma to the external ear, scalp wounds, and a condyle fracture must be differentiated.

Palpation should be done as described previously. In all suspected maxillary fractures the infraorbital rim should be palpated for a bony step, and the lateral orbital rim should be palpated for a separation. If the floor of the orbit is depressed, the eyeball will be lowered, resulting in diplopia. The orbital rims are reasonably easy to visualize on the radiograph, and therefore the presence or absence of a fracture in this region can be diagnosed with certainty. The normally radiolucent frontozygomatic suture line must be differentiated from a traumatic separation.

Treatment
Horizontal fracture

Treatment is directed toward positioning the maxilla in proper relation to the mandible as well as to the base of the skull and immobilizing it there. Since an exact relationship with the mandible is more important, maxillary fractures require intermaxillary fixation. (See Fig. 19-59.)

Concepts of craniomaxillary immobilization have undergone change. Formerly every maxillary fracture was immobilized by wires to a headcap or by internal wires to the nearest superior unfractured bone. These wires often were not tight enough to provide upward traction or they soon became loose and often were not retightened.

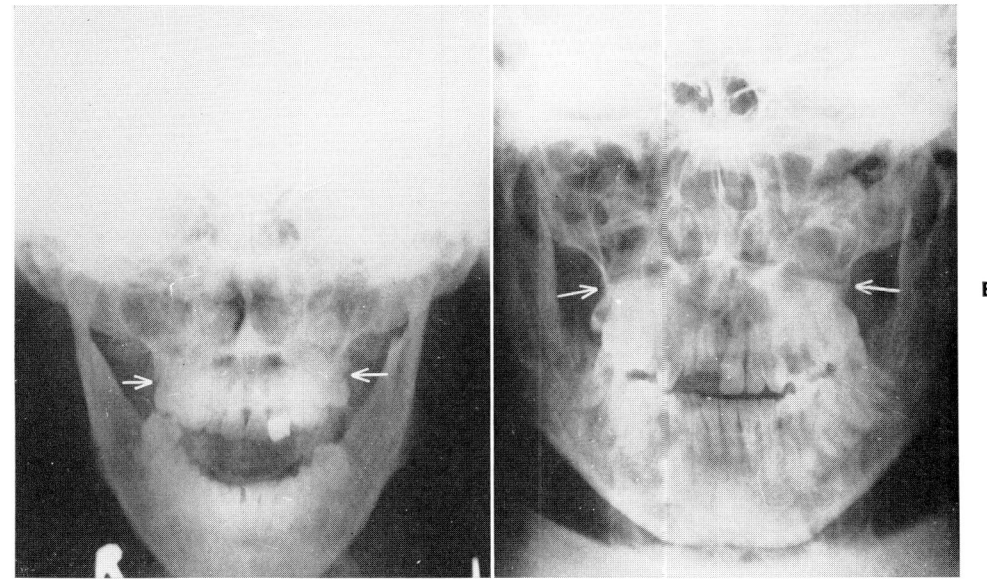

Fig. 19-59. **A,** Horizontal fracture, low level. **B,** Horizontal fracture, high level.

Downward positioning of the maxilla was necessary as often as upward positioning. The fractures healed without much effective aid from the craniomaxillary fixation. The intermaxillary fixation provided the effective immobilization.

A simple horizontal maxillary fracture that is not displaced, or one that can be positioned manually, can be treated with intermaxillary immobilization alone, without craniomaxillary immobilization.

Craniomaxillary fixation is employed in cases of displacement or gross separation to supplement intermaxillary immobilization. The simplest method is that of circumzygomatic wiring. This pulls the separated upper jaw against the base of the skull, and in the case of open bite it pulls the downwardly distracted posterior portion upward while the intermaxillary elastics pull the anterior open bite shut.

If the fracture is high and the fragment is displaced backward, considerable intermaxillary traction with the elastic bands directed downward and forward may be necessary for reduction. Occasionally, extraoral traction is necessary. A plaster headcap can be used for this. A stationary post or a heavy wire is incorporated into the headcap and suspended in front of the maxilla. Elastic traction is placed from the post to the anterior arch bar. When the jaw has been moved forward, usually in 24 to 48 hours, the post is removed and intermaxillary fixation is placed.

An old fracture that has started to heal in malposition sometimes can be separated by manual manipulation or elastic traction. If unsuccessful, open reduction must be performed by raising mucoperiosteal flaps and separating the bones with thin, broad osteotomes.

A few years ago a plaster headcap was placed on all maxillary fractures to position them against the base of the skull. The plaster headcap has several disadvantages. It looks and feels cumbersome, it is uncomfortable and hot, it tends to move or slide around, and it is time-consuming and messy to construct. Many modifications have been made that eliminate the plaster. Many leather headcaps have been made. The Crawford head frame developed by the Navy has three pins that make contact with the outer table of the skull in tripod fashion.

The plaster headcap is made as follows. The head is shaved to the occiput for men and women. The remainder of the hair of women is piled high on the head. Rubber, ¼ inch thick, is taped to the shaved skin over the occipital prominence. A piece of felt ¼ inch thick is placed over the forehead and is removed after the plaster is dry, thereby providing space to prevent pressure necrosis and pain. A piece of stockinet 14 inches long is placed over the head to the level of the chin and pulled slightly upward to arrange the hair in an upward direction. A piece of bandage is tied loosely around the stockinet at the top of the head. A small cut is made in the stockinet above the knot, through which the remaining bandage and the knot are pushed. The upper portion of the stockinet is pulled down over the head. This leaves the crown of the head free, surrounded by the bandage which is used as a purse string to tighten the stockinet. A pencil marks the positions of the ears and the eyebrows. A piece of gauze is placed in the center to protect the hair.

Plaster-of-Paris bandage, preferably one impregnated with melamine resin (which is waterproof, porous, lightweight, cool, and stronger), is wetted with water and wrapped around the head over the stockinet to the penciled lines. Two or three layers are placed. A half roll is laid out on a table so that a piece nine layers thick and 9 inches long is formed. This is placed over the back of the head so that it is closely adapted to the region of the mastoid processes. The excess is cut off. A ready-made appliance such as the Erich attachment or a contrivance previously formed of coat hanger wire is placed. Another roll of plaster is placed around the appliance. The lower border of the stockinet is folded up to the penciled line all around to form a smooth border on the cast, and another layer of plaster bandage is placed over it. A wad of dry gauze is bandaged over the mastoid processes by bandaging around the cast. This provides pressure adaptation to this important area for 18 hours while the cast is drying, after which the gauze is removed. The gauze over the hair at the top of the cast is removed.

The headcap can be attached to the maxillary arch bar by two wires passed through the cheek on a straight needle, one on each side lateral to the infraorbital foramen. Today, however, the wires rarely are passed through the cheek. Internal wiring or circumzygomatic wiring has replaced this technique in many cases. The headcap is used mostly as a traction appliance.

The unilateral maxillary fracture is immobilized by intermaxillary fixation. If satisfactory manual reduction cannot be accomplished, elastic traction is placed. A laterally displaced fracture is treated by an elastic band placed across the palate on attachments anchored to the lingual surfaces of the molars. A medially displaced fracture can be pushed outward by a jackscrew placed across the palate or by a bar attached on the labial and buccal surfaces of the arch and bent away from the displaced fragment. Elastic traction between the bar and the attachments placed on the teeth of the fragment pull the fragment laterally. When correct position has been obtained, the apparatus is replaced by a conventional bar, and intermaxillary fixation is placed all around or on the contralateral side only.

Pyramidal fracture

Treatment of the pyramidal fracture is directed toward the reduction and fixation of a downward displacement of the maxilla

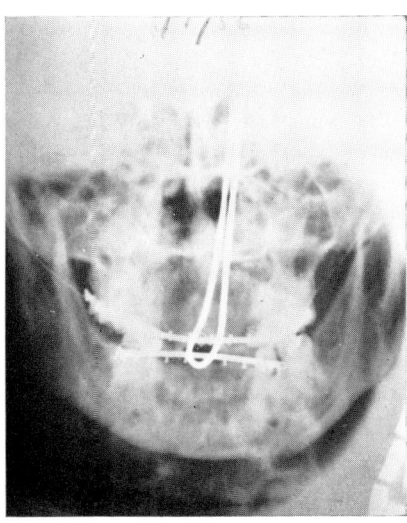

Fig. 19-60. Pyramidal fracture. Bar suspended in front of face, from headcap, was used to pull backwardly displaced maxilla forward. Note circumzygomatic wires.

frequently seen in this injury and reduction of concomitant nasal fractures (Fig. 19-60).

Intermaxillary wires or arch bars are placed. Manual or elastic traction usually reduces the fracture, and intermaxillary immobilization is accomplished. The pyramidal fracture that is severely displaced backward may require manual separation of the lateral portions to disimpact the central pyramidal portion and bring it forward with specially designed forceps. Craniomaxillary fixation then is placed. A head bandage or a headcap may be necessary for extraoral upward traction, particularly in a delayed case, before intermaxillary immobilization is possible. However, internal wiring is used more often. The first intact bone above the fracture is used for suspension on each side. The lateral portion of the infraorbital rim may be used on one side. The lateral margin of the supraorbital rim may be used on one or both sides. Circumzygomatic wiring can be used occasionally, although one or both zygomatic complexes can be involved in this injury.

The nasal fractures are managed by the otolaryngologist or the plastic surgeon. They are reduced by manipulation and shaping, followed by support. The procedure is accompanied by much hemorrhage, which must be managed effectively in the presence of wired jaws. Some clinicians prefer to wait until the maxillary fracture has healed and then perform a submucous resection to reshape the nose. Others prefer to reduce the nasal fractures immediately after the maxillary fractures are reduced. The immediate reduction is done more frequently.

Transverse fracture

Because the zygoma and possibly the zygomatic arch are fractured, the treatment of the transverse fracture is complicated. The circumzygomatic wire cannot be used except in cases of unilateral transverse fracture, in which it can be used on one side. If internal wiring is used, the maxilla is fixed to the first solid bone above the fractures.

A recent fracture that is not complicated by a skull fracture precluding the use of a headcap can be suspended by means of wires through the cheeks.

If the zygoma is depressed, a small skin incision is made on the face at the anteroinferior border. A small hemostat is used for blunt dissection to the bone. A large Kelly forceps is placed under the zygoma and the zygoma lifted upward and outward. The frontozygomatic suture line and the infraorbital rim are examined for position. The zygoma ordinarily will stay in the reduced position. The wound is closed with a silk mattress skin suture. Some type of craniomaxillary fixation is placed.

If the reduction is not satisfactory, or if the zygoma does not stay in place, as determined by examination of the lateral and infraorbital rims, open reduction at one or both of these sites is done.

After the usual preparation the palpating finger locates the frontozygomatic separation at the lateral rim of the orbit. The eyebrows are never shaved. In addition to the general anesthesia, 1 ml. of a local anesthetic containing epinephrine 1:50,000 is injected into the skin for hemostasis. A skin incision 2 cm. long is made under the eyebrow, curving toward the external canthus. It is never carried below the external canthus because the facial nerve branches to the eyelids may be severed. Blunt dissection is carried to bone. A small periosteal elevator is placed medial to the rim to protect the orbital contents. A small hole is drilled in each fragment, preferably directed toward the temporal fossa rather than the orbit,[20] and wires are placed and tightened to immobilize the fracture. At this point it is well to consider internal wire suspension of the maxilla to eliminate the need for a headcap (Fig. 19-61). A long, 26-gauge wire is threaded through the same superior hole in the frontal bone. Both ends of the wire are attached to a long, straight skin needle or a Morin passer and passed into the wound medial to the zygoma to enter the mouth at the crest of the mucobuccal fold opposite the first molar. The wound is closed. The wire is attached later to the maxillary arch bar.

The same procedure is carried out on the opposite side, or if no orbital fracture is found on that side, a circumzygomatic wire can be placed.

If direct wiring on the lateral rim is not sufficient to reduce the step on the infraorbital rim, the latter also should be wired directly. The same general preparation is done. The palpating finger must press through the edema in these fractures, and the finger should be held in place during the incision. A horizontal incision is made down to bone just inside the bony rim. The periosteal elevator is placed to protect the orbit. Two small holes are made and wired together. The wounds are closed.

Since oral contamination associated with passing wire into the mouth may infect the higher areas, it is best to do the lateral

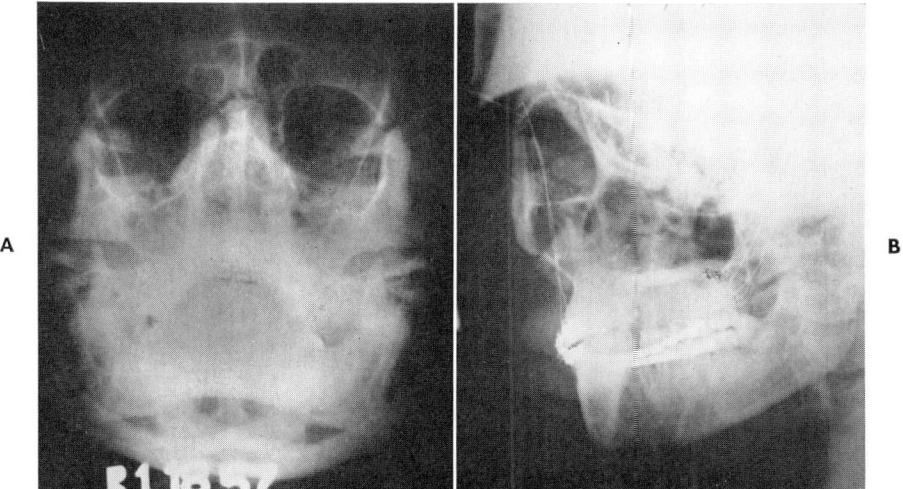

Fig. 19-61. **A,** Transverse fracture complicated by infraorbital rim and zygomatic arch fractures. **B,** Frontozygomatic wiring. Maxillary suspension by means of wire extending from superior hole in frontozygomatic area, medial to the zygoma, to arch bar.

orbital direct wiring first and then the infraorbital wiring if it is necessary. The higher areas are left open. The infraorbital areas are closed. The suspension wire from the frontal bone then is passed downward one one side so that the assistant recovers the needle in the mouth. A new needle is used on the other side without help from the assistant who has recovered the needle in the mouth until the second needle needs to be recovered in the mouth. Closure of the wounds is accomplished after the assistant has changed gloves. Then the wires are attached to the maxillary arch bars in the mouth. The wires are attached to the maxillary arch bar in case the mouth has to be opened hurriedly later. If the teeth are few so that the wiring is poor, the wires are attached to the mandibular arch bar or wiring.

Maxillary fixation is maintained for 4 weeks. At that time maxillary union has usually taken place. Some question exists as to the amount of bony union that actually takes place. The many thin walls may form fibrous unions. At least the thicker pillars of bone heal by direct bony union so that the clinical effect is satisfactory.

The internal suspensory wires are removed under sedation or local anesthesia. They are cut from the arch bar or wiring in the mouth, and a needle holder is placed on each end. The two ends are sawed gently back and forth a few times to determine which end of the wire will move more easily. The other end of the wire is cut as high in the mucobuccal fold as possible. The remaining longer end with the needle holder attached is pulled out. Needless to say, the wires should be placed through the tissues without twisting. The intermaxillary wiring is not removed for at least 6 weeks.

Many combinations of the fractures described above are found, and special procedures for treatment are too numerous to be described here. Then, too, the bones may be comminuted. In instances in which intermaxillary fixation is not a suitable adjunct to craniomaxillary fixation, several techniques are useful. One is skeletal pin fixation between the zygoma and the mandible. Another is the use of the Steinmann pin drilled into the bone across the symphysis of the mandible. The pin is allowed to extend beyond the margins of the bone and through the skin. Traction can be accomplished by the attachment of the free margins of the pin to a headcap arm by elastics or metal attachments. Still another method is the use of a Kirschner pin driven across the maxilla.

Complications

Infection is a possible complication of direct wiring, even under antibiotic therapy.

Malunion or nonunion is not seen often if proper early reduction and fixation are accomplished.[21]

Diplopia may be a complication if the fracture is not reduced soon enough so that proper positioning of the parts is possible. It may result from a depressed orbital floor or an injury to the inferior oblique muscle. In the latter case cartilage under the eyeball will not correct it.[1]

Persistent periorbital edema is a complication that arises occasionally. It may or may not resolve eventually. No treatment is known. It is speculated that this may be the result of a traumatic blockage of the lymphatic drainage of the area.[1]

Poor occlusion, facial disfigurement, damage to the specialized antrum lining, and an improperly functioning nose are possible complications, but they are less frequent if the fracture can be treated early and adequately.

Dimness of vision infrequently increases day by day. It may lead to blindness. This is caused by a hematoma pressing on the optic nerve. Erich decompresses it by removing a little bone from the lateral wall of the orbit.

ZYGOMA FRACTURES

The zygoma is a heavy bone of the face which is fractured rarely. However, its bony attachments and its arch are frequently fractured, often in conjunction with a fracture of the upper jaw. In a series of 134 zygoma fractures at the District of Columbia General Hospital, the zygomaticotemporal suture line on the arch was fractured most frequently, followed by fractures of the suture line on the infraorbital rim and then by the zygomaticofrontal and zygomaticomaxillary suture lines. Fractures of the zygomatic arch may occur without fracture of the other suture lines. The fractures are usually unilateral and frequently multiple, and they may be comminuted, but because of the thick protective muscle and tissue coverings they are rarely compounded. They are displaced primarily by the blow rather than by muscle forces. As a matter of fact, because of the temporal fascia attachment superiorly and the masseter muscle attachment inferiorly, the fractures rarely are displaced upward or downward. The blow usually pushes the parts inward.

Cause of fracture varies somewhat with habits and circumstances. The municipal hospital series finds the largest number (70%) result from fisticuffs and mayhem, whereas the private hospitals show the largest number to be caused by automobile accidents. Frequently the municipal hospital history includes the following statement, "I was standing at the bar, minding my own business, when - - - ." Because of the difficult sidewise angle associated with sudden blows at a bar, the side of the face approach to the zygoma seems to be more prevalent than the direct punch to the nose, even though the latter is the announced purpose. The municipal hospital reports 12% result from automobile accidents, 8% from sports, and 6% from falls.

Time of reduction is important. The man at the bar is collected at once by his friends and rushed to the hospital, where his reduction is accomplished immediately. The automobile victim frequently is fractured in many places, including the skull, and sometimes he is in shock. His zygomatic fracture reduction is delayed until more important structures are treated.

It is difficult to treat a zygoma fracture after 5 days. Earlier than that, the bones frequently snap into place with a sound that can be heard over the room, and they stay in place without fixation. After 1 week they can be reduced, but they will not stay in place. After several months it is almost impossible to reduce them, and no attempt is generally made. Rather, the surrounding structures are treated so that function and esthetics are served.[22]

Diagnosis

The signs of zygomatic fracture are obscured often by edema and lacerations. Swelling of the tissues overlying a depressed fracture can round out the face so that the two sides will be equally full. One unfailing sign of a zygomatic arch fracture, although not always present until edema has subsided, is a dimpling of the skin over the arch. In the presence of moderate edema any or all of the following signs may be present: flattening of the upper cheek and fullness of the lower cheek, hemorrhage into the sclera of the eye, nasal hemorrhage, antrum hematoma, depressed level of the eye, paresthesia over the cheek, and other middle face fractures. When all four suture lines are fractured around the body, the zygoma is depressed downward. When the arch is deeply depressed, mandibular function may be hindered because of impingement on the coronoid process (Fig. 19-62).

Palpation of the arch, the lateral rim, and the infraorbital rim is necessary. Radiographs include the posteroanterior jaw film to show the orbital rims and the "jughandle" view to show the arches. A lateral oblique jaw film sometimes will show the body separations better.

Zygomatic fractures can be considered roughly in two categories: fractures of the suture lines surrounding the body of the zygoma and fractures of the arch.

Treatment

The simplest method of treating the depressed body fracture is to make a stab skin incision beneath the bone and lift upward and outward with a Kelly clamp. If this is unsuccessful an intraoral Caldwell-Luc approach is made into the antrum. The anterior maxillary wall frequently will be found to be comminuted. The gloved finger or a metal urethral sound is used to push the zygoma upward and outward. A rubber bag then is placed into the antrum so that the edge will remain out of the wound for drainage, and it is packed with petrolatum gauze to support the fragments. An inflatable antrum balloon or a Foley catheter can be placed into the antrum to support the reduced parts when inflated with air or even water.[23] The edges of the wound are approximated with sutures, but the central portion is left open for removal of the packing materials. The packing is retained for 2 or 3 weeks, depending upon the tolerance of the patient. Further fixation by direct bone wiring at the orbital rim is necessary occasionally.

An eyelet screw is screwed in the body of the zygoma occasionally and attached to elastic traction from a headcap. This is usually a last resort in delayed treatment

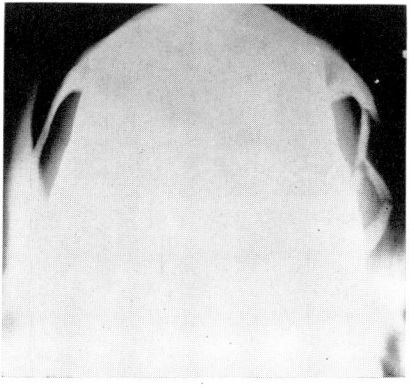

Fig. 19-62. Depressed zygomatic arch impinging upon the coronoid process on the right side.

cases in which manipulation does not succeed or the parts will not stay in place.

The old depressed zygoma can be lifted by means of considerable pull force engendered from an intraoral approach with the help of a large instrument, usually a metal urethral sound.

The simplest method of treating the zygomatic arch fracture is by reduction with a long instrument (for example, a periosteal elevator) through an incision in the mucobuccal fold opposite the second molar (Fig. 19-63). The instrument is passed laterally and superiorly until it reaches the medial surface of the arch. Lateral pressure is then made, avoiding a lever action on the surface of the maxilla or teeth. The fingers of the other hand are placed on the skin over the arch to guide the reduction. Usually no fixation is required. Some operators feel that continued functioning of the mandible may result in displacement of the fragments by action of the masseter muscle. They place an eyelet wire on the teeth in each posterior quadrant, close the jaws with elastic intermaxillary traction, and maintain closure for 10 to 14 days. Clinical healing takes place in 2 weeks.

If the fracture is older and heavy manipulation can free it, reduction will not be maintained by itself in some cases. A large, semicircular needle can be placed under the arch externally. It is placed through the skin inferior to the arch, behind the arch, and back through the skin on the superior side. The attached wires are placed through the meshes of an ether mask, which has been padded on its edges and placed on the side of the face. Reduction is obtained again, and the wires are tightened around the meshes of the mask. This is maintained in place for 3 days.

The Gillies approach for reduction of the arch is an external procedure. A skin incision in the shaved temporal region is made down to the deep temporal fascia. A special instrument is introduced under this fascia in a downward and forward direction to reach the medial surface of the arch. Lateral pressure is generated for reduction.

Following reduction by either method a round gauze "doughnut" is taped to the side of the head, or a tongue blade is taped vertically over a small roll of gauze bandage that has been taped previously to the side of the temple. This is kept in place for several days until the patient becomes trained not to sleep on that side.

These simple methods are not effective after 9 days at most. Special methods may be successful up to 2 weeks, although 2-month fractures have responded to treatment on occasion. Fractures over 2 weeks

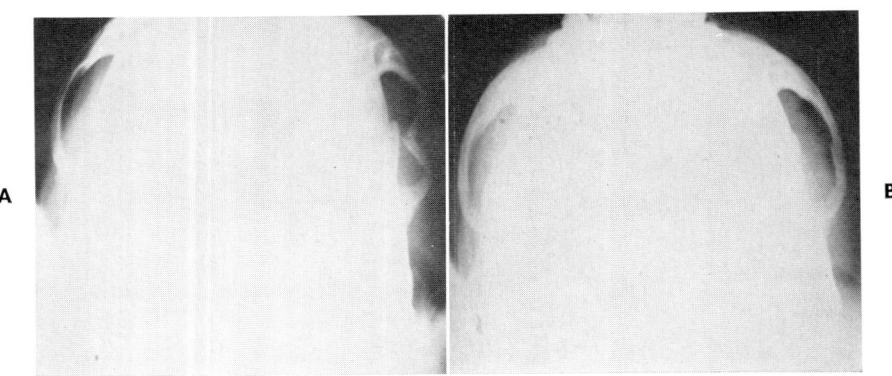

Fig. 19-63. A, Typical depressed zygomatic arch. B, Reduction.

old are commonly considered untreated fractures and are managed as such.

Complications

The treated zygomatic fracture presents few complications. The antrum may be filled with a hematoma, which usually evacuates itself, but it can become infected. Nerve injuries usually subside. Ocular muscle balance may be impaired because of fracture of the orbital process.

One of the considerations in any zygoma body fracture is the possibility of orbital fat herniation through a fractured orbital floor into the antrum. Cloudiness on antrum radiographs may represent hematoma, fat herniation, or both, and differentiation is difficult even with laminagrams. The level of the orbit may not be depressed at early examination because an orbital hematoma props it up. When the hematoma disappears later, diplopia and enophthalmos will be noticed. Examination includes a survey of visual fields. Diplopia may be noticed straight away or when the eyes are turned upward and outward. The possibility of entrapment of orbital muscles should be considered at this time.

If orbital fat herniation cannot be ruled out, the antrum is explored through a Caldwell-Luc opening at the time of fracture reduction. If herniation has occurred, the fat is pushed upward and the antrum is packed with petrolatum gauze. This may be followed by the insertion of a silastic sheet over the fractured orbital floor through an infraorbital incision, although this procedure often is not necessary. If a strong possibility exists that herniation has occurred, the silastic sheet is placed first to protect the globe from possible injury by sharp bony spicules, followed by the antrum packing if necessary.

The untreated fracture creates a marked flatness of the face. The coronoid process may be impinged upon by the depressed fracture so that mouth opening is difficult if not impossible. The coronoid process is removed. The eyeball may be depressed downward with its floor. Rarely is an attempt made to correct an old depressed orbital floor since it cannot be done successfully. Cartilage or bone grafts are placed over the depressed arch and inserted into the orbital floor to prop up the eyeball. Erich[1] advocates a spongiosa paste made from fresh autogenous iliac crest bone for placing in a tunnel over the arch to build it out. It is placed through a temporal incision and molded from the outside. It is firm in 3 days.

REFERENCES

1. Erich, J. B.: Unpublished addresses.
2. Johnson, L.: Unpublished address.
3. Weinman, J. P., and Sicher, H.: Bone and bones, fundamentals of bone biology, ed. 2, St. Louis, 1965, The C. V. Mosby Co., pp. 314-330.
4. Huelke, D. F., and Burdi, A. R.: Location of mandibular fractures related to teeth and edentulous regions, J. Oral Surg. **22:**396, 1964.
5. Fry, W. K., Shepherd, P. R., McLeod, A. C., and Parfitt, G. J.: The dental treatment of maxillofacial injuries, Oxford, 1942, Blackwell Scientific Publications, p. 104ff.
6. Akamine, R. N.: Diagnosis of traumatic injuries of the face and jaws, Oral Surg. **8:**352, 1955.
7. Laing, P. G.: The consultant, J. Oral Surg. **23:**86, 1965.
8. Robinson, M., and Yoon, C.: The 'L' splint for the fractured mandible: a new principle of plating, J. Oral Surg. **21:**395, 1963.
9. Thoma, K. H.: A new method of intermaxillary fixation for jaw fractures in patients wearing artificial dentures, Amer. J. Orthodont. (Oral Surg. Sect.) **29:**433, 1943.
10. MacIntosh, R. B., and Obwegeser, H. L.: Internal wiring fixation, Oral Surg. **23:**703, 1967.
11. Blevins, C., and Gores, R. J.: Fractures of the mandibular condyloid process: results of conservative treatment in 140 patients, J. Oral Surg. **19:**392, 1961.
12. Boyne, P. J.: Osseous repair and mandibular growth after subcondylar fractures, J. Oral Surg. **25:**300, 1967.
13. Caldwell, J. B.: The consultant, J. Oral Surg. **22:**460, 1964.
14. Walker, R. V.: Traumatic mandibular condylar fracture dislocations. Effect on growth

in the macaca rhesus monkey, Amer. J. Surg. **100**:850, 1960.
15. Smith, A. E., and Robinson, M.: A new surgical procedure in bilateral reconstruction of condyles, utilizing iliac bone grafts and creation of new joints by means of non-electrolytic metal. A preliminary report, Plast. Reconst. Surg. **9**:393, 1952.
16. MacLennon, W. D.: Unpublished address.
17. Smith, J. F.: Nutritional maintenance of the oral fracture patient, Oral Surg. **19**:705, 1965.
18. Shira, R. B., and Frank, O. M.: Treatment of nonunion of mandibular fractures by intraoral insertion of homogenous bone chips, J. Oral Surg. **13**:306, 1955.
19. King, A. B., and Walsh, F. B.: Trauma of the head with particular reference to the ocular signs, Amer. J. Ophthal. **32**:191, 1949.
20. Crowe, W. W.: Treatment of zygomatic fracture-dislocations, J. Oral Surg. **17**:27, 1959.
21. Crosby, J. F., and Woodward, H. W.: Autogenous bone graft for repair of nonunion of maxillary fracture: report of case, J. Oral Surg. **23**:441, 1965.
22. Hinds, E. C.: The consultant, J. Oral Surg. **23**:179, 1965.
23. Jarabak, J. P.: Use of the Foley catheter in supporting zygomatic fractures, J. Oral Surg. **17**:39, Jan. 1959.

Chapter 20

THE TEMPOROMANDIBULAR JOINT

Fred A. Henny

The temporomandibular joint has been the subject of considerable interest and scientific investigation for the past 20 years. It is indeed one of the most complex of the facial structures, producing, in its various pathological states, many problems, the correct diagnosis and treatment of which are frequently neither obvious nor easily executed. However, the fact that it is now realized that many forms of therapy advocated in the past were basically incorrect is evidence that much has been learned about the joint in recent years. As understanding of the function and pathology of the joint has progressed, so has the management of its many problems. Today the vast majority of temporomandibular joint problems can be corrected with adequate treatment.

ANATOMY

Since a description of the temporomandibular joint is available in standard texts of anatomy it will not be included in detail here. However, a review of the pertinent points is indicated.

The temporomandibular joint is a ginglymoarthrodial joint differing from most articulations in that the articulating surfaces are covered with avascular fibrous tissue rather than hyaline cartilage. The articular surface consists of a concave articular fossa and a convex articular tubercle.

The fossa terminates posteriorly at the posterior articular lip. This ridge prevents the direct impingement of the condyle on the tympanic bone in posterosuperior displacement of the condyloid process. Bony lips also exist at the lateral and medial borders of the articular fossa, the latter being the more prominent. The fossa continues anteriorly to the articular tubercle (eminentia articularis). The tubercle is markedly convex in its anteroposterior direction and slightly concave mediolaterally. The anterior boundary of the tubercle is indistinct.

Condyloid process. The condyle is of oval shape with its long axis extending in a mediolateral direction. It is more convex in its anteroposterior axis than mediolaterally. The articular surface of the condyle faces in an upward and forward direction, so that, in a lateral view, the neck of the condyle appears to be bent anteriorly.

Articular disk. The articular disk (meniscus) is positioned between the articular surface of the temporal bone (glenoid fossa) above and the mandibular condyle below, dividing the joint into superior and inferior compartments. The disk is oval and fibrous. It is much thinner in its central portion than along the periphery. The posterior border of the disk exhibits the greatest thickness. The upper surface of the disk is concavoconvex, and the undersurface is concave in its anteroposterior direction.

The circumference of the disk is attached to the tendon of the external pterygoid muscle anteriorly; posteriorly the disk continues into a pad of loose neurovascular connective tissue[1] that extends to and fuses with the posterior wall of the articular capsule. The remaining circumference of the disk is attached directly to the capsule.

Capsule. The capsule is a thin, ligamentous structure that extends from the temporal portion of the glenoid fossa above, fuses with the meniscus, and extends below to the condylar neck. The superior portion of the capsule is loose, permitting the anterior gliding movements of normal function, whereas the inferior portion is much tighter where the hinge movements occur.

Synovial membrane. The synovial membrane is a connective tissue membrane that lines the joint cavity and secretes synovial fluid for lubrication of the joint.

Ligaments. The temporomandibular ligament extends from the zygomatic arch inferiorly and posteriorly to the lateral posterior border of the condylar neck. It is the only ligament that gives direct support to the capsule. The sphenomandibular and stylomandibular ligaments are considered accessory ligaments. The former is inserted at the lingula of the mandible, and the latter at the angle of the mandible.

Neural and vascular components. Posterior to the articular disk is a loose pad of connective tissue containing many nerves and the blood vessels.[1] The sensory nerves are derived from the auriculotemporal and masseteric branches of the mandibular nerve and are proprioceptive for pain perception. The vascular network consists of arteries arising from the superficial temporal branch of the external carotid artery.

THE PAINFUL TEMPOROMANDIBULAR JOINT

Considerable attention has been devoted to the diagnosis and treatment of the painful temporomandibular joint since Goodfriend[2] published the original work in 1933, followed shortly afterward by the widely read work of Costen[3] in 1934. As a result of these two contributions and continuing study by oral surgeons, prosthodontists, periodontists, orthodontists, and other interested investigators, much knowledge has been accumulated in this challenging field.[4-7] Many patients with previously undiagnosed facial or head pain have had the benefit of a concise diagnosis and increasingly effective treatment since that time.

Etiology

Temporomandibular arthralgia is usually attributed to one or a combination of the factors listed below:
1. Occlusal disharmony
2. Posterosuperior displacement of the condylar head resulting from a decreased vertical maxillary mandibular relation
3. Psychogenic factors producing resultant habits of bruxism and muscle spasm
4. A single act of trauma
5. Acute synovitis resulting from acute rheumatic fever
6. Rheumatoid arthritis
7. Osteoarthritis

Many of these factors will be discussed later, so it is not necessary to discuss them in detail here. It is important to note, however, that the role of the decreased maxillary-mandibular relation in the production of joint pain has been greatly minimized in recent years. When it is seen clinically, it is usually either in patients wearing full dentures or in individuals who have been tobacco chewers for many years, so that considerable tooth structure has been lost by occlusal attrition. In either circumstance it is not a frequent cause of difficulty per se, and in patients with full dentures the deficiency is usually corrected by simple reestablishment of a proper maxillomandibular space. It must be clearly understood that muscles cannot be extended beyond their normal physiological limit. Any contest that is set up between the muscles of mastication on one side and bone, teeth, and gingiva on the other will always be won by the muscles. Instead of setting up such a contest a precise attempt should be made to adjust the maxillomandibular opening to its normal position. The combination of occlusal disharmony and psychogenic factors (factors 1 and 3 above) are the most common of the etiological agents and are frequently seen together.

Symptoms

The symptoms arising from dysfunction of the temporomandibular joint are varied. All of the various symptoms may occur in one patient, whereas in another only a single symptom may be present. It is, therefore, of importance that the patient be allowed to describe his symptomatology in detail and, if necessary, follow this up with pertinent questions relative to his complaints. The symptoms that are classically present in this syndrome, in the order of their rate of occurrence, are as follows:

1. Pain anterior to the ear, usually unilateral and extending anteriorly into the face; especially marked during use of the jaw
2. Snapping, cracking, or grating sensation in the joint area during mastication
3. Inability to open the mouth normally without pain
4. Pain in the postauricular area
5. Pain in the temporal or cervical areas usually associated with facial pain
6. Inability to close the posterior teeth completely into occlusion on the affected side
7. Rarely pain in the lateral surface of the tongue; usually associated with other more specific joint symptoms

Of the above symptoms the first three are classical and are seen in the vast majority of patients with pain of temporomandibular joint origin. The remainder of the symptoms are usually seen in addition to these three.

Clinical findings

Clinical evaluation is of great importance and must be done with meticulous care. To ensure proper evaluation a routine examination should be developed that is sufficiently inclusive to rule out errors of omission. The clinical signs that are found upon examination, in the order of their rate of occurrence, are as follows.

1. Tenderness over the affected temporomandibular joint during normal opening and closing motions. This is best elicited by placing the examining fingers at the posterosuperior aspect of both condyles and expressing pressure anteriorly during their excursion. This finding is consistent and must be present to justify a positive diagnosis of temporomandibular arthralgia. Some discomfort is usually experienced in the normal joint by the above diagnostic test, but on the pathological side the tenderness is greatly accentuated in comparison to the unaffected joint.

2. Deviation of the jaw to the affected side during the normal opening motion. This is a common finding since muscle spasm frequently accompanies joint dysfunction and, as such, contributes to the pain that ensues. This restricts the motion of the condyle, impairing or completely eliminating the forward gliding motion so that all that remains is a simple hinge action, with the condyle remaining in the fossa. It may also indicate that the joint has degenerated to the point of fibrous ankylosis. It is a significant clinical observation.

3. Crepitation during jaw excursion. Crepitation may be audible, palpable, or both. It is easily discernible with the stethoscope, but is usually noted upon simple palpation directly over the condylar head during the opening movement.

4. Discrepancy in occlusion. Oclusal

discrepancies may be immediately obvious by casual observation or may require careful inspection and study, including the use of articulated models. The common occlusal discrepancies include the following.

Acquired malocclusion. The loss of any tooth or teeth without replacement at an early date is frequently followed by at least a local disruption in occlusal balance by drifting and tipping of the teeth surrounding the edentulous area. This acquired malocclusion disrupts normal occlusal function by producing cusp interference and prematurities of contact that contribute greatly to alteration in joint function and the subsequent development of pain. This alteration, when combined with nervous tension, is the most frequently noted clinical state. Its correction requires treatment that may vary from simple extraction of an extruded maxillary third molar (Fig. 20-1) to extensive occlusal adjustment and so-called equilibration. Such adjustments should be done by someone especially trained and qualified in the procedure of occlusion.

Inherent malocclusion. Many variations are found from the ideal concept of balanced occlusion. Despite the fact that the teeth may be very acceptable cosmetically, either naturally or as a result of orthodontic therapy, cusp interference may be considerable in a dentition in which no teeth have been lost. Here again a nervous tension state is frequently the factor that produces muscle spasm and bruxing habits.

However, purely mechanical factors may also produce joint pain. An example of this is the maxillary third molar that erupts in a posterolateral direction so that it eventually is in the excursion pathway of the anterior border of the ramus of the mandible. This causes deviation of the mandible in order to miss the third molar during normal chewing movements, which may in turn cause a sufficient alteration in physiology to produce an acutely painful joint. Treatment of course consists primarily of extraction of the offending tooth to allow the reestablishment of normal jaw excursion.

Improper dental restorations. When dental structures are repaired or replaced, procedures are frequently done without proper consideration for occlusal function. In the vast majority of the population this is not particularly important. However, in others the end result is either periodontal alveolar bone loss or development of a painful temporomandibular joint. Again, an important contributing factor is nervous tension, with subsequent clenching, clamping, or grinding of the teeth. It is important, therefore, to check the history of in-

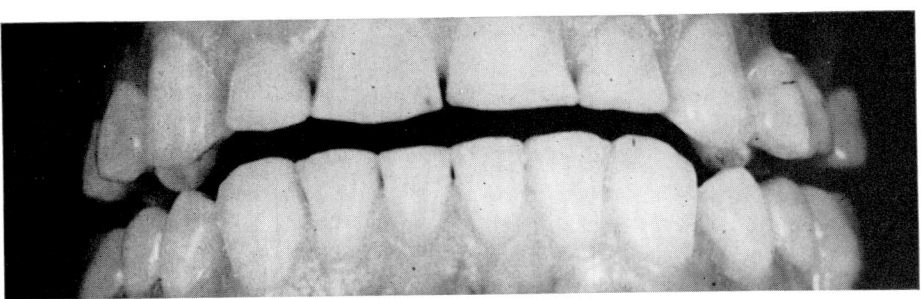

Fig. 20-1. Extruded maxillary third molar that has forced the development of an occlusion of convenience. In centric occlusion the third molar keeps the teeth from coming into proper contact.

sertion of dental restorations or replacements in relation to the onset of joint pain.

5. Nervous tension. This background factor may not be immediately apparent, but it must be recognized as a very active factor in the production of joint pain. Its early recognition as an important factor in a given case may well make the difference between success and failure in treatment. Its importance as an etiological agent can be readily appreciated when it is realized that although great numbers of patients have occlusal disharmonies with cusp interference or even loss of vertical dimension, only a few actually develop joint symptoms. Conversely, those who do suffer with joint pain usually have occlusal disharmonies that are no greater than those of the average population who have no temporomandibular joint problem in any form. The clenching, clamping, and grinding of the teeth are direct results of tension and produce a state of muscle fatigue that in itself may be productive of pain even though the joint may not be involved.

Roentgenographic findings

Proper roentgenographic study should include dental roentgenograms as well as films of the temporomandibular joints (Fig. 20-2). Joint films should be obtained in all cases to classify the type of joint derangement and also to provide a basic record for future reference if the patient develops additional difficulties in the ensuing years. The films should include the normal as well as the painful side to provide proper comparison and should also include both open and closed positions to give an indication of jaw function and possible muscle spasm.

Adequate diagnostic roentgenograms are sometimes difficult to secure. Several techniques are available, and one should be selected that gives the most consistently good results in a given operator's hands.[8] Interpretation of the films is also difficult for the inexperienced observer and requires much patience, persistent study, and correlation of clinical and roentgenographic findings. In viewing them it is important to first become oriented to the position of the condyle and glenoid fossa. Quite often there will be superimposition of other structures over the joint area, further masking the true findings.

The following variations from normal are most frequently noted:

1. Restriction of motion of one or both condyles. This finding is usually unilateral and may indicate either beginning ankylosis or simply muscle spasm. In either event it will immediately verify a clinical impression of joint dysfunction on that side. It is one of the most significant and most frequently seen positive findings.

2. Haziness of the joint space in both the open and closed positions. It is usually indicative of acute inflammation within the joint.

3. Posterosuperior displacement of the condylar head resulting from a decreased vertical dimension. This is difficult to interpret because of variations that may occur in angulation of the films.

4. Erosion or demineralization of the condylar head. This may be a reflection of a generalized metabolic dysfunction, localized osteoarthritis, or may be the result of a localized tumor process. Its presence calls for careful evaluation.

5. Proliferative changes or osteophyte formation, which are portrayed by a diffuse enlargement of the condylar head or by relatively opaque projections from the articular surface into the joint space (Fig. 20-3).

6. Subluxation or luxation of one or both condyles. Relaxation of the supporting ligaments will occasionally allow the condyle to extend anteriorly beyond its normal open position. This may be manifested by true luxation (dislocation) that requires assistance for reduction or it may be merely an overextended excursion anteriorly that is self-reducing (subluxation).

It should be noted that although many pa-

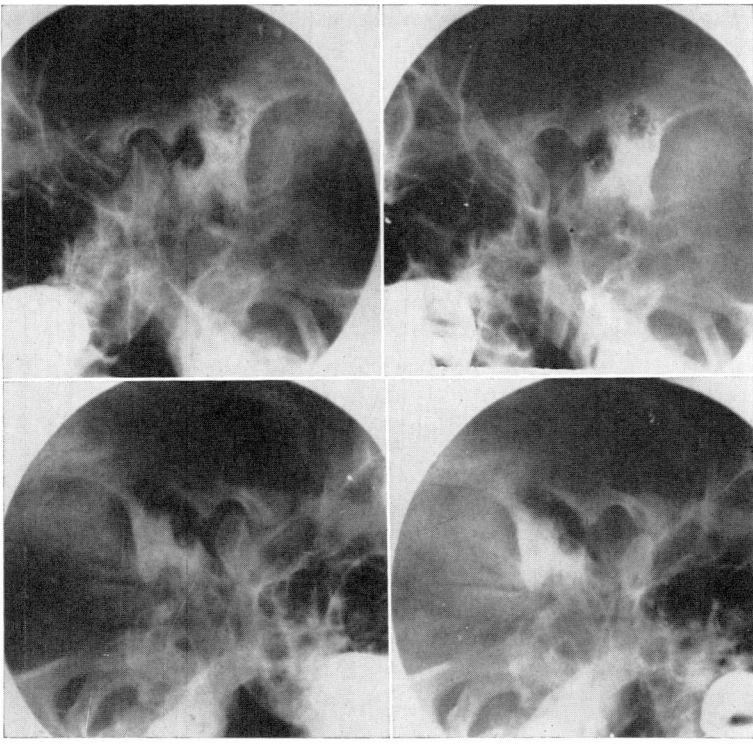

A

Fig. 20-2. **A**, Normal-appearing temporomandibular joint. Outline of glenoid fossa and of condyle is regular and smooth. Excursion of condyle is normal in degree. No hazing of the joint structures is seen. **B**, Bilateral joint dysfunction. In both the closed views (left) and open views (right) there is lack of regularity of outline, with some evidence of demineralization, opacity of meniscus, and inadequate excursion.

tients have demonstrable roentgenographic changes, others may have persistent pain without demonstrable roentgenographic evidence of abnormality. When this circumstance exists, it is usually the result of an early disease process, or the patient may simply have pain of muscle or myofascial origin without true intra-articular involvement.

Treatment

The treatment of temporomandibular joint arthralgia has varied considerably in the past, but in more recent years a relative unanimity of opinion has existed. At present the treatment program should be considered to be in three progressive stages: conservative supportive and corrective therapy; injection therapy; mandibular condylotomy.[9]

Conservative supportive and corrective therapy. Every patient who has temporomandibular joint pain should be placed on a specific program that is designed to reduce local inflammatory changes as promptly as possible. Some points of the program should be continued indefinitely, while others can be discontinued as the patient gradually becomes more comfortable. However, all patients should understand that even though relief is obtained by con-

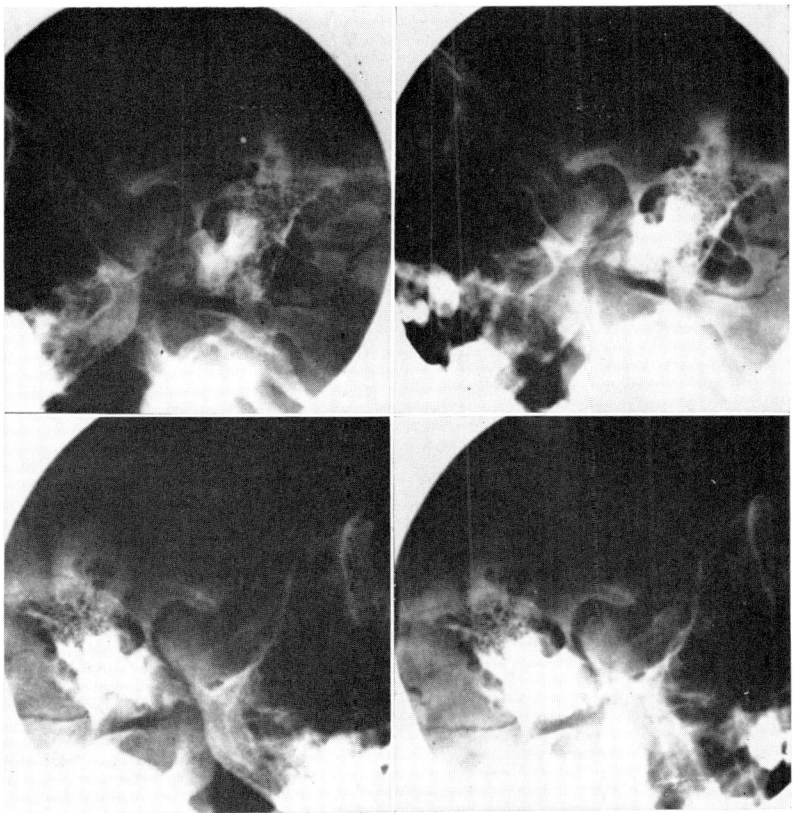

Fig. 20-2, cont'd. For legend see opposite page.

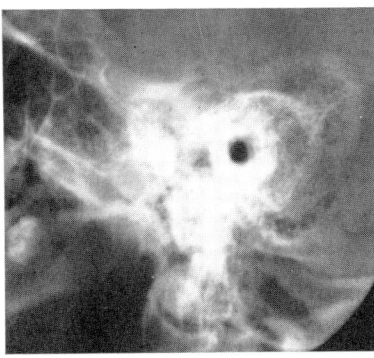

Fig. 20-3. Ankylosis of the temporomandibular joint—condyle no longer identifiable; some indication of outline of the glenoid fossa.

servative treatment the joint may again become painful if it is subjected to undue stress. Because of this they should use the jaw with sensible caution in future years.

Placing the joint at rest. This is accomplished in a relative fashion by placing the patient on a regime consisting of a soft diet and limitation of motion. It is generally unwise to completely eliminate motion by interdental ligation since this may cause an exacerbation of pain by compression of the condyle against the meniscus and periarticular structures, which are already involved in some degree of inflammation, and will not in itself eliminate bruxism that may be present. Voluntary limitation of motion and subsistence on a soft diet allow the joint structures to rest in so far as possible so that the inflammation and edema that is present may gradually recede. Opening of the jaw should be restricted to whatever opening is possible without production of pain. This reduces the stimulus of pain and therefore tends to reduce the accompanying muscle spasm.

Application of heat. Muscle relaxation is also aided by the frequent use of heat to the affected area. An electric heating pad is the most practical form to use, although moist packs may also be of considerable benefit. An electric pad can be used with care at night and early morning when muscle spasms are frequently the most bothersome.

Analgesics. Acetylsalicylic acid, 0.6 Gm. taken four times daily, will do much to eliminate discomfort by its analgesic action, thereby reducing muscle spasm and trismus. It should always be given by prescription with definite directions to maintain the dosage schedule faithfully during the active treatment period. This usually involves approximately 4 to 6 weeks and bears no contraindication unless symptoms of gastric intolerance occur. It is most effective if taken 15 to 20 minutes prior to meals with a full glass of water, with the final daily dose at bedtime.

Sedatives and tranquilizers. Most patients with a painful temporomandibular arthralgia have considerable nervous tension, which is usually a contributing factor to their problem, but on occasions may be secondary to the continuing pain. Mild sedation is therefore in order. Amytal sodium, 60 mg., taken four times daily, is effective and is not depressing. Diazepam (Valium) is a very effective tranquilizing agent and induces muscle relaxation as a side benefit. Dosage varies from 2 mg. four times daily to 5 mg. four times daily in severe cases. It should never be used in association with alcohol since it has a significant potentiating effect.

Regular exercise. Muscle spasm and tension are both relieved considerably by a program of regular daily physical exercise. Out-of-door exercise that is associated with sports is preferable, but not entirely necessary. Daily out-of-door walks or bicycling is excellent and is especially effective for the otherwise sedentary individual. The greater portion of patients of this type are females, and as a group they are prone to naturally refrain from physical exercise. However, they should be urged to adopt a well-balanced physical exercise program and to continue it indefinitely. If the patient is especially tense, an evening walk followed by a warm tub bath and the last of the daily dosage of acetylsalicylic acid and Amytal sodium or Valium will do much to promote a restful night, free of muscle spasm.

Construction of a bite plane. A palatal bite plane should be constructed for those patients who exhibit evidences of bruxism. It should be so designed that only the lower anterior teeth can contact the smooth, shiny surface of the plane so that they cannot be locked into occlusion and thereby permit bruxism (Fig. 20-4). The bite plane should not be considered to be primarily a bite-opening splint, but instead one that will assist the patient in breaking a subconscious habit of clenching and grinding during the sleeping or even the waking hours. It may be necessary for the patient to wear such an appliance continuously for 2 or 3 weeks, but this should be reduced to the night hours as promptly as possible to eliminate the possibility of elongation of the posterior teeth. The bite plane is constructed of clear acrylic, covering approximately the anterior third of the hard palate. The acrylic should be smooth and highly polished. The appliance is held in position by a continuous nonprecious metal wire extending along the labial cervical margins of the maxillary anterior teeth. The appliance should be considered as a temporary splint since it is used primarily to assist the patient in breaking the

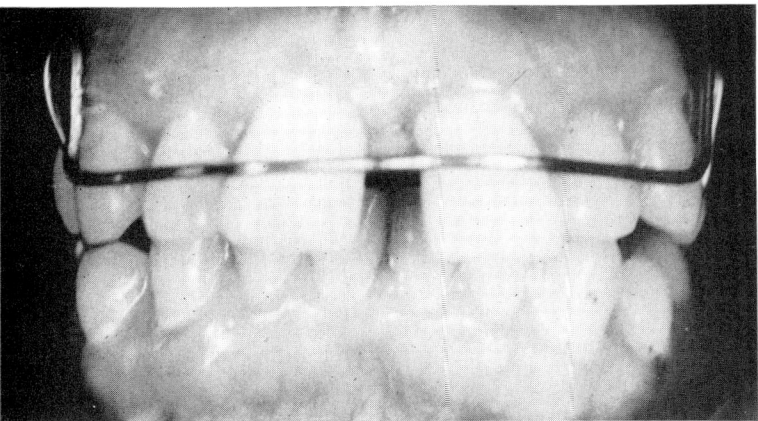

Fig. 20-4. Bite plane in place, allowing contact with the lower incisor teeth only.

bruxing habit. When this has been accomplished, the use of the splint should be gradually discontinued.

Occlusal rehabilitation. Following a conscientious effort by the patient to follow the regimes as outlined above, it is usually possible after 1 or 2 weeks to subject the patient to the indicated occlusal adjustments. The details of this procedure will not be included here. However, the basic objective of occlusal rehabilitation should be the restoration of relatively normal occlusion without premature contacts or cusp interference. This may require extensive occlusal grinding, or it may require a few indicated extractions and restoration of the edentulous areas. The use of carefully articulated models and study of the functioning occlusion are imperative if the objective is to be attained. Ill-fitting restorations that may have been inserted immediately preceding the onset of pain deserve special attention and early correction. Extruded third molar teeth are also of importance since they may cause a subconscious and spontaneous shift in the occlusion that may be sufficient to set up muscle imbalance and subsequent spasm and joint pain. Occlusal equilibration is a subject unto itself, and the interested student should avail himself of proper postgraduate study to develop a proper concept of its execution.

Injection therapy. Injection therapy consists of two types: hydrocortisone compounds and sclerosing solutions.

Hydrocortisone compounds. The intra-articular injection of the hydrocortisone compounds has proved to be very beneficial in reduction of joint pain throughout the body by reduction of the inflammatory process that exists within the joint.[10-12] As a result of recent developments more potent compounds are available. These are Metecortelone acetate (prednisolone acetate) and Hydeltra-T.B.A. (prednisolone tertiary-butylacetate). Rapid and long-acting corticosteroids are combined in Celestone Soluspan, or the two types may simply be combined by mixing rapid and repository drugs prior to intra-articular injection. With either drug beneficial effects can usually be obtained by intra-articular injection into the temporomandibular joint. The following indications for injection should be strictly observed:

1. Joint is so painful that occlusal rehabilitation cannot be started.
2. Pain persists despite adequate conservative and supportive therapy.

Hydrocortisone injections should not be

used routinely, but instead as an occasional adjunct to an over-all treatment program. In those cases in which the onset is sudden and no occlusal complication exists, a permanent cure may result. However, in those patients who have a prolonged history and have occlusal disharmonies and an overlying tension state, relief from injection alone, without additional supportive and corrective treatment, is usually followed by the prompt recurrence of symptoms in 2 to 4 weeks, when the anti-inflammatory action of the drug has disappeared.

Patients in whom roentgenographic evidence indicates extensive proliferative changes within the joint or erosion of the condylar head should, when symptoms persist despite general supportive therapy, be treated surgically. Since both joints are rarely involved simultaneously, the injection is almost invariably given on a single side, although there is no strict contraindication to injecting the drug bilaterally.

The technique of hydrocortisone injection of the joint (Fig. 20-5) is as follows[13]:

1. The injection site must be prepared so that it is surgically clean.
2. The patient's mouth should be opened one third of the normal full distance.
3. When local anesthesia is used, it is deposited through the sigmoid notch and also into the tissues overlying the joint.
4. With the mouth opened one third of the normal full distance, the hydrocortisone injection is done through a 25-gauge needle. The needle is inserted over the lateral surface of the joint and directed at the glenoid fossa.
5. Upon contacting the roof of the glenoid fossa, the needle is withdrawn 1 mm., aspiration is done, and the drug is then deposited.
6. The lower joint cavity can also be injected by directing the needle to the articular surface of the condyle, but this step has largely been abandoned since it does not significantly improve results and may produce additional trauma to the articular surface.
7. The needle is withdrawn, and a small sterile dressing is applied.

Patients who have had such an injection may complain of an increase in symptoms for 24 to 36 hours, but this is almost universally followed by a significant and frequently total reduction in pain and dysfunction. As noted above, the beneficial

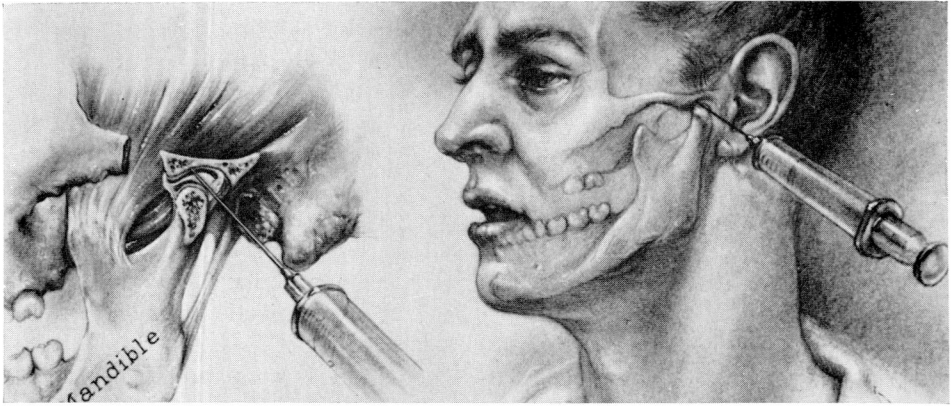

Fig. 20-5. Hydrocortisone injection (25 mg. hydrocortisone or 15 mg. prednisolone acetate or prednisolone tertiary butylacetate) into the superior compartment of the temporomandibular joint. (From Henny, F. A.: J. Oral Surg. 12:314, 1954.)

results will usually persist for a period of 2 to 4 weeks, which is usually ample to carry out most of the occlusal adjustments that are required. It is, of course, always possible to give additional injections if necessary.

Sclerosing solutions. The injection of sclerosing solutions should be restricted to those joints that show demonstrable clinical and roentgenographic evidence of hypermobility (subluxation or luxation). In such a circumstance relaxation of the capsule and temporomandibular ligament permits the condyle to overextend its anterior excursion. Injection of the sclerosing solution should be restricted to the capsule to aid in fibrosis and tightening of that structure. The material used should not be injected into the joint space, such as is done with the hydrocortisone compounds. Usually more than one injection is required, but since a considerable local reaction to the injection may occur, it is wise to space them at intervals of 2 to 3 weeks. The patient should understand that a series of as many as four or five injections may be required.

Mandibular condylectomy. Surgical intervention to eliminate temporomandibular joint pain is indicated only when all other more conservative forms of therapy have failed and roentgenographic evidence indicates extensive proliferative changes or erosion of the condylar head.[9] Psychoneurotic patients should not be submitted to surgery unless the procedure has been approved by a psychiatrist after adequate evaluation. When surgery is indicated, the procedure of choice is a high condylectomy (condylotomy). This approach to the problem has evolved after the failure of earlier methods, which were associated with a high rate of recurrent pain following surgery for meniscectomy.[14] Selection of patients for surgery must be done with care to be certain that the pain is arising from the joint and not the musculature, since if the latter is true, recurrence of pain postoperatively is the rule. The rationale of the procedure is based upon the surgical reduction of the height of the condylar head, thereby relieving the persistent irritation and pressure upon the nerve supply to the joint. This tissue has been described by Sicher[1] to be located posterior to the condylar head and to contain "loose connective tissue rich in blood vessels, nerves and nerve endings" and binding the articular disk posteriorly to the capsule. Although one might normally expect unusual shifting of the mandible in the postoperative state to the side operated on, this does not happen. When deviation does occur it is usually of a relatively slight degree easily correctable by occlusal adjustment. Preservation of the meniscus is of importance since it prevents adhesions that would otherwise form between the stump of the resected mandible and the glenoid fossa, the development of which would cause deviation of the jaw to the affected side. No attempt to restrict motion is necessary in the postoperative state. Instead, the patient should be allowed to gradually resume jaw function as promptly as possible.

The recommended condylectomy procedure (Fig. 20-6) is as follows:

1. The hair is shaved for 1 inch above, behind, and in front of the ear.

2. A local anesthetic solution containing epinephrine is infiltrated into the area anterior to the ear and overlying the condyle.

3. An incision is made immediately anterior to the ear and is extended from its inferior to its superior attachments.

4. A skin flap is undermined for approximately 1 inch anterior to the incision. It is sutured forward to the skin to aid in its retraction.

5. Dissection is begun in intimate contact with the ear cartilage. The dissection actually consists of dissecting the attached soft tissues off from the cartilage of the ear and external auditory canal until the zygomatic arch is reached.

6. The condyle is palpated, and the dissection is carried slightly deeper and then forward until the joint capsule is exposed.

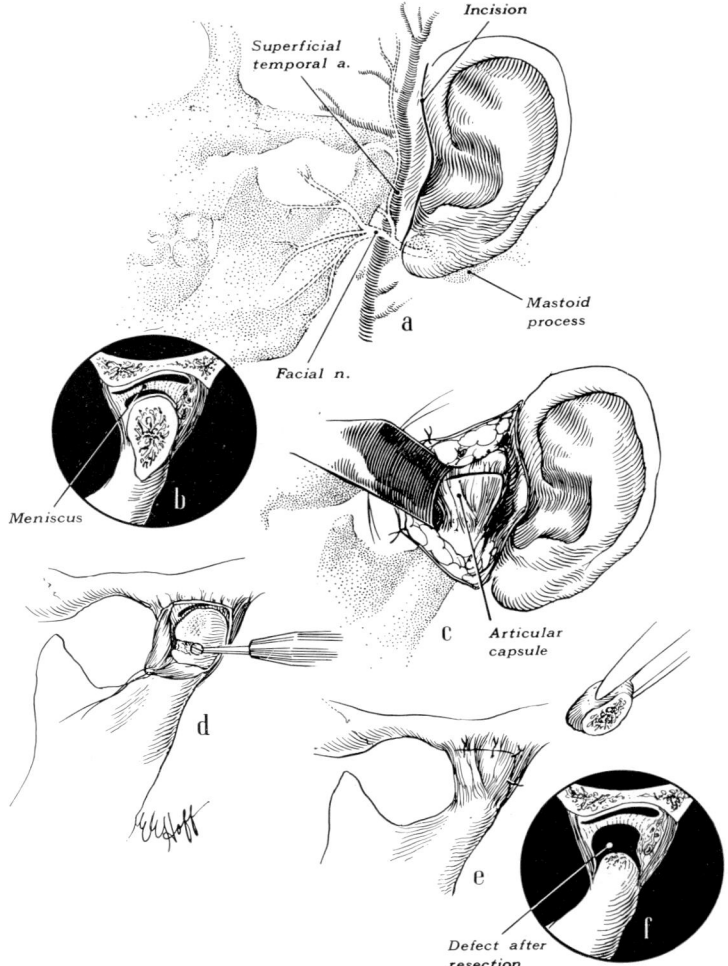

Fig. 20-6. Mandibular condylectomy. **a,** The regional anatomy in relation to the incision and subsequent dissection. It should be noted that by keeping the dissection in contact with the ear cartilage neither the vessels nor the nerve can be damaged. **b,** Cross section of articulation showing relation of meniscus, joint compartments, and neurovascular tissue posterior to the condyle as described by Sicher. **c,** Incision of the capsular ligament. All other overlying tissue has been dissected free and retracted anteriorly. **d,** The condylar head is transected, using a tungsten carbide drill. **e,** Capsule closed with No. 3-0 plain catgut sutures. **f,** Space created by condylar excision. Some rounding off of the resected portions usually occurs. (From Henny, F. A.: J. Oral Surg. **15:**214, 1957.)

7. The capsule is opened through a semilunar incision extending along its posterior and superior borders, but avoiding the meniscus.

8. The condyle is resected 6 to 8 mm. below its superior border. This is accomplished rapidly and easily by means of a small, round, tungsten carbide drill (S. S. White No. 8), driven by a dental engine.

9. The condyle is removed by limited stripping of attaching fibers of the lateral

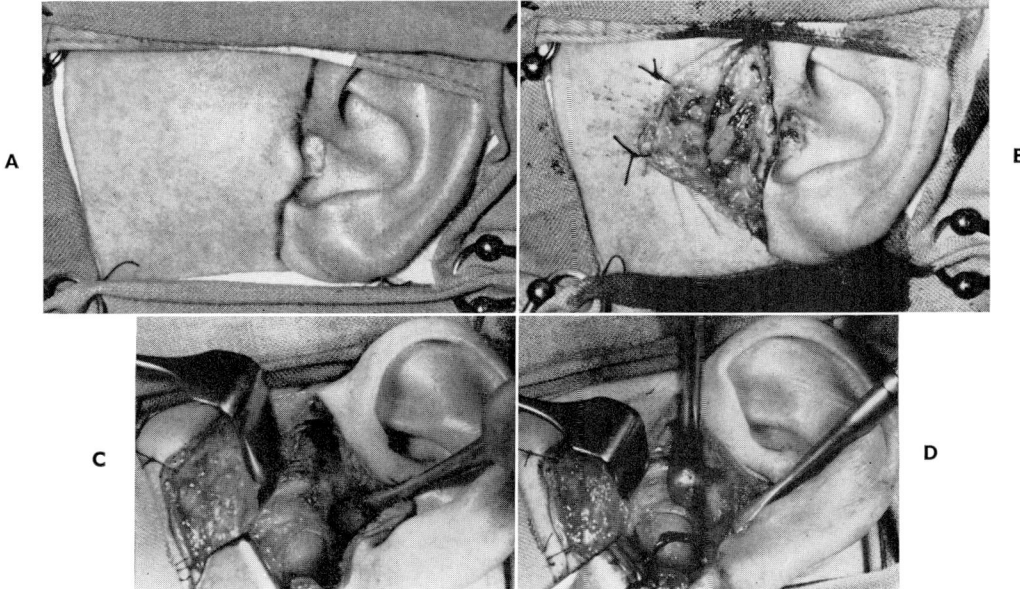

Fig. 20-7. **A**, Outline of preauricular incision. **B**, Skin flap undermined and sutured forward. **C**, Capsule incised and reflected, exposing the condylar head. **D**, Condylar head transected, prior to delivery of specimen.

pterygoid muscle. Most fibers of the lateral pterygoid remain attached above and below the resection site, thus providing good postoperative function.

10. The stump of the condylar neck remaining is smoothed with bone files, and Gelfoam is placed into the defect to control capillary oozing that may be present.

11. The capsule is sutured with fine plain catgut. The balance of the wound is closed in the usual fashion.

12. A generous pressure dressing is applied and is left in place for 48 hours.

13. The patient is urged to use the jaw as soon as possible.

14. Because of the spilling of blood into the external auditory canal, it is usually necessary to irrigate and cleanse the canal postoperatively.

The above technique has several advantages. It allows adequate visualization; also, if the soft tissues are dissected off directly from the ear cartilage as described, it is virtually impossible to damage either the facial nerve or the vessels that richly supply the area (Fig. 20-7).

DISLOCATION

Dislocation (luxation) of the temporomandibular joint occurs with relative frequency when the capsule and the temporomandibular ligament are sufficiently relaxed to allow the condyle to move to a point anterior to the eminentia articularis during the opening motion. Muscle contraction and spasm then lock the condyle into this position so that it is impossible for the patient to close his jaws to their normal occluding position. Dislocation may be unilateral or bilateral and may occur spontaneously following stretching of the mouth to its extreme open position, such as during a yawn or during a routine dental operation. It may also occur when the jaws are forcibly dilated open during general anesthesia.

382 *Textbook of oral surgery*

Treatment

Dislocations can usually be reduced by inducing downward pressure on the posterior teeth and upward pressure on the chin, accompanied by posterior displacement of the entire mandible. It is preferable for the operator to stand in front of the patient. Ordinarily, reduction is not a difficult procedure. However, muscle spasm may occasionally be sufficiently great to disallow simple manipulation of the condyle back to its normal closed position. In such circumstances it is necessary to induce sufficient muscle relaxation to allow proper reduction of the luxated condyle. This can be accomplished by the administration of a general anesthesia supplemented, if necessary, by a muscle-relaxing drug. Johnson[15] has reported the successful spontaneous reduction of dislocations of the temporomandibular joint by infiltration of a local anesthetic solution into the musculature surrounding the condyle. This method requires no manipulation since the muscles become sufficiently flaccid to allow the condyle to drop back into its normal position in the glenoid fossa. It is of interest to mention that Johnson has noted that when the dislocation is bilateral, it is necessary to anesthetize only one side to accomplish spontaneous bilateral reduction.

Occasionally, dislocations of long standing may be present without recognition (Fig. 20-9). Frequently this follows extraction of teeth or tonsillectomy under general anesthesia, the jaw being necessarily forced open. Dislocation may then remain unrecognized if the patient is not examined postoperatively. Frequently dislocations of long standing require open reduction since they have usually had the opportunity of developing a new articulation anterior to the eminentia articularis. Open reduction consists of opening into the joint through a preauricular incision as described previously for mandibular condylectomy, exposing the dislocated condyle, and under deep relaxation medication and direct vision manipulating the condyle back into the glenoid fossa. We have seen two such cases, one of 13 weeks' duration and the other of 8 weeks' duration. Both were bilateral and resisted all efforts to reduce the dislocation by conservative means. Both patients had normal postoperative courses and have had no additional tendency to dislocate since that time.

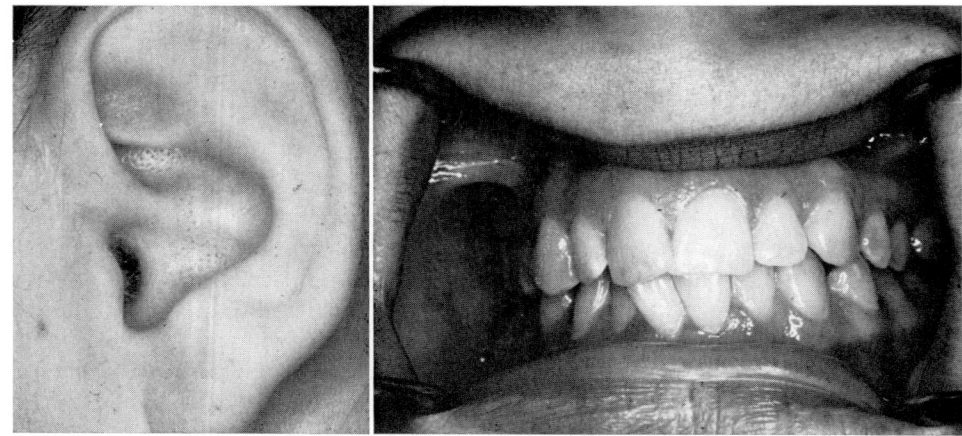

Fig. 20-8. **A,** Postoperative appearance of surgical area 3 years following operation. **B,** Postoperative occlusion 3 years following condylectomy; note midline.

ANKYLOSIS

Ankylosis of the temporomandibular joint (Fig. 20-10, A) occurs with relative infrequency. Loss of jaw function may vary from partial to complete. Surgical correction of the ankylosis is required in all cases to permit proper rehabilitation of the patient. Whereas ankylosis most commonly occurred as a complication of childhood illnesses some years ago, this has rarely been the case since antibiotic medications have been available to control secondary infections. The commonest cause of ankylosis today is trauma. Fracture of the condyle with involvement of the articular surface, hemorrhage, and subsequent elevation of the periosteum followed by clot organization occasionally produces bony union between the ramus of the mandible and the zygomatic arch. Advanced arthritis may also produce proliferative alterations in the condyle, eventuating in ankylosis.

Surgical correction (arthroplasty) involves exposure of the joint area through the previously described preauricular incision. If the condyle area alone is involved

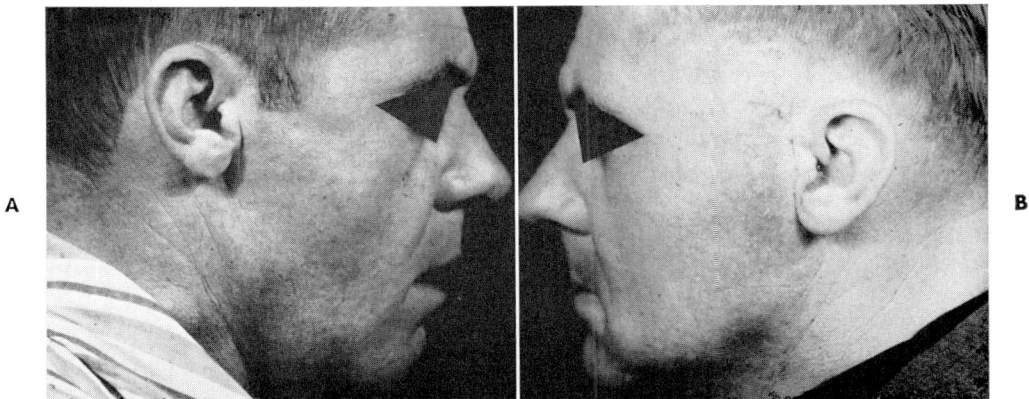

Fig. 20-9. A, Long-standing bilateral dislocation (7 weeks) with repeated unsuccessful attempts at reduction. B, Appearance following bilateral open reduction.

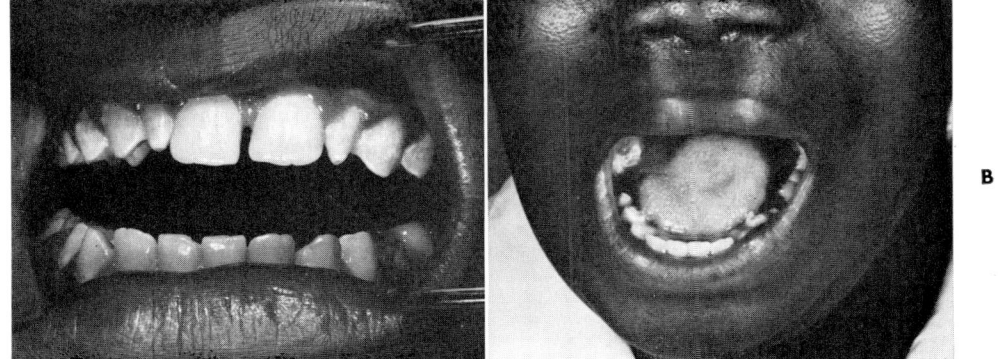

Fig. 20-10. A, Ankylosis of the right temporomandibular joint (see Fig. 20-3) following fracture of the right condyle. B, Jaw excursion following arthroplasty through a preauricular surgical approach and postoperative dilatation.

in the ankylosis it is unnecessary to expose the coronoid process. The arthroplasty is usually first extended across the base of the condylar neck. The condyle is then chiseled loose and is removed. In other circumstances, if the condyle has been fractured and displaced medially, it is necessary to perform a 1 cm. ostectomy at the superior portion of the ramus. This allows visualization of the medial aspect of the ramus and exposure of the malpositioned condyle, which can then be chiseled from the medial surface of the ramus and removed through the wound.

Two principles are involved in developing a successful arthroplasty:

1. Perform an adequate arthroplasty by removing the displaced condyle if one is present and creating 1 to 1.5 cm. space between the superior margin of the ramus and the zygomatic process.

2. Provide early, vigorous, and sustained postoperative jaw dilatation.

An otherwise adequate arthroplasty may fail if the second principle is not carried out with determination. To ensure success it is wise to return the patient to the operating room on the third postoperative day and, under general anesthesia with deep relaxation, forcibly dilate the jaws with a side-action mouth prop. Thereafter, the patient should have forcible daily dilatation with the mouth prop for 2 months following surgery. When this program is followed, postoperative results are universally good, and it is unnecessary to interpose any foreign material at the arthroplasty site (Fig. 20-10, B). Since the dentition of most patients of this type is usually in poor repair, it is important that the patient be encouraged to complete his rehabilitation by undergoing whatever dental procedures may be indicated as soon as is practicable.

Micrognathia may also be a complication of ankylosis because of the lack of the condylar growth center. Surgical correction of this deformity may also be required to develop an acceptable cosmetic and functional result. Although this is not within the scope of this chapter, it should be stated that a combination of surgery and orthodontics yields good results and usually completes excellent rehabilitation of the patient. Bone onlays over the chin area are only rarely indicated and should not be depended upon to mask the jaw deformity, since many of them resorb over a period of time.

REFERENCES

1. Sicher, Harry: Structure and functional basis for disorders of the temporomandibular joint, J. Oral Surg. **13**:275, 1955.
2. Goodfriend, D. J.: Symptomatology and treatment of abnormalities of mandibular articulation, D. Cosmos **75**:844, 1933.
3. Costen, J. B.: Syndrome of ear and sinus symptoms dependent upon disturbed function of the temporomandibular joint, Ann. Otol. **43**:1, 1934.
4. Bauer, W. H.: Osteo-arthritis deformans of temporomandibular joint, Amer. J. Path. **17**:129, 1941.
5. Burman, M., and Sinberg, S. E.: Condylar movements in the study of internal derangements of the temporomandibular joint, J. Bone Joint Surg. **28**:351, 1946.
6. Goodrich, W. A., Jr., and Johnson, W. A.: Roentgen ray therapy of the temporomandibular joint, J. Oral Surg. **14**:35, 1956.
7. Bellinger, D. H.: Internal derangements of the temporomandibular joint, J. Oral Surg. **10**:47, 1952.
8. Doub, H. P., and Henny, F. A.: Radiological study of the temporomandibular joints, Radiology **60**:666, 1953.
9. Henny, F. A.: Treatment of the painful temporomandibular joint, J. Oral Surg. **15**:214, 1957.
10. Thorn, G. W., and others: Clinical and metabolic changes in Addison's disease following administration of compound E acetate (1-dihydro, 17-hydroxycorticosterone acetate), Trans. Ass. Amer. Physicians **62**:233, 1949.
11. Hollander, J. L., and others: Hydrocortisone and cortisone injected into arthritic joints; comparative effects of and use of hydrocortisone as local anti-arthritic agent, J.A.M.A. **147**:1629, 1951.
12. Ensign, D. C., and Sigler, J. W.: Intra-articular hydrocortisone in treatment of arthritis; present status, J. Mich. Med. Soc. **51**:1189, 1952.

13. Henny, F. A.: Intra-articular injection of hydrocortisone into the temporomandibular joint, J. Oral Surg. 12:314, 1954.
14. Dingman, R. O., and Moorman, W. C.: Meniscectomy in treatment of lesions of temporomandibular joint, J. Oral Surg. 9:214, 1951.
15. Johnson, W. B.: New method for reduction of acute dislocation of the temporomandibular articulations, J. Oral Surg. 16:501, 1958.

Chapter 21

CLEFT LIP AND CLEFT PALATE

James R. Hayward

The congenital deformities of cleft lip (cheiloschisis) and cleft palate (palatoschisis) have been known to afflict man since prehistoric time. Efforts to correct these abnormalities have evolved over the centuries with increasing success as scientific knowledge has advanced. It will be seen that oral clefts involve complex, long-range treatment and appear with sufficient frequency to constitute a public health problem. Some form of cleft lip and cleft palate occurs in one out of every 800 live births. Combined clefts of the lip and palate are more frequent than the isolated involvement of either region. With lack of complete knowledge concerning etiology, effective preventive measures are not available to eliminate this deformity. The psychological and socioeconomic handicap of oral clefts may be severe. It is a deformity that can be seen, felt, and heard and constitutes a crippling affliction. Facial deformity with cleft lip involves the structures of the lip and the nose. Further skeletal facial deformity is seen in some forms of cleft palate. The most severe handicap imposed by cleft palate is an impaired mechanism preventing normal speech and swallowing.

The zones involved by common oral clefts are the upper lip, alveolar ridge, hard palate, and soft palate. In a useful classification the normal position of the nasopalatine canal divides clefts of the lip and alveolar ridge (primary palate) from those of the hard and soft palate (secondary palate). Slightly more than 50% are combined clefts of the lip and palate. About one fourth of this number are bilateral. The isolated clefts of the lip and palate constitute the balance of the varieties seen. Clefts of the lip are more frequent in males, whereas isolated clefts of the palate are more frequent in females. Lip cleft involvement is more frequent on the left side than on the right (Fig. 21-1). These phenomena lack explanation and the underlying etiology is incompletely understood. The failure of union of the parts that normally form the lip and palate occurs early in fetal life.

EMBRYOLOGY

The oral cleft problem occurs between the sixth and tenth week of embryo-fetal life. A combination of failure in normal union and inadequate development may affect the soft tissue and bony components of the upper lip, alveolar ridge, and hard and soft palates. The face of the fetus undergoes rapid and extensive changes during the second and third months of development. The embryonic formation of the lip from the nasal frontal and lateral maxillary processes indicates the intimate relation with nasal structures (Fig. 21-2).

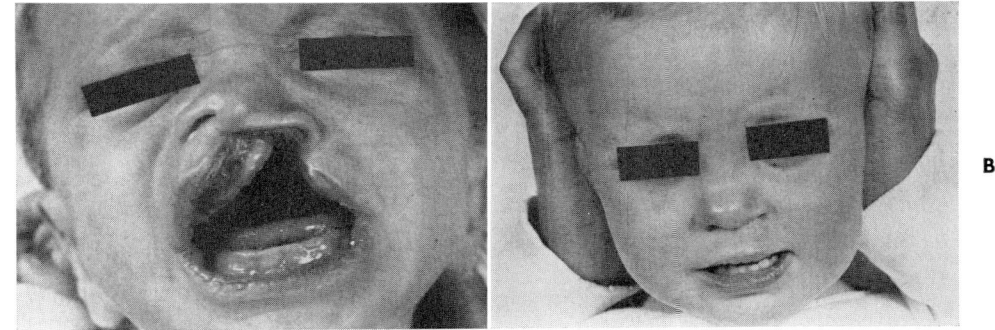

Fig. 21-1. **A,** Unilateral complete cleft of the lip and palate on the left side. Note the deviation of the premaxilla away from the cleft and the associated deformity of the nasal structures. **B,** Postoperative view of the cleft shown in **A,** patient 2 years of age.

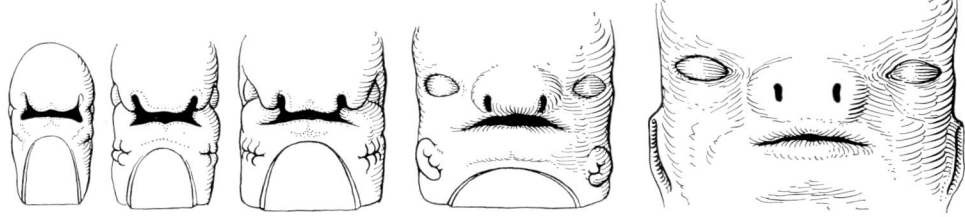

Fig. 21-2. Stages in the embryology of the face. Note that the width between the nostril openings is relatively constant, whereas the remainder of the face expands in development. (Redrawn from Avery, J. K. In Bunting, R. W.: Oral hygiene, ed. 3, Philadelphia, 1957, Lea & Febiger.)

During the sixth and seventh weeks the maxillary processes of the first branchial arch grow forward to unite with the lateral nasal processes and continue to unite with the medial nasal processes, forming the upper lip, the nostril floor, and the primary palate. All structures are developing rapidly, and the tongue is ahead in size and differentiation, growing vertically to fill the primitive stomodeal cavity (Fig. 21-3). The palatine shelves expand medially, and as the face broadens and lengthens the tongue descends. During the eighth to ninth week the palatine shelves further extend medially to contact at the midline and fuse from anterior to posterior for the creation of the palatine partition between nasal and oral cavities (Fig. 21-4). The point of fusion of the future hard palate with the septum is the site for ossification of the future vomer. Normal facial development depends upon a harmonious growth of the parts that are undergoing dynamic changes during this critical period. Asynchronous development and failure of mesodermal proliferation to form connective tissue bonds across lines of fusion are cited as embryological variants involved in cleft formation. Without mesodermal bonding the components of the lip pull apart. Residual epithelial bonds have not been penetrated by mesoderm and are left to span some clefts of the lip and alveolar ridge. The effect of teratogenic influences is seen in a variety of clefts of the palate, incomplete or complete and unilateral or bilateral (Fig. 21-5). Additional

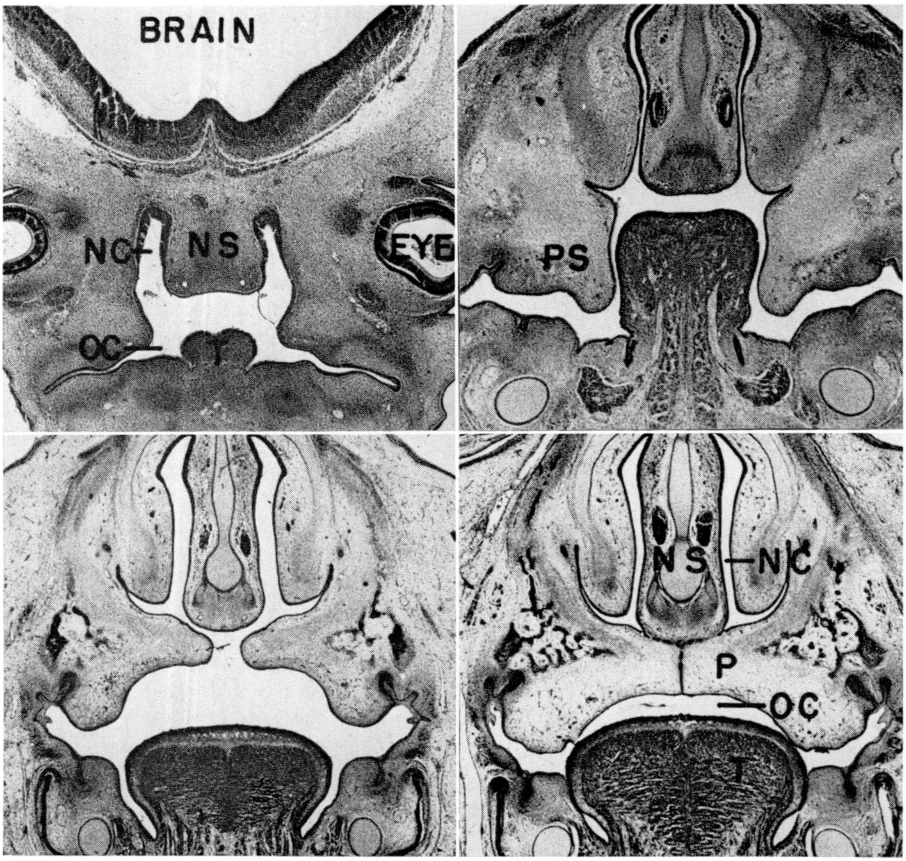

388 *Textbook of oral surgery*

Fig. 21-3. Coronal sections of the developing palate (perpendicular to sagittal). **A,** Six weeks: **NC,** nasal cavity; **NS,** nasal septum; **OC,** oral cavity; **T,** tongue. **B,** Seven weeks: **PS,** palatal shelf. **C,** Eight weeks. **D,** Nine weeks: **P,** palate. (From Avery, J. K. In Bunting, R. W.: Oral hygiene, ed. 3, Philadelphia, 1957, Lea & Febiger.)

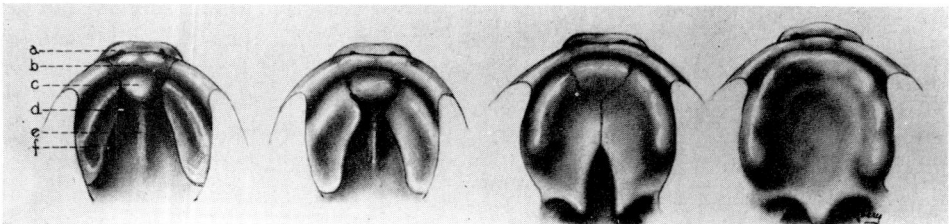

Fig. 21-4. Diagrams of palatal development. Note the fusion of parts and progressive posterior union in stages left to right. (From Avery, J. K. In Bunting, R. W.: Oral hygiene, ed. 3, Philadelphia, 1957, Lea & Febiger.)

Cleft lip and cleft palate

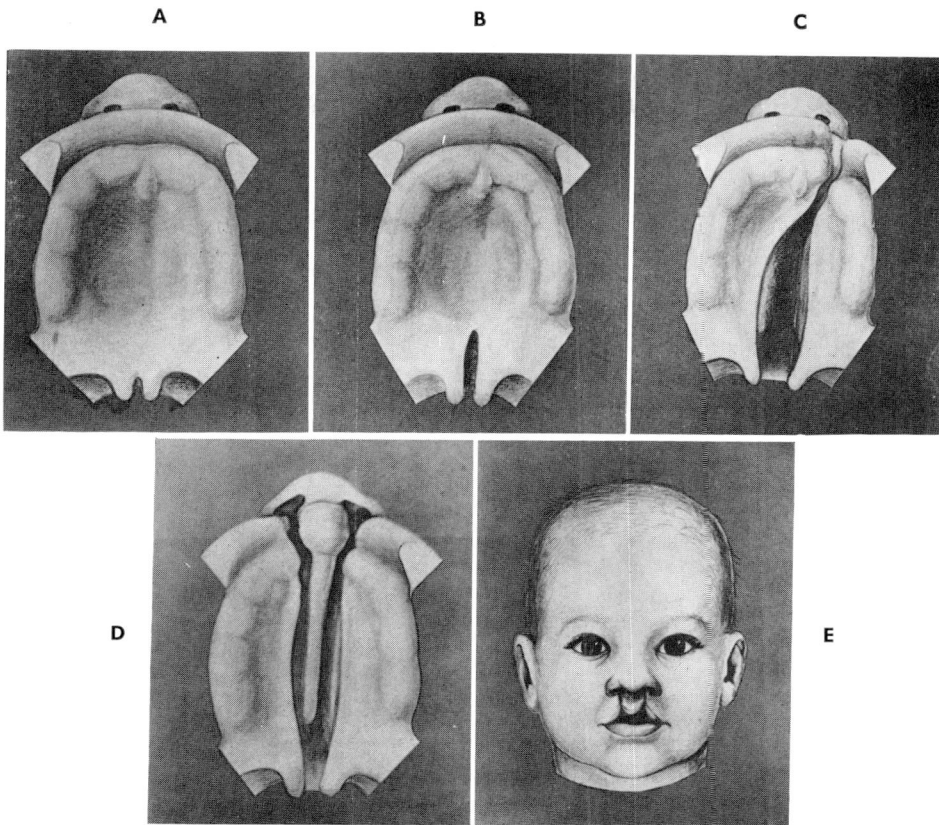

Fig. 21-5. A, The bifid uvula, which may or may not be associated with an occult or submucosal cleft. B, A cleft involving the soft palate only. C, The complete unilateral cleft involving the lip, alveolar ridge, hard palate, and soft palate. D, Bilateral complete cleft of the lip and palate. E, Involvement of structures in the bilateral cleft of the lip.

rare cleft anomalies may involve other zones of the face (Fig. 21-6, A and B).

Progressive central deficiences of the premaxilla and prolabium are seen in the bilateral clefts (Fig. 21-6, C to E). Further decreases in interorbital distance are seen in arrhinencephaly in degrees progressive to cyclopia (Fig. 21-6, F to H). The latter are incompatible with life since midline central nervous system defects and deficiencies are also included. While severe bilateral clefts of the lip and primary palate include deficiencies in midline structure and decrease in interorbital distance, the opposite appears to be true in some isolated clefts of the secondary palate. Here the interorbital space is increased in varying degrees of hypertelorism with or without epicanthial folds.

ETIOLOGY

Heredity. The genetic basis for oral clefts is significant, but not predictable. Hereditary tendency as evidenced by affliction of some known member of the family has been found in 25% to 30% of most reported series throughout the world. Other causative factors obviously must contribute to the production of cleft anomalies. Great variation is seen in the dominant and recessive mani-

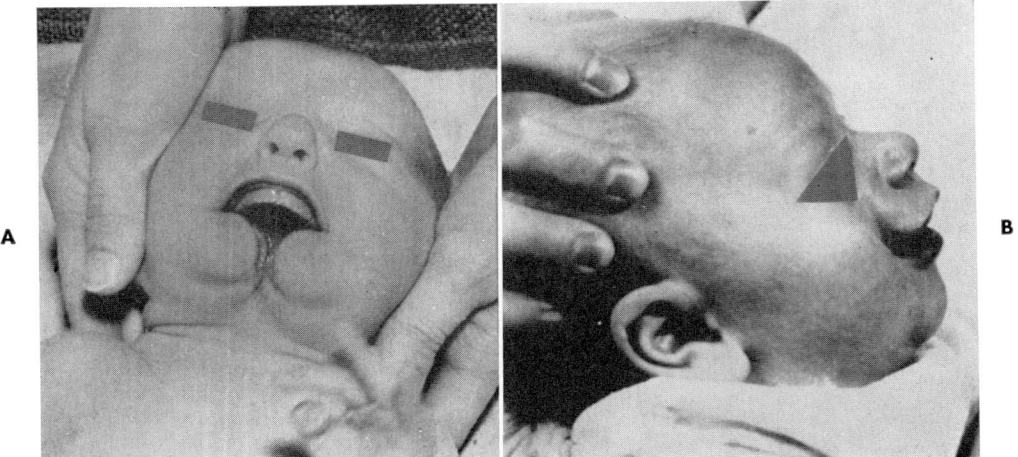

Fig. 21-6. **A**, Congenital cleft mandible. **B**, An oblique facial cleft. **C**, Complete wide bilateral cleft. **D**, Deficiency of premaxilla and prolabium. **E**, Absence of premaxilla and prolabium as well as septum. **F**, Complete absence of central lip, palate, and nasal structures. **G**, Absence of primary palatal and central nasal structures. **H**, Cyclops.

festations of a genetic tendency that fails to conform with common genetic laws. Although the child with an oral cleft is twenty times more likely to have another congenital anomaly than a normal child, no correlation is evident with specific anatomical zones of additional anomaly involvement. Aside from occurrence in certain syndromes of multiple congenital anomalies, oral clefts are related genetically only to congenital lip pits (Fig. 21-7), which appear as depressions in the lower lip associated with accessory salivary glands. The genetic defect for cleft lip and cleft palate is manifest as a lack of potential for mesodermal proliferation across fusion lines after the borders of the component parts are in contact. A fairly common clinical finding of atrophic bands of epithelium across cleft areas and absence of muscle development in the zones of cleft are evidence of mesodermal hypoplasia.

Another theory of cleft production describes an error in transitional shift of embryonic blood supply. Increased maternal age also appears to contribute to embryonal vulnerability to cleft production. The discovery of chromosomal abnormalities as a cause of multiple congenital malformation has directed attention to further genetic background for cleft lip and cleft palate. There seem to be separate genetic disturbances for clefts of the usual type involving the lip and/or palate and those that involve the isolated cleft palate (secondary palate). Several autosomal trisomy syndromes include oral clefts along with other congenital anomalies.

Environmental factors. Environmental factors play a contributory role at the critical time of fusion of lip and palate parts. Investigations with animal studies have directed attention to nutritional deficiency as increasing the incidence of oral clefts. Radiation energy, steroid injection, hypoxia, aspirin and many other drugs, amniotic fluid alteration, and other environmental factors have been shown to increase oral cleft incidence. These factors, however, have been demonstrated to increase cleft incidence when susceptible strains of animals with known genetic cleft tenden-

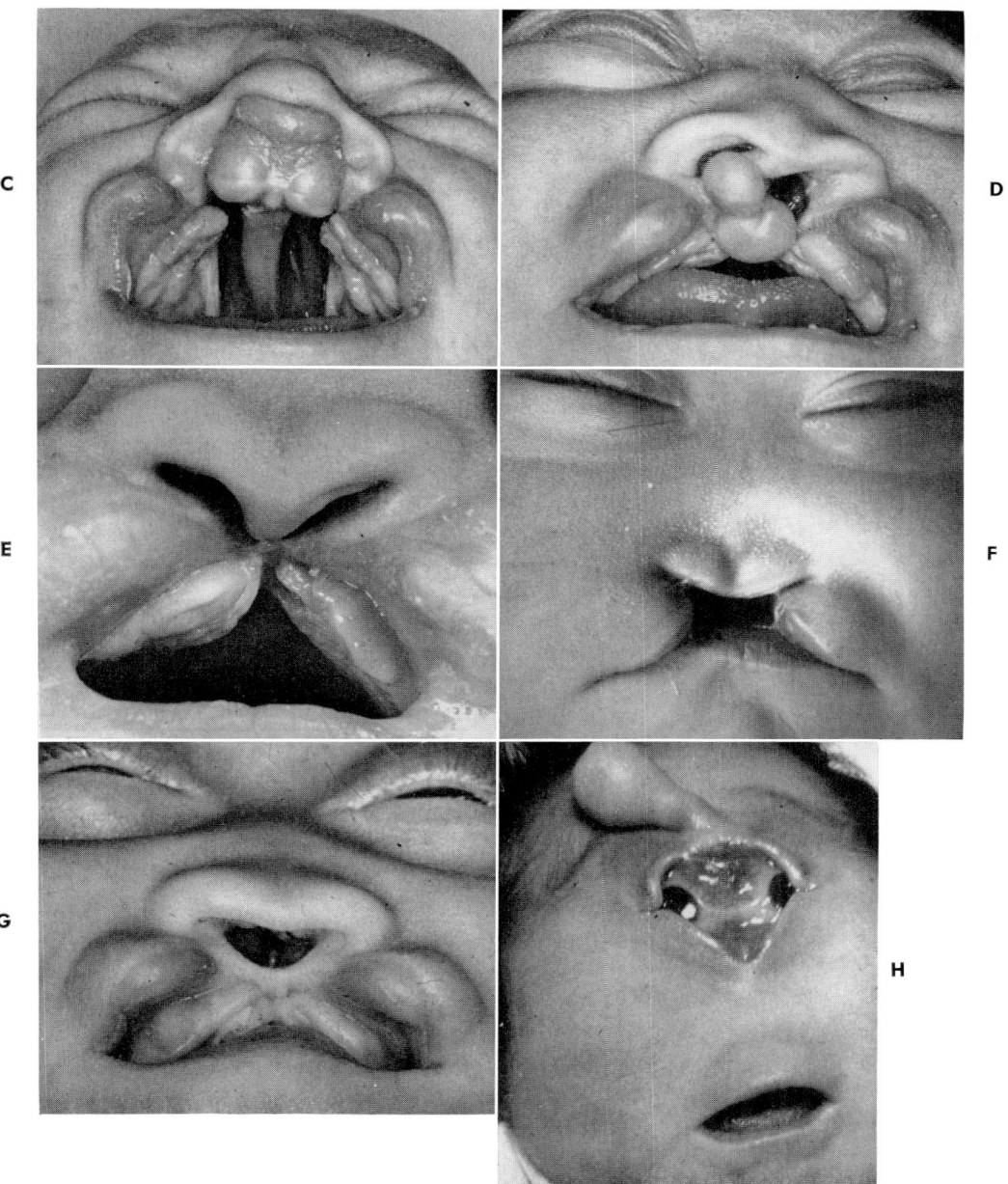

Fig. 21-6, cont'd. For legend see opposite page.

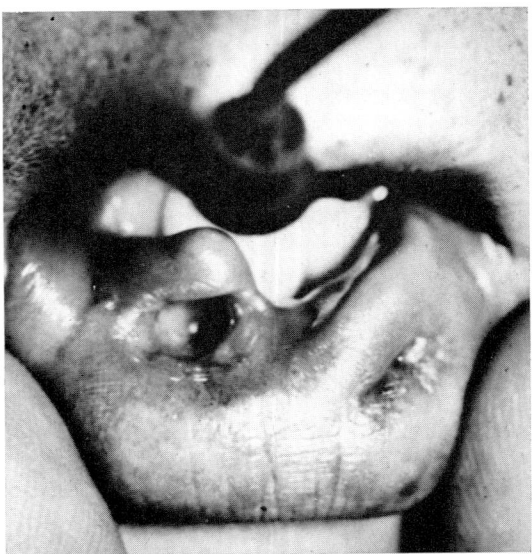

Fig. 21-7. Congenital lip pits. Note that the depression is demonstrated by a stream of compressed air dilating the blind tract.

cies were used. They were less signfiicant in their effect when the strain of animal did not have the genetic tendency. Transposition of maternal malnutrition and other environmental theories to explain the appearance of human oral clefts has not brought consistent or supporting correlation. However, one conclusion can be made. The intensity, duration, and time of action appear to be of greater importance than the specific type of environmental factor.

Mechanical obstruction to the approximating margins of component parts often has been cited as contributory to cleft production. The possible role of an obstructing tongue is suggested in the embryology of the parts. Some asynchronous development or fetal position may cause retention of the tongue and the nasal area between the palatine shelves (Fig. 21-3). The isolated cleft palate, which appears more sporadically and often with less genetic predisposition, suggests this mechanical contributory influence of the tongue on the developing oral structures. Adhesion of one cleft palate margin to the mucosa of the floor of the mouth has been reported as the result of fusion when the palate shelf is blocked by the tongue.

At the present time the etiology of oral clefts appears to depend upon both genetic and environmental factors that are subtle in their expression, and aside from general principles of maternal health they defy known methods of prevention.

SURGICAL CORRECTION

Surgical procedures for correction of cleft lip and cleft palate are always elective. The goals of surgery require that the child be in an optimum state of health before operation is undertaken.

Cheilorrhaphy

Comprehensive pediatric appraisal must find the infant in optimal physical condition for a cleft lip repair. Operation is usually undertaken at 3 weeks to 3 months of age, when a full-term newborn infant has regained original birth weight or approximates 10 pounds. This allows adequate time for manifestation of other possible congenital anomalies of greater significance than the oral cleft. The first problem of feeding has been overcome by careful instruction, using a soft nipple with enlarged opening or a bulb syringe for formula feeding. Structural defects of cleft lip and palate prevent negative oral pressure required for effective sucking. Since larger than normal amounts of air are swallowed, the infant must be fed slowly while held in a head-elevated position and "burped" frequently.

Surgical anatomy. The cleft of the upper lip entails loss of the important orbicularis oris muscle complex. Without the control of this sphincter group of muscles the developing parts of the cleft maxilla deviate to accentuate the alveolar ridge cleft when it is seen at the time of birth. In all significant clefts of the lip a nostril defect is

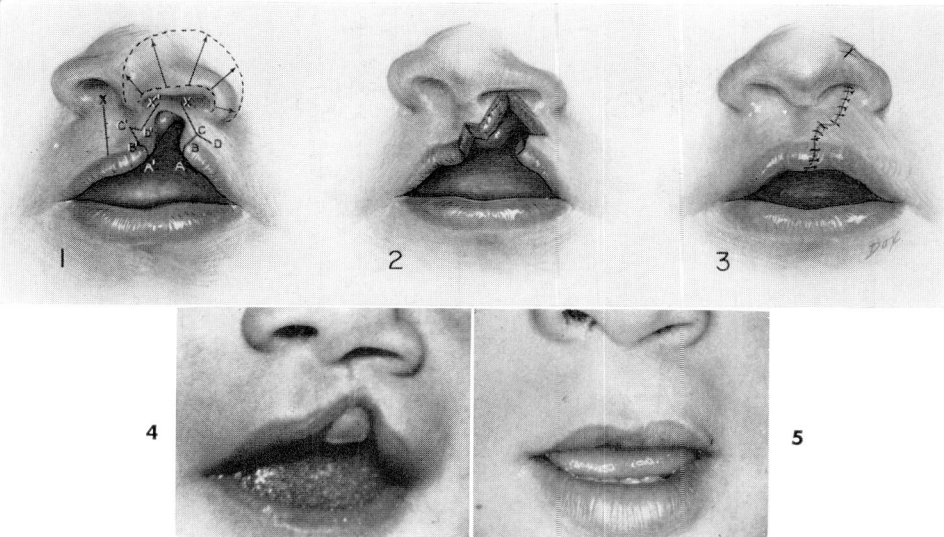

Fig. 21-8. Diagram of the Hagedorn cheilorrhaphy as modified by LeMesurier. 1, Margin incisions mapped out, using uninvolved side for length guide. 2, Prepared margins with flap from full side to insert in notch of deficient side. 3, Closure of margins in three segments (mucosal and muscle closure not shown). 4, Preoperative incomplete lip cleft. Note the nasal asymmetry and groove into nostril floor. 5, View at 22 months after operation in diagrams.

present that ranges from mild nostril asymmetry to absence of nostril floor and gross deformation of nasal alar cartilage and septum. Premaxilla and prolabium are found deviated away from the cleft in unilateral cases and found to project anteriorly in bilateral clefts of the lip and palate. This reflects a difference in the dynamics of growth potential in midline structures as compared with lateral structures, a difference which has had over 6 months to be manifest structurally before birth. Thus the premaxilla that is uncontrolled by the lip deviates to accentuate the cleft in unilateral cases and protrudes monstrously in complete bilateral clefts of the lip and primary palate. Blood supply to all structures is excellent. It is of interest to note that in complete bilateral clefts the nerve and blood supplies to premaxilla and prolabium are distributed along midline structures from the maxillary artery and the inner loop of the trigeminal second division.

Surgical goals and techniques. The safety of cleft lip surgery has been greatly enhanced by the refinements in modern anesthesia using oral endotracheal intubation techniques.

Surgical correction of cleft lip strives to attain a symmetric, well-contoured lip with preservation of all functional landmarks and minimal scar tissue in the result. Since cleft margins are composed of atrophic tissues they must be prepared to provide adequate muscle layers and full-thickness structural definition. Since all scars contract, efforts are made to minimize trauma and sources of inflammation in the procedure and to design the preparation of margins in several planes. This pattern of preparation prevents the linear contracture of a straight-line scar, which would tend to produce a residual notch in the vermilion tissue. All tissue of quality is preserved and utilized in the operation. In unilateral clefts the unaffected side serves as a guide for

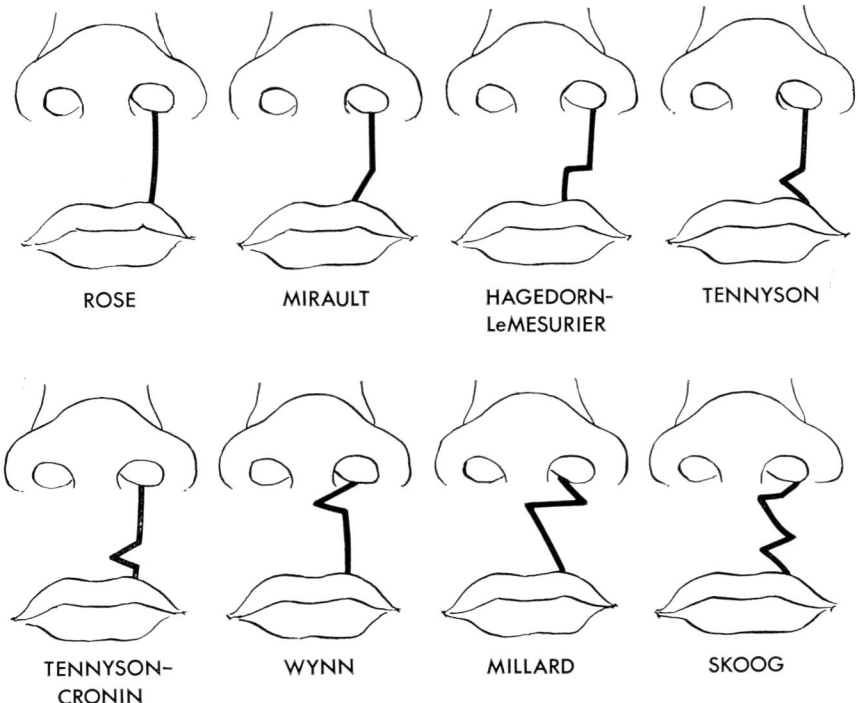

Fig. 21-9. Incision patterns for cleft lip repair. The scar line is broken into segments to achieve greater length in the margins and to offset the contracture of scar tissue into separate planes.

length and symmetry in the restoration of the lip. The preparation of cleft lip margins to gain length, preserve landmarks, and to compensate for scar contracture has developed numerous patterns that are applicable to variations in types of cleft (Fig. 21-9).

Palatorrhaphy

Surgical anatomy. Palate function is necessary for normal speech and swallowing. The hard palate provides the partition between oral and nasal cavities, whereas the soft palate functions with the pharynx in an important valve action referred to as the velopharyngeal mechanism (Fig. 21-10). In normal speech this valve action is intermittent, rapid, and variable to effect normal sounds and pressures by deflecting the air stream with its sound waves out of the mouth. Without this valve action speech is hypernasal and deglutition is impaired. It should be recalled that in addition to their action in the elevation and tension of the solt palate, the levator and tensor muscles effect an opening of the auditory tube. This action is demonstrated when middle ear pressures are equalized by swallowing during changes in atmospheric pressure, such as those experienced in rapid changes in altitude. When this mechanism of tube opening is impaired, greater susceptibility to middle ear infections is experienced. The cleft palate anomaly entails this problem and the additional hazard of lymphoid hyperplasia over the auditory tube orifice in the nasopharynx. It can be appreciated that a combination of hearing loss from middle ear infections added to a defective mechanism for normal speech com-

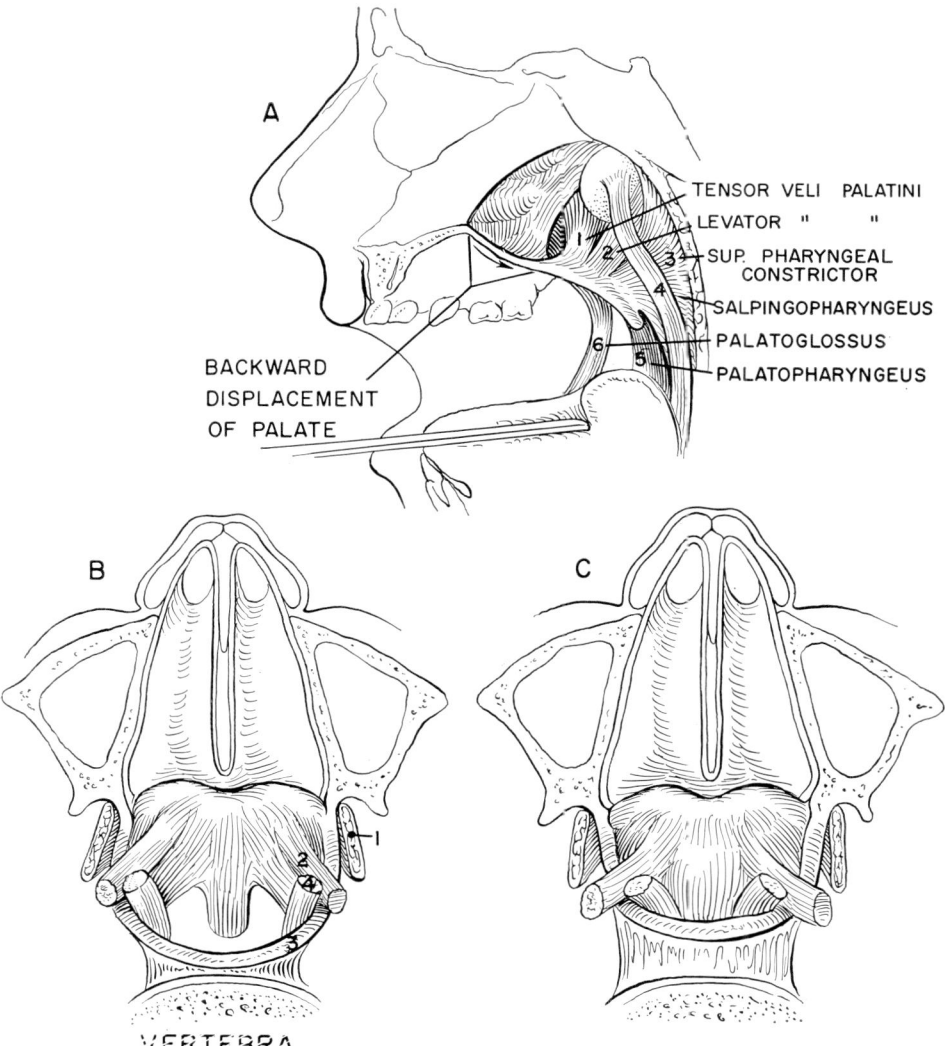

Fig. 21-10. Diagrams of the functional musculature in the velopharyngeal mechanism. **A,** View from sagittal plane to show relations of palate and pharyngeal musculature. **B,** Cross section of soft palate in relaxation, viewed from above. **C,** Muscle position in velopharyngeal closure.

plicates and intensifies the handicap of cleft palate.

Copious blood supply is afforded to the palatal tissues by the major and lesser palatine and nasopalatine branches of the maxillary artery. The ascending palatine branch of the facial artery and branches from the ascending pharyngeal artery contribute further sources of blood supply. Nerve supply to the muscles of the palate and pharynx for motor action arise chiefly from the vagal pharyngeal plexus except for the tensor, which is innervated by the motor branch of the trigeminal nerve, and stylopharyngeus from the glossopharyngeal nerve. Sensory supply for the mucosa in this region arises from the second division of the trigeminal nerve as well as from the ninth and tenth cranial nerve branches of the pharyngeal plexus.

Surgical goals and techniques. The goal of palatorrhaphy is the correction of the embryonal defect to restore palate function for normal speech and swallowing and to accomplish this restoration with minimal disturbance to the growth and development of the maxilla. Cleft palate surgery is always elective, and the child must be free from infection and in optimal physical condition prior to surgery. Because scar tissue defeats the functional goal of a flexible soft palate and, in addition, contracts to deform the developing parts of the maxilla, every effort is made to minimize scar tissue and to establish the functional muscle slings of the velopharyngeal mechanism. Healthy tissues and minimal surgical trauma are required for the operation. Advances in anesthesia with utilization of nasoendotracheal intubation techniques have added to the safety of the operation.

Since a great variation exists in the degree of deformity as seen in cleft width as well as the quality and quantity of tissues, a standard time for best surgical results cannot be stated. However, the majority of cleft palates are corrected surgically between the ages of 18 months and 3 years. Surgeons who advocate palatorrhaphy before 9 months of age emphasize the advantage of muscle development in restored functional position for deglutition, early phonation, and auditory tube action. They point out the hygienic advantages of oronasal partition and the psychological benefits of operation at an early age. Advocates of postponement of surgery until after 6 years of age emphasize the need for avoiding surgical disturbance to the developing parts of the maxilla. They also cite technical advantages of larger and more clearly defined muscle structures for the operation at a later age. The more widely accepted operation for average clefts at around 2 years of age provides a velopharyngeal mechanism before refined speech habits are acquired, with the added psychological advantage of early repair. Although slight disturbances in maxillary development may be induced by surgery at

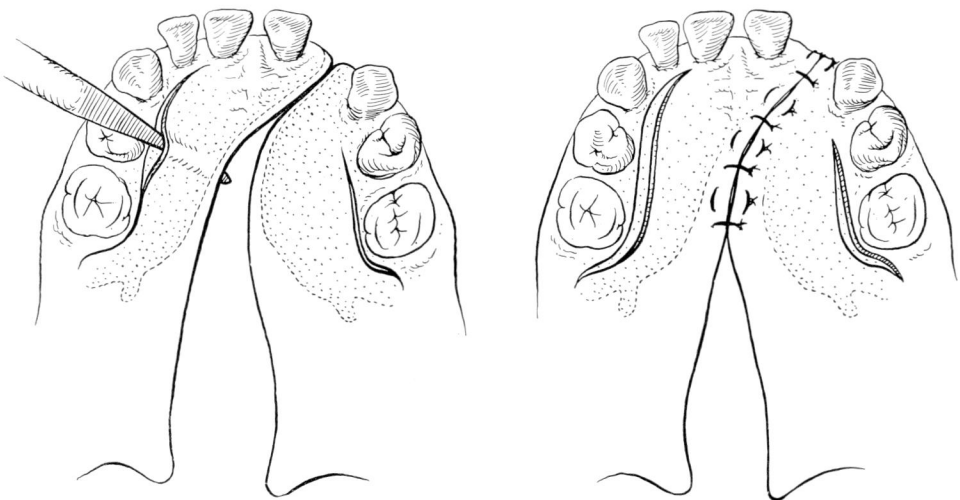

Fig. 21-11. A first-stage palatorrhaphy by the Von Langenbeck method. Elevation of mucoperiosteal flaps mobilized for midline closure. Lateral relaxing incisions heal rapidly.

this age, a correlated and rational utilization of orthodontic therapy may correct constriction tendencies in the maxillary arch. In wider clefts the soft palate may be closed without surgical effort to close the hard palate defect. This area is then obturated by a removable acrylic plastic appliance until possible later repair at an older age.

In techniques of palatorrhaphy a bony union of the hard palate area is not accomplished. Cleft margins are prepared and the tissues are mobilized for approximation in the midline. Preservation of the length and function of the soft palate is of fundamental importance. Closure of complete clefts may be divided into two stages, separated by approximately 3 months, in an effort to prevent scar contracture tending to displace the soft palate anteriorly. Techniques for closure of the hard palate are shown in Figs. 21-11 and 21-12. Soft palate closure (staphylorrhaphy) is shown in Fig. 21-13.

Since the work of Passavant and of others in the late nineteenth century, it has been known that velopharyngeal function depends upon adequate palate length. In addition to adequate length the muscle vector action must displace the soft palate posteriorly and superiorly. The anterior position of the two halves of the palatine aponeurosis attachment found in some clefts is shown in Fig. 21-14. To position the soft palate posteriorly a number of surgical techniques have been devised by Dorrance, Wardill, and others (Figs. 21-15 and 21-16). A superior lining for the extended soft palate, originally advocated by Veau, has been obtained by mobilizing nasal mucosa, from islands of palatal tissue pedicled on the major palatine artery, and from split-thickness skin grafts. The purpose of this lining is to retain flexibility for soft palate action.

INCOMPLETE CLEFT PALATE

The cleft of the secondary palate alone is often termed "incomplete." However, this group includes some very wide involvements and very severe degrees of speech impairment. The aponeurotic muscle attachments seem to be in a more forward position in this type of cleft palate

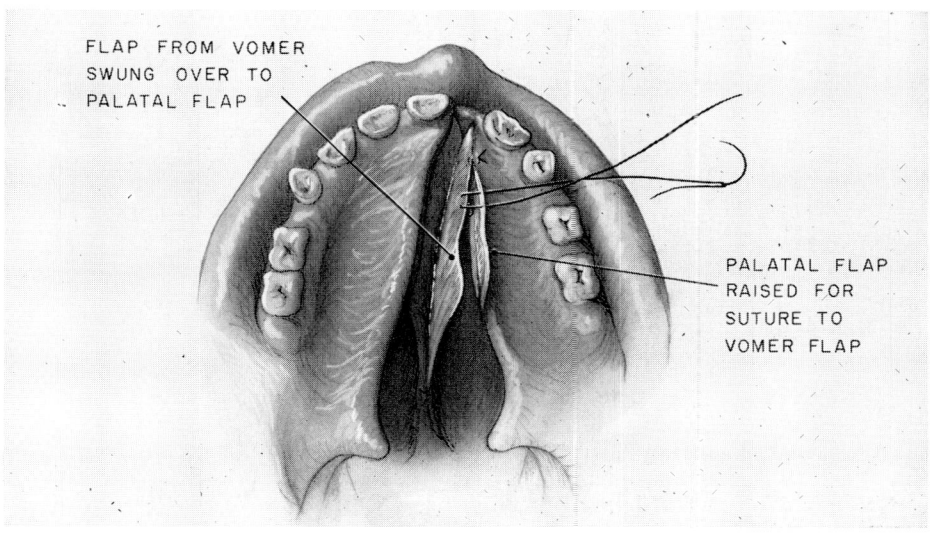

Fig. 21-12. Vomer flap for closure of hard-palate cleft.

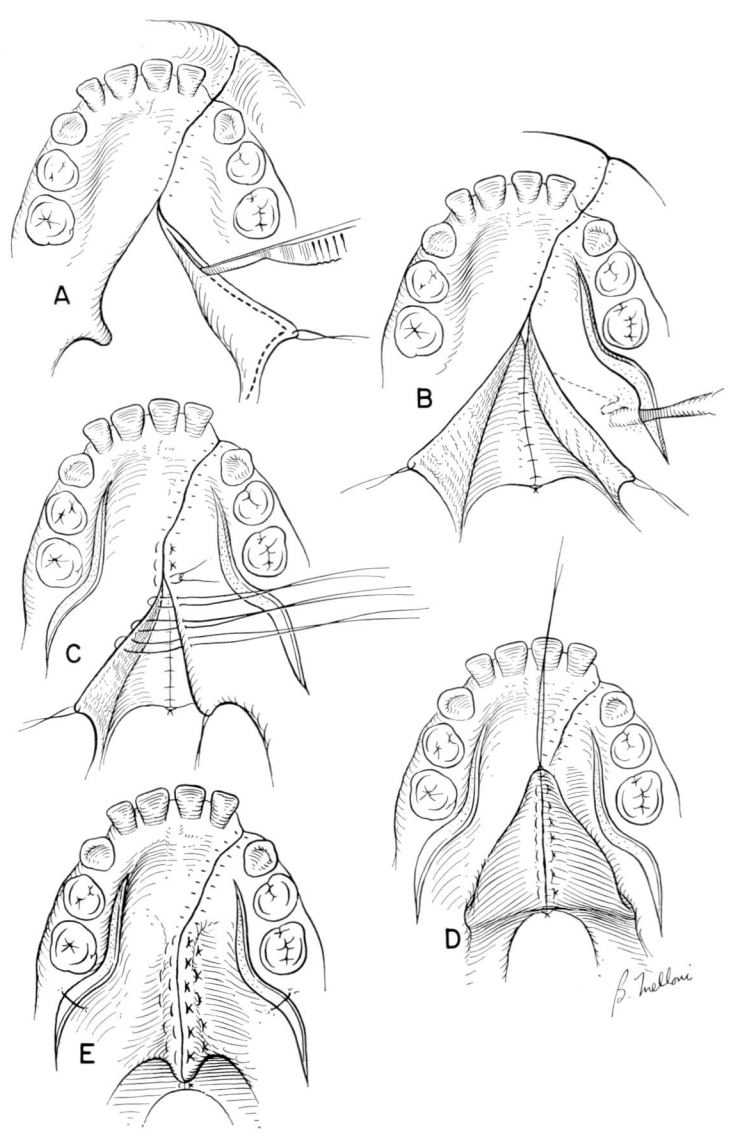

Fig. 21-13. Stages of a second-stage palatorrhaphy (staphylorrhaphy). **A,** Incisions for reflection of nasal mucosa flap. **B,** Broad muscle layer exposed. Nasal mucosal layer closed to form the superior surface. Fracture of hamular processes releases the tendon of the tensor veli palatini muscle. **C,** Vertical mattress sutures close deep muscle and oral mucosa surfaces. **D,** Mucosa closure of posterior uvula seen retracted forward. **E,** Closure completed. Lateral relaxing incisions partially closed.

Cleft lip and cleft palate **399**

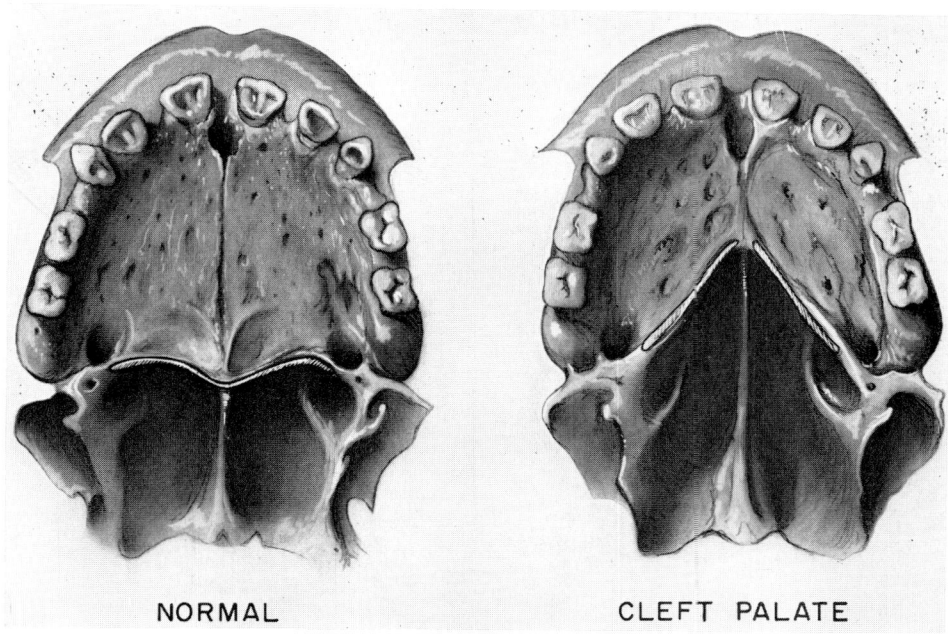

Fig. 21-14. Diagrams showing the normal attachment of the palatine aponeurosis and the site of attachment in some forms of cleft palate. Note that bone defect brings muscle attachment forward.

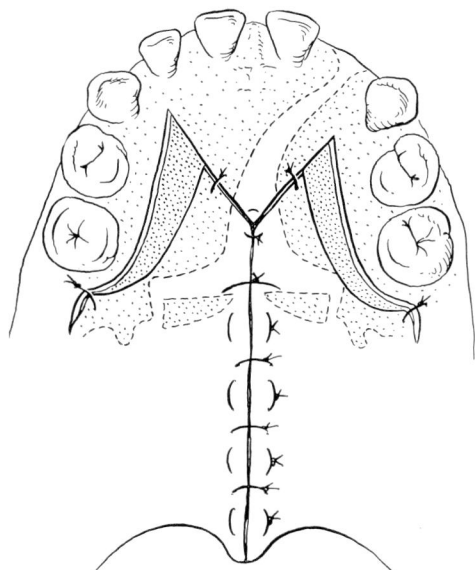

Fig. 21-15. A Wardill "push-back" operation, applicable in cases of complete clefts wherein lengthening is required. Donor sites heal rapidly to cover bone.

and the palate restored by surgery is quite apt to be short (Fig. 21-14). The "complete" cleft involves the alveolar ridge (primary palate) as well as the hard and soft palate (secondary palate). It may be unilateral, bilateral, or have varying degrees of completeness at both poles. The relationship with the vomer and the level of the palatine shelves in comparison with the vomer are quite variable. When the vomer is in good position or attached to one side, it often is utilized in the surgical closure of the hard palate area (Fig. 21-12).

SUBMUCOSAL CLEFT PALATE

In the most minimal variety, the submucosal or occult cleft palate, the muscle slings of the soft palate are not united. No cleft is seen or only a bifid uvula with just a web of mucosa spanning the midline area of the soft palate. At a gag reflex the sides

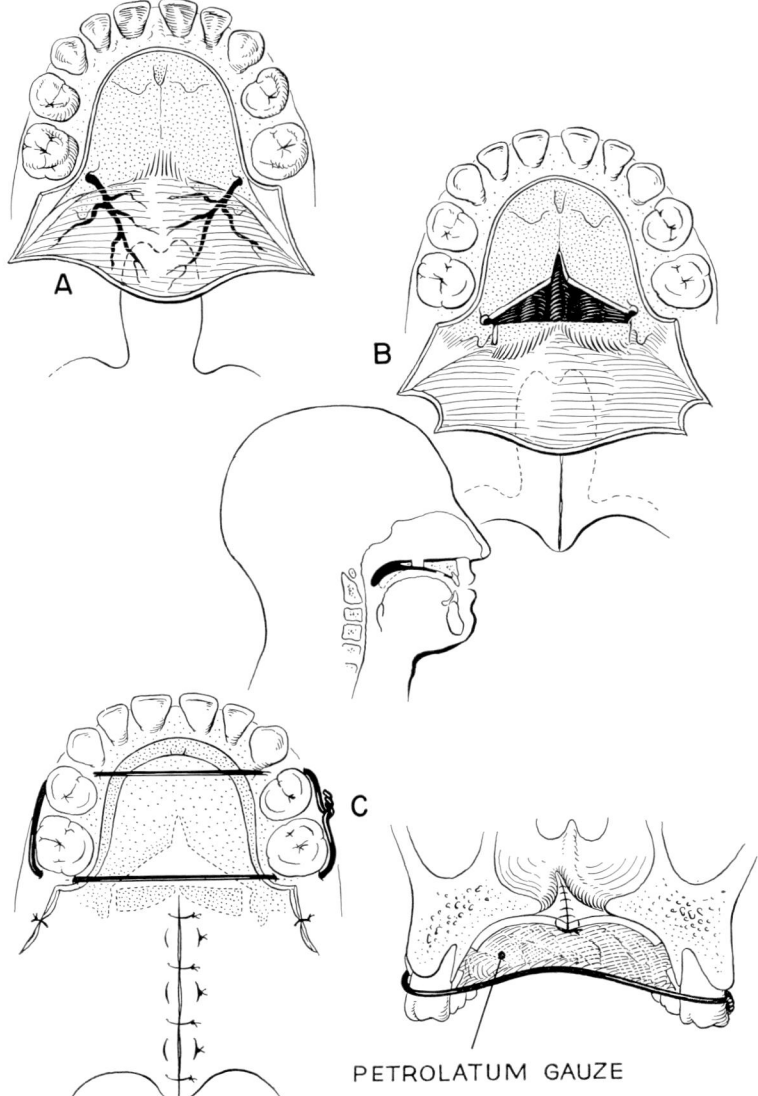

Fig. 21-16. Dorrance "push-back" operation. **A,** Palate mucoperiosteum reflected. Major palatine arteries preserved. **B,** Section of bone flap (Kemper), allowing muscle attachments to retrude. Sagittal diagram of lengthening procedure. **C,** Soft palate structures and flap repositioned posteriorly, with temporary support of gauze pack held with wires during initial healing.

of the soft palate will tend to retract and enlarge, but no lifting action of the soft palate occurs. The speech defect in such a case may be as severe as in the type of cleft that is completely observable. In the submucosal cleft a notch may be palpated at the posterior border of the hard palate where the posterior nasal spine is absent. The bifid uvula does not impair muscle action for soft palate and pharyngeal closure, but it may direct an examiner to the detection of a submucosal cleft.

OTHER HABILITATION MEASURES
Presurgical orthopedics

The fact that the premaxilla in complete clefts has been found in distorted positions influenced by intrauterine pressure pointed out the possible benefit of external pressures before surgery. The width of the alveolar cleft may be reduced by pressure tape over a protruding premaxilla. The restoration of the lip musculature by the cheilorrhaphy repair applies this same molding control; however, the posterior maxillary segment on the cleft side may be deviated by this pressure too far medially to produce a so-called "collapsed arch." Prosthetic devices to prevent this collapse or to correct such contractions by expanding the maxillary parts have been used in treatment. In recent years this expansion in early ages has been combined at a few therapy centers with bone grafts to the alveolar cleft. Such grafts are designed to stabilize the arch and to build up a foundation for the nasal alar base. Long-term results await evaluation in respect to growth potentials and later orthodontic possibilities. Limitations of growth and resistance to arch expansion appear probable.

McNeil has shown not only the early presurgical alignment of the maxillary arch by prosthetic devices in infants, but has influenced the level of the palatine shelves and decreased the width of the hard palate clefts through the influences of prosthetic contact in stimulating growth.

Secondary surgical procedures

The functional potentials of a repaired palate for effective speech can differ from the estimates of morphology that are suggested by the clinical examination. A number of compensatory actions from lateral pharynx contraction and from the existence of adenoid tissue can be involved. Lateral cephalometric radiographs for soft tissue contours and motion picture radiography (cinefluorography) are useful diagnostic aids for estimates of palate function.

If functional soft palate closures have

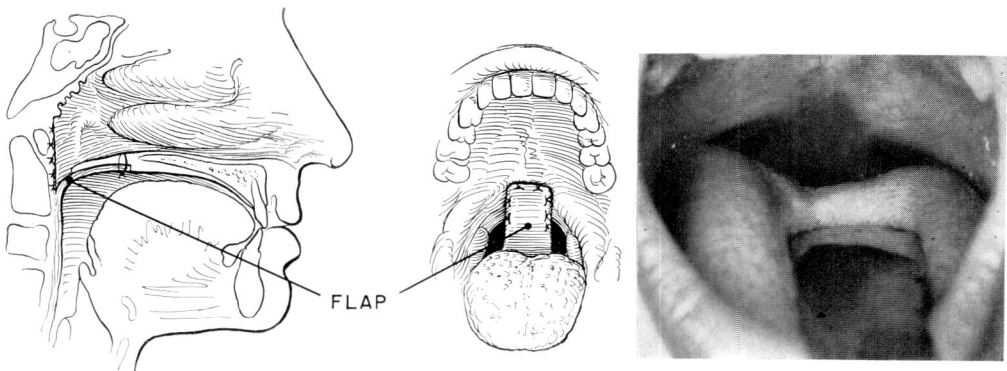

Fig. 21-17. The pharyngeal flap operation to correct velopharyngeal insufficiency (inferior based).

not or cannot be achieved by the methods shown, the procedure known as the pharyngeal flap operation (Fig. 21-17) has been shown to improve velopharyngeal function. Two lateral ports remain between the nasopharynx and the oropharynx. The medial constricting action of the lateral pharyngeal walls produces the intermittent valve action that is desired. Pharyngeal flaps have been based superiorly and inferiorly, but the net result seems to be a combination of holding the soft palate back and up and bringing the posterior of the pharyngeal wall forward. Other pharyngoplasty procedures have been used and materials inserted to advance the posterior pharyngeal wall for this problem of velopharyngeal incompetence.

Prosthetic speech aid appliances

Another solution to the problem of velopharyngeal insufficiency may be accomplished with a prosthesis. Occasionally a cleft palate deformity exceeds the possibility of functional repair through surgery. Postoperative cleft palate results may be deficient in functional potential. In such instances very satisfactory habilitation has been achieved by the skillful construction of a speech aid appliance (Fig. 21-18).

If a palate is reasonably restored, but fails to lift properly to close the velopharyngeal isthmus, a strut can be extended posteriorly from a dental appliance. Often a repaired soft palate is quite insensitive and may tolerate the contact of such an appliance and its extension without a gag reflex. If the palate is deficient in length, a bulb obturator is added to the posterior lift extension. The posterior bulb extension of the appliance affords a partial closure of the velopharyngeal isthmus upon which the pharyngeal musculature may act. The size of the bulb can be gradually diminished as more pharyngeal muscle constriction develops for a better velopharyngeal closure. This type of appliance can be used to develop muscle action before a pharyngeal flap operation is carried out. Such an appliance may also be used to supply missing teeth, to cover hard palate defects, and to add support to the upper lip by means of a "plumping" sulcus flange extension. Retention of the appliance is achieved by anchorage to sound and adequately restored teeth.

Dental care

The importance of preservation of the dentition in the cleft palate patient cannot

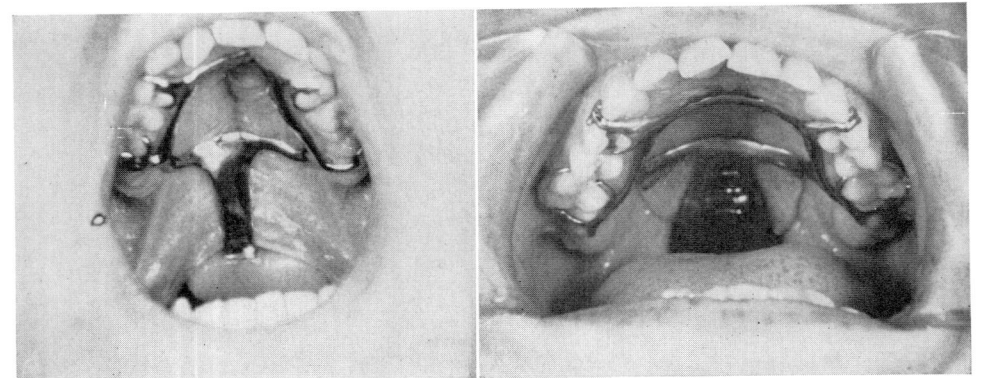

Fig. 21-18. Speech aid appliances for velopharyngeal insufficiency. A, Repaired cleft with insufficiency, showing the speech aid bulb extension. B, Cleft palate that has not been operated on and is treated with obturator for both hard and soft palate areas.

Cleft lip and cleft palate 403

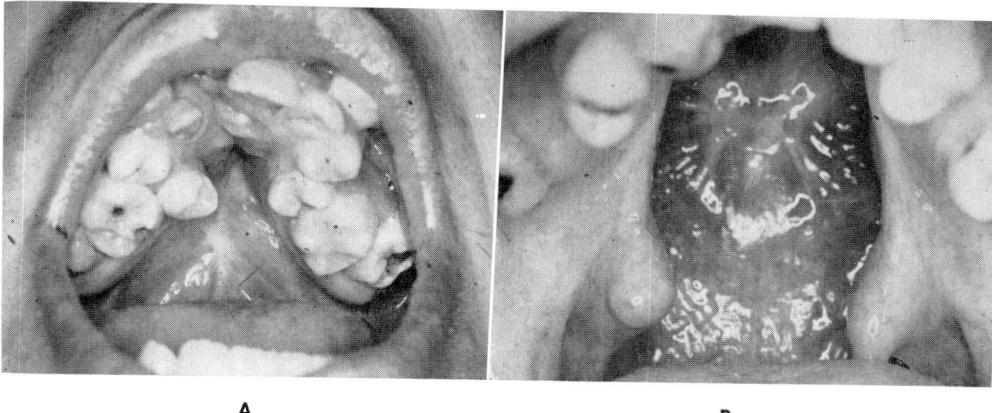

Fig. 21-19. A, Extreme constriction from surgical scar in poorly managed cleft palate. Functional occlusion is lacking and speech is poor. B, Atrophic palate segments where no surgery has been attempted on a wide cleft palate. Anterior arch collapse had been produced by surgical error in amputating the premaxilla and creating a tight lip repair.

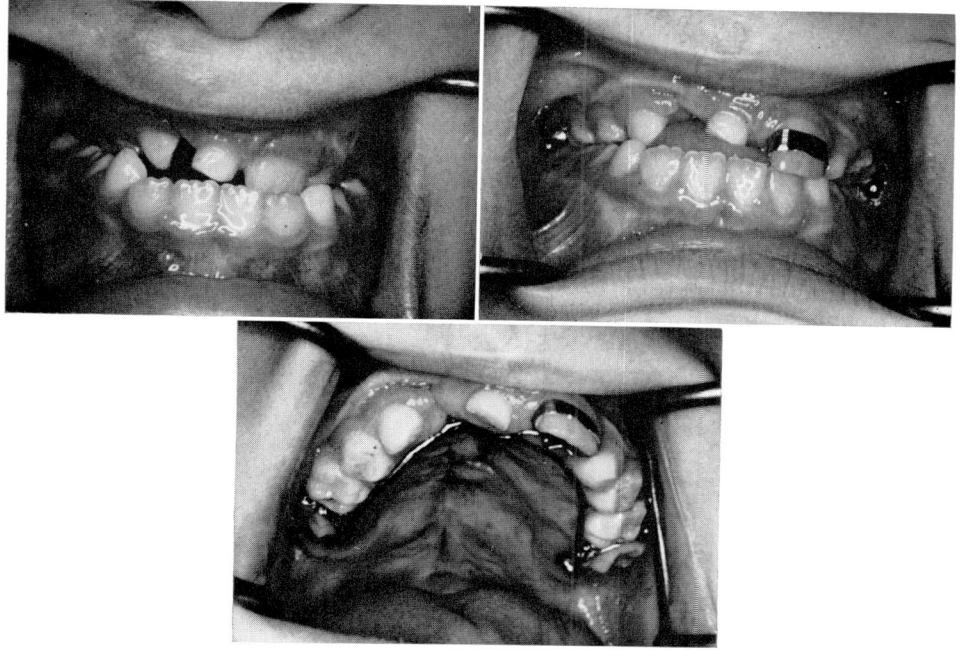

Fig. 21-20. Maxillary collapsed deformity following cleft palate repair and showing orthodontic appliance with "before" and "after" treatment stages. Note the expansion of the maxillary arch.

404 *Textbook of oral surgery*

be overemphasized. Sound teeth are essential to the development of the alveolar process that is deficient in the area of cleft. Teeth are essential to the orthodontic correction of the position of maxillary segments that show tendency for collapse and underdevelopment (Fig. 21-20). All dentists must be aware of the urgent need for preservation and restoration of the dentition for the cleft palate child.

Repair of residual deformities

Residual deformities of the nose and lip may require additional operations for final results. Residual openings into the nose are hazards for escape of dental impression materials. Labial vestibule openings into the nose are sources of irritation and prevent a peripheral seal for denture appliances. A two-layer flap closure lines both the nasal and oral surfaces with epithelium (Fig. 21-21).

Speech therapy

The most exacting criterion of cleft palate habilitation is the accomplishment of normal speech. The basic significance of speech to personality and socioeconomic achievement is appreciated only when one encounters a speech-handicapped individual. Surgery may be able to provide a palate structurally, but speech training usually is required to accomplish its maximum function. The velopharyngeal closure in speech is not a simpler sphincter action, and the refinements of this mechanism are most exacting. In addition to the valve action determinant of nasality in voice quality, many articulatory problems are associated with cleft palate speech. These problems may be complex and require the skill of a competent speech therapist. The status of hypertrophic lymphoid tissue of the adenoids and faucial tonsils often is questioned. Such tissue enlargement may occupy space and compensate for insufficient velopharyngeal closure. A tonsillectomy

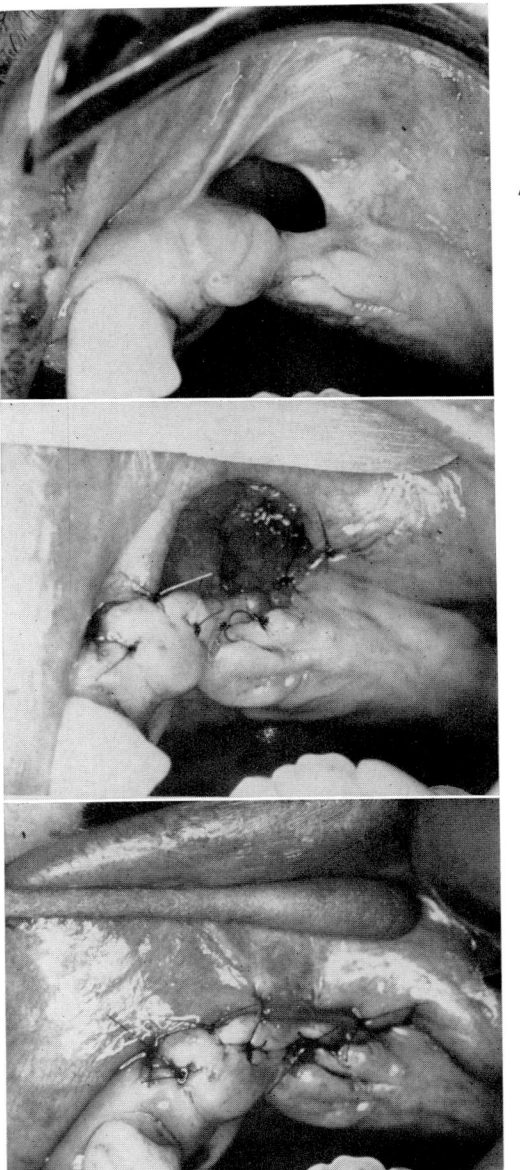

Fig. 21-21. **A**, The residual oronasal fistula in a middle-aged patient requiring complete denture prosthesis. **B**, Nasal mucosal lining turned down from a flap based on the superior edge of the defect. **C**, Oral mucosal coverage from a mobilized pedicle flap completes the two-layer closure.

and adenoidectomy may bring about sudden manifestation of a defective mechanism and marked hypernasality of speech. Lymphoid tissue in these areas undergoes gradual atrophy after puberty, but some workers believe that compensation is more favorable with the lengthened period of atrophy. If diseased adenoids and tonsils are contributing to infections with ear involvement, they must be removed. Careful surgery is required for such procedures to avoid excessive scar tissue, which would further reduce the functional potential of the velopharyngeal mechanism.

Cleft palate team approach

Since the problems of cleft palate habilitation require the services of multiple health care disciplines, centers have evolved to meet the multiple needs. Participants in this effort include the pediatrician, surgeon, pedodontist, orthodontist, prosthodontist, and speech therapist. In addition to the clinical personnel the social workers and public health nurses contribute much to the function of such cleft palate programs. Special problems may require services of psychologists and a number of medical specialists in individual cases. It is logical that centers for the care of the cleft palate child should develop where these services are available. The diagnosis, treatment planning, active treatment phases, recall observation records, and progress reports are accomplished by the conferences and united action of the members of the cleft palate team. The only weakness of the team approach is the danger of an impersonal atmosphere, which can be avoided by good organization and genuine interest in all activities of the group members.

It is evident that surgery is only one link in the chain that is vitally necessary to bring the cleft palate child up to his rightful place in society.

REFERENCES

1. Holdsworth, W. G.: Cleft lip and palate, ed. 3, New York, 1963, Grune & Stratton.
2. Braithwaite, F.: Cleft lip and palate repair. In Battle, R. J. V., editor: Clinical surgery (plastic), Washington, 1965, Butterworths.
3. Steffensen, W. H.: Palate lengthening operations—collective review, Plast. Reconstr. Surg. 10:330, 1952.
4. Longacre, J. J., and deStefano, G.: The role of the posterior pharyngeal flap in rehabilitation of the patient with cleft palate, Amer. J. Surg. 94:882, 1957.
5. Pruzansky, S.: Description, classification and analysis of unoperated clefts of the lip and palate, Amer. J. Orthodont. 39:590, 1953.
6. Hayward, J. R., and Avery, J. K.: A variation in cleft palate, J. Oral Surg. 15:320, 1957.
7. Pruzansky, S.: Factors determining arch forms in clefts of the lip and palate, Amer. J. Orthodont 41:827, 1955.
8. Harvold, E.: Cleft lip and palate morphologic studies of the facial skeleton, Amer. J. Orthodont 40:493, 1954.
9. Subtelny, J. D.: A review of cleft palate growth studies reported in the past ten years, Plast. Reconstr. Surg. 30:56, 1962.
10. Graber, T. M.: A congenital cleft palate deformity, J. Amer. Dent. Ass. 48:375, 1954.
11. Swanson, L. T., MacCollum, D. W., and Richardson, S. O.: Evaluation of the dental problems in the cleft palate patient, Amer. J. Orthodont. 42:749, 1956.
12. Sarnat, D. G.: Palatal and facial growth in macaca rhesus monkeys which surgically produced palatal clefts, Plast. Reconstr. Surg. 22:29, 1958.
13. Woolfe, C. M., and Broadbent, T. R.: Genetic and non-genetic variables related to cleft lip and palate, Plast. Reconstr. Surg. 32:65, 1963.
14. Webster, R. C.: Cleft palate. Part I. (collective review), Oral Surg. 1:647, 1948.
15. Webster, R. C.: Cleft palate. Part II. Treatment (collective review), Oral Surg. 1:943, 1948; 2:99, 485, 1949.
16. McNeil, C. K.: Oral and facial deformity, London, 1954, Pittman & Sons.
17. Pruzansky, S.: Pre-surgical orthopedics and bone grafting for infants with cleft lip and palate: a dissent, Cleft Palate J. 1:164, 1964.
18. Brauer, R. O., Cronin, T. D., and Reaves, E. L.: Early maxillary orthopedics, orthodontia, and alveolar bone grafting in complete clefts of the palate, Plast. Reconstr. Surg. 29:625, 1962.

19. Sesgin, M. Z., and Stark, R. B.: The incidence of congenital defects, Plast. Reconstr. Surg. **27**:261, 1961.
20. Fogh-Anderson, P.: Inheritance patterns for cleft lip and cleft palate. In Pruzansky, editor: Congenital anomalies of the face and associated structures, Springfield, Ill., 1961, Charles C Thomas, Publisher.
21. Schuchardt, Karl: Treatment of patients with clefts of lip, alveolus and palate, Second Hamburg International Symposium, July, 1964. Stuttgart, Georg Thieme Verlag.
22. Fukuhara, Tatsuo: New method and approach to genetics of cleft lip and palate, J. Dent. Res. **44**(supp.): 1965.

Chapter 22

ACQUIRED DEFECTS OF THE HARD AND SOFT TISSUES OF THE FACE

Edward C. Hinds

Deformities of the face have been existent since time began, and attempts at correction have been made almost since the dawn of surgery. However, progress in this field has been very slow, with few outstanding successes until recent years. Early failures resulted from lack of adequate anesthesia and antibiotics and also religious and moral taboos concerning meddling with human features.

Four thousand years ago the Hindus were attempting correction of facial deformities and defects by gluing tissues to the affected part. Evidence also indicates that they were utilizing pedicle flaps from the cheek or forehead to repair defects of the nose or lips. Tagliacozzi (1546-1599), who is given much credit for revival of plastic surgery during the Renaissance, wrote extensively on rhinoplasty, using pedicle flaps from the arm. However, he was severely criticized and ridiculed for his plastic operations because of the religious attitudes of the time. Paré and Fallopius are said to have also criticized Tagliacozzi for introducing his operation. Because of this severe criticism from many sources, the rhinoplasty fell into ill repute and did not become popular again until the early part of the nineteenth century.[69,74]

Von Graefe, Dieffenbach, Lisfranc, and Carpue, in Europe, then began the development of modern reconstructive surgery. Since Reverdin's report on transplantation of skin in 1869, a steady improvement has occurred in methods of reconstructive surgery, facilitated, to a great extent, by the development of modern anesthesia, aseptic technique, and more recently, the use of antibiotics.

According to Peer,[73] König in 1896 was thought to have been the first to use cartilage transplants in man. Ollier studied autogenous bone transplants in animals as early as 1858, but considered such a procedure to be dangerous to human beings.[67,68] Macewen[56] performed the first homologous bone graft in 1878. However, bone grafting did not receive any real impetus until World War I.

SOFT TISSUE REPAIR

Defects of the skin may be repaired by transplantation of free segments of skin or by segments with blood supply maintained by pedicle attachment. Free skin grafts may be in the form of split thickness or full thickness. Pedicle grafts or flaps usually contain considerable subcutaneous tissue along with the skin and may serve to re-

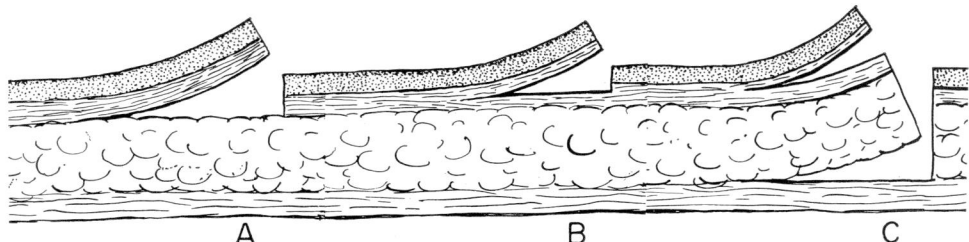

Fig. 22-1. Diagrammatic illustration of free tissue grafts. **A,** Full-thickness skin graft. **B,** Split-thickness skin graft. **C,** Dermal fat graft.

store contour defects as well as surface defects.

Free grafts

Free skin grafts find wide usage in lesions of trauma and neoplasia. Glanz[32] states that one advantage of a free skin graft in management of neoplasms of the face is that the wound may be left open during the time that the permanent pathological sections are being made to determine adequacy of therapy. They can then be covered by a delayed skin graft.

Split-thickness grafts can be taken fairly easily and give good assurance of a "take." A disadvantage of split-thickness grafts is their marked tendency to contract, pigmentary changes, and lack of depth for contour problems. Grafts do not take well in infected areas, over exposed cartilage or bone, or in avascular areas. Split-thickness grafts may be used to convert primary traumatic wounds into closed wounds if there is not enough local tissue. They may also be of value in converting secondary wounds into closed wounds such as in the case of burns or trauma.

Full-thickness grafts are much superior to split-thickness grafts as far as matching face color is concerned, and they have less tendency to contract. They may be quite valuable in various types of lesions of the face particularly if the tissue loss involves skin only. They have been used very successfully in correction of ectropion of the eye and resurfacing of the lip. Perhaps the only disadvantage of the full-thickness graft is the decreased chance of graft survival as compared with the split-thickness graft.

Defects of the oral cavity, nasal cavity, and orbit are best restored by split-thickness grafts. When grafting extensive lesions of the oral cavity, particularly following excision of contractures, the importance of maintaining dilatation by means of some sort of stent must be realized and maintained for several weeks to prevent recurrence of the contracture. One of the most difficult problems in surgery is the management of the badly constricted oral cavity resulting from extensive scar tissue.

In repairing an extensive defect of oral mucosa with skin graft it is best to use a thick, split-thickness graft and to secure it with a stent of gauze or cornish wool saturated in antibiotic solution. This should be left in place 7 to 10 days. These grafts have a marked tendency to shrink; consequently, a generous graft must be used.

The use of skin grafts for extending buccal and labial sulci was originally devised by Esser in 1917, later modified by Waldron, and more recently advocated by Obwegeser.[64] This technique essentially involves the construction of a stent to provide the desired sulcus over which the skin graft is applied, so that the raw surface of the graft is adjacent to the raw surface of

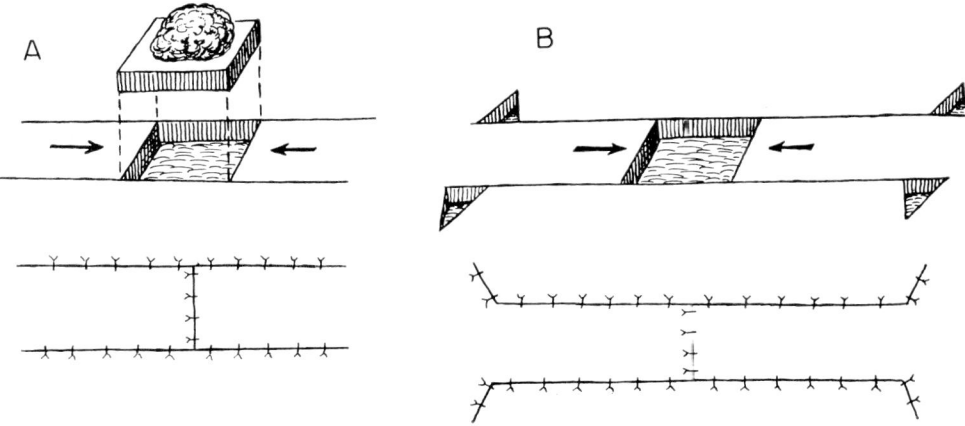

Fig. 22-2. **A**, Advancement flap. **B**, Modification by removal of triangles of skin at base of flap.

the newly constructed sulcus. This is secured in place for 7 to 10 days.

Skin grafts applied to a bony surface such as the alveolar ridge will not shrink, but skin grafts applied to soft tissue will manifest marked shrinkage unless counteracted to some extent by an appropriate stent.

Local flaps

Paletta[70] has very aptly stated that the simplest repair that closely simulates the tissue being reconstructed should be the method of choice. This objective is probably best achieved by use of the advancement or rotation flap wherever possible.

Flaps may be classified as local and distant. Local flaps utilize contiguous tissue and include the following: advancement (Fig. 22-2), rotation, and transposition. Distant flaps are those carried over an area of normal skin on a pedicle that is later sectioned and returned to the donor site. These may be divided into direct and indirect. The indirect flap may be migrated in steps from a distant area to the face or carried on the arm.

The local flap became popularized by a group of French surgeons shortly after Reverdin's description of the epidermic free graft and is sometimes known as the French flap.[74] The simplest form is probably exemplified by undermining the edges of a wound to facilitate closure. The direct advancement flap is created by undermining the skin of one margin of wound defect and creating parallel incisions at the borders of the undermined area for the purpose of closing the defect.

Although the lip shave (vermilionectomy) in the past has been considered a modification of the advancement flap, in recent years we have performed this procedure without a true advancement as follows. The area of altered vermilion tissue to be excised is outlined in an eliptical fashion, beginning anteriorly at the margin of the vermilion. Approximately 5 to 6 mm. of vermilion is included in the elipse near the midline. Posterior and anterior incisions are outlined and brought together near the commissure. Dissection is then carried down to the muscle area, and the entire mucosa and submucosal tissues are excised. The wound is closed directly without undermining the mucosa posteriorly. This allows an ideal closure without the ecchymosis seen when extensive mucosal under-

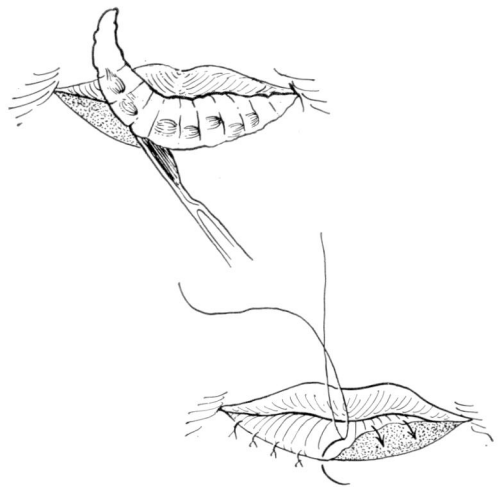

Fig. 22-3. Diagrammatic illustration of lip shave wherein labial mucosa is advanced to form new vermilion after removal of diseased area.

mining is carried out. The slight decrease in fullness of the lip, if anything, is helpful in protecting the lip from the harmful rays of the sunshine. If one area of the lip is more pathological than the rest, a wedge excision of this area should be done in combination with the lip shave.

A rotation flap is created by incising the donor tissue in semicircular fashion to allow rotation into a defect. The advancement flap and the rotation flap may both be facilitated by either the cut-back or a triangular excision of skin (Fig. 22-2, B). A transposition flap is one that is rotated at an angle, jumping an area of normal tissue to reach the defect. Another variety of local flap is the inturned flap in which the margins of a defect are incised, undermined, and turned in to form the back side

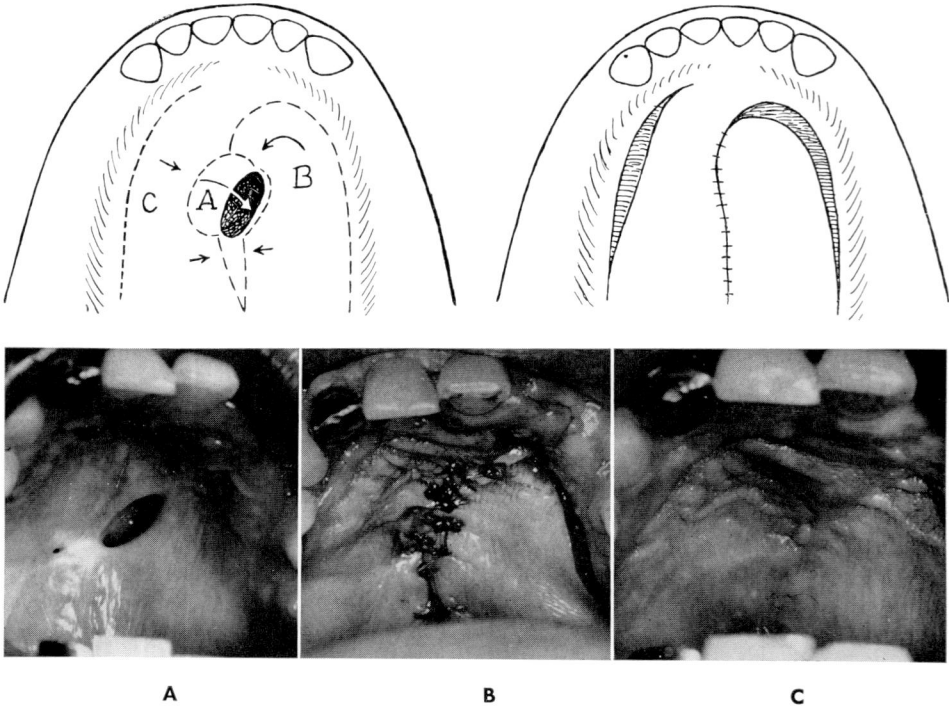

Fig. 22-4. Diagrammatic illustration of use of combination of flaps for closure of traumatic nasal oral fistula: **A**, inturned flap; **B**, rotation flap; **C**, advancement flap. Photographs are of actual case in which the patient was operated upon by Dr. William H. Bell and Dr. Robert R. Debes, Jefferson Davis Hospital.

of the defect if a double lining is required, such as in a nasopalatine fistula or an antral-cutaneous fistula.

Pedicle flaps, in general, have the advantage of possessing subcutaneous tissue as well as skin, thereby providing depth and pliability to the repair. Local flaps have the additional advantages of desirable color and texture as well as simplicity and diminished time requirements. These flaps have wide application, and several variations have been used in closure of oroantral fistulas for many years. Fig. 22-4 demonstrates the use of a combination of local flaps in repairing an oronasal fistula caused by trauma.

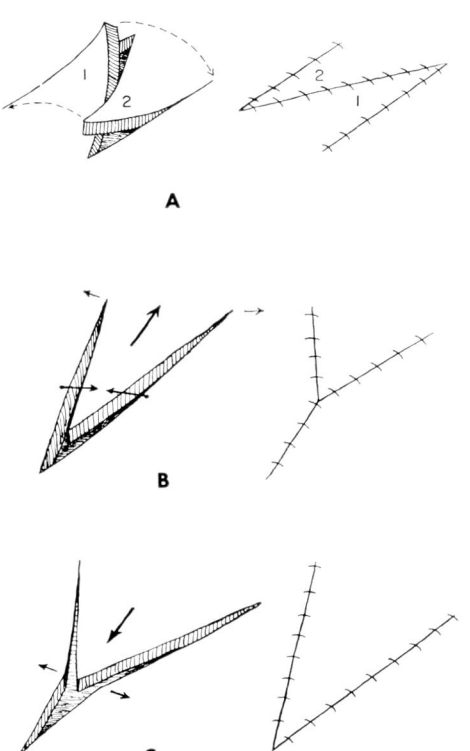

Fig. 22-5. Modification of local flaps. A, Z-plasty for breaking up linear scars or for releasing tension of scar band. B, V-Y procedure for lengthening localized area. C, Y-V procedure for shortening localized area of tissue.

Common modifications of the local flap are the Z-plasty and V-Y flap (Fig. 22-5). The Z-plasty is a double rotation flap and may be used as a series of transposition flaps. It is the most effective method for releasing tension on a linear contracture. The rotation of the flaps allows the direction of tension to be changed with consequent relaxation of the tension of the original axis (Fig. 22-6). It is also applicable if a corner of the mouth or the ala of the nose is depressed or elevated. The V-Y is a type of advancement flap that acts as a lengthening procedure when the incision is made in the form of a V and converted into a Y. It acts as a shortening procedure when made in the form of a Y and converted into a V. This may be particularly useful in repairing notch defects of the lips. It may be carried out by mucosal advancement alone or by full-thickness advancement as described by Gillies and Millard.[31]

The commissure of the mouth may be extended by excising a triangular or arrowhead section of skin, cutting through the orbicularis oris, and undermining and advancing the mucosa to form the new lining of the commissure. Palleta[70] described a simple method for reconstruction of the commissure following excision of lesions in this area, using the principle of advancing mucosal flaps.

Two additional methods for reconstructing the commissure of the mouth are described by Kazanjian and Roopenian.[45] The first involves excision of skin, extension of the line of commissure through the muscle, and advancement of adjacent vermilion lip rather than buccal mucosa (Fig. 22-7). The second involves incision of skin, incision of the orbicularis oris and mucosa, and utilization of upper and lower transposition flaps of buccal mucosa for lining the defect of the vermilion (Fig. 22-8).

Full-thickness losses of the lips are best repaired by local flaps and can usually be carried out by one of the following three methods or a variation of one of these:

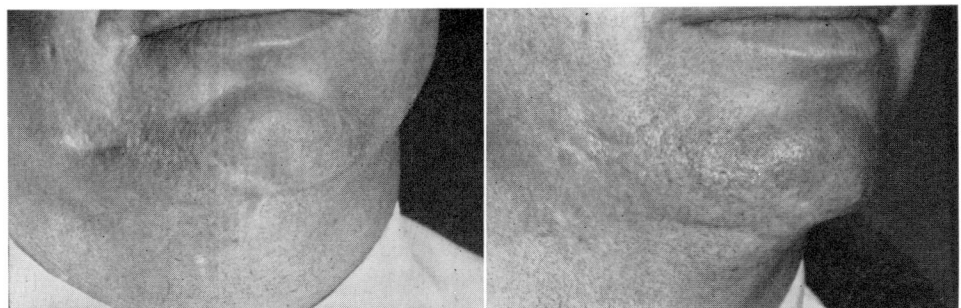

Fig. 22-6. Cicatricial band of segmental area and scar on right side of face corrected by revision and multiple Z-plasty.

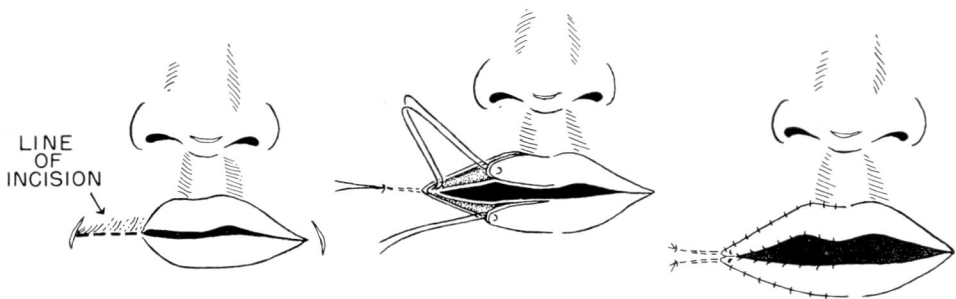

Fig. 22-7. Reconstruction of oral commissure. (Drawn from Kazanjian, V. H., and Roopenian, A.: Amer. J. Surg. 88:884, 1954.)

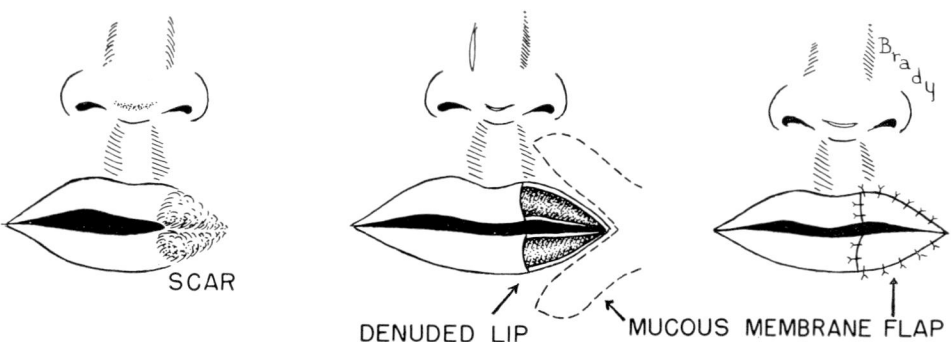

Fig. 22-8. Another method of reconstruction of oral commissure. (Drawn from Kazanjian, V. H., and Roopenian, A.: Amer. J. Surg. 88:884, 1954.)

Acquired defects of the hard and soft tissues of the face 413

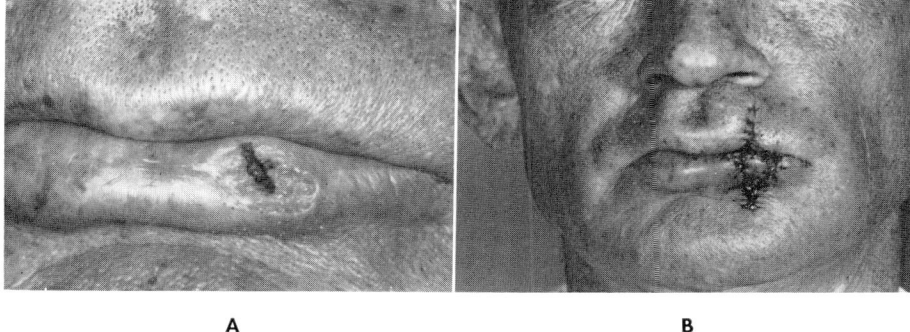

Fig. 22-9. A, Squamous cell carcinoma of lower left lip. **B,** Wedge excision and primary repair with Abbe-Estlander or rotation flap from upper lip. Pedicle detached and revised 18 days following surgery.

1. The Abbe or Estlander flap
2. Straight advancement with triangular excision of skin
3. Transposition flap, such as the nasal labial flap

The most common method for repair of full-thickness losses of the lip is probably the rotation flap from one lip to the other. Although rotation flaps from one lip to the other are associated wth the names Abbe and Estlander, Pietro Sabattini in 1837 repaired an upper lip defect by rotating a lower lip flap through 180 degrees.[91] Stein in 1847 utilized double adjacent flaps from the upper lip to repair a defect in the midline of the lower lip. Estlander in 1865 first repaired a defect of one lip by a pedicle flap from the other and published his procedure in Germany first in 1872. His technique was characterized by a rotation flap consisting of a single wedge of lip substance and, if necessary, a part of the cheek. The pedicle was located at the angle of the mouth, and the operation, as a rule, was completed in one stage. Abbe in 1898 utilized a rotation flap from the lower lip to the upper lip. (See Fig. 22-9.)

In excising lesions of the lower lip it should be remembered that a V-shaped wedge containing up to one third or more

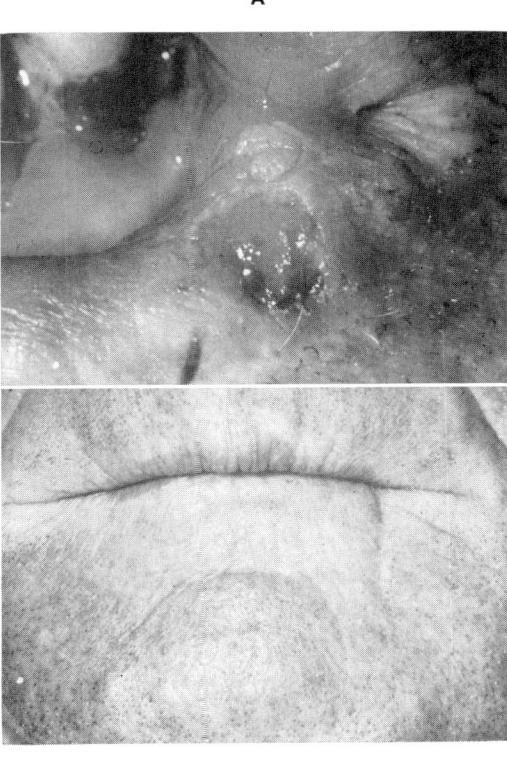

Fig. 22-10. Carcinoma near left commissure of mouth treated by combination V excision and lip shave. **A,** Preoperative photograph. **B,** Postoperative photograph.

of the lower lip may frequently be repaired by primary suture (Fig. 22-10). Recently, a composite V-shaped graft has been transferred from one lip to the other, without utilizing a pedicle, with success.[25] It does not, however, seem advisable to take this added risk when the disability of the pedicle is minimal. Pedicle flaps of mucosa only from one lip to the other may also be used to advantage. Schneider[79] has described a Z closure of a V excision of the lower lip that gives a more normal-appearing lip.

The literature is somewhat confusing on the origin of the closure of lip defects by excising a triangle of skin and advancing the flaps medially. Burow and Bernard are both mentioned in association with this procedure. The methods of Burow and Bernard were both first published in 1853. Burows' method apparently involved excision of lateral triangles from the upper lip and a V excision of the primary lesion from the lower lip, followed by advancement of the lower flaps to recreate the lower lip (Fig. 22-12). Bernard's procedure involved the formation of lateral cheek flaps mobilized from the mandible, allowing greater excision of the primary lesion, which could be rectangular in outline rather than V shaped [57] (Fig. 22-13).

A great variety of lateral rotation or transposition flaps have been used for closure of lip defects. Bruns, Denonvilliers, and Nealton and Ombrédanne were among the first to describe flaps of this type.[91] The possibilities for use of this principle are almost limitless.

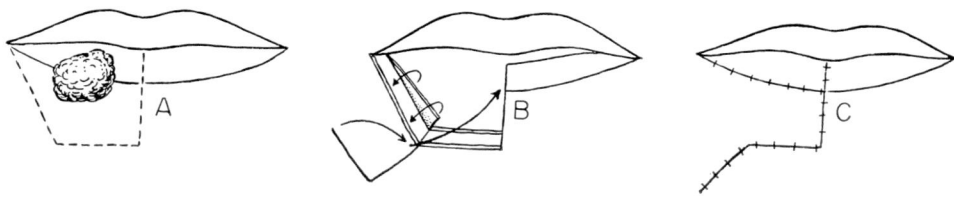

Fig. 22-11. Method of reconstruction of lower lip following wide excision for cancer. **A**, Primary lesion and defect created by excision. **B**, Diagrammatic illustration of method of reconstruction carried out 3 weeks after primary excision. **C**, Closure completed. (Method devised and described by Dr. Richard W. Vincent, New Orleans, La.)

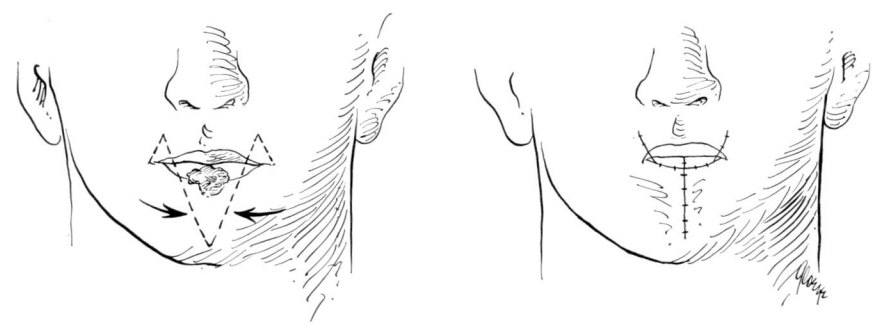

Fig. 22-12. Burow's method of reconstruction of mouth following excision of large lesion of lower lip. (Drawn from Binnie, J. F.: Manual of operative surgery, Philadelphia, 1921, P. B. Blakiston's Son & Co.)

Because of the pliability of the cheek tissue, a large variety of defects can be corrected by rotation, advancement, or transposition flaps. Defects in the anterior portion of the cheek lend themselves to such correction better than defects in the posterior areas. Full-thickness losses of cheek usually require pedicle flaps from a distance for repair.

Distant flaps

Distant flaps are those that are carried over an area of normal skin on a pedicle that is later sectioned and returned to the donor site. It is sometimes difficult to fit all procedures into precise categories. For instance, some local flaps, because of their complexity, might best be included in this group rather than in the previous section on rotation of local tissues. Generally speaking, we may divide pedicle flaps, or distant flaps, into the forehead or scalp flaps, which are supposed to have been developed in ancient India, the open pedicle flap described by Tagliacozzi in Italy, and the tubed pedicle flap developed more recently by Filatov in Russia and Gillies in Great Britain.[74]

A variety of the tube graft is the pillowed or pin-cushioned graft wherein a flap is elevated and turned on itself. Both the tube and the pillowed graft avoid an open wound. The forehead flap, sometimes lined with a free graft, has found wide usage, particularly for extensive repair of the nose. It has also been used for repair of full-thickness defects of the cheek, particularly involving the wall of the antrum. Large flaps from the neck lined with free grafts have also been used for repair of pharyngeal fistulas.

Tubed pedicle flaps seem to have definite advantages over open flaps. Tubing a pedicle flap avoids an open wound, provides better circulation, and may be handled with greater ease, both to the patient and the operator. Pedicle flaps are required for repair if extensive loss of tissue is in-

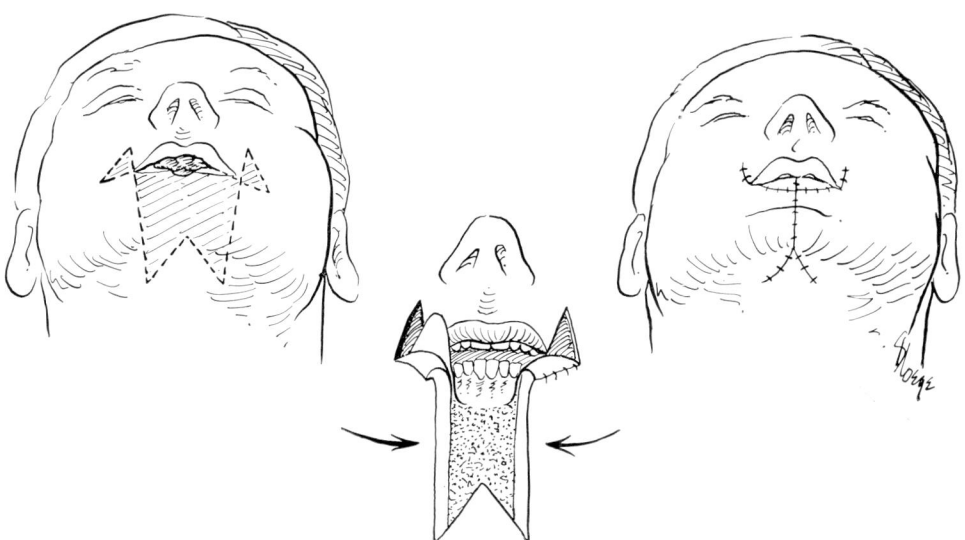

Fig. 22-13. Bernard's method of reconstruction following excision of extensive lesion of lower lip. Triangle of skin removed from upper lip at each lateral margin, saving mucosa for reconstruction of vermilion. (Drawn from Martin, H. E.: Surgery of head and neck tumors, New York, 1957, Hoeber-Harper.)

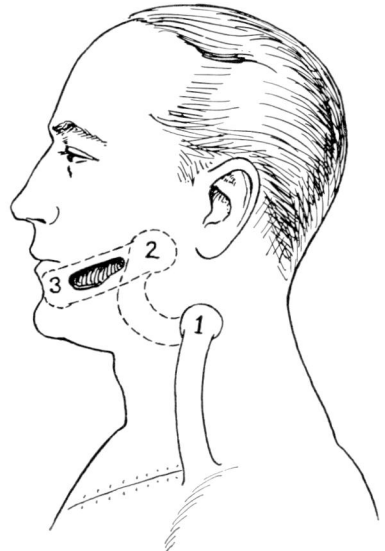

Fig. 22-14. Use of acromiopectoral tube pedicle for repair of full-thickness defect of cheek. Advanced in three stages.

volved or bone grafting procedures are anticipated and soft tissue covering is not adequate. Of the tube pedicles the thoracoepigastric, the acromiopectoral, and the neck pedicle are used most often (Fig. 22-14).

Although most surgeons have felt that repair of radical loss of the maxilla is best handled by prosthetic appliances, some[22,53] have advocated repair of these defects by means of tubed pedicle flaps. Longacre and Gilby[53] state that a prosthesis for an extensive defect is unsatisfactory, and the efficiency of a prosthesis is inversely proportional to the size of the defect. They have reported reconstruction of extensive palatal defects utilizing local flaps as well as tubed pedicle flaps. For perforations and defects not exceeding one half of the hard and soft palates, local mucoperiosteal flaps may be utilized. For more extensive losses they have used tubed pedicle flaps from various donor sites such as the arm, the chest, and the neck.

Edgerton and Zovickian[22] also mention difficulties of retention of prostheses. They make use of a cervical tube inserted through an incision beneath the border of the mandible rather than through the mouth. They also use the bulk of the tube to fill out the defect of the zygomatic area where indicated.

Gillies and Millard[31] have used tubed pedicle flaps for repair of traumatic palatal defects as well as cleft palates. In many instances a combination of local and tube flaps is necessary for a satisfactory reconstruction.

CONTOUR REPLACEMENT
Soft tissue

Lacerations of the cheek frequently leave depressed scars, which may be corrected by excision of the scar, undermining of the skin, and development and imbrication of fat flaps. Free dermal grafts have been used for filling out such soft tissue defects, but have definite limits in regard to the amount of correction that can be made. Peer[72] prefers a free graft containing both dermis and fat (Fig. 22-1, *C*). This is very effective in creating a soft, even contour in the cheek and should be inserted with the dermis placed deep in the wound and the fat superficially facing the skin. These grafts almost universally will show a certain amount of shrinkage, and consequently they must be inserted with overcorrection.

Cartilage

Contour loss of the hard structures of the face is usually repaired by substances of a similar texture. Contour defects characterized by loss or displacement of supporting structure may involve the frontal, mental, or malar prominences, the orbital floor or margins, and the external nose and ear. These defects have been corrected by a variety of substances, including viable autogenous tissue as well as a variety of inert materials. Kazanjian and Converse[46]

Acquired defects of the hard and soft tissues of the face **417**

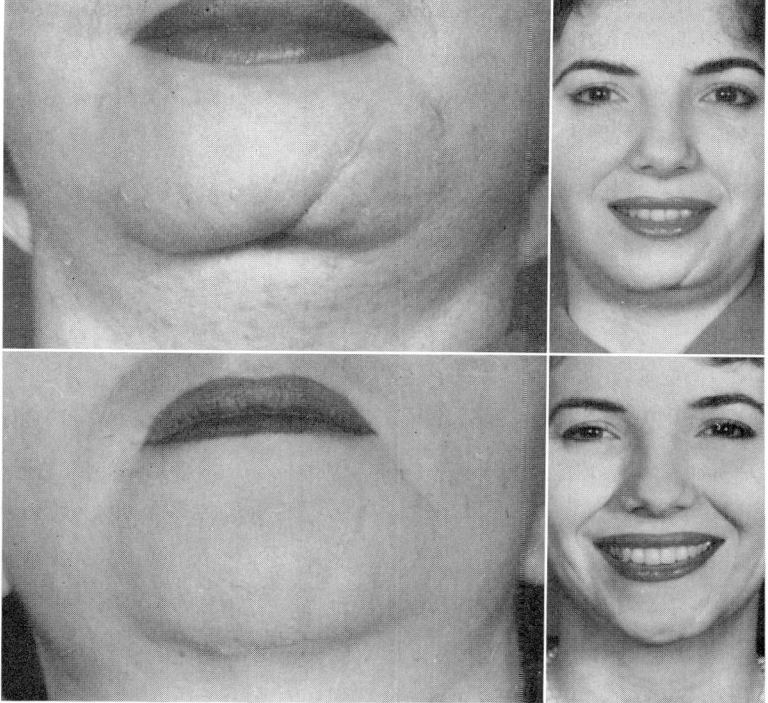

Fig. 22-15. Posttraumatic submental defect corrected by means of dermal fat graft.

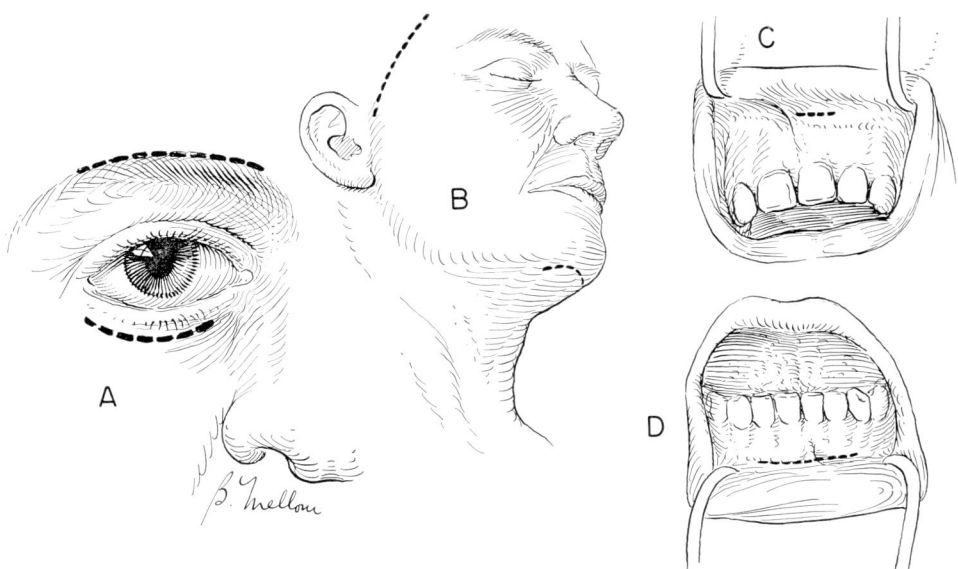

Fig. 22-16. Illustration of routes of approach for implanting filling materials. **A**, Infraorbital and supraorbital. **B**, Temporal and submental. **C**, Intraoral, maxilla. **D**, Intraoral, mandible.

have filled out the prominence of the chin by rotating a fat flap from the neck below the chin, and Gillies and Millard[31] describe the use of a temporal muscle flap for restoration of the malar prominence. These problems are more frequently managed by use of bone or cartilage or an inert material, such as tantalum, Vitallium, or rubber silicone. Good results have been reported with a wide variety of materials, but in some instances this must reflect the amazing tolerance that the tissues sometimes exhibit to any kind of foreign body. A satisfactory implant material by itself will not guarantee success. Meticulous surgical technique must be used, and a satisfactory bed for the implant is necessary as well as adequate skin and subcutaneous tissue covering.

Adequate exposure of the graft bed is essential and requires proper undermining (Fig. 22-16). However, unnecessary extensive undermining is to be condemned. The supraorbital area may be approached through incisions in the eyebrow; the malar bone may be approached through the temporal route, through previous scars, or through an infraorbital incision. The orbital floor is approached via the infraorbital route. The chin prominence may be approached either submentally or through the oral vestibule. With either cartilage or bone the use of preconstructed molds as a pattern for shaping the implant may be of value.

Millard[59] has reported several successful cases of chin implants, utilizing homologous and heterologous cartilage inserted via the oral labial sulcus. An endonasal incision is preferred for nasal restorations. Cartilage grafts are of particular value in nasal and ear reconstructions.

Bone

Bone continues to be popular for correcting contour defects, particularly fresh autogenous bone. As in the case of cartilage, bone grafts have been of three types: autogenous, homogenous, and heterogenous. The physiology of bone growth and bone grafting is one of the most interesting phases of medical science and still a fertile field for new discovery. Excellent historical reviews have been published by Converse and Campbell[17] and by Chase and Herndon.[14]

An overwhelming opinion favors iliac bone for grafting procedures. This apparently results from the fact that the large spaces within the substance of the cancellous iliac bone allow early rapid revascularization with survival of many of the graft cells. Abbott and co-workers[1] report new formation of trabeculae, demonstrated microscopically as early as 10 days, with iliac grafts. They state further that tibial cortical bone is very low in osteogenic power because of the need for resorption and replacement of the increased amount of dense bone that does not survive. They further state that the same is true of rib grafts, although not to such a great extent, and that split-rib grafts compare more favorably with iliac grafts because of the open spaces presented for revascularization.

Mowlem[62] during World War II began correcting facial defects with chip grafts to facilitate revascularization and survival of graft cells. He found that fixation of these grafts was obtained as early as 10 days, using pressure dressing only.

Iliac bone seems to be much more resistant in the presence of infection. Stuteville[83] and more recently Obwegeser[65] have reported the use of homogenous iliac block graft in the presence of infection. It seems evident that the greater the area of graft recipient bone contact, the more certain and more rapid the regeneration. Adequate fixation is essential, although this does not present such a problem in contour defects as it does in full-thickness defects of the mandible. As with all types of implants adequate soft tissue covering is desired, although ultimate healing in the presence of incomplete soft tissue closure has been reported, particularly with iliac chips.

Iliac grafts for facial defects are implanted via similar routes as is done with cartilage in the temporal region, eyebrow, hairline, infraorbital margin, previous scars, and submental area. Ragnell[76] has reported bone implants of the maxillary and nasal areas inserted through an incision in the columella. Adams and associates[2] have applied bone implants to the maxilla through an incision at the alar margin. Converse and Campbell[17] have achieved remarkably good results, inserting iliac grafts to facial defects via the oral cavity.

Block grafts of the ilium are somewhat harder to shape than cartilage. Shaping is done with rongeurs or a Stryker saw. With block grafts a somewhat more extensive dissection is required than with cartilage, and bare bone must be exposed. For this reason Mowlem[62] resorted to chip graft restorations, maintaining that they could be inserted with much less extensive dissection through smaller incision of access, with easier molding and more rapid consolidation.

It may be advantageous to combine a shaped block graft with iliac chips in filling contours. This will aid both in accuracy of restoration and in early consolidation. The block graft may be placed with the cortex external or with the cortex against the graft bed. More accurate shaping usually can be done if the cortex is left toward the external surface. Usually a moderately firm pressure dressing is all that is necessary for fixation, although direct wiring may be utilized. Where large block grafts are use on a curved surface, it may be necessary to cut or fracture the cortex to allow more accurate bending and shaping of the graft.

Some rather extensive defects of the maxilla have been corrected by bone graft. Gillies and Millard[31] have described replacement of the maxilla by graft from malar prominence to malar prominence.

Campbell[12,13] has reported two rather extensive reconstructions of the maxilla. One was a result of trauma, the other an immediate repair at the time of removal of extensive malignant disease. Converse has reported reconstruction of the floor of the orbit and malar bone following extensive excision for neoplastic disease.

Artificial implants

Alloplasts. The use of inert foreign body implants (alloplasts) in surgery continues to be a matter of considerable disagreement. Smith,[81] Peer,[73] and Kiehn and Grino[47] all advised against the use of foreign body replacements. Kiehn and Grino maintained that with slight trauma alloplastic transplants may become infected, absorbed, or extruded and advised use of autogenous tissue transplants whenever possible. In spite of certain apparent objections, there seems to be an increasingly wide usage of such materials, particularly Vitallium and tantalum among the metals, methyl methacrylate, polyethylene, Ivalon, and Teflon among the synthetic resins, and more recently the rubber silicones.

Conley[16] dates the search for a foreign body for implantation purposes back to 1565, when Petronius devised a gold plate for the repair of defects of the cleft palate. Since then many materials have been tried and some, such as ivory and paraffin, discarded because of poor and sometimes harmful results.

In spite of the advantages of cartilage and bone as a filling material, they nevertheless possess certain disadvantages, such as (1) resorption, (2) distortion, (3) difficulty of shaping, (4) problem of additional surgery. For this reason alloplasts continue to be investigated and utilized for purposes of contour reconstruction.

Criteria for a successful alloplastic implant will vary slightly, depending upon its function, particularly with regard to texture of the implant. However, in general, a successful implant (1) should not produce a reaction in body tissues, (2) should not produce tumor, (3) should be easily workable, whether soft or hard, resilient or rigid, according to the individual needs.

Metals. Until the work of Venable and Stuck,[87,88] use of metallic implants was characterized by frequent failure. Venable and Stuck showed that corrosion took place through the process of electrolysis in most of the metals then in use. Their investigations revealed three metals that were sufficiently electropassive to be used in surgery: (1) Vitallium, which is an alloy of cobalt, chromium, and molybdenum; (2) tantalum, a metallic element discovered by Ekeburg in Sweden in 1892; and (3) 18-8-SMO steel, a stainless steel alloy containing 18% chrominum, 8% nickel, and 4% molybdenum. Since then these three metals have been used extensively in bone surgery as plates, screws, wires, and trays.

Tantalum and Vitallium have both been used with success for filling in facial defects. Tantalum is strong and, because of its ductility, can be drawn, stamped, or formed in complicated shapes. It may be machined with ordinary steel tools. It has been used in the form of plates for cranioplasty and is easily adapted to defects, although it tends to leave a dead space on the undersurface.

Perforated tantalum plates are readily adapted for correction of facial deformities. Fig. 22-17 shows reconstruction of the infraorbital floor and rim with a perforated tantalum plate supported by autogenous iliac bone chips. Construction of such a tantalum plate is carried out as follows.

The bony contours of both orbits are

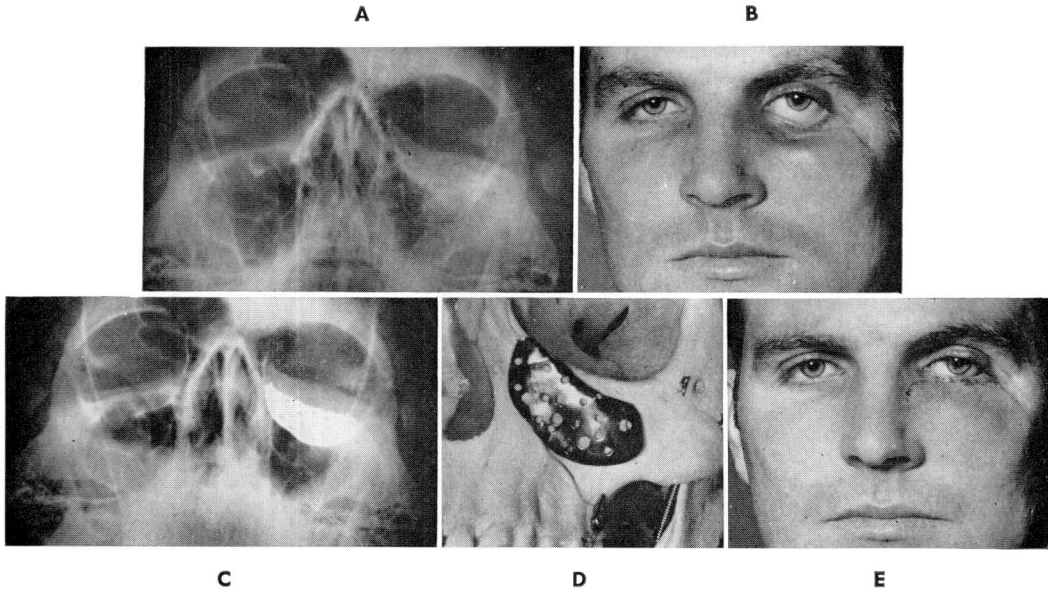

Fig. 22-17. Reconstruction of infraorbital margin utilizing tantalum implant and iliac bone chips. **A**, Preoperative roentgenogram. **B**, Preoperative photograph. **C**, Postoperative roentgenogram. **D**, Contoured tantalum implant adapted to suitable skull. This was the plate used in C. **E**, Postoperative photograph. Note incision beginning at the lateral margin of the nose, carried beneath the margin of the eyelid and laterally along the previous scar to allow reflection of the flap without having the incision lie over the implant.

palpated and marked on the skin with indelible pencil for transferring to the plaster model. Vertical and horizontal dimensions of the uninjured orbit are measured and recorded. The impression is made of the patient's face, using hydrocolloid material, and a cast is poured in plaster. From the actual measurements and x-rays of the facial bones (taken at a 6-foot distance), a skull approximating the patient's dimensions is chosen. Undercuts are eliminated, and a plaster impression is made of that portion of the skull representing the corresponding orbit. The plaster negative is used as a template to restore the orbital margin on the facial cast. The malar portion of the defect is then filled out with Plastiline to correspond to the opposite cheek. From the restored facial cast a stone die and counterdie are constructed, the die extending at least 1 inch beyond the periphery of the involved area in all directions. A tantalum plate, $1/100$ inch thick, is used and perforated with a mechanical drill. The plate to be used is outlined from a tin-foil pattern previously adapted to the defect. It is then swaged and adapted over the defect with a wooden mallet. Final adaption is obtained by swaging between the die and counterdie with a hand press.

Similar replacements may be made using preconstructed Vitallium implants; however, technically this may be somewhat more difficult, and adjustment at surgery is impossible.

Beder[6,7] has performed extensive studies with titanium, a metal characterized by extreme lightness, high degree of strength, resistance to corrosion, and low conductivity. His studies indicate that titanium implants are well tolerated by animal tissues. An additional potential advantage of titanium consists in the fact that it is radiolucent and, when buried in the area of facial bones, will allow satisfactory radiographic evaluation of surrounding and underlying tissues. Tantalum and Vitallium both have the disadvantage of being radiopaque, consequently interfering with postoperative x-ray studies.

Synthetic resins. For contour restoration the synthetic resins have probably found much wider usage than metals in recent years. Ingraham and associates[41] published an excellent review of the use of synthetic plastic materials in surgery. Of the synthetic resins only the thermoplastic products have been used in surgical procedures. A thermoplastic resin can be molded without chemical change, for example, by softening under heat and pressure and cooling following molding. Of these synthetic resins, methyl methacrylate, polyethylene, polyvinyl alcohol (Ivalon), and polytetrafluoroethylene (Teflon) have been used successfully. Ingraham, Alexander, and others caution against the use of synthetic resins containing plasticizers and other foreign irritants. They also point out that controlled experimental studies should be carried out before utilizing new plastic materials.

Freeman[27] has reported on twenty clinical cases, using Ivalon sponge for facial reconstruction. He reported four complications, two of which resulted in removal of the sponge. In one instance the sponge survived "a localized infectious process." Freeman noted that the remaining implants, without complications, maintained in a large measure the desired size, position, and fixation, but were firmer than desired. He further noted that sufficient time had not elapsed to evaluate the effect of friction, trauma, late scar contracture, and carcinogenic stimulation.

Campbell[13] reports the use of polyethylene in a variety of defects of the facial bones over a period of 4 years with satisfactory results. It has not been necessary to remove any of the implants during this period.

In 1956 Quereau and Souder[75] reported on the use of polytetrafluoroethylene (Teflon) in restoring the floor of the orbit and maxillary contour. They refer to the experiments by LeVeen and Barberio,[50] corroborated by Calnan,[11] indicating that Teflon was the least irritating of the plastics to tissue. The material is white, the surface feels waxy, and the plastic can be whittled and shaped with a sharp knife like soft wood. It is the most chemically inert plastic ever developed. It is stable to temperatures up to 620° F. and can be autoclaved. It has a relatively high tensile strength, is flexible, has a memory, and undergoes nearly complete recovery from a deforming load. Nothing will stick to Teflon with any appreciable strength, and water will not wet it.

Rubber silicones. At the present time a rubber silicone (Silastic) is enjoying a high degree of popularity and may prove to be one of the most useful materials yet developed for contour correction. It has several outstanding advantages in that it comes in several different forms and is readily contoured, it can be autoclaved and it is apparently nonirritating.[63] Of particular interest is an injectable form which at present is being used experimentally for elimination of wrinkle lines as well as correction of contour deformities.[23,28]

Unquestionably the use of alloplastic materials must still be considered to be in an experimental stage. However, the eminent surgeon, Sir Harold Gillies, suggested that one of the plastic materials may eventually take the place of all nonautogenous grafts.[31]

Of particular interest is the current trend to intraoral insertion[44] of the alloplastic implants. Apparently with improvement in sterile technique, surgical technique, and use of antibiotics the margin of safety has increased remarkably as far as intraoral procedures are concerned.

Repositioning procedures

Fractures of the mandible may be corrected by open reduction as late as 6 or 8 weeks after injury. Fractures of middle facial bones usually heal in a shorter time. Even after bony union has taken place it is possible in certain instances to perform osteotomies and reposition displaced fragments such as is done in treatment of developmental deformities.

Dingman and Natvig[21] have described such procedures as are particularly applicable to the maxillary and mandibular dentition. Impressions may be made, the models cut, and repositioned for the fabrication of cast splints where indicated. If feasible,

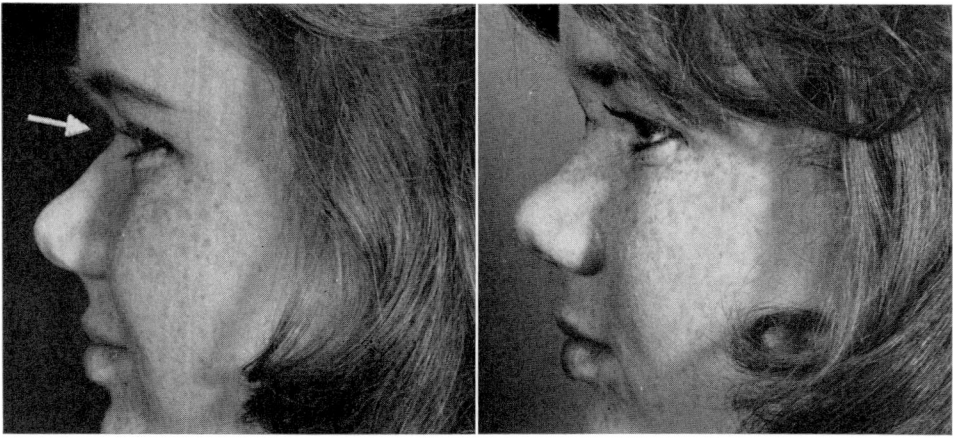

Fig. 22-18. Correction of glabellar defect by means of rubber silicone (Silastic) implant.

Acquired defects of the hard and soft tissues of the face 423

such procedures are preferred to contour corrections or correction by extraction of teeth and construction of prostheses. (See Figs. 22-19 and 22-20.)

RECONSTRUCTION OF THE MANDIBLE

Reconstruction of the mandible presents several problems not found in simple contour restorations, particularly in regard to adequate fixation. Mandibular continuity may be lost because of infection, trauma, or neoplastic diseases and may be restored with alloplastic materials or bone grafts.

Alloplasts

The use of alloplastic materials such as Vitallium, stainless steel, and methyl methacrylate has been largely restricted to restoration of continuity following excision of neoplastic disease, particularly with reference to immediate repair. Prostheses used for restoring the continuity of the mandible may be in the form of intramedullary bars or Kirschner wires or in the form of preformed prostheses constructed of methyl methacrylate or Vitallium.

Maintenance of the continuity of the

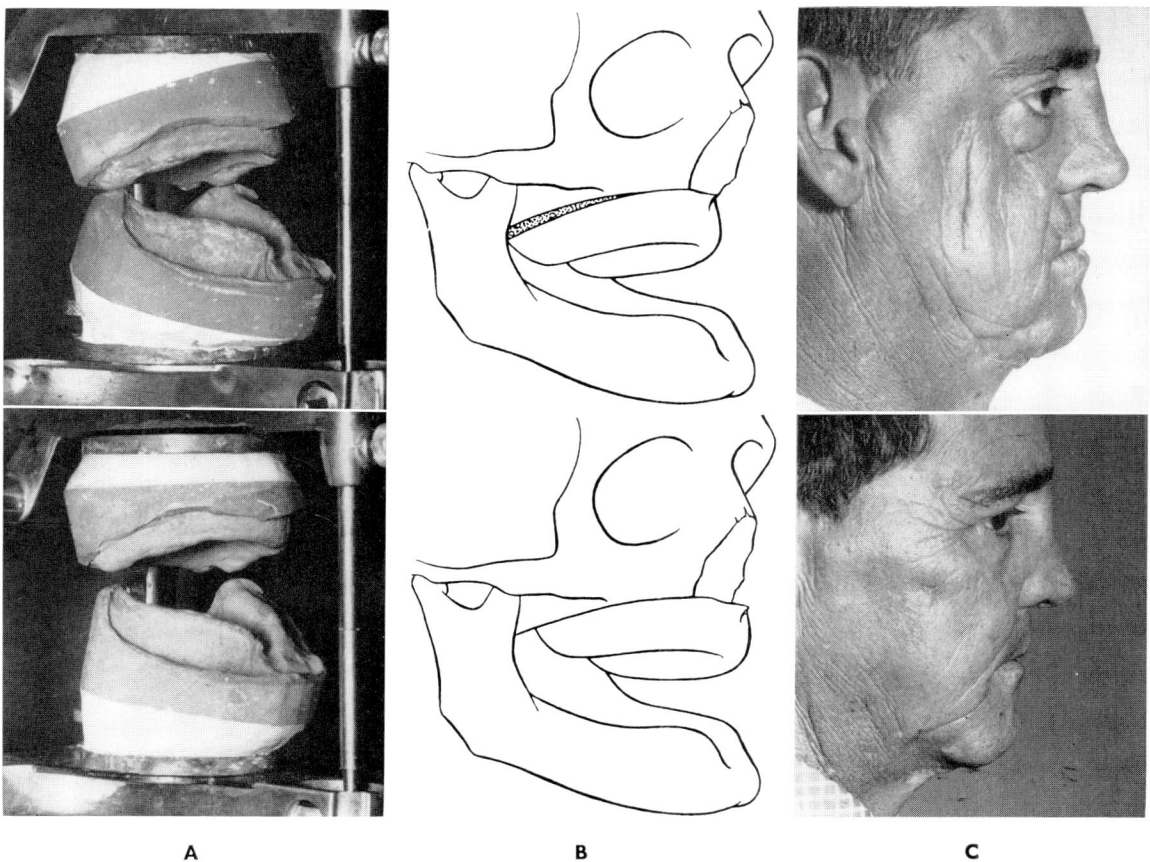

A B C

Fig. 22-19. Repositioning of maxilla 4 years following injury in auto accident. **A,** Preoperative and postoperative study models. **B,** Drawings showing repositioning procedure. **C,** Preoperative and postoperative photographs—patient wearing dentures in postoperative photograph; unable to wear dentures before surgery.

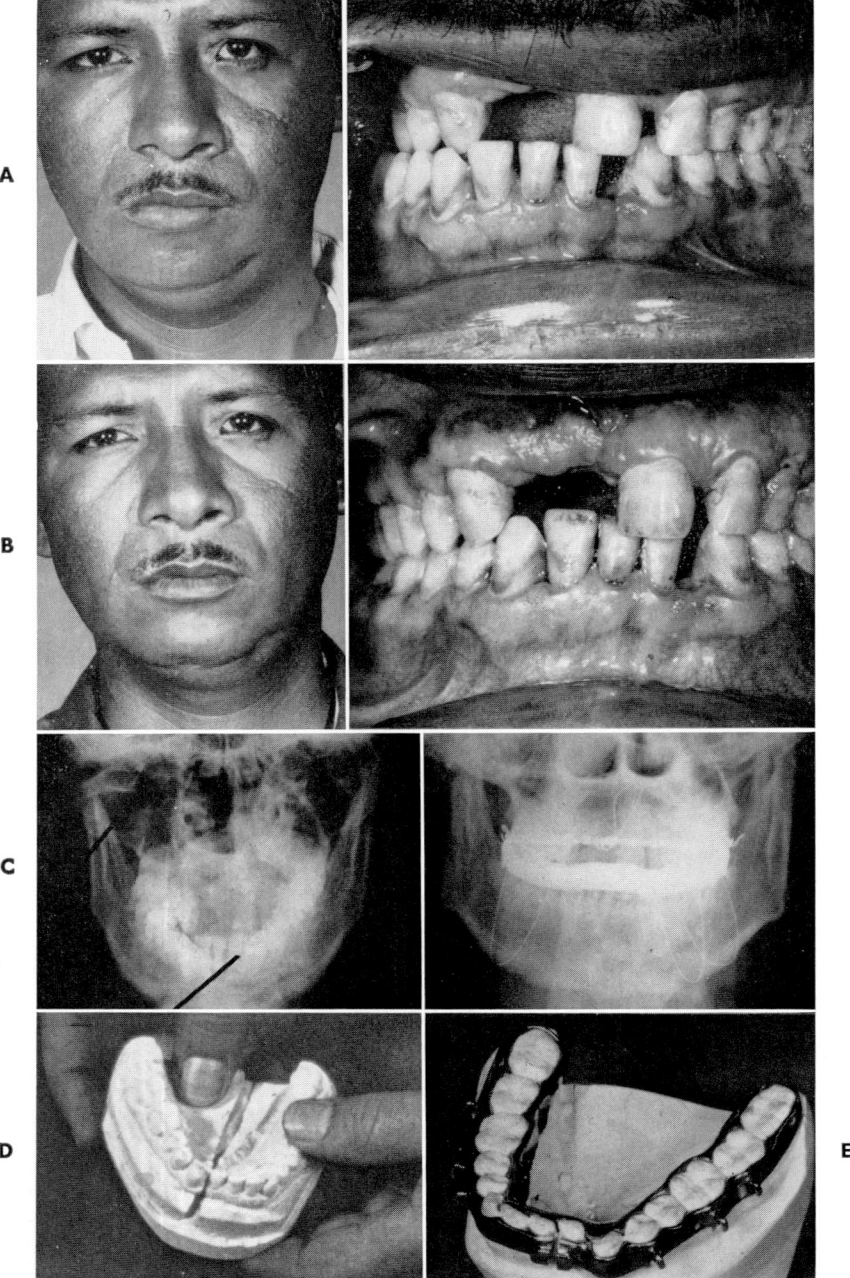

Fig. 22-20. Repositioning of mandible 6 months following injury in auto accident. Initial treatment with headcap and Kirschner wire in malposition. **A,** Preoperative photographs demonstrating crossbite. **B,** Postoperative photographs. **C,** Radiographs showing osteotomy sites and postoperative position. **D,** Correction of crossbite on model. **E,** Construction of splint in corrected position.

mandible is desirable not only from a cosmetic viewpoint, but also to preserve adequate swallowing, speech, and, in some instances, respiration. Losses of the posterior mandible are tolerated much better than losses from the symphysis area. Plates and intramedullary bars may serve the additional function of maintaining the fragments in position until bone grafts can be done, if immediate bone grafting is not indicated (Fig. 22-21).

Full-thickness mandibular segments may be replaced by intramedullary bars or wires, usually of stainless steel. These can be adapted very easily to contour. They present the problem of telescoping, which may be solved by means of threaded pins with flanges or by making L-shaped bends in the pins to prevent further penetration of the marrow cavity. These take up little space and are easily covered with soft tissue. Stainless steel or Vitallium plates, either preconstructed to the individual case or selected from standard kits, may be used. The stainless steel plates are readily adapted to contour. These are secured by means of two screws at each fragment. The screws, ideally, should engage both cortices.

Vitallium replacements of various parts of the mandible may be preconstructed to the individual case, using various sized mandibles as patterns and the patient's x-ray films and actual measurements for selection of proper size. Such replacements have been used on many occasions in the past, and indeed one author[30] has reported complete replacement of the mandible with such a Vitallium prosthesis functioning without difficulty at least 2 years following surgery. Dewey and Moore have recently reported thirteen successful cases wherein varying portions of the mandible were replaced with Vitallium prostheses.[95]

Fig. 22-22 demonstrates an appliance that has remained in place and functioning for 10 years. Matalon[58] has modified Hahn's[35] adjustable Vitallium prosthesis for replacement of segments of mandible lost because of malignant disease. These are cast in ticonium rather than Vitallium, and their chief advantage is their use in more extensive resectioning involving the symphysis area (Fig. 22-23).

Similar replacements may be constructed of methyl methacrylate.[37] These should be somewhat smaller than the original mandibular segment to facilitate soft tissue closure. They should be perforated to allow better fixation and fluid drainage and to allow for muscle attachment. Usually direct fixation is all that is necessary, al-

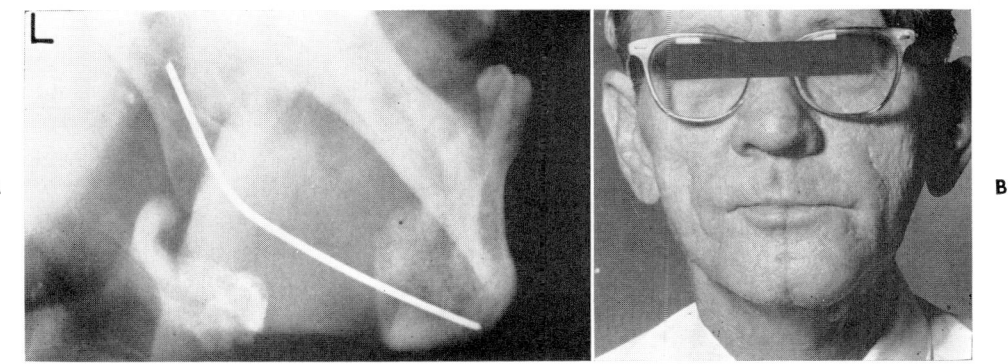

Fig. 22-21. Immediate reconstruction of combined resection of mandible and neck by use of intramedullary bar. **A**, Postoperative roentgenogram. **B**, Photograph showing cosmetic result.

426 *Textbook of oral surgery*

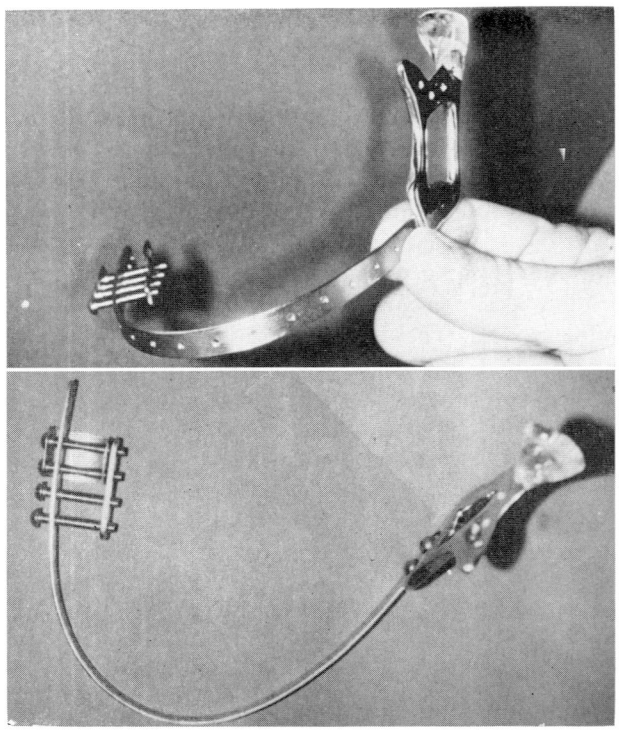

Fig. 22-22. Appliance constructed of acrylic and stainless steel with screw and bolt type of fixation that has been in place and functioning for 10 years. Constructed by Dr. Joe B. Drane and Dr. Duni Miglani, The University of Texas, Dental Branch.

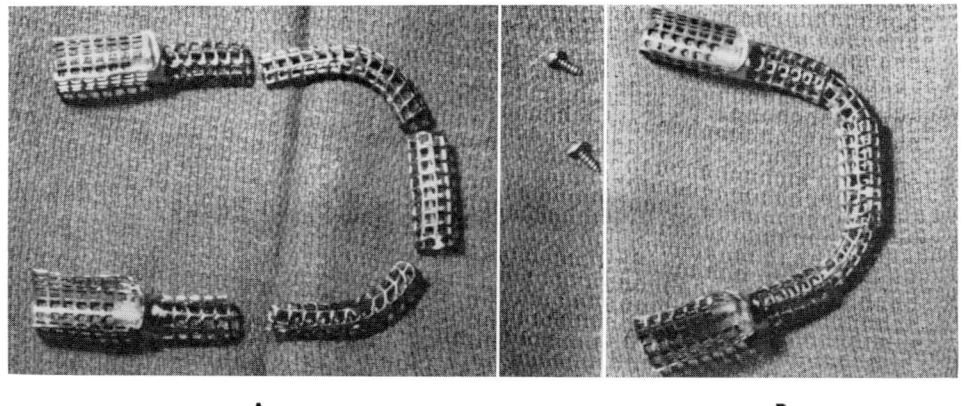

Fig. 22-23. Adjustable cast ticonium prosthesis (Hahn prosthesis modified by Matalon). **A**, Prosthesis dismantled. **B**, Prosthesis assembled.

though fixation can be supplemented with other methods such as external pins. Fixation of these prostheses may be facilitated by use of wedge-shaped attachments at each end that are impacted into the mandible by means of perforated, wedge-shaped attachments placed into the marrow cavity.

In all of these problems greater difficulty is found in replacement of loss as a result of malignant disease than benign, and it is more difficult to replace the symphysis area than more posterior areas.

It has been my feeling that the multiple stresses exerted by the mandible in function would tend to create loosening of most artificial implants, although Freeman noted new bone growth over the screwheads in one implant that had to be removed because of exposure.[26] I have used a Sherman plate as an immediate replacement following excision of a rather large adamantinoma of the body of the mandible. This stayed in place 15 months, but had to be removed because of loosening of the screws at the anterior attachment.

Bone

In spite of the recent successes with alloplastic substances, it is particularly true of the mandible that it is desirable to replace lost tissue with tissue of a similar nature. Hayward and Roffinella[36] have very aptly described the peculiar problems associated with reconstruction of the mandible. They describe the mandible as a mobile functioning unit, influenced to considerable degree by the pull of the adjacent muscles, being shaped and constructed in such a manner as to complicate problems of fixation.

A very excellent review of bone grafting in defects of the mandible was published by Ivy in 1951.[42] Bardenheuer[4] is credited with being the first to perform an autogenous bone graft of the mandible in 1891. This was in the form of a pedicle flap from the forehead, containing skin, periosteum, and bone. Sykoff[84] (1900) is believed to have been the first to employ a free bone transplant to the lower jaw. In 1908 Payr[71] reported on the use of free transplants of the tibia and the rib. During World War I, Lindemann[51] and Klapp[48] began to use the iliac crest as the donor site. Klapp also reported on the use of the fourth metatarsal as a transplant to replace the lost ascending ramus and and condyle. More recently, Dingman[20] has also reported on the use of the metatarsal bone as a replacement for the condyle. Efforts to use this as a growth center graft have not been rewarding.

In spite of the lack of antibiotics and proper metallic fixation of appliances, Ivy[42] reported 76% successful, 7.7% partly successful, and 13.5% failures of 103 bone-grafting operations of the mandible during and immediately after World War I. Broken down into types of grafts, the figures were as follows: 31 cases of pedicle graft, 87%; 38 cases of osteoperiosteal, 71%; 7 cases of crest of ilium, 71%; 17 cases of cortex or tibia, 65%; 6 cases of rib graft, 100% success; 3 cases of sliding ramus graft, 2 of these successful; 1 case of heterologous (ox bone graft), 1 failure. Blocker and Stout,[9] reporting on a large collection of cases from all maxillofacial centers in the United States treating casualties of World War II, reported a total of 1,010 mandibular grafts as follows: 90.7% successful primarily, increased to 97% if regrafts are included. Broken down as to types of grafts, they were as follows: 836 from the ilium, 151 from the rib, and 23 from the tibia.

Indications for bone grafting of the mandible. Bone grafts are indicated in cases of nonunion of fractures of the mandible in which freshening of the fractured ends would result in foreshortening of the mandible. Bone grafts may be indicated in cases of extreme atrophy of the mandible. They may be used for filling out contour defects and for full-thickness loss of mandibular segments resulting from infection, trauma, or excision of neoplastic disease.

Watson-Jones[90] has pointed out that variations are possible in healing time of a fracture and that delayed union does not necessarily mean nonunion. Prolonged and proper immobilization may result in union. In the case of the mandible, because of the absence of weight bearing, osseous union may eventually occur even without immobilization if the patient is maintained on a controlled diet.

All three source types of bone grafts have been used: autogenous, homogenous, and heterogenous. Autogenous bone has been used most widely and is the graft of choice. Preserved homogenous bone has been used both as a block replacement and as chips.

Considerable use has been made of homogenous bone grafts in repair of nonunion for fractures in which defects are small. Here they seem to exert an osteogenetic effect of definite value. Although full-thickness replacements of mandibular defects with homogenous bone have been reported by Converse and Stuteville, its use in such instances appears to be decidedly inferior to autogenous bone.

Grafts may be used in the following forms: (1) block from tibia, rib, or ilium; (2) osteoperiosteal graft, usually from tibia; (3) chip grafts from ilium; (4) pedicle grafts from mandible. The osteoperiosteal graft contains all of the elements necessary for osteogenesis; it is flexible and easily adjustable to size and shape of defect, but is suitable only for small defects. The technique for removal and insertion is simpler than that of any of the other methods. The use of the pedicle graft should also be limited to small defects. Of the block grafts, use of the tibia has for all practicable purposes been discontinued. Most surgeons prefer the ilium; however, the rib still finds favor with some.

The iliac block graft has several definite advantages. It is largely cancellous, it allows rapid transmission of tissue fluids and nutritive elements, and it provides innumerable pathways for ingrowth of growing cells. It may be readily shaped to meet contour and morticing requirements, and because of its cortical layer and bulk it may serve to a great extent as its own fixation appliance. Iliac chips have been used extensively in facial reconstruction since Mowlem's report. He was impressed by their resistance to infection and the rapidity with which vascularization and consolidation took place.[62] In addition to contour defects, iliac chips have found considerable use in the management of nonunions and as an added osteogenetic factor in osteotomies. They are also used to a great extent in combination with larger block grafts for the purpose of filling in minor irregularities and adding to the osteogenetic stimulus. Mowlem's original report described such a technique involving the use of a large cancellous block medially and cancellous chips laterally, the block graft being used to prevent soft tissues from bulging through the mandibular defect and to protect the chips from movement transmitted from the floor of the mouth.

Excellent discussions of the approach to the ilium and the obtaining of the graft are given by Dick[19] and Abbott and associates.[1] The ilium is approached by a transverse skin incision made below the crest to prevent pressure irritation (Fig. 22-24). It is exposed after severing gluteal muscle attachments externally, the external oblique muscle above, and the iliacus medially. Full-thickness grafts may be used, or grafts may be limited to either the outer or the inner plate and medulla.

Chip grafts may be obtained with a gouge after creating a window in the outer cortex, thus leaving the inner cortex undisturbed. I have obtained circular plugs through the outer cortex with an Illif trephine attached to a Stryker saw for repairing nonunions (Fig. 22-25). A circular plug is removed with a No. 7 trephine at the fracture site. The graft is taken with a No. 8

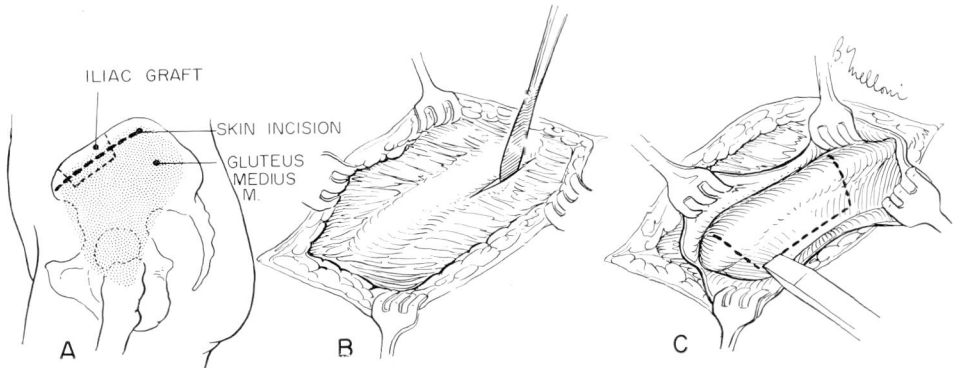

Fig. 22-24. Iliac graft. **A,** Line of incision. **B,** Stripping of muscle and periosteum. **C,** Use of osteotome for outline of graft to be obtained with osteotome.

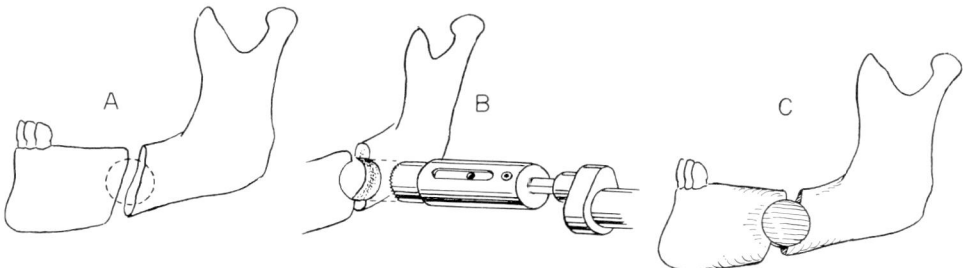

Fig. 22-25. Use of Illif trephine in bone grafting. **A,** Preoperative condition. Site of plug to be removed is diagrammed. **B,** Plug removed from nonunion site with No. 7 trephine. **C,** Graft taken from ilium with No. 8 trephine and inserted into defect. Outer diameter of No. 7 trephine matches inner diameter of No. 8, allowing an accurate fit of graft.

trephine. The outer diameter of the No. 7 trephine matches the inner diameter of the No. 8. The trephine graft is then wedged into the nonunion defect, providing a very precise fit.

Complications following removal of iliac grafts are infrequent, the most common being hematoma formation, which can be prevented to a great extent by careful hemostasis at the time of surgery and the use of fibrin foam or bone wax. However, postoperative pain may be more severe at the iliac site than at the graft site.

Replacement of the angle and entire ascending ramus and placement of large defects of the midline present unusual problems in mandibular bone grafting. Two methods have been used for restoring the angle and ascending ramus. A rib with a portion of its adjacent cartilage may be used, the cartilaginous portion of the graft being placed in the glenoid fossa. The contralateral anterior superior spine, and iliac crest may be adapted very well to the replacement of this portion of the mandible. However, the chances for resorption in such an extensive graft, attached at one end only, are considerable. There may be some advantage in preserving the condylar fragment when possible to facilitate function and regeneration. In such cases the coronoid process should always be removed because of the harmful muscle pull. In most cases in which a large graft must be prepared it is advisable to construct a stent of polymethyl metharcylate that will aid in developing the graft bed and in obtaining a graft of the proper shape and size.

Description of the surgical approach to the restoration of the angle and ascending ramus is difficult to find in the literature. The object is to develop a plane between the masseter and the internal pterygoid muscle. Kazanjian and Converse[46] utilize three nerves as landmarks in developing this plane. These are the lingual, the inferior alveolar, and the mylohyoid nerves. Because of previous difficulties encountered, Rehrmann[77] made a detailed study of the anatomy of this area and described a method for preparing this area with minimum danger to nerves and vessels. He made use of the stylohyoid muscle and process as landmarks in reaching the glenoid fossa.

The symphysis area may be restored with a split-rib graft or a shaped iliac block. It may be restored by a skewer graft as described by Gillies and Millard,[31] consisting of blocks of iliac crest impaled on a Kirschner wire and molded to shape.

Abbott and co-workers,[1] in discussing the merits of cortical and cancellous bone, mentioned the possibility of late fracture in cortical grafts replacing large gaps. Ghormley, in discussing Abbott's paper, stated that cortical grafts, after reaching a stage where they have good circulation, go through a stage of atrophy, during which period some of them may fracture. I have had such an experience with a rib graft (Fig. 22-26). This necessitated replacement with an iliac graft. Because of this problem in large gaps, Abbott has suggested a two-stage procedure wherein cancellous grafts are used initially to establish vascularization, followed by cortical grafts that could then be vascularized throughout their entire length. The necessity for doing this in two stages is not convincing, particularly if one should use split ribs, enclosing cancellous chips for the mandible. The cancellous block, because of its adequate strength, greater bulk, and opportunities for self-splinting, seems more desirable.

Adequate soft tissue covering is of great importance in bone grafting, and, if necessary, grafting should be postponed until soft tissues may be brought in from a distance. Many surgeons advise postponing the graft if the oral cavity is entered during the procedure. In view of the excellent re-

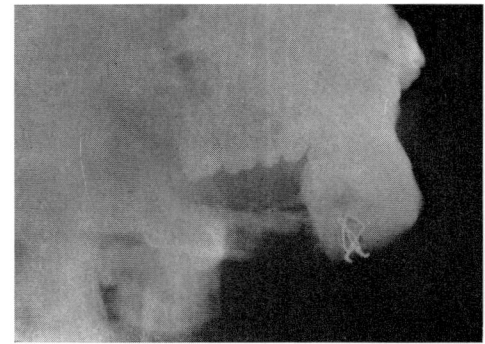 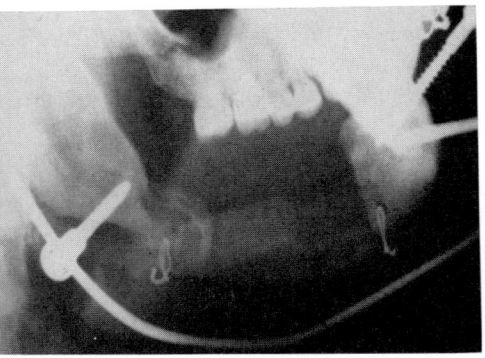

Fig. 22-26. Bone graft. A, Fracture of rib graft following atrophy. B, Same case, with graft replaced with iliac block, showing fixation by direct wiring and external pins. Graft is intact 11 years after insertion.

sults with iliac crest, the work of Converse on intraoral bone grafts, and the present-day trend toward immediate bone grafting, it would seem that contamination from compounding into the oral cavity should not be cause for postponing the procedure. It may be well to remove teeth near the ends of mandibular fragments prior to grafting to avoid cutting through tooth roots when freshening the mandibular stumps.

In spite of the fact that many reports of grafting in the presence of infection have been published, most present-day surgeons feel that it is advisable to eliminate all infection and allow a waiting period of from 2 to 6 months. At the present time with the use of cancellous iliac bone and antibiotics, it is felt that defects resulting from gunshot wounds and other trauma may be grafted soon after injury, provided adequate soft tissue covering is present. Such early repair facilitates the grafting procedure because of minimal scarring and distortion of fragments. The mandibular stumps should be cut back to an area of good vascularity. Graft and stump should be corticated in areas of contact. The wider the area of contact, the better the chance of "take." Avascular scar tissue should be removed from the muscle bed also.

Probably the most important factor in bone grafting, next to the use of the proper type of graft, is fixation. In mandibular grafts in which teeth are present, intermaxillary fixation is the method of choice. The problems of fixation arise in relation to edentulous fragments and to proximal fragments posterior to the last tooth.

Watson-Jones[90] has pointed out that immobilization serves two significant purposes: (1) control of position of the fragments and (2) protection of growing cells,

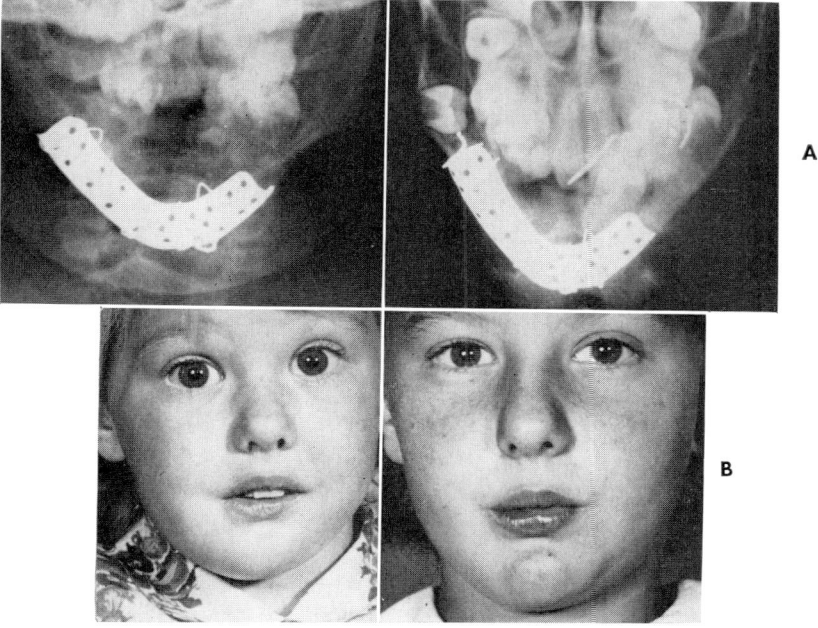

Fig. 22-27. Through-and-through deformity of mandible resulting from excision of atypical fibrous dysplasia corrected by autogenous rib graft fixed with tantalum tray at age 5. **A,** Radiographs at ages 5 and 12, demonstrating symmetrical facial development over 7-year period. **B,** Photographs, ages 5 and 12.

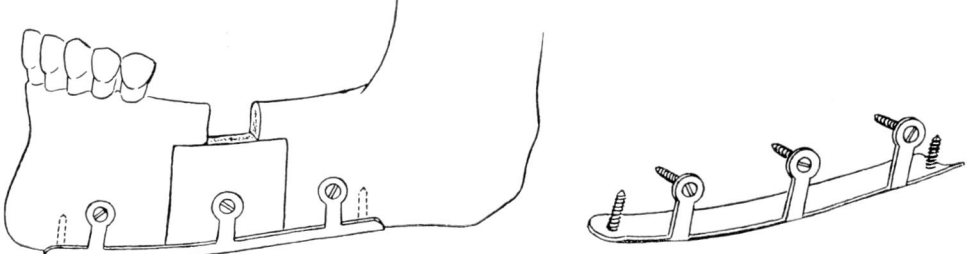

Fig. 22-28. Type of stainless steel splint described by Smith and Robinson.[82]

preventing delayed union and nonunion. Fixation may be obtained by tantalum trays, by stainless steel, tantalum, or Vitallium plates, by external pin fixation, by intramedullary pins, or by a modified gunning splint–type appliance (Fig. 22-28). In addition, direct wiring with 24-gauge stainless steel is advisable and may in itself provide sufficient fixation. A mattress suture should be used. Decortication and mortising at the graft junction will enhance the opportunities for primary union. Mortising may be accomplished by holding the graft in a bone forceps or vise and cutting with a Stryker saw. Decorticating a portion of the body of the graft will aid in revascularization, although some cortex should be maintained for strength (Fig. 22-29).

All of these methods have been used with success, and it should be emphasized that perhaps more important than method is the exercise of sufficient care in technique. In using the gunning splint principle, I prefer the two-piece modification shown in Fig. 22-30. Walden and Bromberg[89] have avoided pressure necrosis with this method by constructing the splint larger in all dimensions over the graft area to allow for the pressure of postoperative edema. The upper splint may be wired directly to the alveolar ridge, the piriform fossa, the zygomaticomaxillary pillar, or to the infraorbital margin. The lower splint is fixed by means of circumferential wires, and intermaxillary fixation is instituted by means of rubber traction or wires.

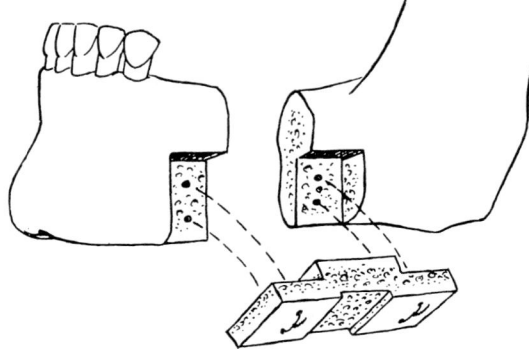

Fig. 22-29. Mortising of iliac block and partial decortication to facilitate revascularization. Fixation by direct wiring.

The criticism of bone plates is that they hold fragments apart and prevent osteogenesis by compression. This does not seem to be valid from the many reports of successful results. It would seem advisable to use screws that engage both cortical plates. Our personal preference has been for direct wiring of the graft with fixation augmented by tantalum trays or direct wiring. Fig. 22-27 shows a graft supported by a tantalum tray, inserted at age 5, with subsequent normal and symmetrical development of the mandible over a 7-year period. Intermaxillary fixation, when used, should be maintained for a period of from 8 to 12 weeks. Antibiotics should be used routinely and the patient's general health and nutrition maintained at an optimum level.

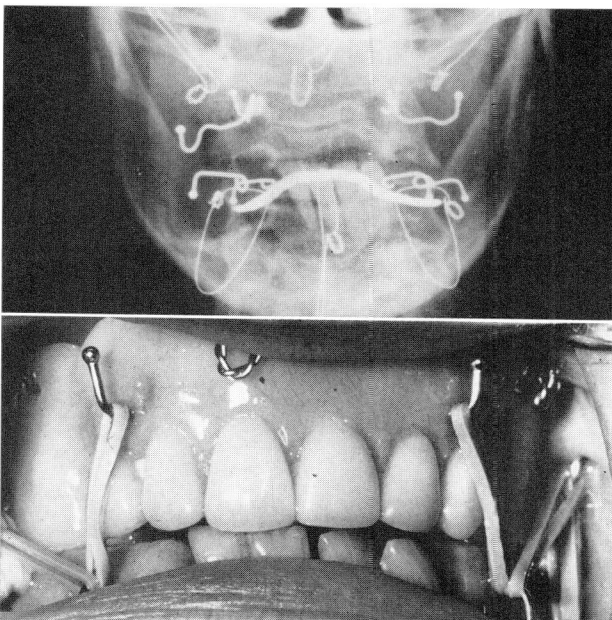

Fig. 22-30. Roentgenogram and photograph illustrating fixation by modified two-piece gunning splint in which the upper piece is wired directly to the zygomaticomaxillary pillar and the lower is fixed by means of circumferential wires.

External pin fixation and intramedullary pins may serve both to retain fragments in position at the time of original loss of mandibular structure as well as for immobilization when the graft is performed. Henny[38] has obtained excellent results in such cases with a threaded Steinmann pin containing washers and bolts for additional stabilization.

The insertion of alloplastic implants, bone grafts, and other surgical procedures upon the mandible and maxilla are being increasingly performed through the oral cavity and oral mucosa rather than the extraoral route with remarkable success for reasons already cited.

The factors must commonly associated with graft failure seem to be mobility, infection, and inadequate soft tissue coverage.

Alveolar ridge

Restoration of the edentulous alveolar ridge may be the area of greatest promise for the future as far as reconstruction with autogenous bone is concerned. It is true that such efforts in the past have frequently proved unrewarding, but some authors are reporting successes.

Genest[30] has reported several successful cases using split autogenous ribs and limiting reconstruction to the posterior portion of the alveolar ridge. Obwegeser[66] reports good results utilizing an extensive incision over the alveolar crest with incision of the periosteum and detachment of the muscles to allow extensive relaxation and advancements of the mucosal flaps. He has used both iliac crest and rib with success.

Such a case is illustrated in Fig. 22-31, in which an atrophic alveolar ridge was reconstructed with autogenous iliac crest shaped and contoured from a preconstructed acrylic template. Fixation is accomplished by circumferential suture of No. 1-0 mersilene. A vestibuloplasty must be performed as a secondary procedure.

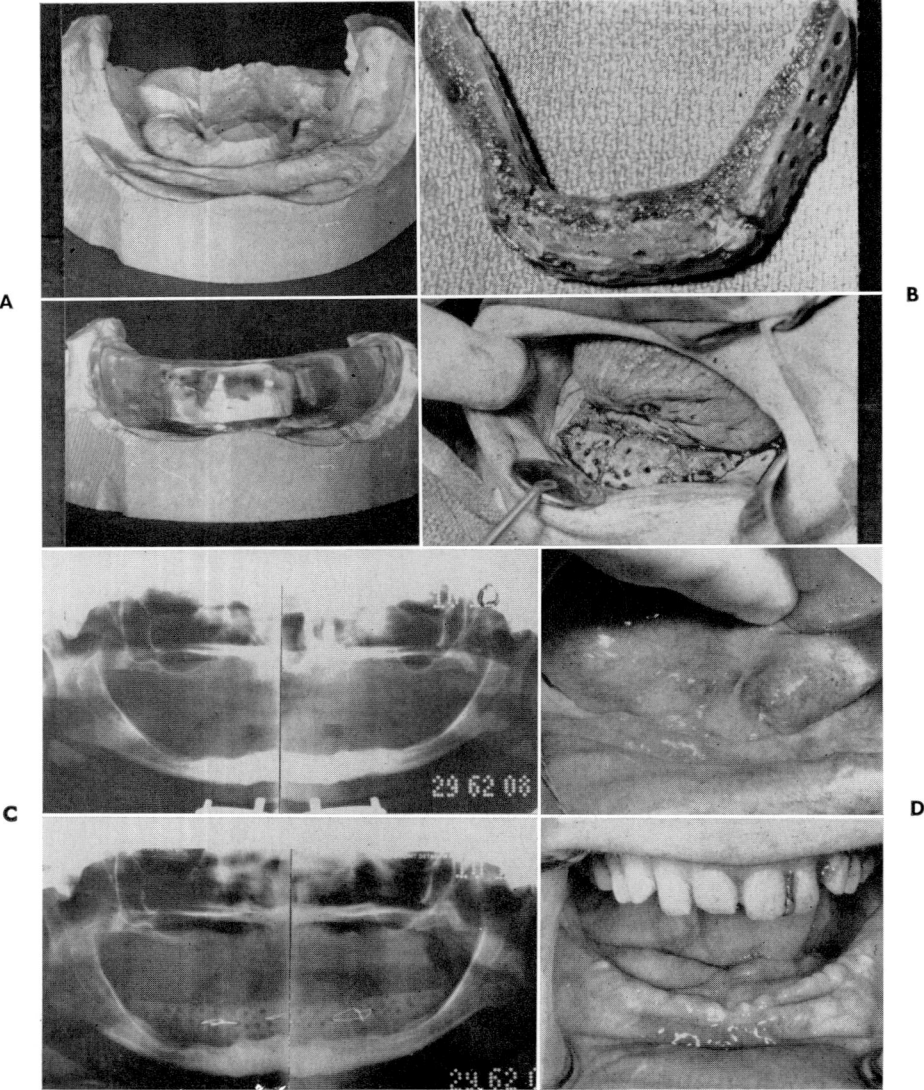

Fig. 22-31. Reconstruction of alveolar ridge with autogenous bone graft. **A**, Preoperative model and template. **B**, Iliac graft after contouring and after insertion. **C**, Preoperative and postoperative radiographs. **D**, Preoperative and postoperative photographs of ridges.

IMMEDIATE REPAIR OF COMPOUND DEFECTS RESULTING FROM CANCER SURGERY

The trend toward immediate repair of extensive wounds created by removal of malignant tissue, noted on the occasion of the initial publication of this text, not only seems to be surviving, but becoming even more popular, as evidenced by recent articles.[3,15,29,39,52,60] These procedures involve methods previously discussed, including use of free bone grafts, skin grafts, utilization of adjacent pedicle flaps in skin, mucosa, or muscle, and stabilization of mandibular fragments with metallic pins. Such reconstruction done at the time of resection allows optimum exposure while preventing contraction of tissues and degeneration of morale. Whether such a philosophy may compromise adequate surgery or hide recurrent disease remains somewhat controversial.

REFERENCES

1. Abbott, L. C., Schottstaedt, E. R., Saunders, J. B. deC. M., and Bost, F. C.: The evaluation of cortical and cancellous bone as grafting material, J. Bone Joint Surg. 29:381, 1947.
2. Adams, W. M., Adams, L. H., and Jerome, A. P.: Iliac bone graft for correction of maxillary retrusion in cases of cleft palate, J. Int. Coll. Surg. 27:384, sect. 1, 1957.
3. Bakamjian, V., and Littlewood, M.: Cervical skin flaps for intraoral and pharyngeal repair following cancer surgery, Brit. J. Plast. Surg. 17:191, 1964. Vol. XVII, No. 2, April 1964.
4. Bardenheuer: Verhand. Deutsch. Ges. Chir. 1:69, 1892.
5. Bauer: Ueber Knochentransplantation, Zbl. Chir. 37:(Beilage: 20-21), 1910.
6. Beder, O. E., and Eade, G.: An investigation of tissue tolerance to titanium metal implants in dogs, Surgery 39:470, 1956.
7. Beder, O. E., Eade, G., Stevenson, J. K., Jones, T. W., Ploger, W. J., and Condon, R. E.; Titanium metal in alloplasty, J. Dent. Res. 45:1221, 1966.
8. Bell, W. H.: Personal communication, 1958.
9. Blocker, T. G., and Stout, R. A.: Mandibular reconstruction, World War II, Plast. Reconstr. Surg. 4:153, 1949.
10. Bush, L. F.: The use of homogenous bone grafts. A preliminary report on the bone bank, J. Bone Joint Surg. 29:620, 1947.
11. Calnan, J.: The use of inert plastic material in reconstructive surgery, Brit. J. Plast. Surg. 16:1, 1963.
12. Campbell, H. H.: Reconstruction of left maxilla, Plast. Reconstr. Surg. 3:66, 1948.
13. Campbell, H. H.: Surgery of lesions of the upper face, Amer. J. Surg. 87:676, 1954.
14. Chase, S. W., and Herndon, C. H.: The fate of autogenous and homogenous bone grafts, J. Bone Joint Surg. 37A:809, 1955.
15. Coleman, C. C.: Surgical treatment of extensive cancers of the mouth and pharynx, Ann. Surg. 161:634, 1965.
16. Conley, J. J.: The use of Vitallium prostheses and implants in the reconstruction of the mandibular arch, Plast. Reconstr. Surg. 8:150, 1951.
17. Converse, J. M., and Campbell, R. M.: Bone grafts in surgery of the face, Surg. Clin. N. Amer. 34:375, 1954.
18. Conway, H., and Goulian, D.: Experiences with and injectable Silastic RTV as a subcutaneous prosthetic material, a preliminary report, Plast. Reconstr. Surg. 32:294, 1963.
19. Dick, I. L.: Iliac-bone transplantation. Preliminary observations, J. Bone Joint Surg. 28:1, 1946.
20. Dingman, F. O., and Grabb, W. C.: Reconstruction of both mandibular condyles with metatarsal bone grafts, Plast. Reconstr. Surg. 34:441, 1964.
21. Dingman, R. O., and Natvig, P.: Repair of residual deformities. In Surgery of facial fractures, Philadelphia, 1964, W. B. Saunders Co.
22. Edgerton, M. T., and Zovickian, A.: Reconstruction of major defects of the palate, Plast. Reconstr. Surg. 17:105, 1956.
23. Farrior, F. T.: Synthetics in head and neck surgery, Arch. Ophthal. 84:82, 1966.
24. Fischer, W. B., and Clayton, I.: Surgical bone grafting with cultured calf bone, Quart. Bull. Northwestern Univ. M. School 29:346, 1955.
25. Flanigin, W. S.: Free composite grafts from lower to upper lip, Plast. Reconstr. Surg. 17:376, 1956.
26. Freeman, B. S.: The use of Vitallium plates to maintain function following resection of the mandible, Plast. Reconstr. Surg. 3:73, 1948.
27. Freeman, B. S.: Complications following subcutaneous insertion of plastic sponge, Plast. Reconstr. Surg. 15:149, 1955.
28. Freeman, B. S., Bigelow, E. L., and Braley, S. A.: Experiments with injectable plastic, Amer. J. Surg. 112:534, 1966.
29. Gaisford, J. C.: Reconstruction of head and neck deformities, Surg. Clin. N. Amer. 47:295, 1967.
30. Genest, A.: Vitallium jaw replacement, Amer. J. Surg. 92:904, 1956.
31. Gillies, H., and Millard, D. R., Jr.: The principles and art of plastic surgery, vol. 2, Boston, 1957, Little, Brown & Co.
32. Glanz, S.: Skin grafting in reconstructive surgery, Texas J. Med. 52:242, 1956.
33. Gonzales-Ulloa, M., Stevens, E., and Noble, G.: Preliminary report of subcutaneous perfusion of Polysiloxane to improve regional contour, read before the meeting of the American

Association of Plastic Surgeons, Chicago, May, 1964.
34. Guillemient, M., Stagnara, P., and Dubost-Perret, T.: Preparation and use of heterogenous bone grafts, J. Bone Joint Surg. 35B:561, 1953.
35. Hahn, G. W.: Vitallium mesh mandibular prosthesis, J. Prosth. Dent. 14:777, 1964.
36. Hayward, J. R., and Roffiella, J. P.: Iliac autoplasty for repair of mandibular defects, J. Oral Surg. 13:333, 1951.
37. Healy, M. J., Jr., Sudbay, J. L., Niebel, H. H., Hoffman, B. M., and Duval, M. K.: The use of acrylic implants in one stage reconstruction of the mandible, Surg. Gynec. Obstet. 98:395, 1954.
38. Henny, F. A.: Personal communication, 1957.
39. Hoopes, J. E., and Edgerton, M. T.: Immediate forehead flap repair in resection for oropharyngeal cancer, Amer. J. Surg. 112:527, 1966.
40. Inclan, A.: The use of preserved bone graft in orthopaedic surgery, J. Bone Joint Surg. 24:81, 1942.
41. Ingraham, F. D., Alexander, E., Jr., and Matson, D. D.: Synthetic plastic materials in surgery, New Eng. J. Med. 236:362, 402, 1947.
42. Ivy, R. H.: Bone grafting for restoration of defects of the mandible, Plast. Reconstr. Surg. 7:333, 1951.
43. Judet, J., Judet, R., and Arviset, A.: Banque d'os et heterogreffe, Presse Med. 57:1007, 1949.
44. Junghans, J. A.: Profile reconstruction with Silastic chin implants, Amer. J. Orthodont. 53:217, 1967.
45. Kazanjian, V. H., and Roopenian, A.: The treatment of lip deformities resulting from electric burns, Amer. J. Surg. 88:884, 1954.
46. Kazanjian, V. H., and Converse, J. M.: The surgical treatment of facial injuries, Baltimore, 1949, The Williams & Wilkins Co.
47. Kiehn, C. L., and Grino, A.: Iliac bone grafts replacing tantalum plates for gunshot wounds of skull, Amer. J. Surg. 85:395, 1953.
48. Klapp, R., and Schroeder, H.: Die Unterkieferschussbrüche, Berlin, 1917, Hermann Muesser.
49. Kreuz, F. P., Hyatt, G. W., Turner, T. C., and Bassett, A. L.: The preservation and clinical use of freeze-dried bone, J. Bone Joint Surg. 33A:836, 1951.
50. LeVeen, H. H., and Barberio, J. R.: Tissue reaction to plastic used in surgery with special reference to teflon, Ann. Surg. 129:74, 1941.
51. Lindemann, A.: Ueber die Beseitigung der traumatischen Defekta der Gesichtsknochen. In Behandlung der Kieferschussverletzungen, vol. 4, Wiesbaden, 1916, p. 6.
52. Longacre, J. J., deStefano, G. A., Holmstead, K., Leichliter, J. W., and Jolly, P.: The immediate versus the late reconstruction in cancer surgery, Plast. Reconstr. Surg. 28:549, 1961.
53. Longacre, J. J., and Gilby, R. F.: The problem of reconstruction of extensive severely scarred palatal defects in edentulous patients, Plast. Reconstr. Surg. 14:357, 1954.
54. Losee, F. L., and Hurley, L. A.: Successful cross-species bone grafting accomplished by removal of the donor organic matrix, Naval Medical Research Institute Project NM 004 006.09.01, p. 911, Dec. 5, 1956.
55. Losee, F. L., and Hurley, L. A.: Bone treated with ethylenediamine as a successful foundation material in cross-species bone grafts, Nature. (London) 177:1032, 1956.
56. Macewen, W.: Observations concerning transplantation of bone, illustrated by a case of inter-human osseous transplantation, whereby over two-thirds of the shaft of a humerus was restored, Proc. Roy. Soc. 32:232, 1881.
57. Martin, H. E.: Cheiloplasty for advanced carcinoma of the lip, Surg. Gynec. Obstet. 14:914, 1932.
58. Matalon, Victor: Personal communication, June, 1967.
59. Millard, D. R.: Chin implants, Plast. Reconstr. Surg. 13:70, 1954.
60. Millard, D. R., Jr.: A new approach to immediate mandibular repair, Ann. Surg. 160:306, 1964.
61. Mohnac, A. M.: Surgical correction of maxillomandibular deformities J. Oral Surg. 23:393, 1965.
62. Mowlem, A. R.: cancellous chip bone-grafts, report on 75 cases, Lancet 2:746, 1944.
63. Mullison, E. G.: Silicones in head and neck surgery, Arch. Otolaryng. 84:91, 1966.
64. Obwegeser, H.: Surgical preparation of the maxilla for prosthesis, J. Oral Surg. 22:127, 1964.
65. Obwegeser, H.: Simultaneous resection and reconstruction of parts of the mandible via the intraoral route in patients with and without gross infections, Oral Surg. 21:693, 1966.
66. Obwegeser, H.: Personal communication, June, 1966.
67. Ollier, L.: Recherches experimentales sur les greffes osseuses, J. de Physiol. de l'Homme et des Animaux 3:88, 1860.
68. Ollier, L.: Traite experimental et clinique de la regeneration des os et de la production

artificielle du tissu osseux, Paris, 1867, Victor Masson et Fils.
69. Padgett, E. C., and Stephenson, Kathryn L.: Plastic and reconstructive surgery, Springfield, Ill., 1948, Charles C Thomas, Publisher.
70. Paletta, F. X.: Early and later repair of facial defects following treatment of malignancy, Plast. Reconstr. Surg. 13:95, 1954.
71. Payr, E.: Ueber osteoplastischen Ersatz nach Kieferresektion (Kieferdefekten) durch Rippenstücke mittelst gestielter Brustwandlappen oder freier Transplantation, Zbl. Chir. 35:1065, 1908.
72. Peer, L. A.: The neglected "free fat graft," its behavior and clinical use, Amer. J. Surg. 92:40, 1956.
73. Peer, L. A.: Transplantation of tissues, vol. 1, Baltimore, 1955, The Williams & Wilkins Co.
74. Pick, J. F.: Surgery of repair, vol. 1, Philadelphia, 1949, J. B. Lippincott Co.
75. Quereau, J. V. D., and Souder, B. F.: Teflon implant to elevate the eye in depressed fracture of the orbit, Arch. Ophthal. 55:685, 1956.
76. Ragnel, A.: A simple method of reconstruction in some cases of dish-face deformity, Plast. Reconstr. Surg. 10:227, 1949.
77. Rehrmann, A.: Autoplastic repair of the ramus mandibulae, avoiding a lesion of the facial nerve and of large blood vessels, Plast. Reconstr. Surg. 17:452, 1956.
78. Reynolds, F. C., Oliver, D. R., and Ramsey, R.: Clinical evaluation of the merthiolate bone bank and homogenous bone grafts, J. Bone Joint Surg. 33A:873, 1951.
79. Schneider, P. J.: V-excision with Z-closure for carcinoma of the lower lip, Plast. Reconstr. Surg. 18:208, 1956.
80. Sherman, P.: The open method of skin grafting, Amer. J. Surg. 94:869, 1957.
81. Smith, F.: Plastic and reconstructive surgery, a manual of management, Philadelphia, 1950, W. B. Saunders Co.
82. Smith, A. E., and Robinson, M.: Individually constructed stainless steel bone onlay splint for immobilization of proximal fragment in fractures of the angle of the mandible, J. Oral Surg. 12:170, 1954.
83. Stuteville, C. H.: A new concept of treatment of osteomyelitis of the mandible, J. Oral Surg. 8:301, 1950
84. Sykoff, W.: Zur Frage der Knochenplastik am Unterkiefer, Zbl. Chir. 35:881, 1900.
85. Tucker, E. J.: The preservation of living bone in plasma, Surg. Gynec. Obstet. 96:739, 1953.
86. Tulffier, T.: Des greffes de cartilage et d'os humain dans les resections articularies, Bull. Mem. Soc. Chir. Paris 37:278, 1911.
87. Venable, C. S., and Stuck, W. G.: Three years' experience with vitallium in bone surgery, Amer. Surg. 114:309, 1941.
88. Venable, C. S., and Stuck, W. G.: General considerations of metals for buried appliances in surgery, Int. Abstr. Surg. 76:297, 1943.
89. Walden, R. H., and Bromberg, B. E.: Recent advances in therapy in maxillofacial bony injuries in over 1,000 cases, Amer. J. Surg. 93:508, 1957.
90. Watson-Jones, R.: Fractures and joint injuries, ed. 4, vol. 1, Baltimore, 1955, Williams & Wilkins Co.
91. Webster, J. P.: Crescentic peri-alar cheek excision for upper lip flap advancement with a short history of upper lip repair, Plast. Reconstr. Surg. 16:434, 1955.
92. Wilson, P. D.: Experience with a bone bank, Ann. Surg. 126:932, 1947.
93. Brown, J. B., Fryer, M. P., and Ohlwiler, D. A.: Study and use of synthetic materials such as silicone and Teflon as subcutaneous prosthesis, Plast. Reconstr. Surg. 26:263, 1960.
94. Parkes, M. L.: Chin implants with a newer plastic compound, Arch. Otolaryng. 75:429, 1962.
95. Dewey, A. R., and Moore, J. W.: Mandibular repair after radical resection, J. Oral Surg. 20:34, 1962.

Chapter 23

DEVELOPMENTAL DEFORMITIES OF THE JAWS

Jack B. Caldwell

Developmental deformities of the jaws are those deformities that present malocclusion of the teeth, malrelation of the jaws, and associated facial disfigurement. They are thought of most often as congenital in origin, but they may also result from other causes.

The surgical correction of these deformities is one of the most challenging and intriguing aspects of all oral surgery. Helping persons so afflicted is also one of the most gratifying services that it is possible to render.

Individuals with developmental deformities of the jaws are invariably self-conscious of their abnormal facies and usually have reflected personality problems. Their primary concern is their appearance. However, when correction of these deformities is contemplated, more than esthetic improvement must be considered. Correction of functional deficiencies is equally as important, and this factor must be fully considered in treatment planning. In almost every instance personality inadequacies are eliminated automatically following corrective surgery.

For the sake of simplicity deformities of the jaws will be discussed in their basic forms, namely, prognathism, micrognathia, and apertognathia. It must be understood that many variations do occur and that the primary deformity may be in the maxilla as well as in the mandible, or it may be coexistant in both jaws. A complete knowledge of surgical procedures applicable to the basic deformities should enable the oral surgeon to deal properly with all deformities.

Definition of terms applied to developmental deformities of the jaws is necessary for an understanding of the problem. *Prognathism* is defined as an abnormal projection forward of one or both jaws, whereas *micrognathia* is defined as a smallness of the jaws, especially the underjaw. *Apertognathia*, or open bite, is a condition in which a space remains between the maxillary and the mandibular anterior teeth when the posterior teeth are in contact.

One cannot be fully appreciative of the age in which we live today until he takes the time to read of the experiences of earlier surgeons who dealt with facial deformities. The details of case histories reported by pioneers in this field are truly fascinating to study. We are fortunate, indeed, that men such as Hullihen and Blair had the basic knowledge, imagination, and courage to attempt the surgery that they describe so vividly. Many of the original contributions in this field of corrective surgery are the basis for standard operations today. Refinements in surgical technique, better understanding of physiology and anatomy, and the addition of modern methods of anesthesia and drug therapy have eliminated or minimized the hazards that were so great a few short years ago.

Dr. S. P. Hullihen[1] of Wheeling, Virginia (now West Virginia), can be credited with the first operation for correction of malrelation of the jaws. The patient he described in 1849, aged 20 years, had been severely burned on the neck and lower part of the face 15 years previously. The "cicatrix produced a deformity of the most dreadful character. Her head was drawn forward and downward with the chin confined to within an inch of the sternum. The underjaw was bowed slightly downward and elongated, particularly its upper portion, which made it project about one inch and three-eighths beyond the upper jaw."* Dr. Hullihen studied his patient's problem and resolved it surgically by "sawing out" a V-shaped segment of bone from the upper "elongated portion three-fourths of the way through the jaw" and then completing the section forward horizontally, thus allowing "that portion of the jaw and teeth which before projected and inclined outward" to return to its "proper and original place."

Probably the most important early contributions came from Dr. Vilray P. Blair[2] of St. Louis, Missouri, who was a great philosopher and author as well as a great surgeon. In 1907 Dr. Blair wrote "While surgeons for centuries have expended every talent and energy upon the correction of deformities of almost all kinds, from clubfoot to malrelation of the teeth, both for cosmetic and utilitarian reasons, yet little study or work seems to have been done to alleviate those distressing conditions that arise from excessive asymmetry of the dental arches. Where this deformity was too great to be corrected by orthodontic appliances, the victims have, so far as I can determine, with the exception of a few isolated cases, been compelled to go through life without relief."* Furthermore, Dr. Blair recognized and classified facial deformities much in accordance with present-day concepts. He stated that ". . . the malrelation consisted either in a disproportionate growth in the length of the body of the lower jaw, in the lack of development of the upper jaw, in a lack of development of the lower jaw, [or] in a bending downward of the lower jaw at or in front of the angle . . . ."*

Typical of his optimism was the statement "We have to deal with an upper solid jaw and a lower one that is a hoop of bone *capable of almost any kind of adjustment*, and it is upon the latter that our efforts must be expended."* He described ostectomies and osteotomies for correction of prognathism, open bite deformities, and micrognathia. He recognized "three distinct problems: (1) the cutting of the bone, (2) the placing of the jaw in its new position, and (3) holding it there." This classical paper was written sixty years ago, but should be prescribed for reading and study today by anyone who contemplates performing surgery for correction of these deformities.

Articles and single case histories describing various operations for correction of these deformities appeared in the literature intermittently thereafter. Among them were many outstanding contributions. The difficulties were many until more recent years, and probably the failures went unreported, whereas successful cases were well documented. Much of the difficulty encountered earlier was eliminated with the

---

*Hullihen, S. P.: Case of elongation of the under-jaw and distortion of the face and neck, caused by burn, successfully treated, Amer. J. Dent. Sc. 9:157, 1849.

*Blair, V. P.: Operations on the jaw-bone and face, Surg. Gynec. Obstet. 4:67, 1907.

advent of antibiotics and the increased publicizing of cases and techniques. Refinement of certain techniques has led to their acceptance as standard procedure, the operative details of which will be discussed.

GROWTH AND ORTHODONTICS

Detailed experimental and clinical studies have been made of the growth of the mandible, and it is unnecessary in this chapter to go into a comprehensive review of this subject as it relates to deformities.[3-7] Normal growth of the mandible occurs in two ways: (1) appositional at all of its borders except the anterior border of the ramus and (2) epiphyseal-like growth of the condyles. No definite etiological factors account for prognathism. Although heredity and endocrines must influence the development of this deformity, it may be a result of hyperactivity of the growth center in the mandibular condyle. Clinically, I have observed that practically all excessive prognathic development of the mandible has occurred someplace in the vertical ramus. This observation is based almost entirely upon the preoperative relating of study models. Invariably the dental arches relate to a satisfactory degree, but occlusion may not be ideal.

Conversely, micrognathia is usually a result of an interference in the condylar growth center by systemic or local causes. Trauma at child birth or during infancy or early childhood is the most commonly observed etiological factor. Growth interference may be unilateral or bilateral, resulting in asymmetrical or symmetrical deformity.

Prior to surgical correction of jaw deformities the surgeon must establish the fact that the condition is in a static state and that it is not the result of endocrine disturbances such as giantism and acromegaly resulting from pituitary dysfunction. Tumors and ordinary hypertrophy should be recognized in differential diagnosis also.

Whether surgery should be adjunctive to orthodontics or vice versa is debatable. I have seen patients with extreme prognathism who were treated by orthodontics for 3 or 4 years with no benefit or retardation of the progressing deformity. I have also seen patients with prognathism who were treated surgically at an absurdly early age. Of a certainty, developmental deformities must be dealt with at a proper time, and the best interests of the patient are served if the oral surgeon, orthodontist, and speech therapist combine their knowledge on a cooperative basis. Surgical correction and orthodontics should not be undertaken in mandibular prognathism until maturity is reached and maximum growth is attained. Depending on conditions and the operation contemplated, micrognathic mandibles may be corrected surgically at younger ages. Open bite deformities should not be corrected surgically until a speech therapist has controlled tongue thrusting habits. It is sometimes difficult to come to an understanding with younger patients, or more especially the parents, because of the patient's personality problems.

SELECTION OF AN OPERATIVE PROCEDURE AND PREOPERATIVE PLANNING

No specific operative procedure is applicable to correction of jaw deformities. A correct solution is available to each individual deformity problem, but it must be obtained through utilization of every diagnostic adjunct available. Adhering to a fixed preoperative "work-up" as outlined below will clearly indicate surgical methods adaptable to any case that may present.

Roentgenographic survey. A complete dental roentgenographic survey is necessary as a diagnostic procedure prior to surgery to (1) rule out periapical or periodontal pathology, the treatment of which might require mobilization of the jaw following surgery, and (2) aid in the determination of the stability of teeth in the supporting tis-

Developmental deformities of the jaws **441**

sue and their ability to withstand the stresses of fixation devices and immobilization.

Study models. Study models of artificial stone are necessary for preoperative studies of occlusal relationship:

1. One set indicating the exact preoperative occlusion is desirable for file, should any question ever arise subsequent to surgery as to the improvement achieved (Fig. 23-1, A).

2. One set is needed in cases in which preoperative adjustment of occlusion is indicated. When the lower complement of teeth is moved as a unit at the time of surgery, the new occlusion should be determined and well established preoperatively. Although this preoperative occlusal "equilibration" is arbitrary, it is an exceedingly important procedure. When the study models are occluded into the desired relation, prematurities will be found, but they usually are not excessive, and minor occlusal adjustment will provide normal function. Occasionally orthodontics will be necessary after healing as an adjunctive measure for good functional occlusion.

Preoperative equilibration is accomplished by trimming one inclined plane on a single tooth on the study model at a time. The same degree of adjustment is done in the mouth on the same tooth. Equilibration is thus carried out from one tooth to another until a fairly stable occlusion has been secured on all teeth. Final definitive equilibration is accomplished when the jaws are mobilized after healing is completed. This equilibrated set of study models should be taken to the operating room to be used as a guide to the placement of occlusion when the surgical movement of the jaw is accomplished (Fig. 23-1, B).

If it is decided to correct the deformity by ostectomy in the body of the mandible, study models are needed for preoperative sectioning. In the planning of ostectomy for correction of prognathism, measured sections of each side of the ridge are cut out to determine occlusal and jaw relation (Fig. 23-1, C). The same planning applies when osteotomies are contemplated in correction of micrognathia (retrusion of the mandible).

Extraoral roentgenographic survey. Di-

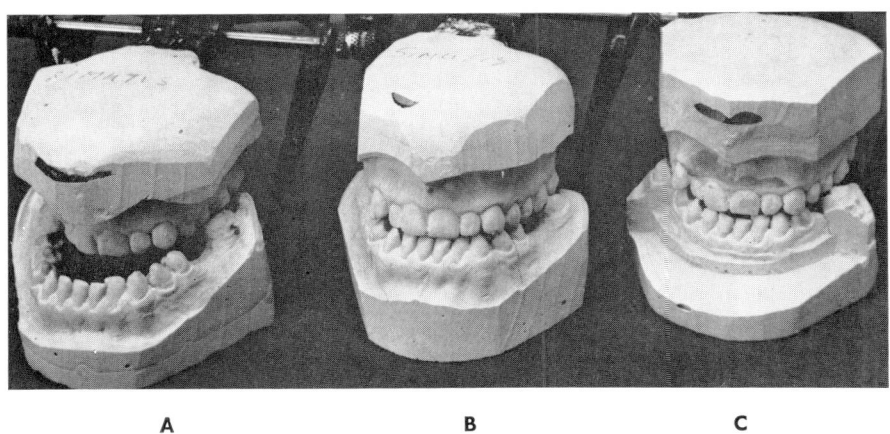

Fig. 23-1. Study models are necessary for permanent record, study of jaw relation and occlusion, determination of operation indicated for correction, and for preoperative occlusion equilibration. **A,** Preoperative occlusion. **B,** Osteotomy in vertical ramus. **C,** Ostectomy in horizontal ramus. (U. S. Army Photograph; Letterman Army Hospital.)

rect lateral skull roentgenograms (cephalograms), including the mandible, are essential for preoperative evaluation in all patients regardless of the type of deformity. Cephalometry, primarily utilized in the study of craniofacial growth and orthodontic analysis, is most helpful in the determination of the precise location of jaw deformities and in selection of proper operative sites for surgical correction. The practical application and value of cephalometric techniques are well documented;[8-11] however, these studies are adjunctive and must be correlated with clinical observations to arrive at a proper conclusion.

If a cephalometer is not available, a lateral skull roentgenogram properly made will suffice. For this projection a 5-foot target to film distance is recommended, using a technique of 300 milliamperes, 70 kilovolts, and 1/10 second exposure. The central ray should be directed at absolute right angles to the midsaggital plane through the mandible at the gonial angle (Fig. 23-2). As the exposure is made, the patient should be instructed to take his teeth out of occlusion just enough so that mandibular and maxillary occlusal planes are not superimposed (Fig. 23-3). One exposure should also be made with the teeth

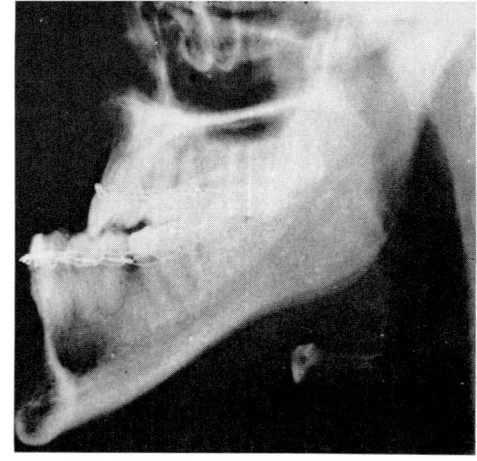

Fig. 23-2. Comparison of cephalogram and direct lateral skull roentgenogram. A, Lateral cephalogram. B, Direct lateral skull roentgenogram of the same patient, used for diagnostic studies when a cephalometer is not available. The quality of the roentgenogram and its adequacy for this study purpose is equal to the cephalogram. These roentgenograms accurately record actual size of skeletal structures and are valuable adjuncts to treatment planning. (U.S. Army Photographs; Letterman Army Hospital.)

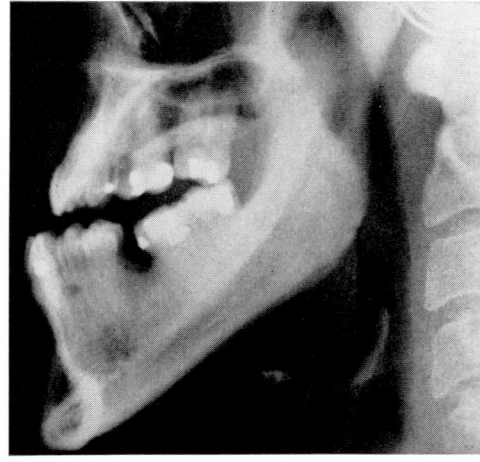

Fig. 23-3. One lateral roentgenogram should be taken with the mandible in rest position so that the mandibular and maxillary occlusal planes are not superimposed. Tracings for study purposes are thus facilitated. (U. S. Army Photograph; Letterman Army Hospital.)

Developmental deformities of the jaws **443**

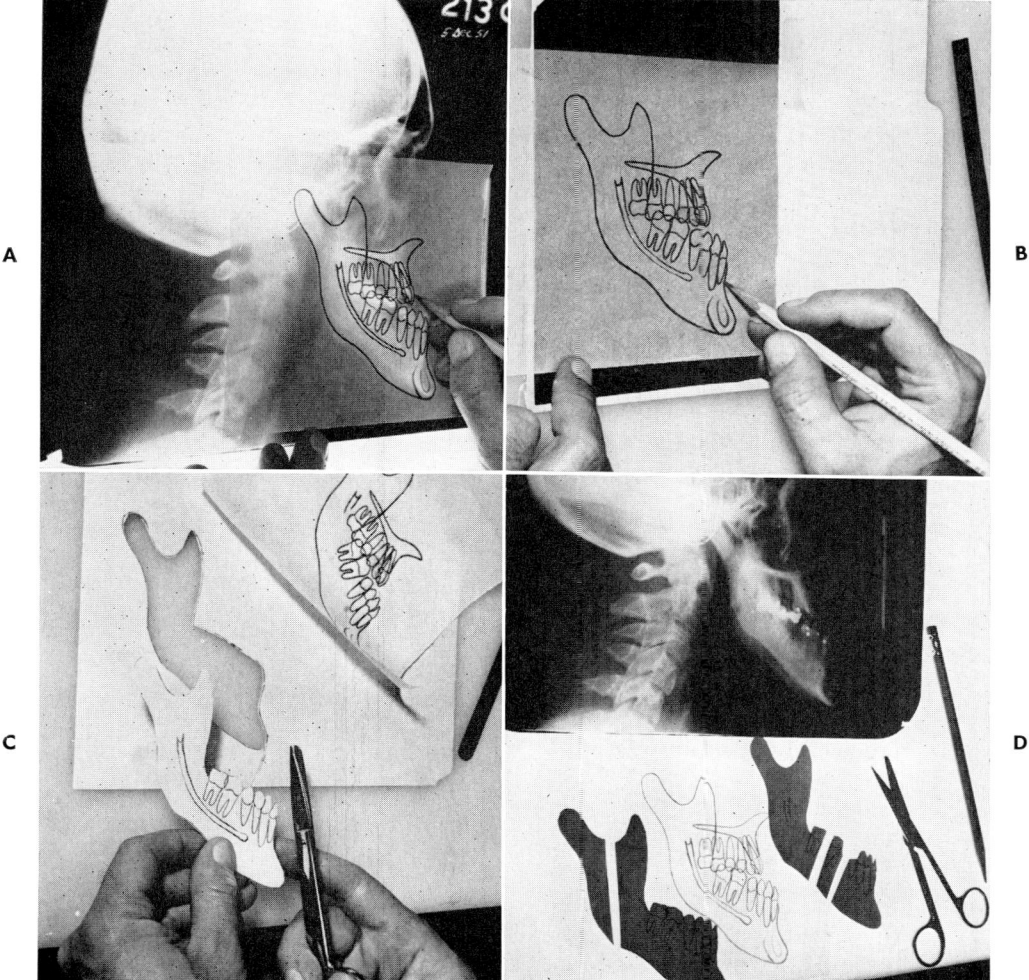

Fig. 23-4. Preparation of diagnostic templates is very enlightening in planning an operation for correction of any jaw deformity. **A**, The skeletal profile of the mandible and maxilla is traced onto transparent paper. **B**, The tracing of the mandible is transferred with carbon paper to thin cardboard. **C**, The cardboard "template" is then cut out. **D**, "Trial sections" aid in selecting an operation suitable for correcting the deformity. The roentgenogram and tracings are quite accurate reproductions of actual size, and measurements are therefore reliable. (U. S. Army Photographs; Letterman Army Hospital.)

in occlusion so that true degree of retrusion, protrusion, or open bite can be measured.

With the use of tracing paper the skeletal profile of the mandible and maxilla is traced. Superimposition of one side onto the other makes accurate definition of the occlusal surfaces of the teeth impossible. The occlusal planes can be followed when one roentgenogram has been made with the jaw in rest position. Location of the mandibular and mental foramina and the mandibular canal should be recorded on the tracing also (Fig. 23-4, *A*).

This profile tracing is then transferred with carbon paper to thin cardboard (Manila letter file holder) (Fig. 23-4, *B*), and the resulting outline is then cut out, thus producing cardboard templates (Fig. 23-4, *C*). From these templates "trial sections" can be made until a desirable location for osteotomy or ostectomy is found (Fig. 23-4, *D*). The cut sections of the template of the mandible are then fitted back to the tracing in the desired occlusal relation. The section containing the condyle is overlaid in its precise "preoperative" position, whereas the other section is "occluded" and otherwise adapted for the study. This is a very helpful and enlightening diagnostic procedure.

Measurements. The amount of protrusion measured in millimeters in prognathic mandibles is not necessarily indicative of the amount of correction necessary. Measurements vary. Occasionally the degree of Class III malocclusion measured in the first molar region will be unequal bilaterally. This measurement cannot be correlated exactly to the incisal edge discrepancy. Therefore, measurements should be standardized in every clinic. In our clinic the amount of protrusion is calculated from the incisal edge of lower central incisors to a point lingual to the maxillary incisors where ideal incisal relation is estimated to be.

PREPARATION OF THE PATIENT FOR SURGERY

Routine procedures. Routine procedures required for any patient undergoing a general anesthetic and major surgery should be accomplished the day prior to surgery. These are as follows:
1. Preoperative physical examination
2. Routine laboratory work:
    a. Urinalysis
    b. Hematology
    c. Typing and cross matching for blood replacement
    d. Chest roentgenogram

Miscellaneous preparations. In addition to the routine procedures, a number of other preparations are considered to be essential in these cases. These are as follows:

1. *Shave and skin preparations.* Most male patients are instructed to shave closely the night before surgery. Those with heavy beards should shave early the morning of surgery. Male patients are shaved over the temporal and lateral occipital areas and instructed to get fresh haircuts the day before surgery.

Female patients are instructed to put their hair up in "curlers" or braids the night before surgery so that it can be easily controlled under the drapes.

All patients are ordered to take "lather" showers and shampoos with antiseptic surgical soap the night before surgery. Their instructions are to lather from head to toe out of the shower for 5 minutes (by the clock), rinse, relather for 5 minutes, rinse and dry.

2. *Antibiotics.* Antibiotics are optional and are ordered only upon specific indication or at the discretion and judgment of the surgeon in charge of the case.

3. *Fixation appliances.* These should be placed prior to the day of surgery since most of the corrective surgical procedures are time-consuming, and anything that can be accomplished ahead of time should be done. If orthodontics is to be done adjunctive to surgery, it is good planning to have the necessary appliances in readiness prior to surgery and utilize them during the period of immobilization.

4. *Oral hygiene.* Prophylaxis should be accomplished if indicated. Any inflammatory conditions of the gingiva or oral mucous membranes should be treated and eliminated.

Anesthesia

Choice of an anesthetic is a matter for consideration by both the surgeon and the anesthesiologist. The latter must thoroughly understand the problems related to surgery about the jaws and the need for protection of the airway during the recovery period. The selection of anesthetic agents should take into account the possibility of nausea and related complications that may develop with the patient's mandible immobilized and fixed to the maxilla.

Nasoendotracheal intubation is routine, and the airway is maintained until the patient has reacted from the anesthetic. The stomach is emptied by suction during surgery and the recovery period via a Levin tube, thus controlling the incidence of vomiting in most cases.

Skin preparation and draping the patient

The patient should be placed in a supine position on the operating table with his head well extended (Fig. 23-5, A).

After he is intubated and asleep, two small, towel-wrapped sandbags are placed under his shoulders from either side of his head. They are directed together under the shoulders, which permits further extension of the head and makes the submandibular area accessible to light and surgery. The sandbags lying alongside the head also serve to stabilize it when it is repositioned during surgery (Fig. 23-5, A).

The anesthesiologist should be placed at the head of the table to permit direct access to the airway and thus good control of the anesthetic. At the same time the surgical team has ample access to both sides of the patient (Fig. 23-5, A).

An antiseptic surgical soap is routinely used in preparation of the skin of the operative field. A wide area of skin is lathered for 3 to 5 minutes, wiped free of lather, and relathered for another 3 to 5 minutes. The preparation is started in the immediate area of the incision and circled outward to the perimeter.

Proper draping of the patient is exceedingly important in the maintaining of a clean surgical field, in prevention of postsurgical infection, and in savings in operative time. Step procedure recommended is as follows:

1. After the skin is prepared, the entire body is covered with sterile sheets to a point just above the clavicles (Fig. 23-5, B).
2. A towel and folded sheet arrangement is utilized to drape the head. Both are carried across the table under the patient's head as it is raised by the anesthesiologist or a circulator, care being exercised that the scrubbed area of the face is not contaminated (Fig. 23-5, B).
3. The head towel is secured over the nasoendotracheal tube with Backhaus towel forceps (Fig. 23-5, B).
4. Another towel is draped over the head towel with the folded edge carried across the upper lip. It is secured to the head towel on both sides with towel forceps (Fig. 23-5, C).
5. A single towel is then placed on each side over the patient's neck, with the folded edge about 2 inches below the lower border of the mandible and parallel to it on each side (Fig. 23-5, C). These two towels are clipped together as they cross at the midline above the sternum as well as to the head towels on each side. All towels are sutured to the skin with No. 4-0 silk at intervals of 1½ inches (Fig. 23-5, D).
6. A drape sheet is then placed over the patient's head, secured to the head towels with towel forceps and to I. V. standards on each side of the table, thus "draping out" the anesthesiologist (Fig. 23-5, D).
7. One more towel is now placed across the patient's mouth with the folded edge just below the lower lip and draped toward the head, thus "draping out" the mouth (Fig. 23-5, E). It is also secured on each side with towel forceps and to the skin with sutures at intervals of about 1 inch. It should be sutured to the skin just below the lower lip so that the whole chin is exposed, permitting visualization of areas innervated by the mandibular branch of the facial nerve. Thus, as the nerve is stimulated during surgery, it can be identified. This last towel drape is an important one and a timesaver. It protects the extraoral

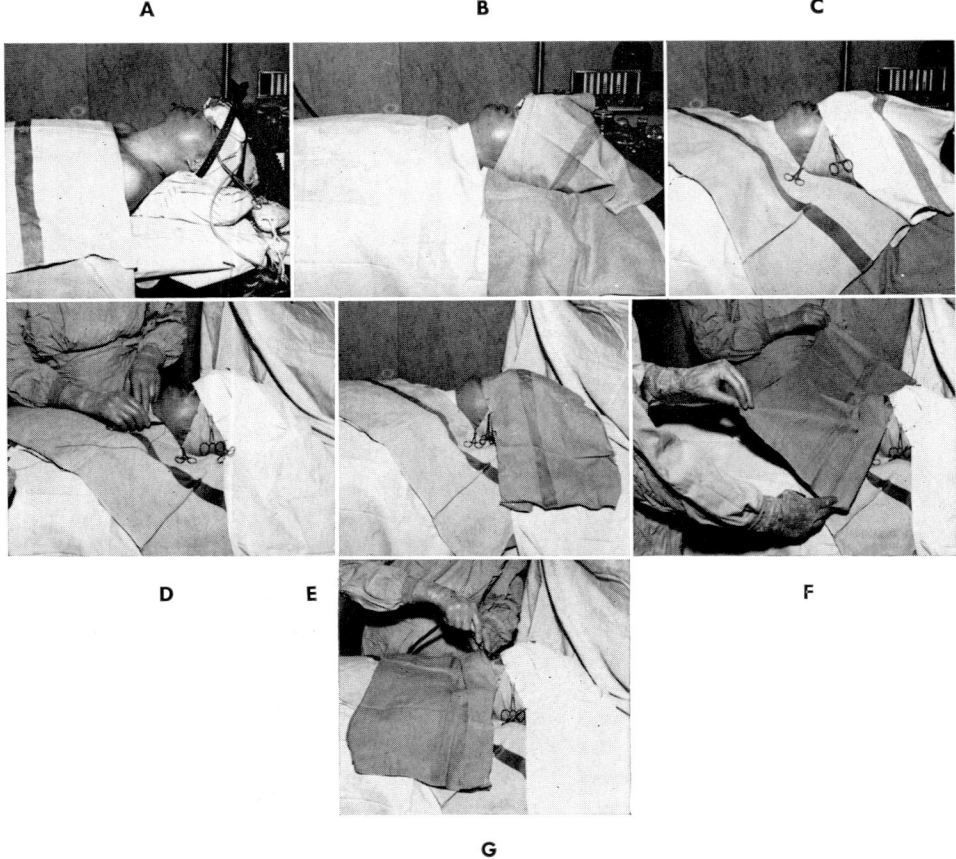

Fig. 23-5. Draping for operations for correction of deformities must be adequate to ensure against contamination. Entering the mouth, turning the patient, and other factors tend to defeat aseptic technique. To cope with these problems and at the same time effect a savings of operative time, draping technique is illustrated. **A,** Position of the patient with the anesthetist at the head of the table. **B,** The entire body is covered with sterile sheets and the head drapes are placed. **C,** The nasoendotracheal tube is covered and towels are also placed on each side of the face. **D,** A sheet is placed over the patient's head, "draping out" the anesthetist. The towel edges at the perimeter of the surgical field are sutured to the skin to prevent shifting of drapes when the patient is repositioned during surgery. **E,** A *"curtain" drape* is sutured across the face, covering the mouth but exposing the chin as well as the surgical field. **F,** The "curtain" drape is adjustable and is a timesaver, permitting access to the mouth with the least possibility of contaminating the sterile surgical field. Before it is turned down to expose the mouth, the surgical area is covered with a sterile towel. **G,** After the mouth has been entered, gloves are changed before reentering the surgical field. (U. S. Army Photographs; Letterman Army Hospital.)

surgical field from oral contamination during surgery and yet provides access to the oral cavity, since it can be turned down over the surgical wound (Fig. 23-5, *F*). Thus, following occlusion adjustment and fixation of the appliances, the surgeon's gloves are changed, this adjustable "curtain" drape is replaced over the mouth, and surgery is continued (Fig. 23-5, *G*).

Suturing the drapes to the skin at the periphery of the surgical field is important since the patient's head must be moved from side to side during the surgery. Unless so secured the drapes tend to shift and loosen, with contamination sure to occur.

TECHNIQUE OF SOFT TISSUE SURGERY

The standard technique for exposing the inferior border of the mandible through the soft tissue is used (see Chapter 2). However, to ensure success certain parts of the technique are worthy of emphasis since the ease with which bone surgery is accomplished is directly dependent upon adequate access. This is especially true in access to the ramus for osteotomy.

Location of the incision must be given careful attention to be sure that deeper anatomical structures come to view in proper relation. Positioning of the patient can alter the relation of the incision to the lower border of the mandible as much as an inch. The proposed incision lines should be marked with the sharp end of a broken applicator stick which has been dipped in one of the aniline dyes. The patient's head should be centered and not extended so that both sides can be marked symmetrically and the incision lines can be made in proper relation to the lower border of the mandible. Landmarks such as the gonial angle and the mandibular notch are then palpated and dye marks made on the skin, identifying their location. In locating the incision line for surgery to correct prognathism it must be remembered that an obtuse gonial angle is characteristic and a part of the deformity. Also to be remembered is that when corrected, ideally, a more pronounced angle should be developed. This being the case, it is often desirable to have the incision line somewhat lower than normal toward its posterior aspect for a good esthetic result. It should also be kept in mind that with the patient relaxed under anesthesia, the mouth may hang open an inch or so, resulting in a changed relation of skin to border of mandible. Therefore the mandible should be held in a closed occluded position as incision lines are located.

PROGNATHISM (MANDIBULAR)

Significant progress in this field of surgery has occurred since the first edition of this textbook. Notable contributions in the literature indicate a marked trend to surgery in the ramus for correction of prognathism in preference to the body of the mandible. Basic operations commonly employed in recent years include (1) osteotomy through the neck or at the base of the condyle (Fig. 23-6, *A*), (2) modification of the earlier horizontal osteotomy[2,36,37,39,40] by intraoral sagittal splitting according to Obwegeser, (3) subcondylar (or oblique) osteotomy in the ramus (Fig. 23-6, *C*), (4) vertical osteotomy in the ramus (Fig. 23-6, *D*), and (5) ostectomy in the body of the mandible (Fig. 23-6, *E*). (*Osteotomy* is the surgical cutting of bone, while *ostectomy* is the excision of a bone or a portion of a bone.) Operations in these locations will be discussed in detail in the following text. The first three (ramus) procedures employ the principle of repositioning the entire body of the mandible, whereas the body of the mandible itself is shortened in the latter. Osteotomy through the neck of the condyle has been popular with a few oral surgeons for a number of years. More recently, oblique osteotomies below the neck of the condyle (subcondylar) have become quite popular. Definition of osteotomy by direction, that is, oblique, vertical, or horizontal is difficult; for ex-

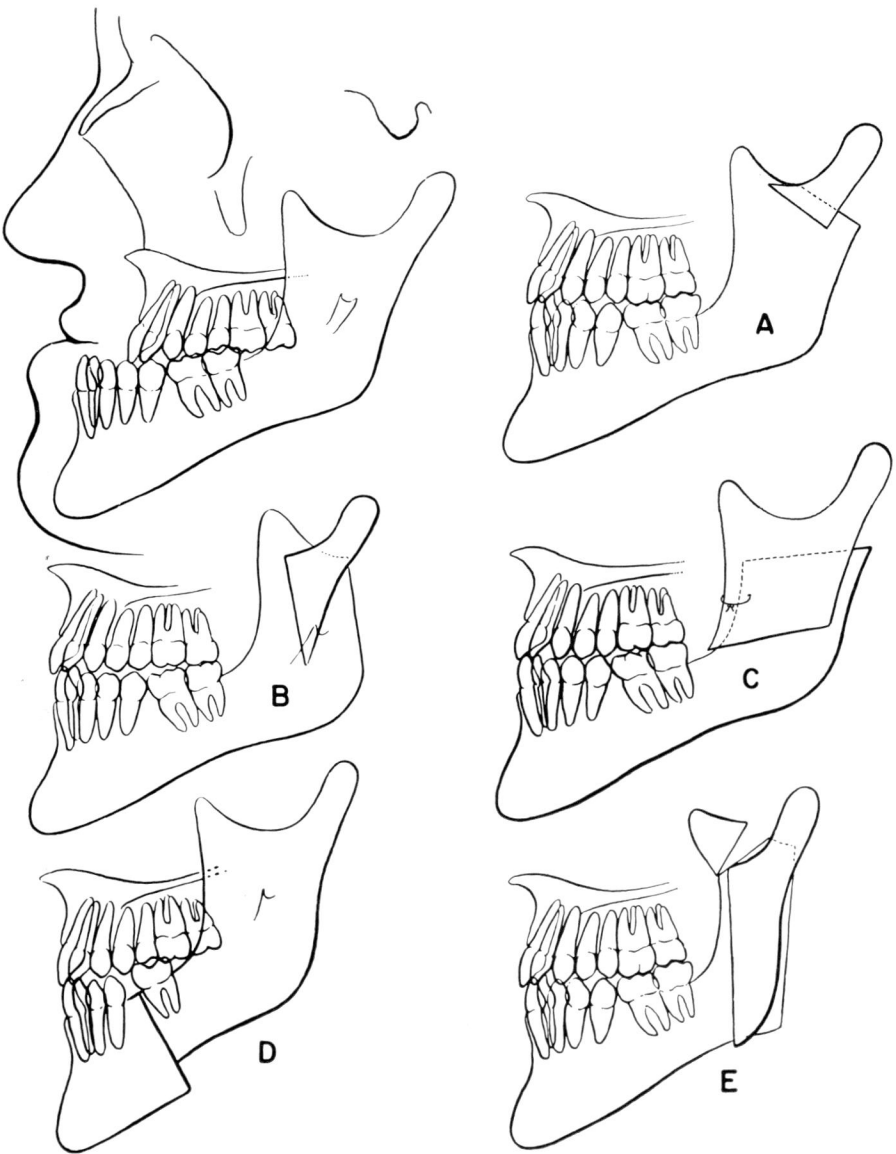

Fig. 23-6. Basic operations employed in correction of prognathism. A 16 mm. protrusion of mandible. **A,** Osteotomy through the neck or at the base of the condyle. **B,** Subcondylar (or oblique) osteotomy in the ramus above the angle. **C,** Modified intraoral osteotomy by sagittal splitting. **D,** Ostectomy in the body of the mandible. **E,** Vertical osteotomy in the ramus.

ample, an "oblique" subcondylar osteotomy in which the section is carried to a low point on the posterior border of the ascending ramus may well be in a vertical direction. The term *oblique* osteotomy as used in this text originally included all subcondylar osteotomies or those below the condyle head extending from the sigmoid notch to the posterior aspect of the ramus. For the sake of clarity and definition, ramus operations to be described herein will be referred to as (1) osteotomy in the condylar neck, (2) subcondylar osteotomy (oblique and below the neck or base of the condyle), and (3) vertical osteotomy to the gonial angle or anterior to it.

Few are the indications for ostectomy in the body of the mandible since a disparity between the mandibular and maxillary arches is rare. We have seen but three patients out of more than 200 who could not be operated by one of the ramus procedures. Hinds[12] found only one out of 20 patients where ostectomy in the mandibular body was indicated. Mohnac[11] states "In my series of more than 100 cases, I have rarely found a Class III malocclusion in which the tooth-bearing alveolar region of the mandible was not in proportion with that in the maxilla." Improved surgical techniques and a broader knowledge of operative procedures have also led to greater use of ramus procedures, which now seem less formidable than a decade ago.

Osteotomy in the condylar neck

Osteotomy in the condylar neck is most commonly accomplished by utilizing the Gigli saw in a "blind" section. It may also be performed via a preauricular incision, a Risdon incision, or by an intraoral approach. The objective is surgical section of the neck of the condyle, creating bilateral surgical fractures with repositioning of the whole mandible to normal occlusal and jaw relation. In rare instances bony union may not occur or even may not be expected, but a satisfactory functional pseudoarthrosis is hoped for.

History of this condyle site for osteotomy dates back to 1898, when Jaboulay and Berard[13] reported destroying the condyle "piece by piece," "with the aid of gouge tooth-forceps" by way of a preauricular incision. Duformental[14] in 1921 also advocated condylectomy as a means of correcting "a protruded lower jaw." Pettit and Walrath[15] in 1932 were the first to suggest osteotomy through the neck of the condyle. Their "bow back" operation was based on the principle of interposing temporal fascia and the creation of a pseudoarthrosis or flail joint as had been a standard arthroplastic procedure in treatment of temporomandibular joint ankylosis.

The first refinement to operations in this site came in 1940 when Smith and Johnson[16] suggested the removal of a "parallelepipedonal" section of bone from the region below the sigmoid notch. This was followed by horizontal osteotomy from that point posteriorly below the neck of the condyle to permit posterior repositioning of the mandible. Subsequently, Smith and Robinson[17] reported fifty-seven cases in which the patients were treated successfully by this subsigmoid notch ostectomy.

"Subsigmoid" notch ostectomy and condylotomy suggested by Smith and associates[16,17] offers no advantages over the blind osteotomy in the condylar neck. This method has never been popular because of the surgical anatomy involved and the technical difficulties of the operation. In any open surgical procedure via a preauricular incision the hazards of injury to the facial nerve are almost as great as by the blind Gigli saw method. The delicate excision of a measured section of bone from the subsigmoid notch area, as suggested by Smith, is a tedious procedure to contemplate because the depth of the wound is great and retraction of adjacent tissues must be limited.

In 1955 at the Los Angeles meeting of the American Society of Oral Surgeons, Moose suggested osteotomy at the neck of the condyle through an intraoral approach similar to that used for horizontal "sliding" osteotomy in the ramus. He recommended establishing an incision line in the bone with drill penetrations followed by surgical fracture with chisel and mallet (Fig. 23-7). I assisted with one such operation on a patient with only 7 mm. of protrusion. Healing occurred in 6 weeks, and a good result was obtained. He reports favorable results using this method in the correction of prognathism in fourteen patients.[18] In several other operations he found it impossible to adequately visualize the ascending ramus at a proper height for subcondylar osteotomy and resorted to the "ramus bisection" operation (horizontal osteotomy in the mandibular ramus above the mandibular foramen). This plus other disadvantages suggest that candidates for this procedure must be carefully selected.

Dr. E. R. Reiter[19,20] of Cleveland was one of the foremost proponents of operations in this region of the condyle and is said to have performed more than seventy-five such operations, but no published reports are available to date as to the successful results in his cases. He used a "blind" Gigli saw technique originally suggested by Kostecka[21] for correction of open bite and performed by Schaefer[22] for correction of prognathism. Verne, Polachek, and Shapiro[23] studied fifty-two cases in which essentially the same techniques were employed. Their published results are impressive.

Technique for blind Gigli saw condylotomy (Fig. 23-6, B). The steps are as follows:

1. An incision approximately 1 cm. in length is made through the skin at the posterior border of the ramus, somewhat below the base of the condylar neck, or about halfway between the lobe of the ear and the angle of the mandible.

2. The bone is reached by blunt dissection to prevent injury to the facial nerve or its branches.

3. A curved aneurysm needle is then passed in constant contact with the medial surface of the ramus below the neck of the

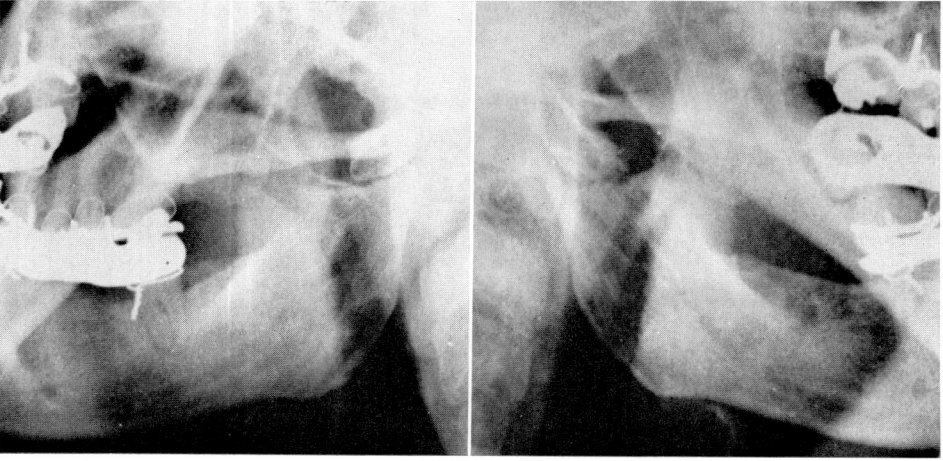

Fig. 23-7. Right and left postoperative roentgenograms of osteotomy at the neck of the condyle by intraoral bur and chisel section (Dr. Sanford Moose). (U. S. Army Photographs; Letterman Army Hospital.)

condyle in an angular direction upward and obliquely forward until it slides out over the sigmoid notch (Fig. 23-8, 2).

4. As the skin is elevated by the emergence of the needle over the sigmoid notch, another short incision is made to permit exit.

5. At this point the Gigli saw is attached to the needle and carried through the tissues to position for the osteotomy (Fig. 23-8, 3).

6. It is recommended that "funnellike" cannulas be placed into both wounds with the wire saw passed through them for protection of vital soft tissue components (Fig. 23-8, 3).

7. With osteotomy completed and the saw removed, one or two sutures are placed in both incisions to close the skin.

8. The mandible is repositioned to the desired occlusal relationship, and intermaxillary fixation is applied to previously placed arch bars.

Advantages

1. The operation is a simple one to perform.

2. The operating time is short (30 minutes to one hour).

3. It may be done as a clinic or office procedure, although this is not recommended.

4. Instruments required for the operation are available commercially.

5. Fixation appliances need not be elaborate since immobilization should not require more than 6 to 8 weeks.

6. External scarring is negligible.

7. Teeth need not be sacrificed, nor is edentulous alveolar ridge area for future denture coverage lost.

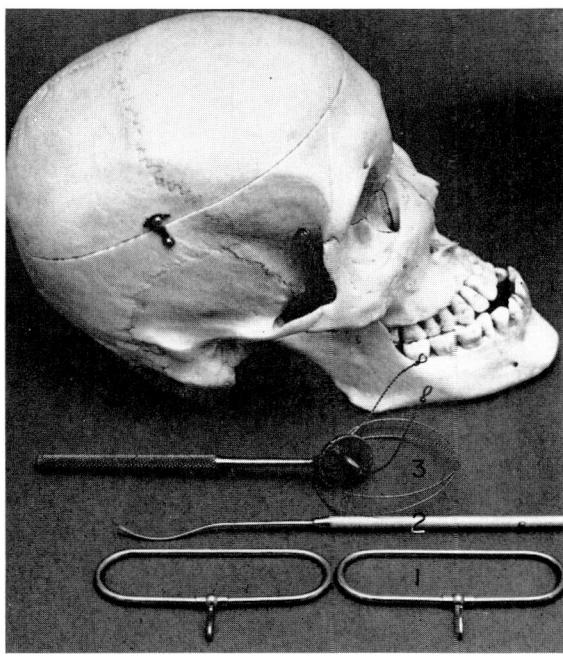

Fig. 23-8. Gigli saw used in oblique subcondyloid osteotomy. *1*, Handles for Gigli saw; *2*, aneurysm needle used to pull wire saw blade into position; *3*, Gigli saw threaded through cannula used in wound to protect soft tissues as section is made with the saw. (U. S. Army Photograph; Letterman Army Hospital.)

452 Textbook of oral surgery

8. Injury to the mandibular nerve is not likely.

Disadvantages

1. A blind procedure in this area carries the hazards of:

    a. Injury to branches of the facial nerve, with permanent facial paralysis as a possibility

    b. Deep hemorrhage resulting from severance of the maxillary artery, one of its larger branches, or the posterior facial vein and hematoma formation

    c. Injury to the parotid gland or its capsule and formation of a salivary fistula

2. Lack of control of fragments occasionally results in a nonunion with "flail" joint (Fig. 23-9, *B*).

3. Open bite is a distinct potential.

4. This latter potential increases with every millimeter of correction required beyond 10 or 12 (this results almost entirely from the strong bipennate temporalis muscle, which prohibits posterior movement of the coronoid process more than about 10 mm.).

5. Based on Nos. 3 and 4 above, this operation is not suitable for patients with more than a moderate degree of prognathism.

6. Kaplan and Spring[24] reported seven occurrences of gustatory hyperhidrosis associated with subcondylar osteotomy in fourteen patients. They admonish the surgeon to understand and recognize the phenomenon as a relatively frequent complication. It is related to the misdirected regeneration of cut secretory and vasodilator fibers of branches of the auriculotemporal nerve, which results in postoperative sweating and flush of the skin during mastication.

Vertical osteotomy in the rami

Vertical osteotomy in the rami for correction of prognathism is an extraoral operation accomplished through a submandibular approach. The objective is vertical section of the ramus in a line from the lower aspect of the mandibular notch vertically downward over the mandibular foramen, or just posterior to it, to the lower border of the mandible at the angle. By decortication of a portion of the distal fragment (ramus, anterior to the vertical section), overlapping of the proximal fragment, and thus creation of a morticed overlay, the whole body of the mandible is repositioned posteriorly to a normal occlusal and jaw relation. It is an operation that is ideally suited to correction of extreme prognathism (anything in excess of 10 to 12 mm. (Fig.

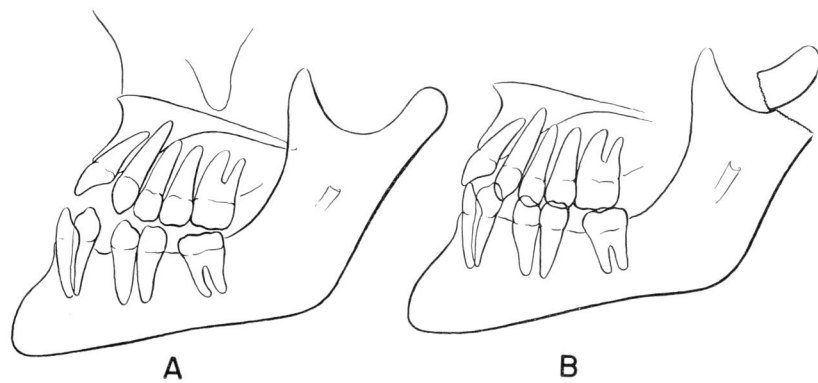

Fig. 23-9. Tracings of cephalograms. **A,** Preoperative. **B,** Postoperative, after correction of 7 mm. protrusion by blind Gigli saw osteotomy; a good result was achieved after 7 weeks' immobilization, despite poor apposition of bone cut ends.

23-10) and produces excellent results in fully or partially edentulous patients. Details of this operation were described by Dr. Gordon S. Letterman and this author in 1954.[25] A follow-up study of the original cases was made in 1965, 10 years after surgery. Functional and cosmetic results were excellent at that later date.[26] We had used the procedure since 1952 and had operated upon eight extreme deformities when the original article reporting three cases was finally published. In 1954[27] I also recommended this operation for selected patients in military facilities, since it had been established that healing time was short and need for immobilization did not ordinarily exceed 4 weeks. We have performed this surgery for approximately 160 patients, with generally excellent results. The Walter Reed Army Hospital group under Shira's direction has also operated upon a large number of patients using this method, with equally successful results.[28]

Technique for vertical osteotomy in the

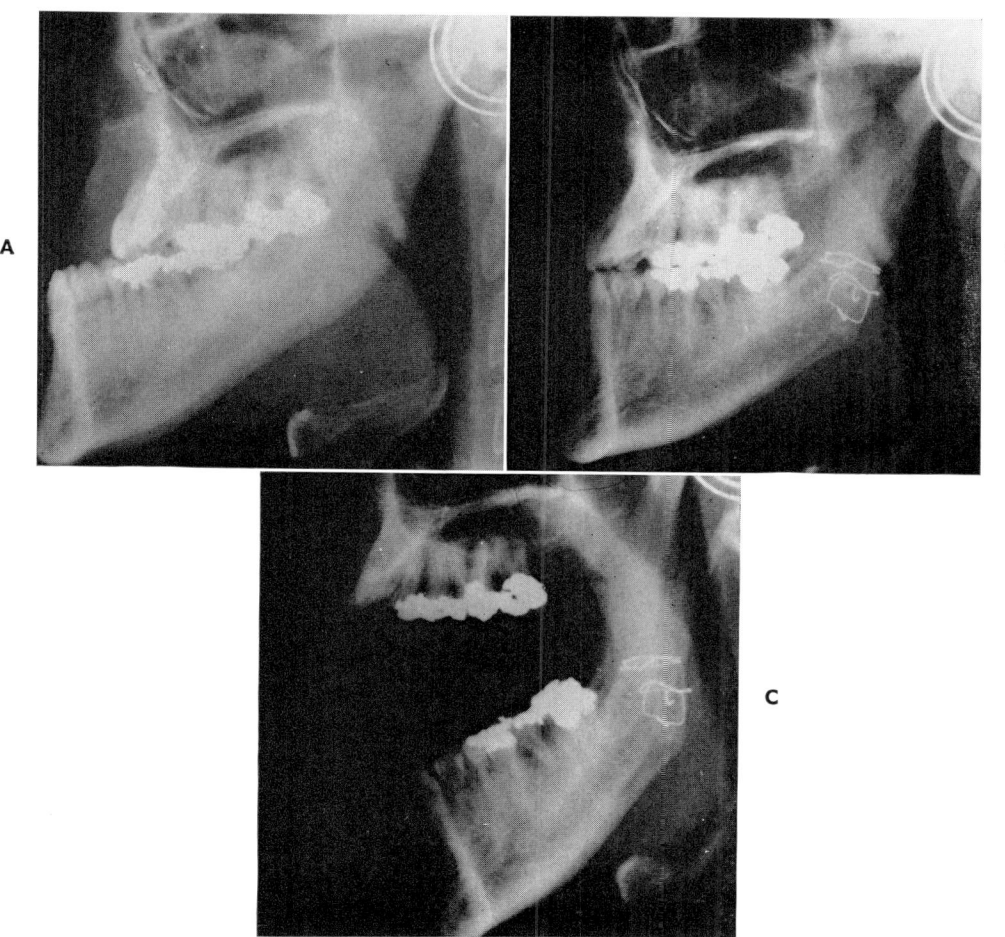

Fig. 23-10. Cephalograms of a patient with extreme prognathism (20 mm.), which was corrected by vertical osteotomy in the rami. He was immobilized for 28 days. **A**, Preoperative. **B**, Postoperative. **C**, Functional result. (U. S. Army Photographs; Letterman Army Hospital.)

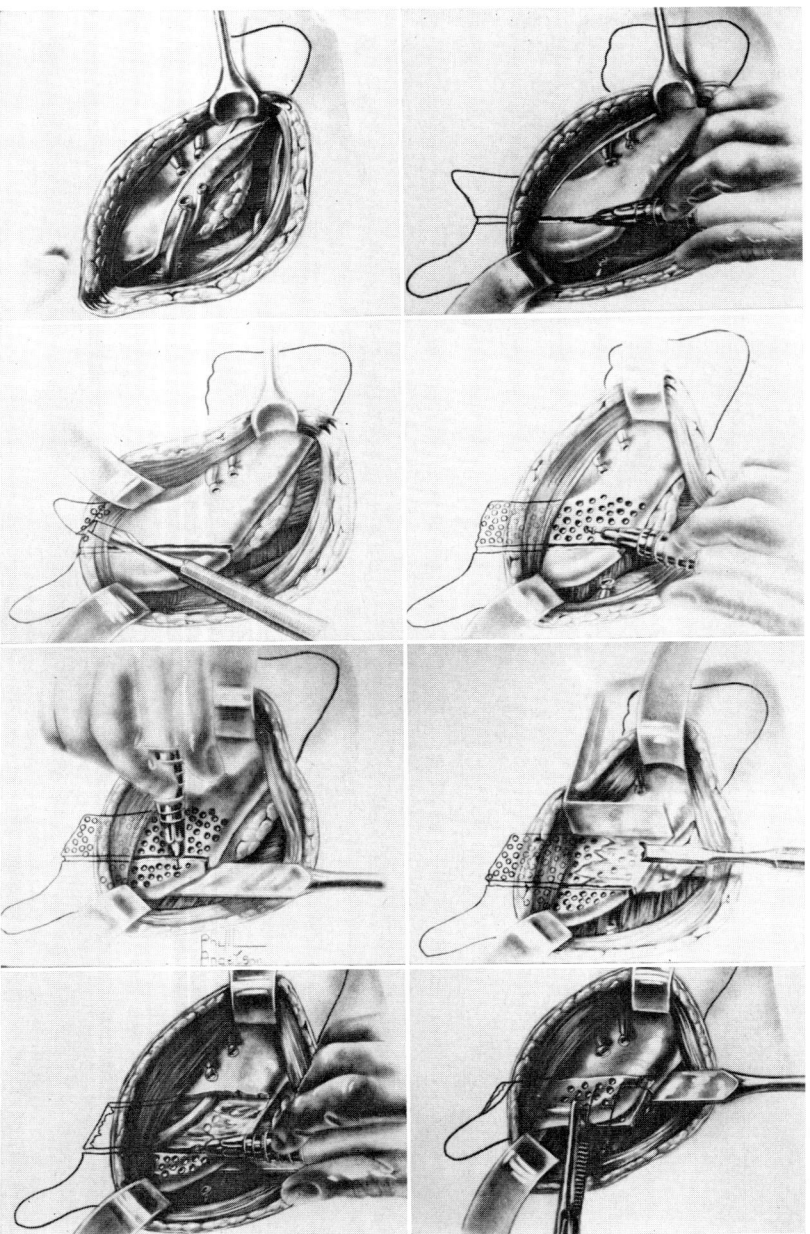

Fig. 23-11. Original vertical osteotomy. In recent years drill holes have not been placed routinely in the proximal (condyle) fragment. Also, the line of vertical incision in the bone may vary, but usually ends at some point in the angle of the mandible. (Original drawings by Phyll Anderson.) (From Caldwell, J. B., and Letterman, G. S.: J. Oral Surg. 12:185, 1954.)

rami. Certain modifications and improvements have been made in the technical procedure of vertical osteotomy since it was first reported in 1954 (Figs. 23-11 and 23-12).

1. Soft tissue surgery has been described previously.
2. The lateral aspect of the ramus is exposed to the mandibular notch. Muscle attachments on the medial aspect of the ramus are not disturbed at this time.
3. The prominence overlying the mandibular foramen is identified.
4. A straight line is drawn from the lowest point of the mandibular notch to the lower border of the mandible at the angle passing over the prominence of the mandibular foramen or slightly posterior to it. This line may be scratched onto the surface of the bone with a sharp instrument. The pointed end of an applicator stick soaked in an aniline dye is used as a marker, and a metal rule is used as a straight edge.
5. Exposure is ample with the second assistant elevating and protecting the soft tissue with a pair of Army-Navy retractors.
6. A No. 703 taper fissure carbide bur in a straight high-speed handpiece, powered by a Jordan-Day or Emesco, autoclavable, explosion-proof engine is used to make the initial vertical cut in the lateral cortical plate. Either engine runs at about 13,000 rpm, ample speed for safe, accurate bone cutting.
7. The first assistant maintains a constant flow of water on the bone as cuts are made, aspirating at the same time to prevent soaking the drapes.
8. This initial cut is made with extreme care in the area of the foramen to avoid complete penetration of the lateral cortex and thus avoid injury to the nerve as it enters the bone (Figs. 23-11, upper right, and 23-13, B).
9. The coronoid process is sectioned if indicated. It may be left undisturbed in less pronounced protrusion, but if a correction of more than 8 to 10 mm. is anticipated, it must be sectioned free to obtain unrestricted movement of the jaw pos-

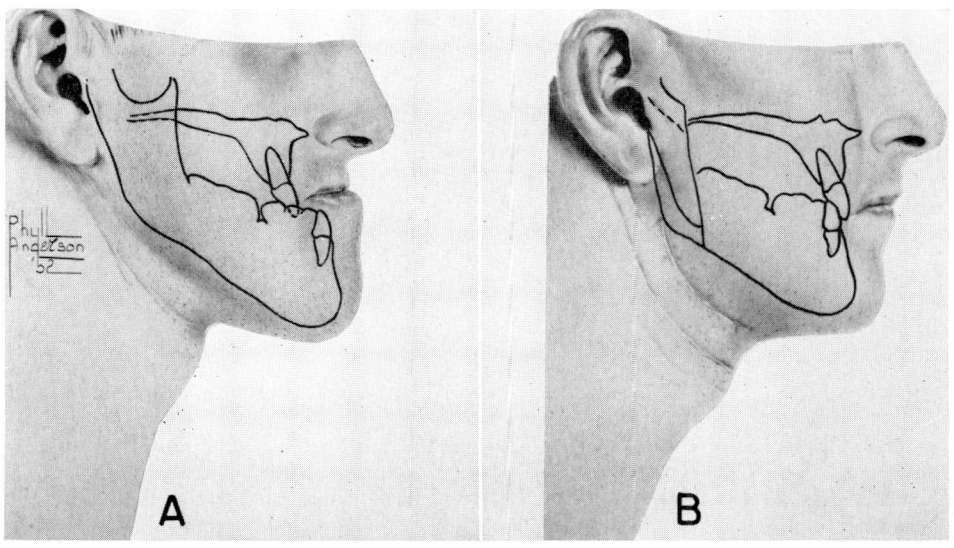

Fig. 23-12. Vertical osteotomy. (From Caldwell, J. B., and Letterman, G. S.: J. Oral Surg. 12:185, 1954.)

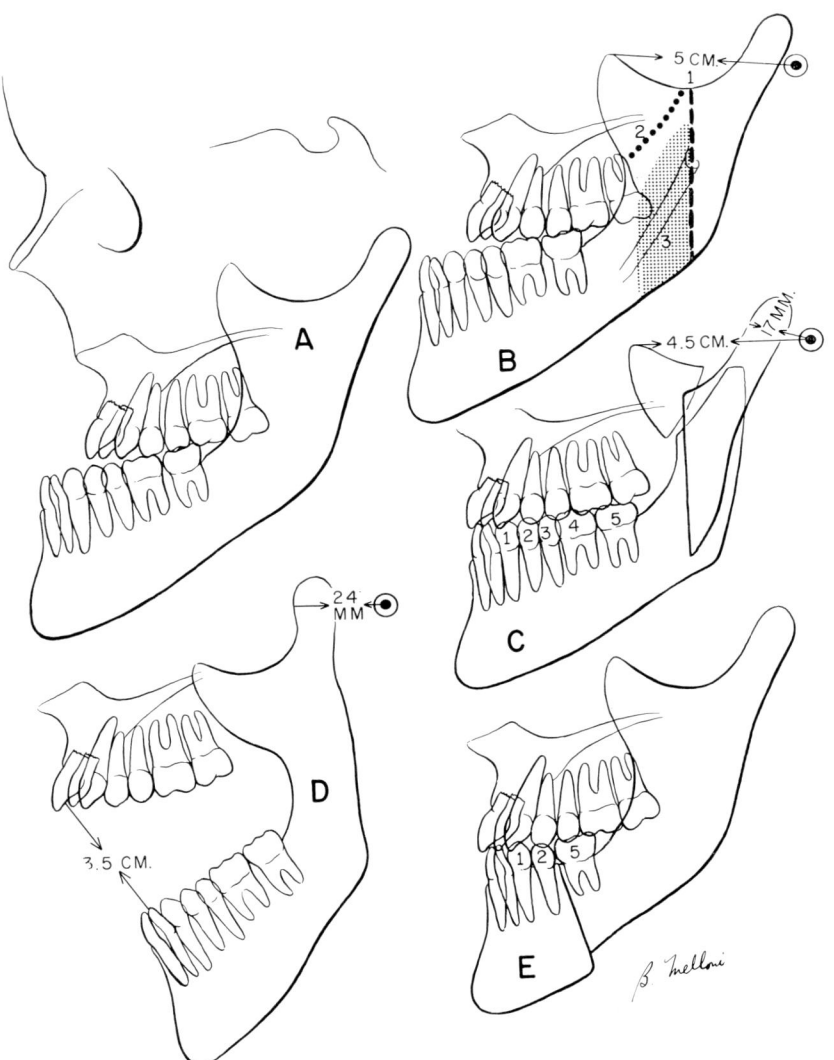

Fig. 23-13. Tracings of cephalogram of patient described in Fig. 23-28. **A,** Preoperative tracing. **B: 1,** Vertical line of cut; **2,** bur penetrations for coronoidotomy; **3,** shaded area of decortication. **C,** Postoperative tracing from Fig. 23-28, *B,* showing measured distances of coronoid movement as they can best be determined. **D,** Tracing of vertical opening of jaw and condyle excursion. **E,** The hypothetical operation of ostectomy in the body of the mandible applied to this patient (operation actually was vertical osteotomy). Note loss of two teeth and no change in obtuse gonial angle.

teriorly. (See discussion in Relationship of musculature to surgical correction of jaw deformities.)

10. Sectioning the coronoid is simple. Closely spaced drill penetrations are made obliquely from the sigmoid notch to the anterior border of the ramus using a No. 15 bone drill. An imperceptible medullary space is present here, so as soon as the high-speed bur no longer meets resistance, adequate penetration has been achieved. The section is then completed by sharp chisel and mallet. Three or four firm, short, sharp blows with the mallet usually suffice. (See Fig. 23-11, second from left top, and Fig. 23-13, B, 2.)

11. Similar drill penetrations are made from the notch vertically downward to a safe level above the foramen. The character of bone here is the same as in the coronoid process, thin and without medullary space.

12. Drill penetrations are made into the cortical plate for a measured distance (amount of correction required) anterior to the already placed vertical cut. Care must be exercised not to completely penetrate the lateral cortex over what is judged to be the route of the inferior alveolar canal. *The extent of these drill holes superiorly need not be further than the convexity just above the foramen since decortication above that level is not necessary* (Fig. 23-13, B, 3).

13. Using a sharp, long-beveled, broad, flat chisel (Stout's No. 3 is ideal), the drill-weakened cortex is shaved off in thin layers until the medullary bone comes to view and the neurovascular bundle is visualized and its course identified. Importance of tracing the course of the nerve cannot be over emphasized, for once this is accomplished the vertical section can be completed with impunity and without fear of injury to the nerve.

14. At this point, while the first side is still intact, the patient is turned to the other side and steps 1 through 13 are repeated.

The operation on the second side is then completed as follows:

15. A sharp Molt No. 4 curet is used to initiate elevation of the periosteum and anterior attachment of the medial pterygoid muscle, starting at the inferior border.

16. Once started, a broad, blunt periosteal elevator is used to push off soft tissue to an approximate level of the lower margin of the mandibular foramen. *Troublesome bleeding may be caused if sharp elevation is used or if these medial attachments are raised too far at this time.* A No. 9 Molt periosteotome is recommended.

17. With this broad, protecting elevator in position on the medial aspect of the vertical cut, the incision through the bone is completed from the inferior alveolar nerve (which is already in view) to the lower border, through the medial cortex of the ramus. Use of water and suction during all bur cuts in bone permits clear vision of structures encountered and protects the bone from injury.

18. The vertical section above the nerve is completed in the same manner with a No. 3 chisel and mallet, fracturing through the drill holes to the mandibular notch. Occasionally the No. 703 bur can be used to facilitate the completion of the osteotomy at this level.

19. The ramus posterior to the vertical section is clamped with a large Kocher forceps, and the Lane periosteotome is inserted into the vertical cut. By gentle manipulation the thin remnants of uncut bone immediately around the nerve at the foramen are fractured.

20. With the Kocher forceps still applied, the posterior section is rotated slightly, and periosteum on its medial surface is elevated posteriorly.

21. Drill penetrations may be made through both cortices of this fragment for 2 to 4 cm. up from the angle to assure early union when the parts are overlapped (not done routinely).

22. Irregularities along the vertical cut

are planed away with a chisel or removed with rongeur until acceptable adaption of the medial surface of the posterior fragment can be anticipated when it is lapped onto the anterior decorticated surface.

23. At this point the patient's head is turned back to the first side and steps 15 through 22 are repeated.

24. Both wounds are now covered, and the "curtain" drape is turned down over the surgical fields, exposing the mouth. *Upon oral examination and when the jaw relation is inspected the mandible should be hanging posteriorly in a completely free and unrestricted relationship, and it should be possible to relate the teeth into a predetermined occlusion without forceful effort. If this is not the case, coronoidotomy is indicated.*

25. The jaw is manipulated until desired occlusion is secured and intermaxillary elastic ligatures are generously placed. Firm fixation is necessary to prevent displacement as transosseous wiring of the osteotomy is accomplished.

26. The "curtain" drape is replaced to its previous position, instruments used in the mouth are discarded, gloves are changed, and the surgical field is reentered.

27. The posterior fragment is lapped

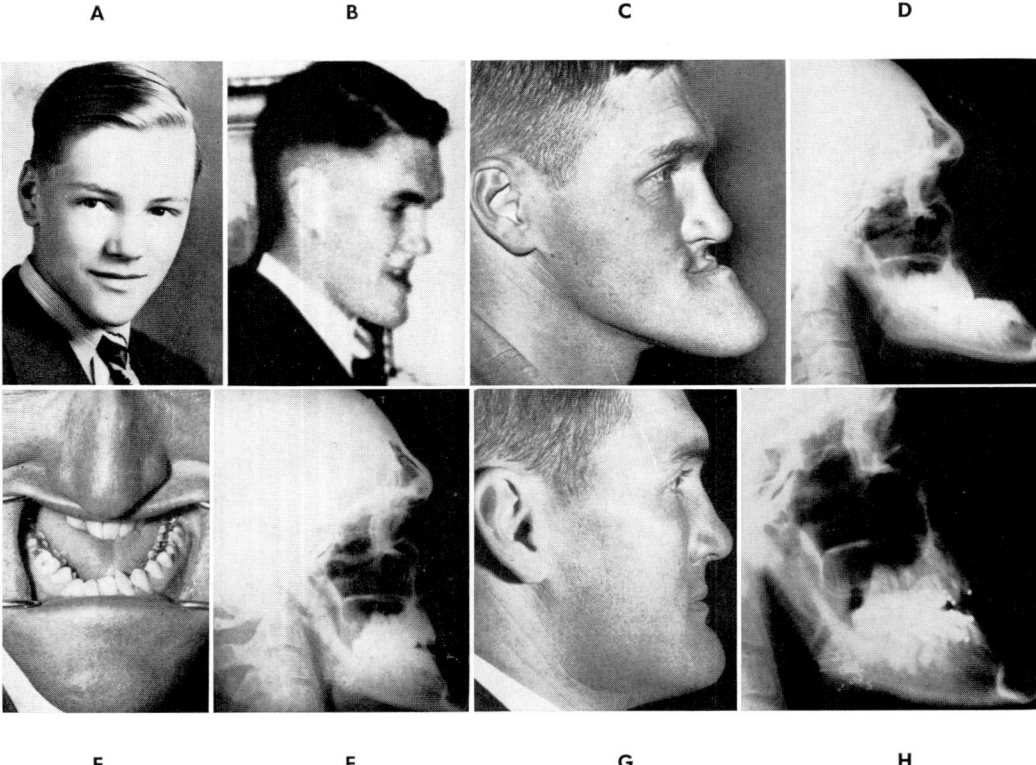

Fig. 23-14. **A**, At age 14 there was only slight suggestion of chin prominence. **B**, Pronounced prognathism was present at age 20, but minimal when compared to that at age 33. **C**, At age 33 with extreme prognathism, the patient was 6 feet 8 inches tall and weighed 265 pounds. **D**, From this preoperative cephalogram a required 32-mm. correction was confirmed. **E**, The mandible completely encircled the maxilla without any occlusion prior to surgery. **F**, Postoperative cephalogram. **G**, Profile of patient after *modified vertical osteotomy*. **H**, Appearance 4½ years postoperatively.

Developmental deformities of the jaws 459

onto the decorticated area anterior to the vertical osteotomy in a relationship visualized on the templates preoperatively. Both parts are held firmly, and small holes are placed strategically for security of the wiring. *The posterior fragment (proximal or condyloid part) should lap onto the decorticated part freely and without binding or bowing. If it does not, recheck step 22. It may be necessary to excise portions of medial cortex at points of impingement—the posterior fragment may be rotated outward somewhat to accomplish this. Occasionally that thin portion of ramus below the mandibular notch, above the mandibular foramen, requires sectioning. It need not be removed, simply depressed medially. See Figs. 23-14 and 23-15, E and F.*

28. Double 0.018- or 0.016-inch stainless steel wire is threaded through the holes, carried around the margins, divided, and twisted down individually. Three or four single-wire fixations are adequate (but at least one should be carried back through anteriorly to prevent rotation of the posterior fragment with resulting malrelation in the temporomandibular joint).

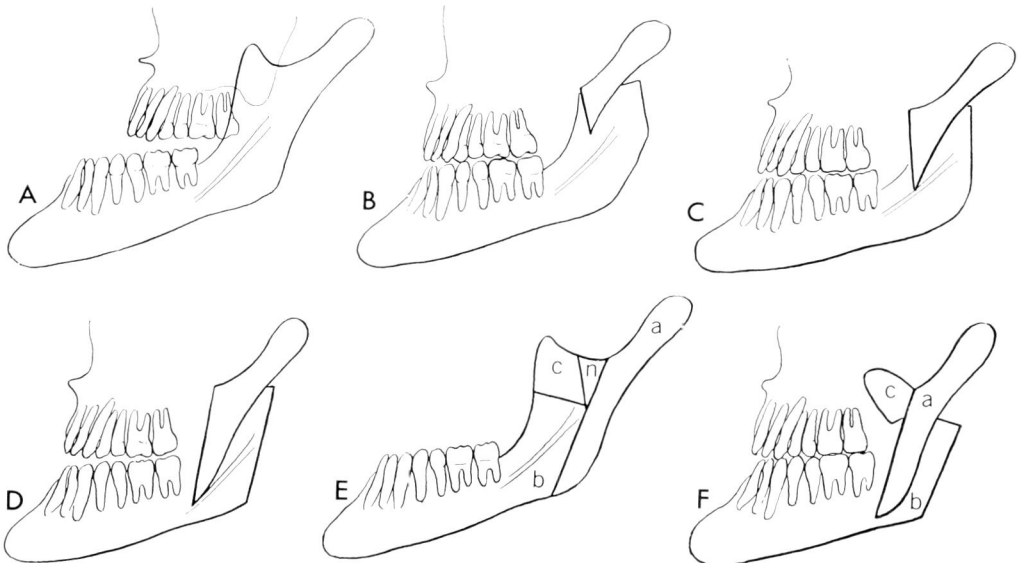

Fig. 23-15. **A,** From a preoperative cephalogram, tracings and numerous cardboard templates were made. **B,** Relationships if condylotomy had been the surgical method employed (Reiter, Verne). Obviously the ramus would have been retruded excessively, resulting in functional impairment of the jaw—and the *coronoid process cannot be retruded 32 mm.* **C,** Relationships if subcondylar (oblique) osteotomy had been employed (Hines, Robinson). The same problems are evident as in **B** with condylotomy. **D,** Vertical osteotomy (Caldwell, Letterman) required *modification* as shown in cutouts **E** and **F. E,** The lines of *modified vertical* osteotomy as planned. The vertical cut was made more nearly parallel to the posterior border of the ramus. A V-shaped segment below the mandibular (sigmoid) notch, labeled **n**, was sectioned free and depressed medially, permitting complete freedom of movement of the mandible posteriorly and eliminating interference in overlapping of the proximal portion (segment **a**) onto the distal part (segment **b**). Good mortising is frequently interfered with in the area of segment **n**. At the same time this V-shaped segment, **n**, resulted in a decreased anterior-posterior dimension and eliminated any chance of impingement posteriorly as in **B** and **C** above. *Coronoidotomy* was essential in this case, as it is in all surgery for extreme prognathism.

29. The tendinous attachments of the masseter and medial pterygoid muscles are picked up and closed together. The masseter muscle, which may have been entirely elevated, and the pterygoid, partially or often completely elevated, are readily reapposed in their normal anatomical position. Their relationship to the bone that was moved may be changed, but reattachment in harmonious functional position occurs.

30. Closure of soft tissue is completed according to the technique described in Chapter 2. Careful attention is given to reapposition of tissues in proper anatomical relation, to ensure a good cosmetic and functional result.

31. Pressure dressings are avoided, but semipressure inhibits excessive swelling and is desirable. Kerlix gauze or cotton elastic bandage applied according to the Barton method is preferable.

Discussion. The necessity for sectioning the coronoid process has been a point of controversy. Our attitude toward the inelasticity of the temporalis muscle explains why we consider this essential for the perfect results obtained in correction of moderate to severe prognathism. If one remembers that the central tendinous attachment of the temporalis muscle extends for a considerable distance downward along the anterior border of the ramus and also broadly over the medial surface of the coronoid process, the effect of this sectioning should be clear. The effect created is that of a hinge. As the body and anterior portion of the ramus are repositioned in the posterior direction, the coronoid process swings forward, with its tip remaining to a large degree in its original position. Its base anteriorly, still attached below and medially by the tendon of the temporalis, is the joint of the hinge. The strong fibers of this tendon's attachment act much the same as the old-fashioned leather barn door hinge. Finally bony union of the coronoid occurs as illustrated (Fig. 23-13, *C* and *D*).

Another point deserving clarification is application of the technique of vertical osteotomy in slight to moderate degrees of prognathism. Results have been equally good in all patients who have been operated upon, but the technical details of the operation are more difficult to accomplish in patients requiring less than 10 to 12 mm. of correction than in the more severe cases. There are two reasons for this: (1) decortication of a more narrow area anterior to the vertical line is more tedious than the broader area needed in extreme cases, and the nerve is usually deeper, probably because the ramus may be thicker (mediolaterally) than the longer, more obtuse rami, and (2) the overlapping and morticing procedure, which is more important. The proximal (posterior portion) of the ramus does not overlap as precisely, and this fragment tends to "bow out." This can only be overcome by partial decortication of its medial surface and other "fitting" bone adjustments as morticing is accomplished following step 21 of the technique. For these reasons our operating time in minimal prognathisms is longer than in more extreme cases; however, as technique and operative skills have improved, our operating time never exceeds 4 hours and frequently is less than 3 hours, including coronoidotomy, decortication, and transosseous wiring. For these reasons we favor vertical osteotomy in more extreme prognathic surgery and *subcondylar osteotomy* in less severe cases.

In application of the "vertical osteotomy" technique for edentulous patients, careful preparation of the template from the cephalogram and measurements of its relationship are adapted arbitrarily in the osteotomy. Positive, firm, intraosseous wiring of the sectioned parts usually provides adequate fixation and intraoral "Gunning" splinting is not essential.[29] Shira[30] uses preoperatively fabricated and arbitrarily related splints, the lower of which he has secured by circumferential wiring to the mandible. Either procedure is satisfactory,

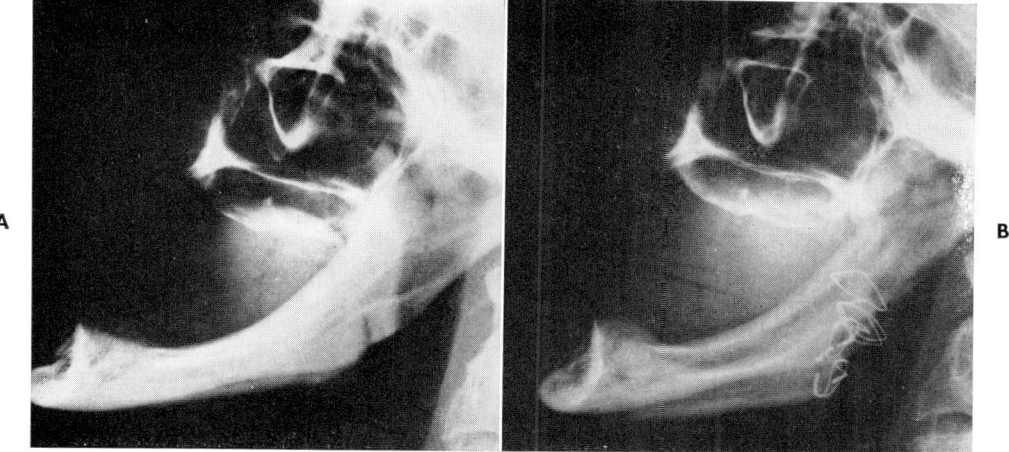

Fig. 23-16. Cephalograms of a completely edentulous patient who had a moderate degree of prognathism. He was treated by vertical osteotomy without benefit of fixation appliances. Dentures were initiated 3 weeks postoperative and inserted 2 weeks later. **A,** Preoperative. **B,** Postoperative. (U. S. Army Photographs; Letterman Army Hospital.)

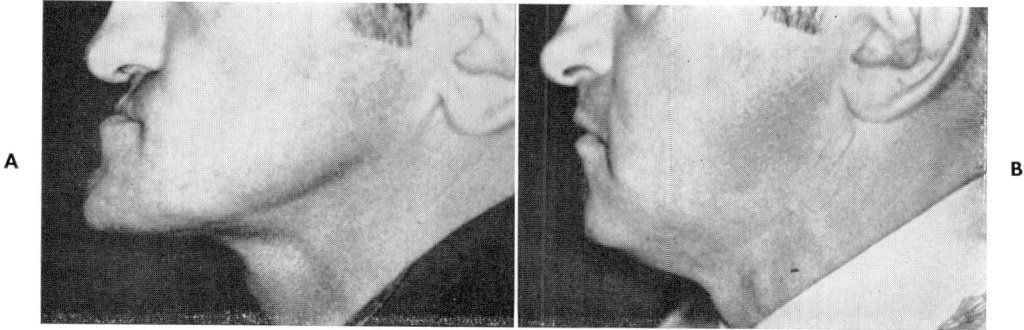

Fig. 23-17. Photographs of the patient described in Fig. 23-16. **A,** Preoperative. **B,** Postoperative. (U. S. Army Photographs; Letterman Army Hospital.)

and healing is such that dentures can be initiated 3 to 4 weeks after surgery (Figs. 23-16 and 23-17).

Advantages

1. Although almost universally suitable for correction of all cases of this deformity that we have observed over a 20-year period, the procedure is especially applicable in cases of severe prognathism. It produces ideal results in patients requiring 10 mm. or more of correction.

2. Clinically, union occurs in 3 to 4 weeks and relapse or nonunion has not occurred.

3. Simple fixation appliances suffice, eliminating a need for orthodontic banding, elaborate splinting, or arch bars. (We use Ivy loop or multiple-loop intradental wiring in the large majority of cases.)

4. As a result of points 2 and 3 above, teeth are not extruded or damaged by protracted stress.

462 Textbook of oral surgery

5. Standard, commercially available instruments are used entirely.

6. Injury to the inferior alveolar and facial nerves can be completely avoided.

7. The body of the mandible is not shortened anteroposteriorly, and no teeth need be sacrificed as in ostectomy.

8. In addition to preservation of the alveolar ridge, the vertical dimension is positively assured in partially or completely edentulous patients, and dentures can be provided at an early date (initiated within 3 to 4 weeks) (Figs. 23-16 to 23-18).

9. Normal temporomandibular joint relation is also assured, and no joint malfunctional sequelae should occur in patients treated by this method (Fig. 23-13, *D*).

10. In addition to excellent functional results which are so very important, the cosmetic result is also excellent in every instance. The characteristic obtuse angle de-

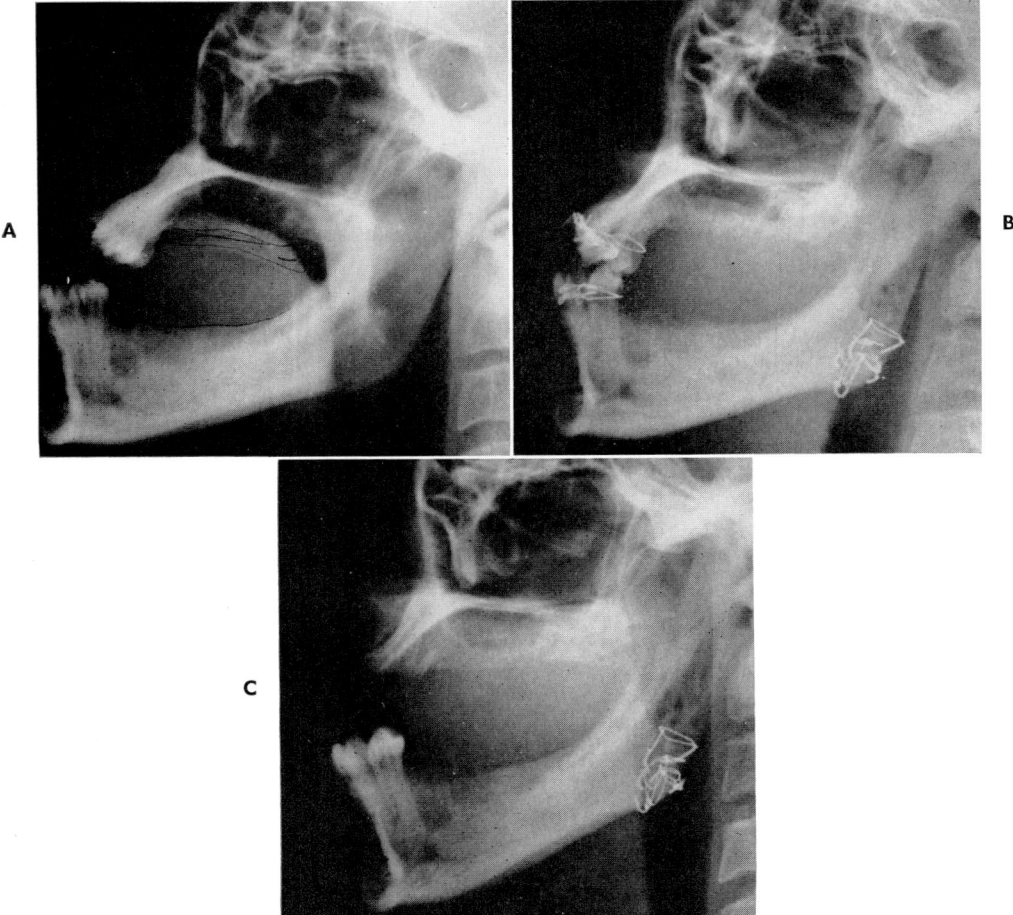

Fig. 23-18. Cephalograms of a partially edentulous patient with moderate prognathism treated by vertical osteotomy. **A**, Preoperative. **B**, Postoperative. Immobilization was maintained for 21 days postoperatively. **C**, Later the patient's remaining maxillary teeth were removed and a complete upper denture and partial lower denture were furnished. (U. S. Army Photographs; Letterman Army Hospital.)

Developmental deformities of the jaws   **463**

formity is corrected at the same time a good profile result is achieved, in contrast to the result obtained in ostectomy (Fig. 23-13, *E*). Also, since bony union is positively assured, no "open-bite deformity" (which is observed occasionally following other operations for correction of extreme protrusion) occurs. Examples of normal facial contours achieved by vertical osteotomy in the rami are illustrated (Fig. 23-19).

Disadvantages

1. Operating time, which is ordinarily 2½ to 4 hours, is not considered excessive, but to many this constitutes a disadvantage.
2. External scarring is minimal, but is objected to by some patients.

Subcondylar osteotomy (oblique)

Subcondylar osteotomy for correction of mandibular prognathism was reported by Robinson[31,32] (1956-1958) and Hinds[33,34]

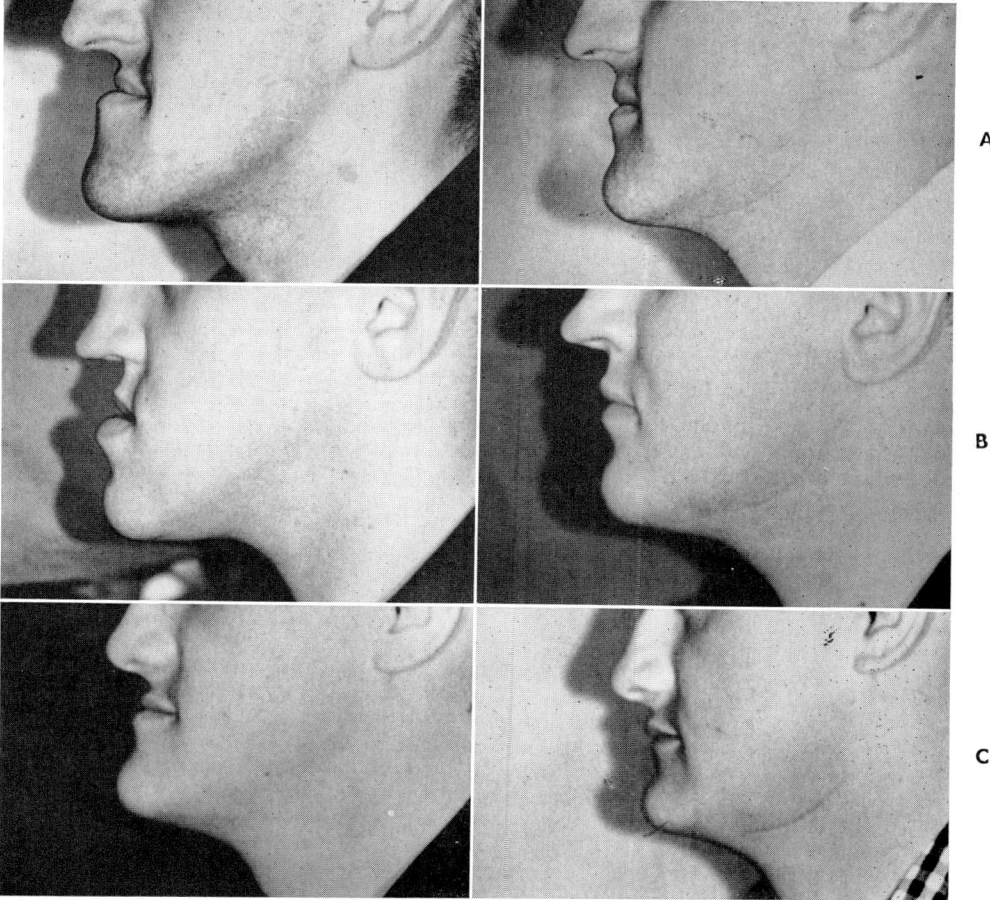

Fig. 23-19. Three patients, all with 15 mm. or more of prognathism, treated by vertical osteotomy in the rami have good profiles, normal-appearing gonial angles, and negligible scarring. None was immobilized in excess of 4 weeks. **A,** Two months postoperative. **B,** Two months postoperative. **C,** Six weeks postoperative. (U. S. Army Photographs; Letterman Army Hospital.)

(1957-1958) from independent endeavors. Both writers described open procedures with the line of osteotomy almost identically placed in the ramus (Fig. 23-6). Robinson used a nasal saw to perform the osteotomy; Hinds made drill holes, used a No. 8 round bur to cut a connecting groove along the line of holes, and then completed the osteotomy with an osteotome. Both operated through short incisions (2.5 to 4 cm.), and neither saw a need for transosseous wiring. Robinson referred to his operation as *vertical subcondylotomy,* and Hinds as *subcondylar osteotomy.* Thoma[35] refers to the same procedure as *oblique osteotomy.* He believes it to be the ideal method by which a great many, if not most, of the occlusal problems may be solved. All of these osteotomies were in essentially the same location anatomically and all were reminiscent of "vertical osteotomy" (Caldwell and Letterman), the difference being that the line of bone incision was somewhat posterior to the mandibular foramen, no decortication or morticing was done, less hazard existed to the mandibular nerve, and the entire procedure was greatly simplified. Subcondylar osteotomy (oblique) is a very acceptable operation for correction of mandibular prognathism, especially when protrusion is not extreme. It is a more desirable procedure than vertical osteotomy in minimal cases (less than 10 or 12 mm. correction). It is definitely not the operation of choice in extreme cases (Figs. 23-14 and 23-15), and therefore preoperative appraisal must *never* be neglected. Subcondylar osteotomy must not be utilized simply because it is technically easy. Its use must be limited to cases in which it is indicated. The need for a simplified, standard subcondylar technique was recognized by Robinson, Hinds, Thoma, Kruger, and many others, and this method has been an answer.

Technique for subcondylar osteotomy (oblique). This operation follows the same general technique as described for vertical osteotomy except for a few modifications.

1. The incision may vary in length from 2.5 to 4 cm.

2. The line of osteotomy is scribed from the lowest point in the mandibular notch "obliquely" (it may be a "vertical" line, depending on the obtuse angle of the mandible) downward to a point on the posterior border of the ramus, 1 to 2 cm. above the angle of the mandible (Fig. 23-6, C).

3. The osteotomy may be accomplished using a nasal saw (Fig. 23-20, A) or a No. 703 carbide taper fissure bur. In either case care must be exercised to avoid injury to soft tissues on the medial surface of the ramus. However, injury to the inferior alveolar nerve or vessels is not expected since the line of osteotomy is posterior to the mandibular foramen.

4. Musculature and periosteal covering must be elevated sufficiently to permit lateral placement of the posterior (proximal) fragment and unrestricted movement of

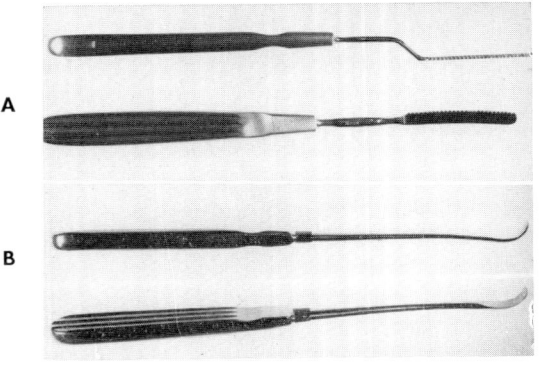

Fig. 23-20. A, Nasal saws are preferred by many surgeons for performing oblique or vertical subcondylar osteotomy in the rami. A shorter incision and more modest reflection of soft tissues is possible when these instruments are used. B, A deeply hooked side-cutting periosteal elevator (Obwegeser), essential for elevation of periosteum and muscle attachments in performance of intraoral sagittal osteotomy and necessary to permit unrestricted movement of the sectioned jaw either anteriorly or posteriorly.

the body (distal) fragment posteriorly to a satisfactory degree.

5. Decortication of the lateral surface just anterior to the line of osteotomy is usually not contemplated, but, if it is desirable to obtain better bone apposition of the parts, it may be accomplished with a bur or a double-action rongeur.

6. Transosseous wiring may or may not be used, but wire ligatures should not be applied as a means of overcoming a tendency of the proximal fragment to "bow out" or displace posteriorly. If either situation exists, the meticulous surgeon will correct it to a necessary degree by decortication as indicated.

7. The rule governing coronoidotomy applies in subcondylar osteotomy also. If posterior movement of the jaw is limited, regardless of the measurement of correction, the coronoid process must be cut free from the distal (body) fragment.

8. The teeth are placed in occlusion as already described (vertical osteotomy). However, immobilization should be accomplished by use of well-adapted arch bars or splints—for 6 to 8 weeks, to ensure against unnecessary injury to the teeth (extrusion), as may occur if ordinary intradental wiring is used for this period of time.

Advantages and disadvantages are about the same as enumerated for vertical osteotomy except:
1. Longer immobilization period required (6 to 8 weeks as opposed to about 4 weeks)
2. Probably more suitable for minimal to moderate deformities
3. Shorter operating time (1½ to 3 hours as opposed to 2½ to 4 hours for vertical osteotomy)

Horizontal osteotomy in the rami
(Fig. 23-20)

Horizontal osteotomy in the rami for correction of mandibular prognathism is performed at a level just above the mandibular foramen. It may be accomplished by "blind" section with a Gigli saw, by an open operation intraorally, or by an extraoral operation.

Blair[2] first proposed the principle employed in this operation in his original article on the subject of developmental deformities. Many have been proponents of this method, but there is rarely an indication for this operation today. As originally conceived this was what appeared to be a simple procedure and consisted of passing a long, curved Blair needle or a Gigli saw guide through a short skin incision at the posterior border of the ramus, introducing the Gigli saw to the medial surface of the ramus above the foramen, and making the section. The hazards are numerous, many of them beyond control since no one, regardless of experience, can ensure against them in this blind procedure. Foremost among the hazards are (1) injury to the branches of the facial nerve, resulting in temporary or permanent facial paralysis, (2) hemorrhage resulting from severance of the maxillary artery, (3) severance of the inferior alveolar nerve, which may not regenerate, resulting in permanent anesthesia to the teeth and lower lip of the injured side, and (4) injury to the parotid gland or its capsule, with formation of salivary fistula.

Because of these hazards "blind" horizontal osteotomy has been discarded by most oral surgeons. One of the first modifications of the "blind Gigli saw" procedure was offered by Hensel[36] in his appraisal of deformities of the mandible in 1937. Based on photognathostatic studies, he specifically located the ramus osteotomy on an oblique line from high on the coronoid process downward and posteriorly to the posterior border of the ramus, passing through a central safe area midway between the sigmoid notch and the mandibular foramen. He advocated a direct surgical approach to ensure a correct line of osteotomy.

Moose[37] in 1945 proposed an intraoral direct visualization osteotomy, which he performed with an orthopedic, power-driven, short-stroke, cross-cut saw (designed by Dr. E. A. Cayo of San Antonio, Texas). By utilizing the intraoral route the hazards of "blind" osteotomy were minimized. The Cayo saw has been modified somewhat since 1945 to make it more adaptable for this operation. Moose has also indorsed a hand saw suggested by Sloan[38] in 1951. It is a specially designed saw with a "clamp on" guide adapted to intraoral ramus osteotomy (Fig. 23-21). To overcome the disadvantages of "vertical collapse in the ramus" and "open bite," Sloan also suggested wiring the sectioned parts in apposition by looping a strand of stainless steel wire over the sigmoid notch and tying the proximal fragment down to the anterior border of the distal fragment of the ramus through a drill hole previously placed. Skaloud[39] also recommended this method of fixation, although he performed the osteotomy using a Gigli saw.

In 1941 Kazanjian[40] advocated horizontal osteotomy above the mandibular foramen via an extraoral Risdon submandibular approach and accomplished the section using a surgical bur. Later, in 1951,[41] he recommended an incision through the bone on an angle using a sharp osteotome. "Beveling in this fashion allows for a greater area of contact of the cut ends, promoting early consolidation."

If osteotomy in the ramus on a horizontal plane is indicated as the method for correction of mandibular prognathism, the intraoral method of Moose and Sloan may be utilized. The disadvantages of this horizontal osteotomy in the mandibular ramus by any method so heavily outweigh the advantages that it is not recommended as an acceptable site or technique for osteotomy —to correct either prognathic or retrognathic deformities. Principal among these disadvantages are the following:

1. The tendency to open bite anteriorly is great, especially when correction in excess of 10 to 12 mm. is necessary. This is the result of several factors, chief of which are (1) the thinness of ramus and the tendency of the sectioned ends to disengage and override as a result of (2) the tremendous power of the masseter and the medial pterygoid muscles and the pull of the de-

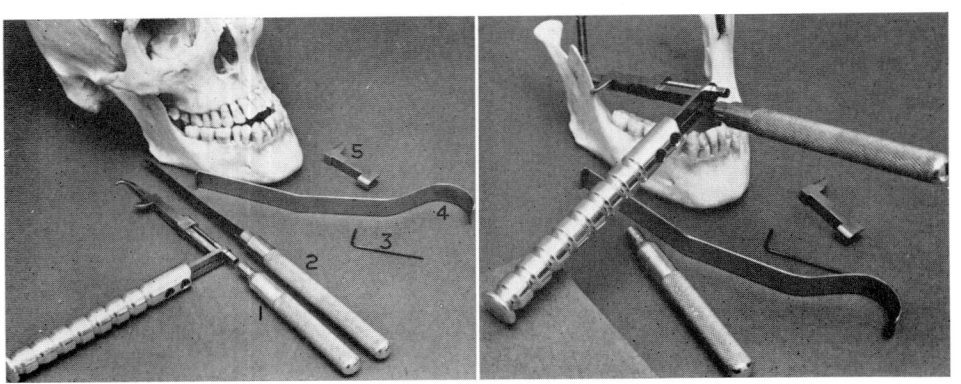

Fig. 23-21. A, Instruments specially designed for intraoral horizontal sliding osteotomy in the ramus (Dr. A. C. Sloan): 1, adjustable clamp with two handles, handle on left for surgeon to hold during the section, handle on the right (middle of picture) used to tighten clamp onto ramus (it is removed during procedure; see B); 2, detachable saw blade in handle; 3, L-shaped key to tighten setscrew onto saw blade; 4, retractor (Moose); 5, interchangeable clamp for left ramus. B, Application of clamp to ramus with saw placed in guide groove of clamp. (U. S. Army Photographs; Letterman Army Hospital.)

Developmental deformities of the jaws 467

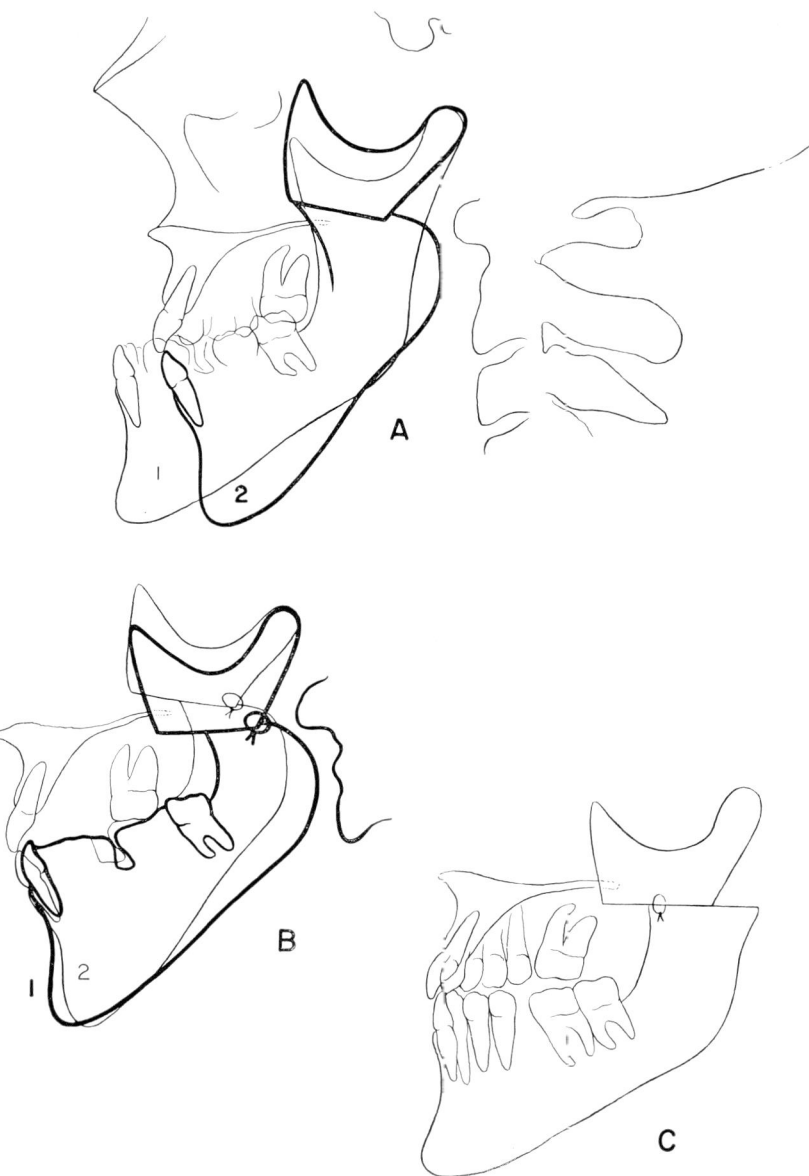

Fig. 23-22. Tracings of cephalograms of patient with 15 mm. protrusion corrected by extraoral horizontal sliding osteotomy with direct wiring posteriorly. A: 1, Preoperative tracing; 2, final postoperative tracing 7 months after surgery. The tip of the coronoid process has been distracted superiorly 15 mm. and the point of the mandible (menton) has been retruded 23 mm., whereas the incisal edges of the lower anterior teeth have been retruded only 13 mm. B: 1, Tracings made from cephalogram 1 month postoperative; 2, tracing, 3 months postoperative, when union was present clinically and immobilization was discontinued. C, Results possible by intraoral osteotomy, with transosseous wiring anteriorly preventing the open-bite tendency and resisting the distracting force of the temporalis muscle.

Continued.

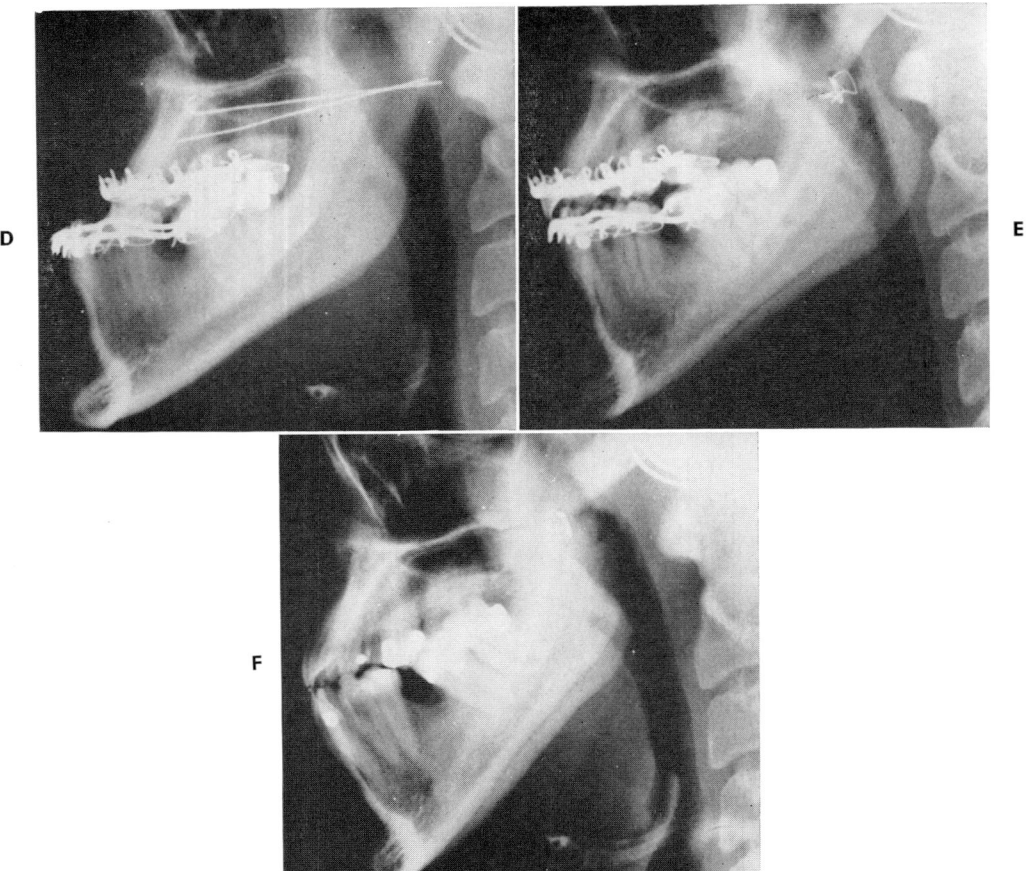

Fig. 23-22, cont'd. Cephalograms of the postoperative course; 15 mm. of protrusion corrected by horizontal sliding osteotomy. D, Preoperative. E, One month postoperative. F, Follow-up, 7 months postoperative. (U. S. Army Photographs; Letterman Army Hospital.)

pressor group, all of which combine to create a Class I lever with the posterior teeth as a fulcrum.

2. Concurrently with this tendency to open bite is the possible complication of nonunion. The action of the temporalis muscle tends to rotate the proximal fragment superiorly by its coronoid attachment, thus separating the cut bone ends, which may prevent bony union.

3. Healing may require excessive periods of immobilization. At the level of the prescribed cut through the ramus the bone is very thin, composed almost entirely of cortical bone, which by the very nature of its dense structure tends to delay union even though the cut ends are wired directly. The greater the correction, the less will be the contact of the cut bone ends, another contributing factor to delayed union and prolonged fixation. (See Fig. 23-22.)

Sagittal osteotomy, ascending ramus (Obwegeser)

Intraoral operations for correction of various deformities of the jaws are often indicated or desirable. Obwegeser[42] described a method of splitting the ramus sagittally

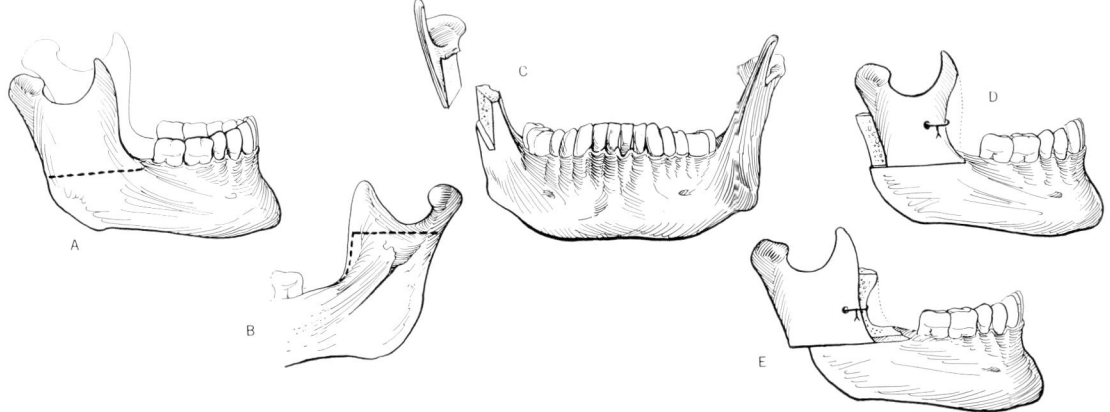

Fig. 23-23. Intraoral osteotomy in the ramus results in a steplike splitting on the sagittal plane suitable for correction of both prognathism and retrognathia. **A,** Line of cut in lateral cortex when prognathism is to be corrected. Line may be directed obliquely to the gonial angle from the retromolar area when retrognathia is corrected and the mandible advanced forward. **B,** Line of horizontal cut in medial cortex for correction of either prognathism or retrognathia. This should be as low and as close to the mandibular foramen as possible without chancing injury to the inferior alveolar nerve. **C** to **E,** Sagittal splitting with broad mortised surface in either an advanced or retruded repositioning. Note that an oblique cut in the lateral cortex (**E**) would have preserved a prominent gonial angle when the retruded jaw is advanced (DalPont's modification). (Modified from Obwegeser, H.: Oral Surg. **10:**677, 1957.)

(Fig. 23-23). This is in some respects reminiscent of Moose's[37] original horizontal osteotomy via intraoral approach and Kazanjian's[40] modification; however, Obwegeser's vertical sagittal splitting overcomes many disadvantages of these earlier operations. Later, DalPont[43] described a modification that Obwegeser endorses as an improvement, especially when the operation is used to correct retrognathia. As modified, a more pronounced gonial angle is obtained, which is desirable in correction of retrognathia.

Technique for intraoral sagittal osteotomy

1. The incision is made through mucosa and periosteum on the anterior border of the ascending ramus from well up toward the coronoid process downward along the external oblique line. To facilitate accurate accomplishment, soft tissues are compressed medially and laterally with retractors or the index and middle fingers as the incision is made firmly to bone.

2. With an assistant retracting the cheek the operator retracts the soft tissue medially and elevates the periosteum with a sharp, broad-bladed elevator. Exposure of the ramus on the medial aspect is obtained to the sigmoid notch superiorly, to the border of the ramus posteriorly, and to the lingula over the foramen inferiorly. The mandibular nerve is displaced medially in the soft tissues as they are elevated.

3. A retractor of the type specially designed by Dr. Sanford Moose is inserted and engaged around the posterior border of the ramus so that soft tissues are protected during osteotomy (Fig. 23-21).

4. Soft tissues on the outer or lateral surface of the ramus are now elevated, exposing the bone. In cases of correction for prognathism, exposure of bone is above the attachments of the masseter muscle for the most part and extended to the posterior

border. For correction of retrognathic cases the exposure of bone laterally is carried downward to the lower border of the mandible and anteriorly to the masseter muscle attachments.

5. The periosteum must be elevated fairly generously over the posterior border of the ramus and angle of the mandible to permit unrestricted movement of the sectioned jaw either anteriorly or posteriorly. A deeply hooked, side-cutting, periosteal elevator suggested by Obwegeser is used for this purpose and is quite essential to the operation (Fig. 23-20, *B*).

6. A horizontal incision in the bone is then made just above the mandibular foramen, but only through the medial cortical plate of bone. The bone becomes quite thin a bit higher, so it is wise to stay as low as possible without chancing injury to the inferior alveolar nerve. A Lindemann bur is preferable for this purpose, although Hu Friedy's long-shank, cross-cut drill is quite satisfactory also. The tendency of bleeding in the cut line usually indicates when cortical bone has been penetrated (Fig. 23-23, *B*).

7. Incision in the bone on the lateral surface is now made. In prognathic jaws the cut is made in a horizontal direction also and as parallel as possible to the cut made on the medial surface. In retrognathic correction this cut is made obliquely downward and back toward the lower border of the mandible anterior to the angle. Here again the incision in the bone is made through the cortical plate only (Fig. 23-23, *A*).

8. The medial and lateral bone incisions are now connected on the anterior border of the mandible using a No. 703 carbide taper fissure bur.

9. The next step is the critical one—splitting anterior-posteriorly between the medial and lateral cuts in the cortical plates. A thin, broad (at least 1 cm wide), long-beveled osteotome is necessary. It is inserted into the vertical cut on the anterior border of the ramus with the bevel to the medial. As it is gently inserted deeper and deeper posteriorly the sharp edge is kept firmly contacting the lateral cortex. Although Obwegeser suggests twisting the osteotome (and he uses one 2 cm. wide), such leverage may result in undesirable fracture, especially at the horizontal level above the mandibular foramen. Splitting is effected through the posterior border of the ramus in a desirable vertical direction if gentle but firm malleting is applied to the osteotome, at varying levels (Fig. 23-23, *C*).

10. When splitting is completed, the sectioned parts are adjusted as desired for the problem at hand. With completely mobilized segments very little problem is encountered in maintaining relationship of the parts. Transosseous wiring may be used, but it is difficult to place drill holes properly for wiring, and it has been our experience that the irregularities in the contacting medullary surfaces seem to impact and engage onto each other and maintain desired placement (Fig. 23-23, *D* and *E*).

Comments

1. This operation has been used by us in females only.
2. It is not dependable in patients with small skeletal framework since potential of undesirable fracture is present.
3. Trauma to the inferior alveolar nerve is to be expected, but injury has not resulted in permanent anesthesia in our experience.
4. No more than minimal to moderate correction should be expected or planned.
5. Relapse has not been observed, and clinical union may be expected in about 5 to 6 weeks.
6. Our principal problem with the operation, except splitting the bone itself, has been to completely free and mobilize the soft tissue sling to permit free movement of the fragments in repositioning. It would be quite difficult without an instrument

such as the side-cutting, sharply hooking periosteotome described previously.

Ostectomy in the body of the mandible

Ostectomy, when performed for correction of prognathism, consists of the excision of a measured section of the body of the mandible to establish normal relation of the anterior teeth and correct protrusion of the lower jaw. It may be performed by an intraoral approach, an extraoral approach, or a combination of both in one or two stages.

Blair[2] described this operation first in 1907. He used a hand saw for removal of bone in the bicuspid or molar region. In 1912 Harsha[44] reported a case in which he had corrected prognathism by excision of a rhomboid section of bone from the third molar area. The section removed was wider above than at the lower border of the mandible in an effort to increase the angle from the obtuse deformity, which is characteristically observed in prognathism. He used "bone-cutting forceps and rongeurs" to accomplish the excision of bone and then placed "wire sutures to maintain apposition of bone during healing." New and Erich (1941)[45] favored ostectomy in the bicuspid or first molar regions and preferred to accomplish the surgery by an "open" method "in which the mandible is exposed both externally and from within the mouth." Excision of bone was accomplished by a combination of a motor-driven circular saw, chisel, Gigli saw, and rongeurs in an effort to preserve the continuity of the mandibular nerve. In 1948 Dingman[46] made a comprehensive review of the literature on the subject of prognathism and also made a detailed appraisal of various methods utilized for its surgical correction. He had previously described in 1944[47] a two-stage method of ostectomy in which he overcame the disadvantages of compounding the extraoral surgical wound intraorally and at the same time avoided injury to the mandibular nerve. These articles were classics and served to popularize ostectomy in treatment of prognathism. Ostectomy, or the "Dingman two-stage operation," as it is frequently referred to, was probably the most widely used of all the methods 10 or 12 years ago. Preference for this oper-

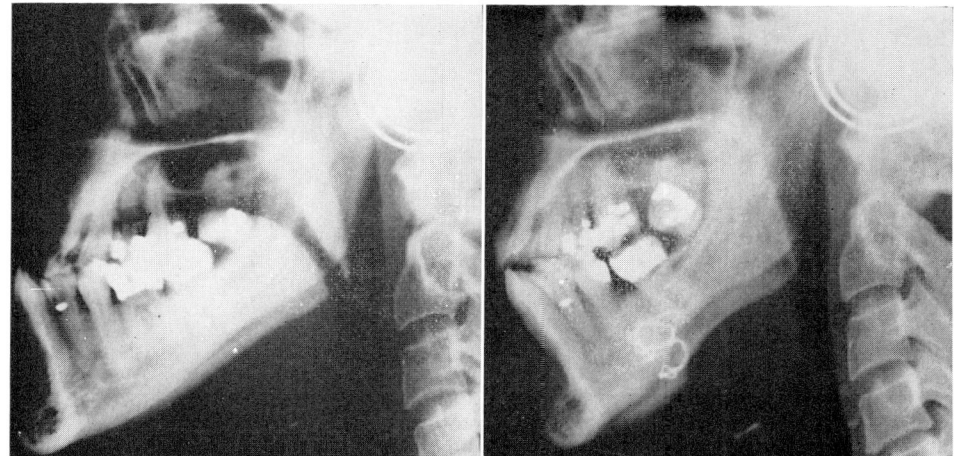

Fig. 23-24. Lateral cephalograms of a patient with 10 mm. of protrusion corrected by ostectomy in two stages. **A**, Preoperative. **B**, Postoperative. (U. S. Army Photographs; Letterman Army Hospital.)

472 *Textbook of oral surgery*

ation is easily understood because technically it is not difficult to accomplish. Thoma[48] describes intraoral ostectomy accomplished by utilizing bone drills and osteotomes.

Technique for ostectomy in the body of the mandible. When correction of prognathism by ostectomy is indicated, it may be accomplished at one operation or in two stages (Figs. 23-24 to 23-26). In our opinion the two-stage approach is rarely indicated. Complete ostectomy in a single operation is much more desirable. In operations such as this that are open and directly communicate to the oral cavity, antibiotic prophylaxis starting the day prior to surgery is indicated.

1. The patient is especially prepared for the initial part of the operation by thorough washing of the face with surgical soap and scrupulous cleansing of the oral cavity. Draping is standard for operations in the mouth.

2. Incisions are made into the interdental papillae adjacent to the site of the ostectomy and also through the mucoperiosteum at the crest of the edentulous ridge, if a tooth has been removed previously.

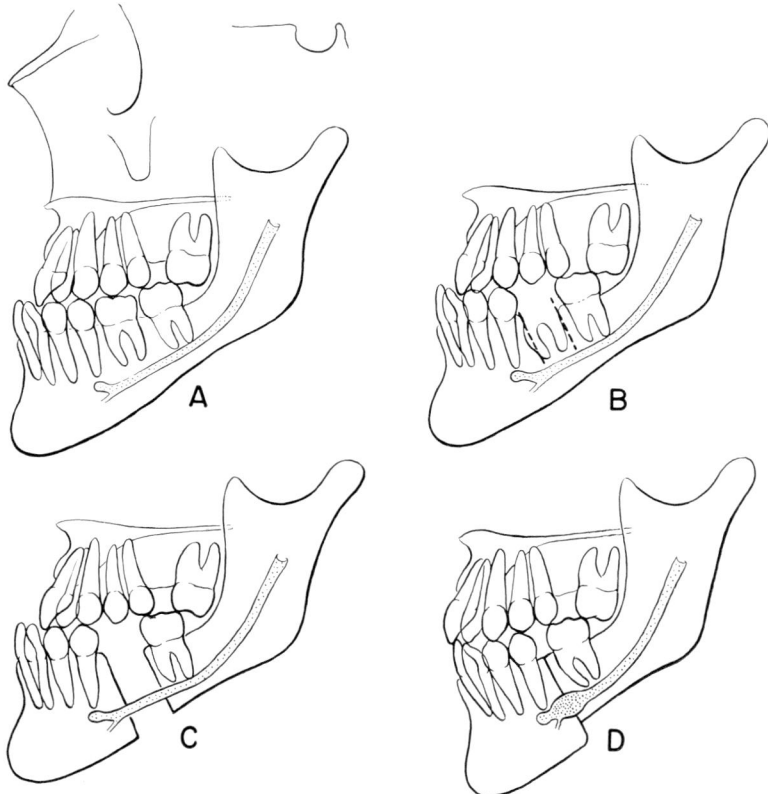

Fig. 23-25. Tracings of cephalogram in Fig. 23-24. **A,** The gonial angle was not markedly obtuse in the preoperative tracing, a satisfactory case for this operation. **B,** Intraoral first stage of bone incisions. **C,** Uninterrupted continuity of inferior alveolar nerve after second-stage ostectomy. **D,** Tracing of cephalogram 9 months postoperative. Clinical union was present after 10 weeks of fixation by splinting of the teeth. This was a good result of ostectomy, usually observed in patients with no more than 10 to 12 mm. of correction necessary.

3. An incision should be carried obliquely anteriorly and downward into the buccal vestibule, one or two teeth anteriorly to the site of ostectomy.

4. Since no such oblique incision should be made on the lingual aspect of the mandible, it is usually necessary to incise papillae as far forward as the cuspid or lateral incisor, to permit detachment of the lingual periosteum without tearing.

5. The mucoperiosteal flap on the buccal aspect intraorally is then elevated from the bone. Caution is exercised to protect the mental nerve. For flap retraction intraorally, I prefer a smaller periosteotome (Molt No. 9) and use both the No. 2 and No. 4 Molt curets for periosteal detachment and elevation.

6. The lingual flap is raised in a similar manner down to the mylohyoid muscle. It need not be detached at this time.

7. For precise bone incision, a caliper or measured metal template is used to guide the bone cuts.

8. Vertical cuts across the alveolar ridge are accomplished with a No. 703 fissure bur in an 18,000 rpm engine and handpiece to a safe level above the course of the mandibular nerve. They are extended as low as possible into both buccal and lingual cortices, and the alveolar portion of bone is removed by rongeur and chisel and mallet. The inferior alveolar nerve may or may not be seen at this time.

(If the operation is to be completed in one stage, the intraoral wounds are covered with moist gauze sponges, but not closed. If a delayed "second stage" is planned the following steps 9, 10, and 11 are carried out.)

9. The soft tissue flaps are closed as each side is completed, and the wounds are permitted to heal for 3 to 5 weeks before the second stage of ostectomy is undertaken.

10. During this interim period between the two surgical procedures, the fixation appliances (splints or orthodontic appliances) are prepared and inserted.

11. Local anesthesia may be utilized for all of the preparatory work, including the first surgical stage. The patient need not be hospitalized unless a specific unusual reason makes this necessary.

12. The skin of the face and neck is again prepared by washing with soap and draped for the extraoral surgery, and the versatile "curtain" draping technique is used since the mouth must be entered later in the operation.

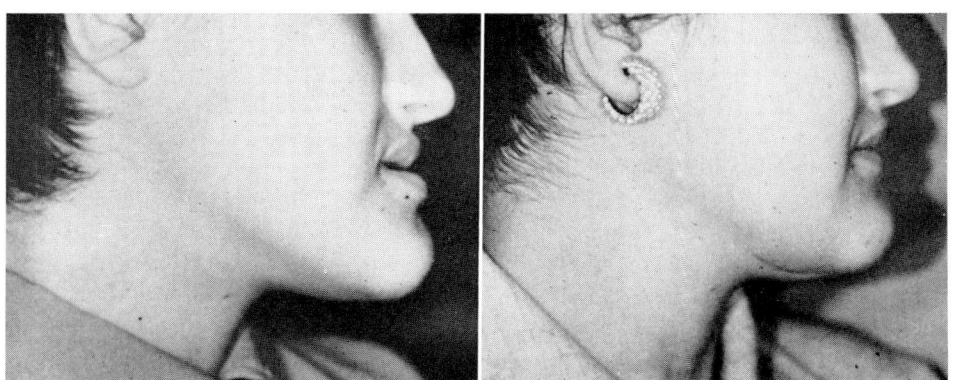

Fig. 23-26. A 20-year-old girl with only 8 mm. of protrusion that was corrected by two-stage ostectomy in the body of the mandible with excellent functional and esthetic results. **A**, Preoperative. **B**, Postoperative. (U. S. Army Photographs; Letterman Army Hospital.)

13. The soft tissue dissection extraorally is carried out as previously described.

14. When the lower border of the mandible is reached, the periosteum is incised sharply and then, using a Lane periosteotome in the left hand for retraction of soft tissue, the periosteum is elevated sharply with a Molt No. 4 curet.

15. The mental foramen will come to view quickly on the lateral aspect of the mandible, and elevation of the periosteum is carried superiorly beyond it, due caution being exercised to protect the mental nerve. Blunt spreading of soft tissues around the nerve with a curved mosquito forceps will gain relaxation of the flap as it is elevated and prevents damage to the nerve. The cuts in the lateral cortex will be visualized for orientation of the final phase of ostectomy.

16. Periosteum on the medial aspect is elevated in the same manner and with no more difficulty until the attachments of the mylohyoid muscle come into view.

17. Both the lateral and medial surfaces of the bone should be exposed for a distance of 4 to 5 cm. for adequate access for bone excision without injury to soft structures.

18. A No. 703 carbide bur is used to complete the previously made bur cuts down to the lower border of the mandible. These cuts on the lateral aspect of the mandible are made through cortical bone only. The shape of the bone segment outlined by the bur cuts has been determined by previous careful measurement.

19. When both vertical cuts through the cortex are completed, they are connected anteroposteriorly at the lower border of the mandible with the No. 703 carbide bur. (All bone cutting with the bur should be irrigated with sterile saline solution to prevent thermal damage to bone.)

20. A broad, flat-bladed periosteotome is now placed into the anteroposterior connecting cut at the lower border of the mandible and turned, thus elevating off the lateral cortex.

21. The mandibular nerve is exposed and identified by removal of cancellous bone with curets.

22. The medullary bone is removed in this manner until the dense substance of the lingual cortex is reached. The cortical plates anterior and posterior to the cuts are undermined slightly by scooping out more medullary bone in order to create space into which the nerve and vessels may coil when the ends of the bone are approximated.

23. The inferior alveolar neurovascular bundle is protected with a blunt retractor (Molt No. 9), and the soft tissues lingual to the mandible are guarded with a broad Lane periosteal elevator.

24. Assuming that transosseous wiring is planned, drill holes to accomodate it are made at this time using a No. 14 bone drill in the handpiece or a No. 52 twist drill point in the Smedberg hand drill.

25. With protection afforded as in step 12 the ostectomy is completed through the lingual cortex using the No. 703 carbide bur at 18,000 rpm under saline irrigation. As this plate of bone is removed the mylohyoid muscle attachments must be sharply dissected free to avoid tearing.

26. Lingual ostectomy on the first side may be left incomplete until the second side is finished, to afford stability of the jaw as the surgery progresses.

27. When the lingual ostectomies are completed, the transosseous wires are placed in both sides, but they should not be tightened completely at this time, merely enough to hold the parts in approximate relation with some movement still possible.

28. The mouth is now entered. Intraoral soft tissue flaps are replaced and sutured. Previously placed fixation appliances are secured and intermaxillary immobilization is accomplished with the teeth in the desired new occlusal relationship.

29. Gloves are changed, and the extraoral wound is again entered.

30. If the ostectomy was properly planned and executed, the bone ends should now be in close apposition. The wire

sutures are twisted down tightly to add to the stability of the mandible during healing.

31. The wound is closed in anatomical layers as previously described, but a small rubber dam drain should be placed from deep in the wound to the outside. Since we routinely keep our dressings on for 4 days, the drain is not removed until the fourth day, when the sutures are also removed.

Technique for intraoral ostectomy. The intraoral ostectomy suggested by Thoma requires more extensive reflection of buccal and lingual mucoperiosteal flaps intraorally. In fact, the buccal exposure must be to the lower border of the mandible, a procedure difficult to achieve and still protect the mental nerve. The operation should be done under general anesthesia, for complete relaxation is essential. Its application is somewhat limited, and patients with big mouths and pliable, tractable tissues are most suitable for it.

The excision of bone is achieved in the same manner as described previously, using No. 703 carbide burs in a handpiece, driven by an 18,000 rpm engine, with removal of the lateral cortex, exposure and identification of the mandibular nerve, and then excision of the medial or lingual cortex. Thoma prefers to use long-shanked Henihan drills in a contra-angle handpiece since they are long enough to penetrate both cortices of the bone. I have more difficulty controlling the progress of the bone incision with a contra-angle handpiece and, furthermore, I am never positive as to the exact location of the nerve until I can uncover it laterally. I have also found it difficult to perform the cuts in the precise direction desired, even when the facial muscles are completely relaxed. I much prefer to complete the ostectomy from an extraoral approach, unless the patient is absolutely and unalterably opposed to an external scar.

Advantages of ostectomy. The advantages are few:

1. Dissection through the soft tissue to the lower border of the mandible at the midportion of the body can be accomplished quickly, and adequate access to the site of ostectomy is acquired without difficulty.

2. Excision of bone can be done without injury to the mandibular nerve, and if the nerve is damaged, it tends to recover.

3. Immobilization of the sectioned bone is possible when stable teeth are available in both fragments and the parts are secured by intraoral splinting or orthodontic appliances augmented by transosseous wire ligatures.

4. A good cosmetic result is achieved in slight to moderate cases of prognathism (Figs. 23-25, D, and 23-26).

5. The operation may be performed in two stages, with the final extraoral surgery accomplished without communication into the mouth and possible contamination of the surgical wound.

Disadvantages of ostectomy. Following are the disadvantages to be considered:

1. Although a good profile can be produced in every case, a good cosmetic result is not attained in moderate to extreme cases of protrusion for the very simple reason that the obtuse angle of the mandible is not corrected by the surgery. The excision of bone in the body merely shortens the length of the bone, and the obtuse gonial angle deformity is often accentuated (Figs. 23-27 and 23-28).

2. If it becomes necessary to remove more than one tooth, the sacrifice of functional surfaces is too great to contemplate this method, thus contraindicating the procedure in moderate to extreme prognathism. When two teeth per side are sacrificed, the difference in the transverse distance between the two second molars and the two first bicuspids is excessive, and the degree of medial rotation of the proximal fragments is unduly great (Fig. 23-29). Also to be considered is the loss of area that is left available to the prosthodontist if the patient subsequently becomes edentulous.

3. Nonunion, though not a common oc-

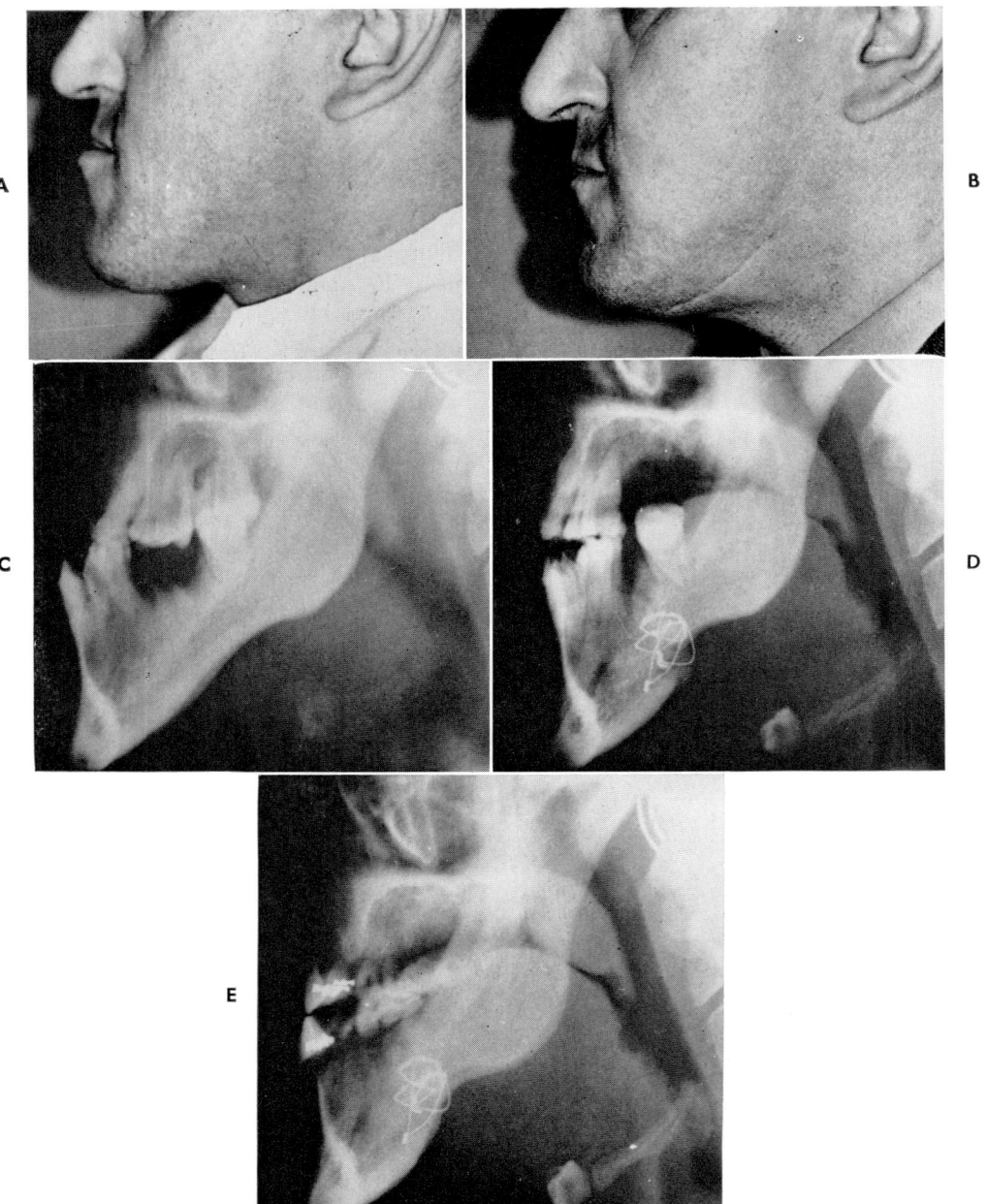

Fig. 23-27. A, This patient had 15 mm. of protrusion. B, After correction by a single or one-stage ostectomy in the body of the mandible there appears to be a disproportionate vertical length of his face compared to the short anteroposterior length. Although he has a good postoperative profile, he does not have a desirable correction of the gonial angle. C, Preoperative cephalogram. Moderately advanced periodontal disease was present, indicating complete extractions and dentures after surgical correction of prognathism. D, Postoperative cephalogram showing downward tilt of anterior portion of mandible caused by action of depressor group of muscles, permitted by unstable periodontally involved teeth, despite interdental splints and intramaxillary immobilization. E, Poor skeletal profile with pronounced obtuse gonial angle present in final cephalogram. These poor results are commonplace following ostectomy in extreme prognathism. (U. S. Army Photographs; Letterman Army Hospital.)

Developmental deformities of the jaws 477

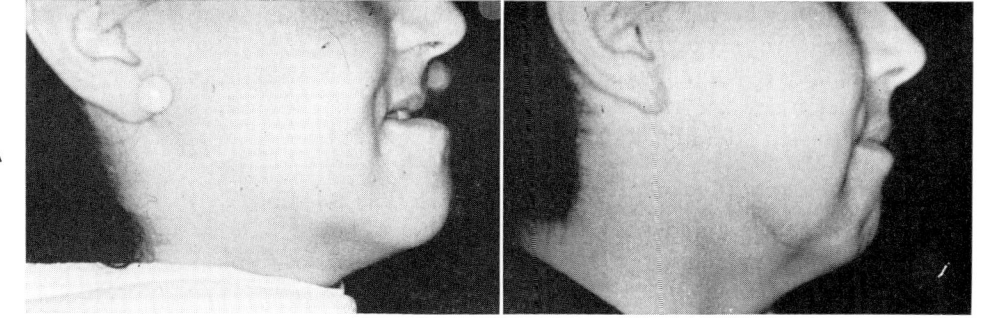

Fig. 23-28. **A,** Another patient (prognathism measuring 13 mm.) was treated by ostectomy in the body of the mandible. **B,** The complication of nonunion occurred on one side; the angle of the mandible was not improved; scarring was conspicuous because of "bunching" or "folding" of soft tissues when the mandible was shortened. (U. S. Army Photographs; Letterman Army Hospital.)

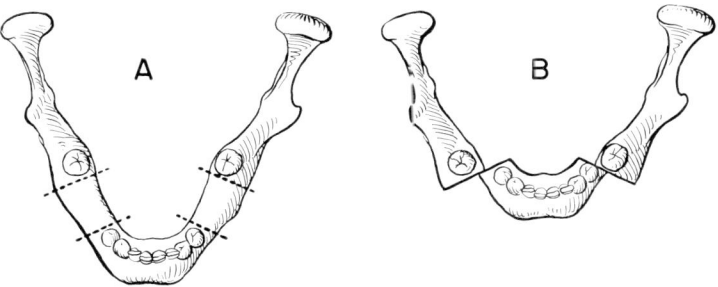

Fig. 23-29. Removal of a large segment of bone from the body of the mandible (ostectomy) results in imperfect bone end apposition, **B,** or excessive medial rotation of the proximal (ramus) fragments.

currence, is a complication to be considered. The potential is in direct proportion to the degree of bone end approximation and postoperative immobilization, discounting the possibility of contamination from the oral cavity and possible postoperative infection. If, through miscalculation in bone excision, the bone ends are not in direct apposition, nonunion may occur. If as much as 2 to 3 mm. of space exists, nonunion is sure to result. Absolute immobilization of the parts is also essential if union is to be assured.

4. Firm clinical union cannot be expected in much less than 8 weeks in the most favorable cases and may not be attained for up to 3 months or more.

5. It is cited as an advantage by advocates of ostectomy that the muscles of mastication are not interfered with; however, no mention is made of the action of the depressor muscles and their continual action tending to produce open bite. If this does not occur, there is the tendency of the anterior teeth to be extruded because of this muscle action. Preoperative tongue thrust habits may add to these complications.

6. External scarring is an objection unless ostectomy is done intraorally. This should not be objectionable if the incision

is well below the lower border of the mandible and closure is carefully accomplished; However, occasionally resulting from an excessive bulk of soft tissue, an irregular scar with "folding" is observed (Fig. 23-28).

Supportive and postoperative care

The details of supportive and postoperative care must be governed by the extent of surgery and the requirement of the individual patient.

With the mandible immobilized by intermaxillary elastic ligatures, it is routine practice to pass a Levin tube through the unused nostril to the stomach so that it can be emptied by suction during or immediately upon completion of surgery. This does much to eliminate nausea, and if vomiting does occur, it is of such minimal proportion that no hazard to the airway develops.

When the patient is ready for transfer from the operating room to the recovery room he should be placed on the litter or his bed *on his side* to ensure dependent drainage of fluid from the mouth. He should be moved from one side to the other occasionally until he is finally reactive. It is also wise to impress on the patient that when he awakens from anesthesia his jaw will be fixed closed so that he will not fight against the appliances or become panicky. From this time on emergency instruments—scissors and wire cutters—should be immediately available at the bedside to permit immediate access to the oral pharynx in case of airway obstruction.

Fluid requirements must be met. When the patient has been deprived of fluids for several hours prior to surgery, the daily requirements must be furnished by intravenous infusion during the day of surgery. The type of replacement must be calculated individually. If an excessive blood loss has occurred, part of the replacement should be in the form of whole blood. If the patient has lost fluids through the skin (perspiring) a part of the replacement may be in the form of saline infusion. The bulk of fluid replacement, however, is usually in the form of 5% glucose in distilled water.

Patients undergoing this type of surgery may require antibiotics to protect against infection, but this is a matter of judgement in each individual case.

Pain can be controlled by administration of appropriate opiates or analgesics.

Ordinarily if the patient has not voided within 6 to 8 hours after returning to the recovery ward, catheterization is indicated.

If normal bowel movements have not occurred by the third day, an enema should be ordered.

Early ambulation hastens recovery. The patient is permitted bathroom privileges on the first postoperative day, and activity is encouraged thereafter.

The initial dressings are left in place until the third or fourth postoperative day, at which time all sutures are removed, but the skin is immobilized with collodion gauze strips for another week or more.

Relationship of musculature to surgical correction of jaw deformities

In appraisal of various surgical methods of correction, authorities on the subject invariably consider the effect that musculature has upon the healing of the jaw and the influence that this musculature may exert in causing relapse or a tendency to reversion of the part to its former malrelation. Formerly, if the cosmetic objective was achieved, the result was considered to be satisfactory even when function was impaired or bony union had not occurred. This philisophy is no longer tenable. Complete repair and good function must be expected.

The complexities of this matter of muscle balance, abnormal stresses, and imbalance resulting from surgery are variable with the extent of repositioning and the operations performed in surgical correction. The compensatory powers of the musculature are often adequate to reestablish normal function after corrective surgery, though the direction and functional length of muscles are changed. However, certain limitations to the adaptability of the musculature must be recognized and due cognizance taken when a method of surgical correction is selected.

Foremost of the muscles that potentially mitigate against good results is the temporalis. It is a "bipennate" muscle, which, according to Batson,[49] "accounts for the *short length of the muscle fibers* and for the strong pull that this muscle exerts." Batson's description of the muscle, its attachments, action, and function explains certain difficulties encountered in surgical correction of jaw deformities, especially prognathism. He states that "from anatomic evidence the temporal muscle is capable of lifting the coronoid process some fifteen millimeters and retracting it seven or eight millimeters."

Probably the difficulty most frequently encountered is the tendency of the coronoid process to tip superiorly following horizontal (sliding) osteotomy above the mandibular foramen. This is a direct response to the strong pull of the temporalis muscle and has two effects: (1) displacement of cut bone ends from apposition, resulting in questionable bony union, and (2) shortening the functional length of the temporalis muscle fibers, undoubtedly weakening the effectiveness of this muscle as one of the principal masticators. This upward displacement of the coronoid process seems to be in direct proportion to the amount of repositioning attempted, practically no displacement occurring in minor corrections but moderate to extreme displacement in repositioning of 12 mm. and over.

Clinically we have observed that the temporalis muscle places a definite restriction on the posterior repositioning of the mandible in operations in which the coronoid process is carried back with the body of the mandible (osteotomy in the condylar neck, subcondylar or oblique osteotomy and vertical osteotomy in the ramus). This places a definite limit on the amount of correction that may be successfully achieved by blind osteotomy through the neck of the condyle. I am positive of this restriction imposed by the temporalis muscle because in vertical osteotomy via the open surgical method, I have been unable to obtain adequate posterior movement in certain instances after the vertical section has been completed until I have sectioned free the coronoid process with its muscle attachments. About 1 cm. seems to be the limit of repositioning freely obtainable without coronoid section.

The lateral pterygoid muscle is probably least affected of all of the muscles of mastication in any of the operations for correction of prognathism. It probably also has the least effect or interference with the reestablished positions of the mandible. It may tend to distract the head of the condyle after osteotomy through the condylar neck, and nonunion may result.

The medial pterygoid and masseter muscles, because of their overpowering strength, possess a great potential to cause overriding of cut bone ends after horizontal (sliding) osteotomy above the mandibular foramen, especially if direct transosseous wiring has not been accomplished. This tendency plus the action of the hyoid depressor group of muscles creates a forceful muscle action, with the posterior teeth acting as a fulcrum, and accounts for the tendency to open bite in the anterior part of the mouth. According to Reiter the reason that open bite does not occur in condyle osteotomy due to these same factors is the counteracting action of the temporalis muscle. However, bilateral traumatic fracture-dislocations of the condyles that are untreated surgically have posed many plaguing problems of open bite. On this basis it seems that the entire musculature would also operate to produce open-bite complications following osteotomy in the condylar neck.

The effect on the action and function of the medial pterygoid and the masseter muscles following vertical osteotomy in the ramus is negligible. This is because the masseter muscle is elevated intact from its mandibular attachments and the medial pterygoid is partially elevated. After the sectioning of the bone is completed and the parts repositioned, the muscle attachments are returned to essentially their original relationship, and their detached stumps are sutured together under the lower border of the newly established gonial angle. Thus, healing and reattachment may occur in normal functional position as a result of shifting the location for the muscle insertions.

The depressor or suprahyoid musculature functions in harmony with the principal muscles of mastication and also the infrahyoid muscles. This "group action" common to muscles throughout the body may be disrupted following traumatic injury or surgical ostectomy. Interruption in unity of the body of the mandible bilaterally is followed by a tendency to distraction of the anterior segment (distal fragment) inferiorly. Thus, in addition to the part played by these muscles in contributing to the open-bite tendency following osteotomy in the ramus, they also exert considerable influence toward separation of the bone ends following ostectomy in the body of the mandible and open bite anteriorly. Though not great, this effect is present and must be combated by proper fixation appliances.

The complex musculature of the tongue is another factor worthy of comment. This powerful group of muscles, by virtue of uninhibited or uncorrected "habit," is a potent factor in the tendency of the mandible to return to a preoperative protrusive or open bite relationship. Added to the actions of the depressor group, it has considerable displacing effect following osteotomy or ostectomy. This plus the action of the major muscles of mastication may constitute the total force needed to overcome fixation appliances following any corrective jaw surgery. Direct transosseous wiring cannot be relied upon under these conditions either. The combined force of all of these muscles places a tremendous stress on the teeth bearing the fixation appliances, and over long periods of immobilization, even though this musculature may relax from trismus and compensate to a degree to new relations and length, there is undoubtedly a great potential for irreversible damage to the teeth and supporting structures. Examples of poor results for these reasons are seen in Figs. 23-22 and 23-27.

In addition to unfavorable thrusting habits the tremendous bulk of the tongue in patients with extreme protrusion has been a matter of considerable concern since conceivably it could result in mechanical obstruction of the oral pharynx, since the tongue, in its entirety, is also repositioned posteriorly when the mandible is retruded to desired occlusal relationship. Added to the mechanical factors is the potential of edema. Ample precautionary postoperative observation is necessary.

Fixation appliances and immobilization

Arch bars (Fig. 23-30) or custom-made cast labial splints (Fig. 23-31) are indicated for fixation of the mandible following any corrective surgery in which immobilization is expected to extend beyond 4 weeks. They should be well adapted to afford protection to the teeth against movement or extrusion over protracted periods of immobilization.

Cast, sectional, wing type, screw lock splints (Fig. 23-32), as advocated by McCarthy and Burns[50] for war injury cases, are ideal for immobilization following ostectomy, or osteotomy for advancement of a retruded mandible, since connecting devices are adjustable. However, an appliance of the type suggested by Kazanjian[51] may be preferred. Since it is technically difficult to remove a section of bone with absolute accuracy of measurement (as in ostectomy), some type of adjustable appliance should be planned. Many surgeons obtain orthodontic banding for this reason even if

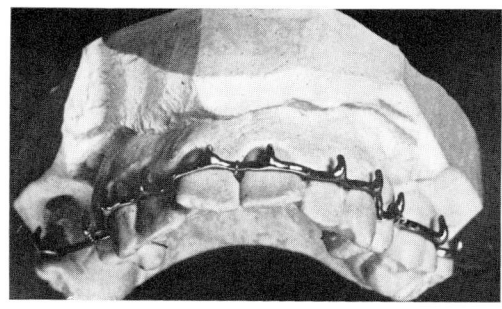 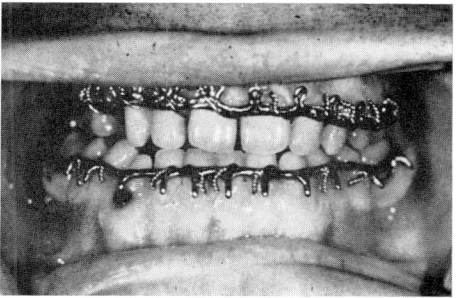

Fig. 23-30. **A**, Individually fabricated arch bar. Fourteen-gauge half-round clasp wire is adapted to a stone model and 18-gauge round wire lugs are soldered or welded onto it. **B**, Mandibular individually or custom-made arch bar. Maxillary arch bar of the commercial type. Arch bars should be adapted to stone models unless they are made of malleable metal and are readily adaptable. Otherwise they are likely to cause tooth movement or extrusion when not perfectly adapted. (U. S. Army Photographs; Letterman Army Hospital.)

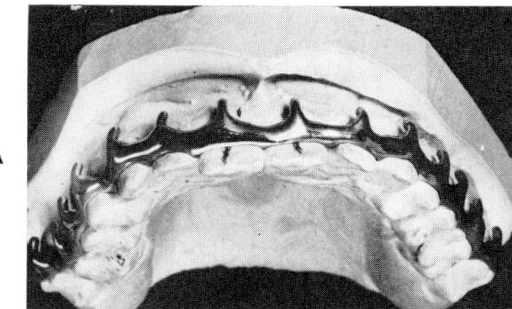 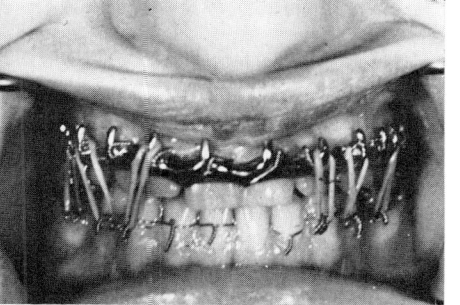

Fig. 23-31. **A**, Cast labial splints are more reliable than arch bars, especially when immobilization is expected to be necessary for a long time (more than 8 to 10 weeks). **B**, This appliance actually splints and protects the teeth against stresses of intermaxillary fixation. (U. S. Army Photographs; Letterman Army Hospital.)

orthodontic treatment is not contemplated, and this may be the most practical and dependable appliance.

The simple expediency of Ivy loop or multiple-loop wiring should not be utilized except when fixation is needed for only a short period of 3 to 5 weeks. This type of fixation is preferred in vertical osteotomy since the desired occlusion can be established with greater accuracy (Fig. 23-33).

Robinson[31] is a strong advocate of the use of an intermaxillary splint (clear acrylic "wafer") interposed between the teeth at the time of surgery to ensure postoperative occlusion. Use of such a splint is highly desirable when many teeth are missing and a relation cannot otherwise be positively assured (Fig. 23-34). Routine use of the intermaxillary splint is not desirable or recommended, especially if good jaw relation and reasonably good occlusion are anticipated.

Van Alstine and Dingman[52] recommended use of an acrylic splint and circumferential wiring to supplement transosseous wiring in edentulous patients corrected by ostectomy. Cameron and Stetzer[53] reported an

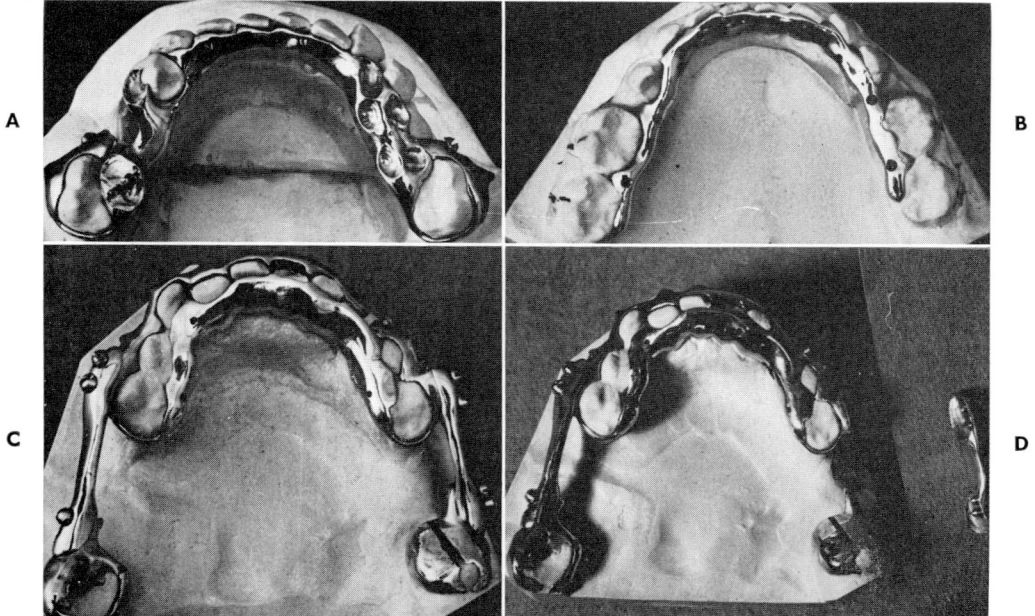

Fig. 23-32. Cast sectional screw lock splints used for stabilization after ostectomy for prognathism or micrognathia. **A,** Lingual wing-type screw lock with occlusion built on to afford rest position during the recovery period. Used for fixation following correction of prognathism. The anterior segment of the mandible is moved back to proper relation, and the teeth in this fragment are then wired into the splint. **B,** Simple cast lingual splint that is used in the same manner. It may also be placed preoperatively and teeth of anterior part of mandible wired onto it after the section is completed. **C,** Sectional splint with connector bars used for either prognathism or micrognathia. The posterior overlay crowns and anterior splint are placed prior to surgery. **D,** The connector bars can be made ahead of time also and screwed to place immediately following ostectomy. They can also be made after the jaw is repositioned and stabilized by intermaxillary fixation by taking impressions of the connector seats and casting the connector subsequent to surgery. They are not as complicated as they may appear to be. (U. S. Army Photographs; Letterman Army Hospital.)

extreme case of prognathism in an edentulous patient, which they treated by ostectomy. They stabilized the bone during healing by means of a tantalum saddle tray adapted to the lower border and wired circumferentially to the bone. Since this metal is well tolerated ordinarily, it would appear that this means of stabilization would be much more preferable than that of an intraoral acrylic splint. As previously stated, it is my experience that edentulous patients with prognathism can be treated by vertical osteotomy in the ramus without benefit of intraoral splinting or immobilization, provided that firm transosseous wiring is inserted. No doubt dentures or Gunning type splints wired to place give added stability and insure correct jaw relation during healing.

Discussion

As previously stated, no single operation is universally applicable to all deformities of prognathism. Before undertaking the surgical correction of these deformities the problem must be evaluated thoroughly

Developmental deformities of the jaws 483

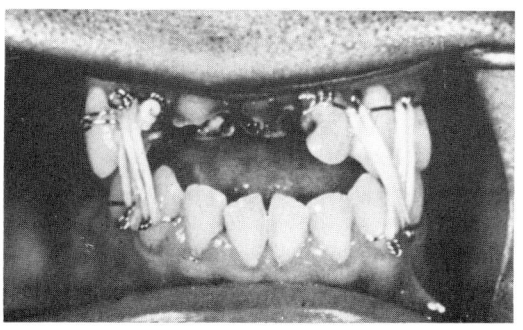

Fig. 23-33. Simple Ivy loop or multiple-loop wiring is adequate for immobilization following vertical osteotomy in prognathism. This example of wiring used on the few remaining anterior teeth is typical of the simplicity of fixation in this particular operation. (U. S. Army Photograph; Letterman Army Hospital.)

by all adjunctive diagnostic means available. Preoperative planning and selection of a proper technique for correction of any given case of prognathism cannot be overemphasized. When several acceptable techniques are available, the surgeon should select the method most suited to the problem. Size of individuals is variable, and it is possible that a tiny female with 1 cm. of protrusion of the mandible would be considered as having extreme prognathism while a large man needing 1 cm. of correction might be considered as slightly prognathic. As an average, vertical osteotomy is recommended in cases requiring correction in excess of 1.5 cm.

Modification of any standard operation

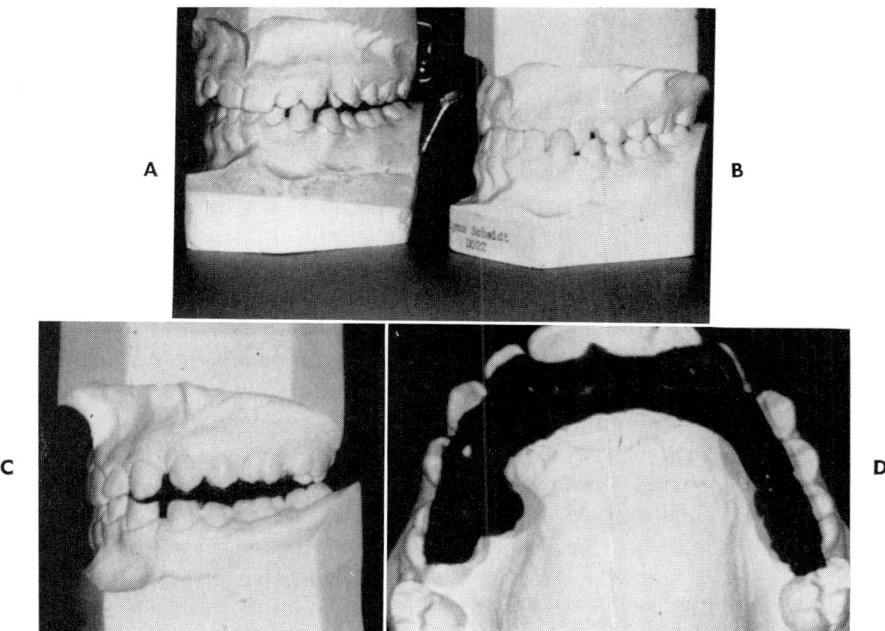

Fig. 23-34. A, A clear acrylic "wafer" interposed between the teeth at time of surgery should be used when the jaw and occlusion are insecure in the new position or if it is desirable to block the teeth from extrusion or other shifting during the period of immobilization. B, Study casts show lack of occlusion in bicuspid and molar areas. C, Study casts with interposed "wafer" to prevent extrusion of teeth that will be moved by controlled orthodontic management later. D, When many missing teeth make a stabilized occlusion doubtful at the time of surgery, a modified Gunning type of splint should be planned to guide the repositioning and ensure proper jaw relation through the healing period.

is often needed. For example, we have varied the vertical technique that we reported in 1954 many times since then, and in 1963 the most severe prognathism in the author's experience was treated by a modified "vertical" operation.[54] The patient was a 33-year-old man whose prognathism measured 32 mm. No occlusion of teeth was present because of the gross size of the mandible and its complete encirclement of the maxilla (Fig. 23-14). It was quite evident that correction of the problem could only be achieved in the ramus. Osteotomy at the base of the condylar neck, subcondylar (oblique), and vertical osteotomy were all considered, but none of these procedures appeared to be acceptable (Fig. 23-15, B to D). A modified "vertical" operation was planned and used with good results (Fig. 23-15, E and F). *Decortication, coronoidotomy*, and transosseous wiring were necessary to achieve the correction. It was also necessary to obtain access through a fairly generous submandibular incision and to elevate all involved musculature to permit unrestricted posterior repositioning of the mandible. It must be concluded then that simplified techniques have a place in corrective jaw surgery, but that the more difficult technical procedures must be mastered also.

Another lesson of importance is that no infallible rule exists regarding the correct age to operate on prognathic patients. The patient illustrated in Figs. 23-14 and 23-15 grew 2 inches in height from age 20 to 28, and he is certain that his mandible grew more after age 20 than during his teenage years. He was a rare exception and should not influence criteria for surgical scheduling. However, all prognathic patients should be advised of this possibility, and most physically mature teenage patients should be deferred and measured cephalometrically for at least 1 year before surgery is provided. We generally believe that prognathic deformity attains its maximum when full body growth and development is attained.

In boys this is usually age 16 to 18, and in girls about 2 years younger. Psychological problems and poor social adjustment often justify earlier consideration of surgery.

MICROGNATHIA AND RETROGNATHIA

A distinction should be made between *micrognathia* and *retrognathia*. Micrognathia is defined as abnormal smallness of the jaw, especially the lower jaw, while retrognathia simply implies a retruded position (Angle's Class II) of the mandible without diminution. Another term deserving definition is *microgenia*, or abnormal smallness of the chin. Surgical correction of the micrognathic mandible has always been a more difficult undertaking than correction of prognathic deformities. Two principal reasons account for the difficulty: (1) bony substance in which to perform osteotomy is minimal, and (2) availability of investing soft tissue to cover the surgically elongated jaw may also be critical.

An ideal surgical technique for correction of mandibular micrognathism should provide (1) improved acceptable occlusion of the teeth into Angle's Class I relation, (2) cosmetic benefits, including mental prominence and pronounced gonial angle, (3) psychological benefits, (4) improved phonetics, and (5) technical feasibility including (a) adequate bone contact at site of osteotomy to ensure bony union, (b) minimal or no injury to important anatomical structures such as contents of mandibular canal, (c) surgical repair and closure assuring no permanent disruption of function, and (d) reasonable operating time.

Innumerable operations have been suggested for the correction of this deformity. Blair,[2] in his article published in 1907, advocated oblique section of the ramus at the level of the mandibular foramen. In 1909[55] he reported two cases treated in that manner. In 1928 Limberg[56] reviewed the literature on this subject. At that time a number of methods had already been advocated for osteotomy and forward repositioning of the mandible in micrognathia. He proposed a "step" operation in the body of the mandible with the addition of a rib graft. He credited Pehr Gadd (1906) with the original conception of the principle of "step" sliding osteotomy, which has been commonly employed in correction of micrognathia or retrognathia. In 1936 Kazanjian[57] described an L-shaped sliding osteotomy that is suitable for correction of the deformity also. If teeth are present in the ridge posterior to the proposed location for osteotomy, the L-shaped incision in the bone is preferable since bony contact can be assured. Obwegeser[42] suggested vertical (sagittal) splitting of the posterior body of the mandible anterioposteriorly through the lower portion of the ramus and gonial angle. Caldwell and Amaral[58] and Robinson[59] modified the vertical ramus osteotomy used in prognathic cases and added iliac bone to permit advancement of the mandible. This mortised inlaid onlay of autogenous bone provides desirable additional substance. The procedure is indicated in selected cases and will be discussed in further detail. Thoma[35] suggests using a rib graft instead of iliac bone. When more prominence at the gonial angle is desirable, he recommends securing the rib with attached cartilage from the costochondral junction since projecting cartilage at the gonial angle will not resorb as does bone. Robinson and Lytle[60] reported fourteen micrognathic patients surgically corrected by the same vertical (or oblique) section in the ramus, but did not add bone. Wire sutures were inserted to ensure bone contact and union. This is similar to the procedure that Limberg[61] reported in 1925 for correction of "open bite" deformity. In view of the newer improved vertical L or C osteotomy (Caldwell, Hayward, Lister) this simple vertical osteotomy of Robinson's is not recommended because of the very minimal bony contact and loss of gonial angle. Caldwell, Hayward, and Lister[62] present a new approach to this difficult problem, and by the method have eliminated to a great extent many of the shortcomings and technical difficulties encountered heretofore in the generally accepted standard operations. Details of the surgical technique will be described later in the text. This new technique more nearly satisfies criteria for an ideal surgical approach for correction of either micrognathia or retrognathia.

Preparation for surgery

Planning surgery for the correction of micrognathia must be meticulous and detailed. The "work-up" should follow the outline found on p. 440. Use of the cardboard templates made from cephalometric type of roentgenograms and sectioned study models affords a great deal of help (Fig. 23-35).

Since the body of the mandible in micrognathia is smaller than normal, if osteotomy is contemplated in this area it must be determined that a sufficient bulk of bone exists between the apices of the teeth and the cortex of the lower border of the mandible to assure apposition of bone and union. The mandibular notch anterior to the gonial angle is often very accentuated, and it is the vertical dimension from this area to the apices of the molar teeth above that may be limited. The size of bone is best determined by the cephalometric type of lateral roentgenograms (Fig. 23-35, A). Routine oblique lateral roentgenograms of the mandible are misleading because the image of the bone may be enlarged appreciably.

Apposition of bone along the horizontal cut can be assured as the mandible is moved forward in step or L osteotomies in the body of the mandible if no teeth are located posterior to the vertical incision in the alveolar ridge. However, if teeth in the posterior (proximal) portion occlude with maxillary teeth, an appreciable space may result between the cut fragments (Fig. 23-36, B). Plans for a step operation should be discarded if it is evident that bony contact

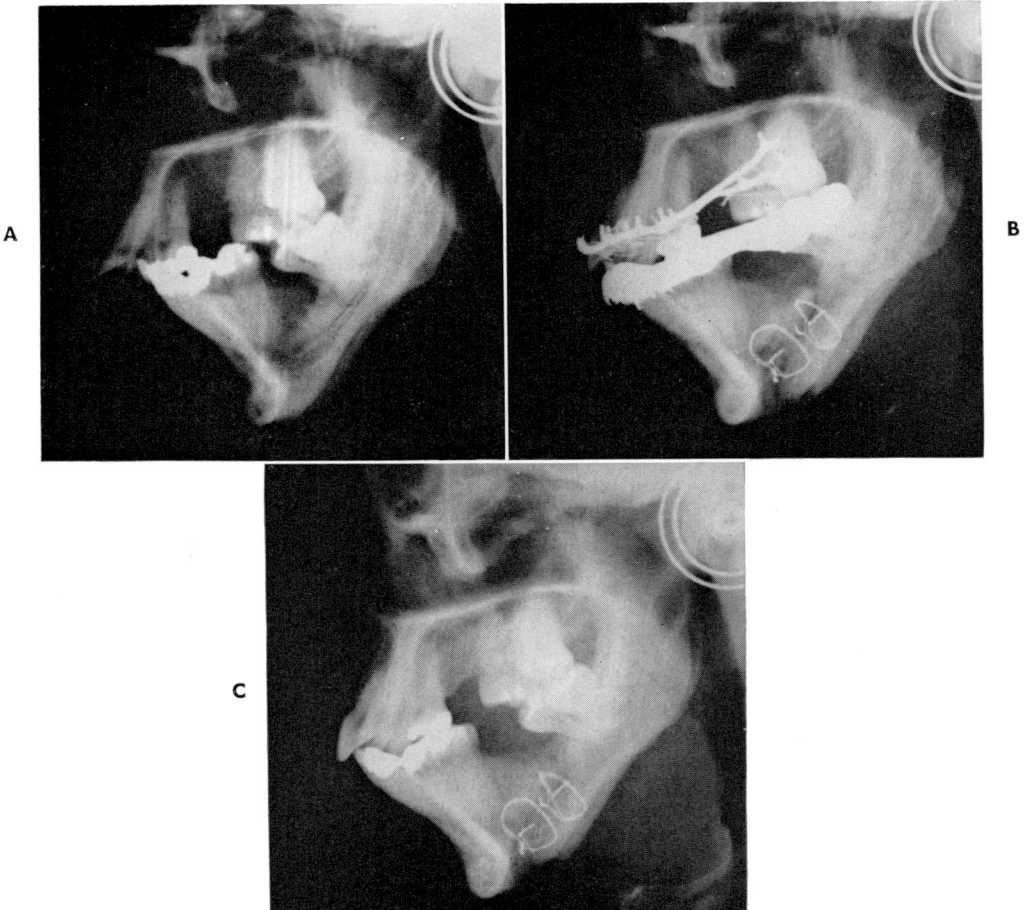

Fig. 23-35. **A**, Cephalogram of patient with micrognathia, requiring 11 mm. of forward movement. **B**, Corrected by step sliding osteotomy and addition of autogenous bone chips; fixed with sectional screw lock splints (Fig. 23-32, *C*). Splinting was supplemented by intermaxillary fixation for 1 month. **C**, After 3 months of intradental splint fixation union had occurred. (U. S. Army Photographs; Letterman Army Hospital.)

between the cut sections will be inadequate for union to occur. Addition of autogenous bone chips from the ilium affords one solution; however, selection of another operation is better. Step operations in the body of the mandible should generally be confined to use in the retrognathic cases in which bulk of bone is ample.

If the lower third of the face is exceptionally tiny, ramus osteotomy with addition of iliac bone or rib should be considered. If the bulk of the bone seems to be adequate, the new vertical L or C osteotomy in the rami is no doubt the method of choice.

Technique for step sliding osteotomy. It has been suggested that this operation be done in two stages on the premise that there is less likelihood of creating a compound wound into the oral cavity and that chances for injury to the mandibular nerve are minimized.[46] This is a suggestion worthy

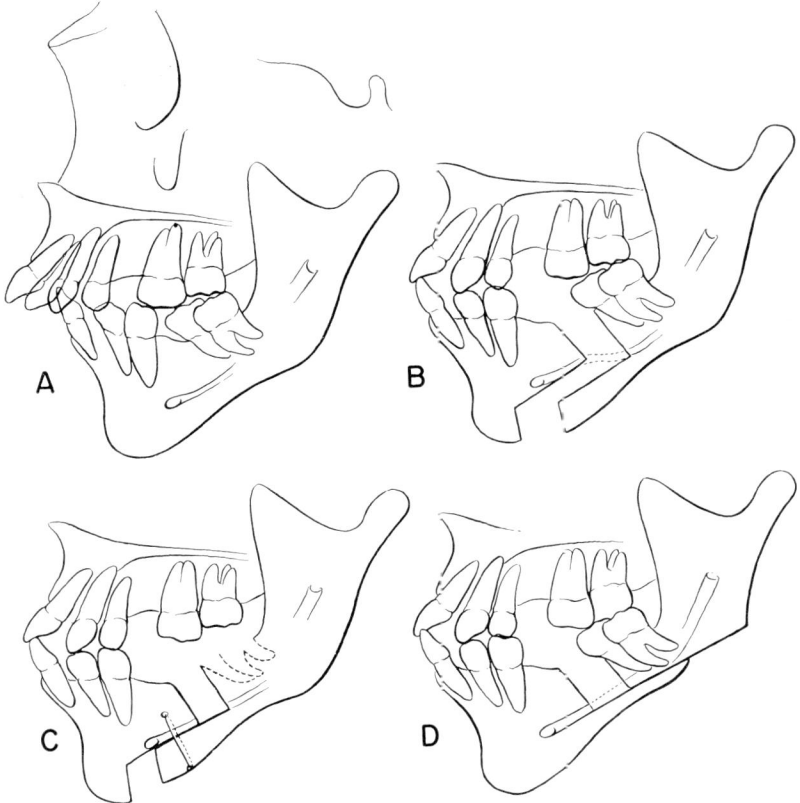

Fig. 23-36. The value of tracings of lateral cephalograms in planning sliding osteotomy in the body of the mandible is illustrated (case shown in Fig. 23-35). **A,** The lack of adequate medullary space between the apices of the teeth and the relatively thick lower cortical border make section without injury to the neurovascular bundle technically impossible. **B,** The deformity was corrected by step sliding osteotomy in an effort to protect the contents of the canal, but voids thus created had to be filled with bone chips to assure union (see Fig. 23-35, B). **C,** Had there not been teeth in the proximal (posterior) fragment, contact on the horizontal plane could have been attained, but fixation of one part to the other would have been by transosseous wiring only. **D,** L sliding osteotomy would definitely have violated the mandibular canal and would have provided inadequate bony contact; the cosmetic result would be poor, with practically no gonial angle.

of consideration even though it is exceedingly difficult to avoid injury to the mandibular nerve. Also, because periosteum is inelastic it is inconceivable that the mandible can be elongated in this "step" sliding osteotomy without interrupting the continuity of the oral soft tissues at some point, either by frank laceration or detachment of gingival margins. It is recommended that step sliding osteotomy be performed in one operation following essentially the same technique as described for ostectomy in correction of mandibular prognathism (p. 472). Exceptions to that technique and other considerations include the following:

1. As a rule the whole procedure can be accomplished via an extraoral submandibular approach; however, preparation of skin and draping should include the oral cavity and "curtain draping" since splinting

and intermaxillary immobilization must be attended to when the osteotomies are completed.

2. If no edentulous space is present it may be necessary to sacrifice a tooth to accomplish the vertical cut through the alveolar ridge. If indicated, the extraction is done prior to the extraoral surgery.

3. The incision must be of sufficient length to permit generous access without undue trauma to the soft tissues. Because of the need for space to manipulate instruments, this exposure should be 6 to 8 cm. in length.

4. A Luc orthopedic oscillating saw or No. 702 carbide fissure bur is utilized to make the vertical cut from the lower border of the mandible upward in the region of the cuspid or first bicuspid to a level just below the mental foramen.

5. A horizontal cut is then carried posteriorly, paralleling the plane of occlusion. The Luc saw or burs are employed here too. The line of this cut cannot be accurately gauged, but a close estimate of its proper direction can be ascertained preoperatively by the use of cardboard templates and measurements. A sterilizable metal template is helpful for this determination. If no attempt is to be made to preserve the continuity of the inferior alveolar nerve, this horizontal cut can be made through both the lateral and medial cortical plates at the same time with the oscillating saw since its narrow blade is long enough to penetrate. Many surgeons favor this practice, believing that accuracy of the horizontal cut is more important than other factors. Operating time is also saved, and the inferior alveolar nerve usually regenerates.

6. The posterior vertical cut through the alveolar margin is completed with long shank bone bur perforations, which are connected using a thin-bladed sharp chisel.

7. Final separation of the bone through the cuts may be facilitated with a thin, flat chisel and mallet or simply by placing the edge of a Lane periosteal elevator into cuts and prying the bone apart gently. Frequently incompletely severed areas can be freed in this manner.

8. At this point the mouth is entered and the teeth are fixed into occlusion, which has been previously determined. It is essential that splints or orthodontic appliances be planned. The connections that have been arranged are placed to stabilize the sectioned dental arch. (I prefer to use a sectional screw lock splint with screw lock connector bars as illustrated in Figs. 23-32, C, and 23-35, B.)

9. The intraoral instruments are discarded, gloves changed, the "curtain" drapes readjusted to expose the surgical field, and the paralleled edges of the horizontal cuts are wired together.

10. Closure and dressings are as previously described. The technique is illustrated in Figs. 23-35, 23-36, B and C, and 23-37.

Horizontal L sliding osteotomy (Fig. 23-36, D). Horizontal L sliding osteotomy is a variation of the "step" operation that has just been described, and it is performed in essentially the same manner. The incisions and approach to the bone are the same as described for vertical osteotomy in the ramus for correction of prognathism since L sliding osteotomy is somewhat more posterior than step sliding osteotomy. A vertical cut is made through the lateral cortical plate from the alveolar ridge down to a point below the level of the mandibular canal. This bone incision is connected at right angles to a horizontal cut, which is carried back to the posterior border of the ramus. Again, the inferior alveolar nerve is jeopardized, but its location can be estimated roughly and an effort made to direct drill penetrations away from its general vicinity as the lingual cortex is weakened. Final section is accomplished with a chisel and mallet. It is more expedient to make the horizontal cut with a Luc oscillating saw and

Developmental deformities of the jaws **489**

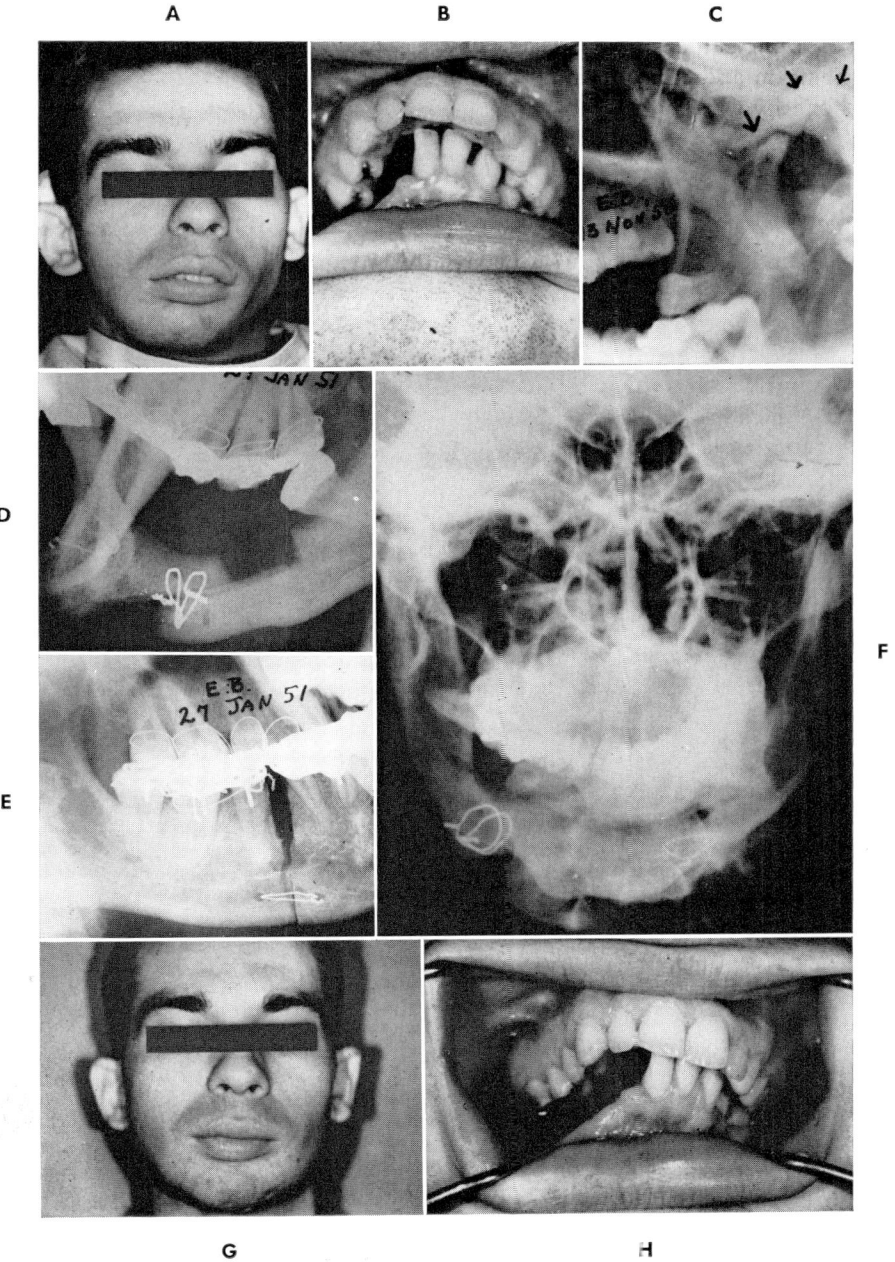

Fig. 23-37. **A,** Unilateral facial deformity caused by osteomyelitis, with loss of much of the right ramus and mandible at 6 years of age. **B,** Class II malocclusion resulting. **C,** Pseudoarthrosis of right temporomandibular joint (false joint indicated by lowest arrow, glenoid fossa above and posteriorly). **D,** Right mandible lengthened by step sliding osteotomy. **E,** Left mandible sectioned to permit "swinging" advancement of right side. **F,** Union of bone with bilateral symmetry. **G,** Unaffected left side of face was contoured with a cartilage onlay implanted for final facial symmetry. **H,** Improved occlusion. (U. S. Army Photographs; Letterman Army Hospital.)

sacrifice the nerve, an acceptable procedure under these circumstances. It is easier to establish occlusion and still obtain approximation of bone by this L type of osteotomy than by the step procedure. After occlusion has been established the approximated bone cuts are wired together.

Step and L sliding osteotomies have many practical applications. In Fig. 23-37 one side of the mandible is lengthened by a step sliding procedure while the advancement is permitted by hinging on the other side via a straight osteotomy. *Step sliding osteotomy* may be accomplished posteriorly and down to the lower border of the mandible, with better chance for bone approximation (Fig. 23-38). This is actually a modification of *horizontal L sliding osteotomy,* but has the advantage of retaining the gonial angle for cosmetic benefit.

The principle of step operations to secure elongation of the mandible may also be utilized to correct other abnormalities in jaw relationship. As an example, the patient illustrated in Fig. 23-39 had a Class I jaw relation, but with no occlusion of teeth. The entire mandibular arch was in lingual version to the maxillary arch with contact of buccal surfaces of the lower teeth to lingual surfaces of the upper teeth. At one time he had gross anterior maxillary protrusion, but when we first saw the patient an effort had been made to correct this cosmetic problem with a six-tooth anterior bridge. The step operation was used in this case to *widen* the mandible.

Anterior segmental osteotomy

Hofer[63,64] proposed an operation designed to advance the entire anterior portion of the mandible, including the teeth in their alveolar bone, but excluding the lower body of the symphysis itself (Fig. 23-40). Köle[65] modified Hofer's operation to permit "elongation of the mobilized mucosa and allow the protrusion of the osteotomised bone and not merely its tilting." Both have performed this operation intra-

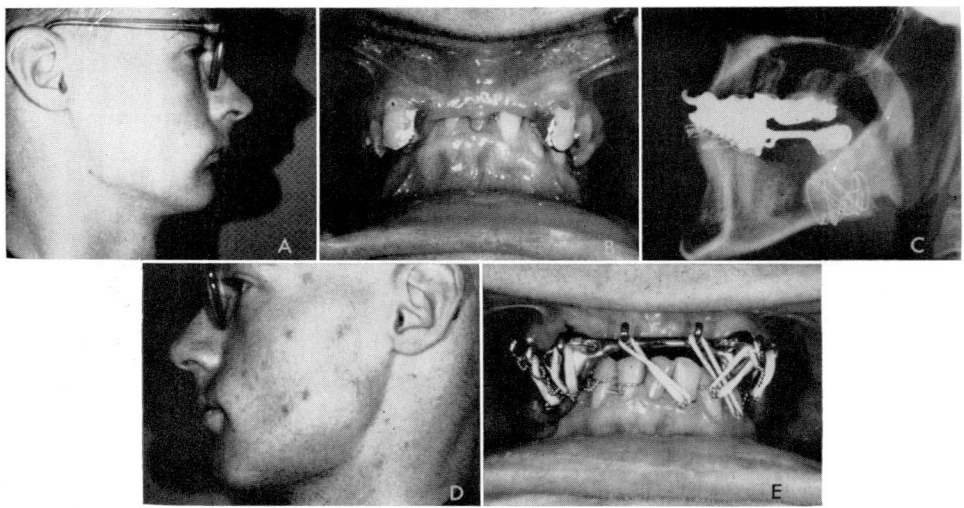

Fig. 23-38. **A,** Young adult male with retrognathia. **B,** Nonrestorable dentition resulting from Class II malocclusion with complete lingual version of all mandibular posterior teeth on the right side. **C,** Postoperative profile roentgenogram shows step sliding osteotomy and prominence of gonial angle retained. **D,** Stronger appearance of jaw and face with improved lower lip relation. **E,** Improved occlusion permitted dental rehabilitation.

Developmental deformities of the jaws 491

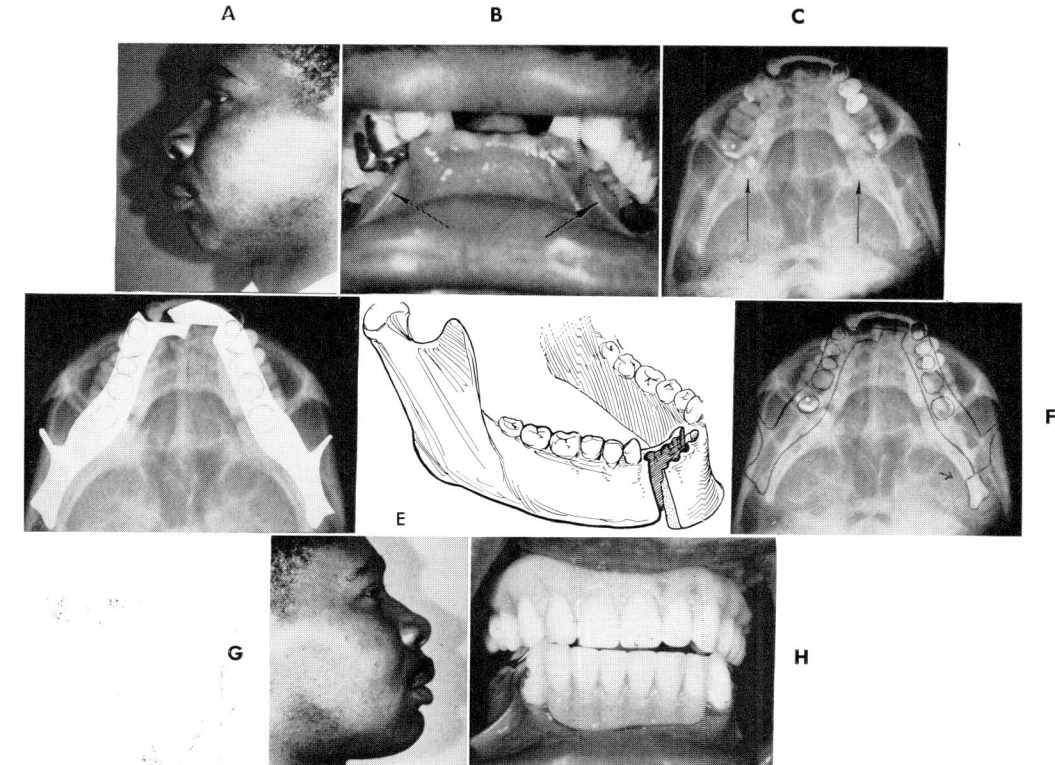

Fig. 23-39. **A**, The profile view of a patient who appears to have a receding lower jaw gives a *false* impression. **B**, Anteroposteriorly the teeth are in Class I relation, but buccolingually there is *no* occlusion—the whole lower arch closes into the palate of the maxilla. **C**, A submentovertex roentgenogram clearly shows the mandibular teeth in ligual version to the maxillary teeth. **D**, A paper cutout traced from the roentgenogram was "step" cut to show how expansion of the mandible could be obtained to establish proper occlusal relation in the posterior teeth. However, if the whole body of the mandible is moved laterally on each side, the *condyle* also moves laterally from the glenoid fossa. **E**, Via extraoral submental approach, the step expansion of the mandibular symphysis was done by osteotomy through the labial cortex in one lateral incisor area, across the midline, and out through the lingual cortex in the other lateral incisor area. The lower four incisor teeth had been removed to allow for the procedure. There was no problem maintaining the symphysis in the expanded relation using a cast metal lingual splint (see Fig. 23-32, *B*), but there was a tendency to relapse posteriorly with collapse medially as healing progressed. **F**, A line tracing on the roentgenogram shows that the problem in **D** was overcome by subcondylar oblique osteotomy bilaterally (arrow). **G**, The final result was excellent cosmetically. **H**, A full upper denture was furnished to replace the upper natural teeth since the lingual alveolar bone support was entirely destroyed by trauma from the relation of the lower teeth preoperative. Six lower incisors were needed to replace the four lower natural teeth that had been sacrificed to allow for symphysis expansion.

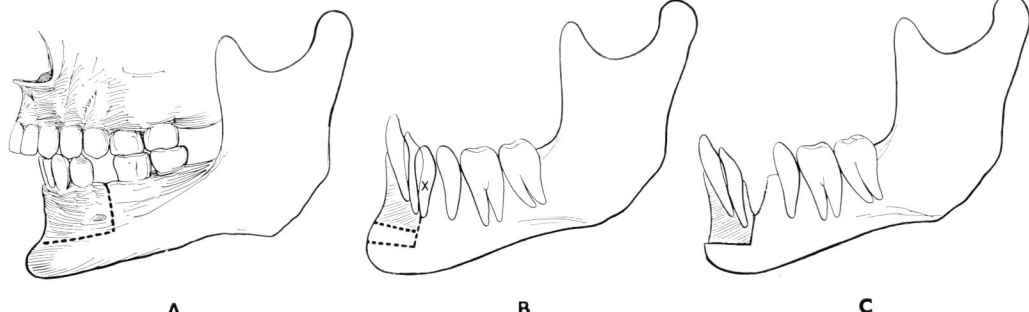

Fig. 23-40. **A,** Hofer's operation for advancing the anterior portion of the mandible, excluding the lower border of the symphysis. **B,** A tracing made from the preoperative profile roentgenogram of the case shown in Fig. 23-41 gave evidence of the lower incisors relating high in the palate back of the protruding maxillary anterior teeth. A line drawing made from the profile roentgenogram illustrates *anterior segmental* osteotomy (Hofer and Köle). **C,** Both lower first premolars were removed, osteotomy was extended apically, and a wedge ostectomy was accomplished from the symphysis horizontally back to the vertical cut. Thus the entire anterior segment of the mandible, excluding the lower border, was tipped down and forward.

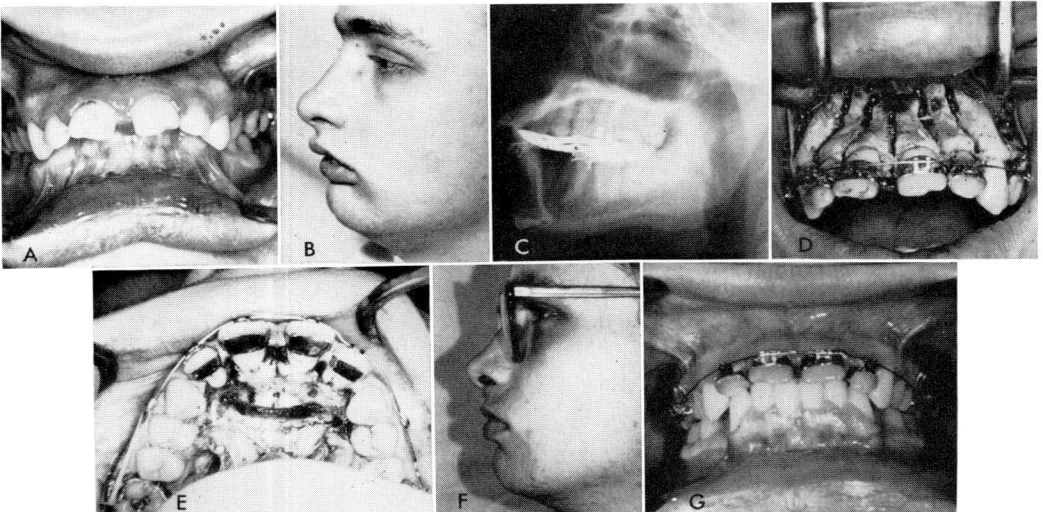

Fig. 23-41. **A,** Young adult male had severe Class II malocclusion with the lower incisors relating high in the palate with maxillary diastema and anterior maxillary protrusion resulting. **B,** The patient's appearance was typical of that seen with this type of occlusion—the lower lip rolled out over a deep crease between it and the chin, and at rest, the lips were apart. **C,** In a postoperative profile roentgenogram results of the mandibular segmental osteotomy are observed and the protrusion of the anterior maxilla is still noted. **D,** Corticotomy to facilitate orthodontic movement of protruding anterior maxillary teeth and close the diastema. **E,** Portions of cortical bone were also excised on the palatal aspect of ridge as suggested by Köle. **F,** The results of combined orthodontic and surgical treatment after 6 weeks. Retainers must be furnished after active orthodontic movements are finished. **G,** Appearance after all active treatment was completed. The mandibular surgery was accomplished on April 4, 1962, orthodontic banding April 14, maxillary operation April 18, and active treatment completed May 10, 1962—a total treatment period of about 5 weeks.

orally. In our experience, this procedure is useful in the correction of Class II anterior malocclusion when the anterior teeth relate high on the palatal mucosa posterior to the maxillary incisor teeth and it is desirable to tilt the anterior alveolar portion of the mandible containing the lower teeth downward as well as forward (Fig. 23-41). To accomplish this it is more expedient to operate via a combination intraoral and extraoral approach and perform a horizontal wedge ostectomy using a Luc orthopedic saw. This Hofer principle also has excellent application in cases of anterior Class III malocclusion if the posterior occlusion is functionally acceptable and the patient has minimal but not unfavorable prognathic appearance. The operation can usually be done via an intraoral approach.

Discussion. Step sliding osteotomy and variations of the principle are standard acceptable operations for surgical correction of micrognathia or retrognathia. However, it must be understood that the problems here are much different from those encountered in prognathism. Although results are generally good so far as improved appearance and function are concerned, the operations are more tedious to perform and more difficulties are encountered. Specifically, these difficulties are (1) making the horizontal incision for the "slide" without injury to the inferior alveolar nerve, (2) making this incision in a plane that assures approximation of the bone, (3) maintaining the patient immobilized for a sufficient time to assure bony union, and (4) avoiding compounding of the surgical wound intraorally.

Injury to the nerve is not a serious objection since it usually recovers in a reasonable time. Nor is compounding of the surgical wound intraorally a serious problem. In fact, with antibiotic coverage these operations can be performed in one stage with little risk of infection or complicating sequelae. Absolute apposition of bone along the horizontal incision is essential for union, or autogenous bone chips must be added. Emphasis, then, must again be placed on preoperative planning.

Vertical osteotomy in the rami with bone grafting

In 1954 we[25] predicted that modification of vertical osteotomy as it is utilized in correction of prognathism would also make possible correction of micrognathia. In 1960 the technique was completely described.[58] The principles of vertical section in the ramus, coronoidotomy, and decortication are applicable in this operation. The objectives are (1) separation of the ramus vertically from the mandibular notch to the lower border of the mandible at the angle in a line over or just posterior to the mandibular foramen (Fig. 23-42, *B*), (2) angular section of the coronoid process from the mandibular notch obliquely downward and forward to the anterior border to permit forward repositioning of the distal fragment (body and anterior ramus) without interference (Fig. 23-42, *B*), (3) decortication of the lateral cortex over a broad area of the lower aspect of the ramus as a recipient area for bone graft (Fig. 23-42, *D* and *E*), (4) movement forward of the distal (body of the mandible) fragment to the desired occlusal relation (Fig. 23-42, *B* and *F*), and (5) interposition between the fragments and onlay into the decorticated area of a measured full-thickness block section of bone from the crest of the ilium (Fig. 23-42, *G* and *I*).

Technique for vertical osteotomy in the rami with bone grafting. The basic approach is similar to that for prognathism.

1. The patient is prepared and draped in the manner already described. In addition, the pubic area is shaved the day previously, and the iliac donor site is prepared and draped for the removal of the bone for grafting.

2. The lateral aspect of the ramus is exposed in the manner already described, and

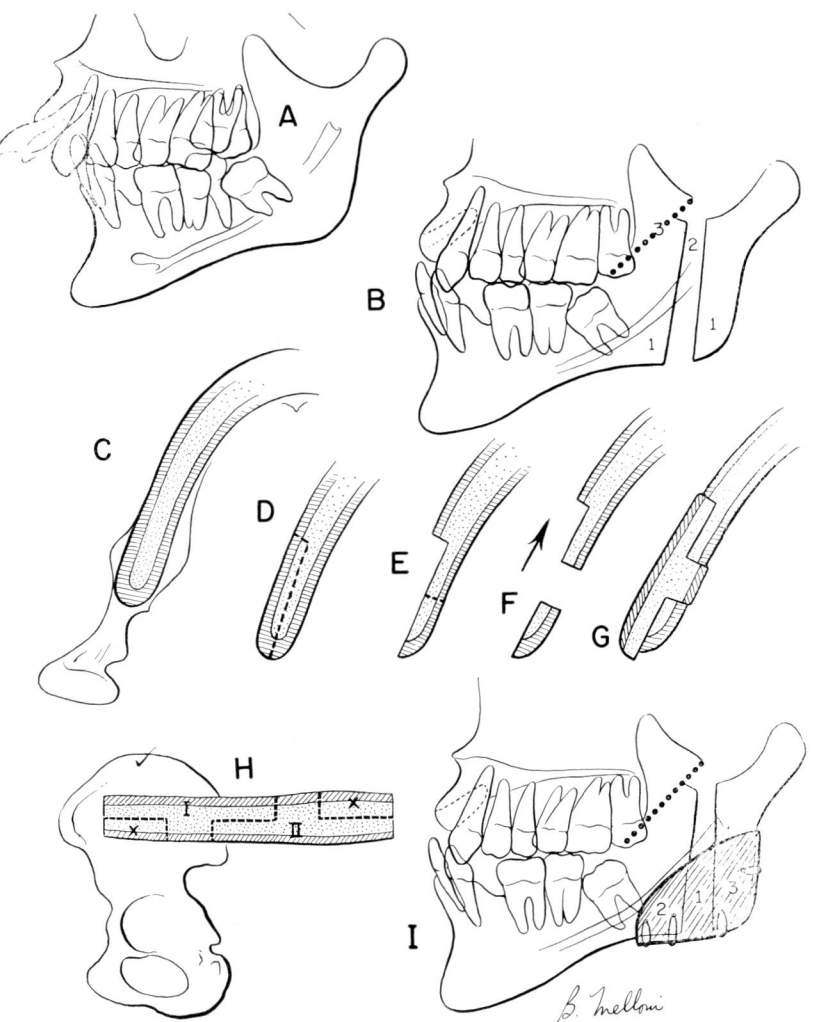

Fig. 23-42. Tracings of lateral cephalograms of micrognathia corrected by *vertical osteotomy* with bone graft. **A,** Protrusion of maxillary anterior teeth and retrusion of the mandible. One centimeter of discrepancy in incisal relation corrected by removal of maxillary anterior teeth and moderate alveolectomy, and 1 cm. of discrepancy corrected by movement of the whole mandible forward. **B,** Technique of procedure: **1,** areas decorticated on lateral aspect of ramus; **2,** vertical section of ramus over mandibular foramen; **3,** oblique section of coronoid process to permit it to remain in proper relation with temporalis muscle as mandible is moved forward. **C,** Mandible viewed from below; lined areas represent lower border and lateral and medial cortices. **D,** Heavy broken line indicates extent of decortication on lateral aspect of ramus as viewed from below. **E,** Lateral cortex removed and vertical section made (dark dotted line). **F,** Body of mandible moved anteriorly the desired distance. **G,** Bone graft from ilium onlaid onto decorticated lateral aspect of ramus with full-thickness graft filling void created by forward movement of mandible. **H,** Iliac graft viewed from the crest of ilium showing method of sectioning graft for both sides of mandible: **I,** graft for left side; **II,** graft for right side; **X,** shaved-off medullary bone for use as filler chips. **I,** Bone graft wired into place: **1,** full-thickness graft in void; **2** and **3,** split thickness of ilium onlaid over decorticated surfaces.

the prominence of the mandibular foramen is identified.

3. A vertical cut is made from the mandibular notch to the lower border of the mandible as described for vertical osteotomy in prognathism, and the coronoid process is also detached in the same manner.

4. The course of the mandibular canal from the foramen downward and anteriorly is estimated and so marked with a dye stick.

5. Multiple drill penetrations are made into the lateral cortex from the mandibular foramen and the estimated level of the mandibular canal to the lower border of the mandible. They are extended from the posterior border to a point approximately 2 cm. anterior to the vertical cut in the ramus (Fig. 23-43).

6. The lateral cortex is removed from this broad area with the flat, long-beveled Stout No. 3 chisel, creating a flat surface onto which the bone graft will subsequently be fitted. Due care should be taken not to injure the inferior alveolar nerve during the decortication, but it should be identified so that it can be avoided when the vertical section is completed.

7. The wound is packed, the patient's head turned, and the above procedure repeated on the other side.

8. By this time the surgical team that is to obtain the graft should be started.

9. The procedure on the second side is completed except for fitting and placement of the graft.

10. The vertical sections are completed on both sides following the technique described for the treatment of prognathism.

11. It will be found that the mandible and anterior portion of the ramus are easily repositioned anteriorly. The mouth is entered and intermaxillary elastic ligatures are placed to fix the teeth into desired occlusion. Arch bars wired to all teeth should be utilized because heavy traction must be placed to ensure maintenance of teeth in proper occlusion during the manipulation necessary to inlay the bone graft.

12. The length of the section of bone needed can be measured with accuracy by calculating the replacement as graphically illustrated in Fig. 23-42, *H* and *I*. It can be cut accurately, also, if an assistant holds it securely on a wood block while the surgeon sections it to the desired size with the Luc oscillating saw. The full-thickness portion of the graft must be tapered to a lesser width to fit superiorly since the void to be filled is less superiorly than at the lower border (Fig. 23-42, *I*). The full thickness of the graft with both cortices remaining serves to maintain the elongation of the

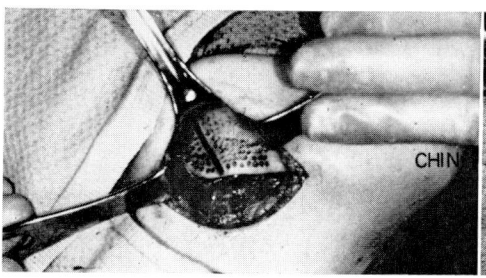
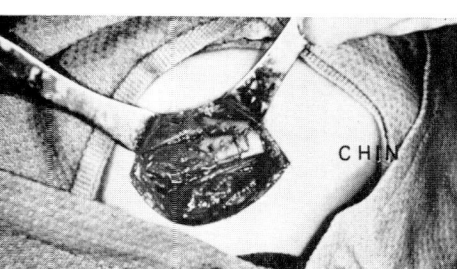
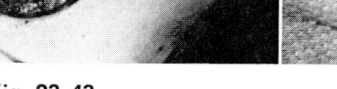

Fig. 23-43. Exposure of the ramus, the vertical cut, and drill holes for vertical osteotomy and bone grafting. (U. S. Army Photograph; Letterman Army Hospital.)

Fig. 23-44. Onlay of bone graft over lateral surface of ramus for correction of micrognathia. (U. S. Army Photograph; Letterman Army Hospital.)

496 *Textbook of oral surgery*

mandible, and union of the well-mortised graft occurs in about 8 weeks.

13. Once fitted into the voids, the graft is wired onto the decorticated bed with fine stainless steel wire sutures (0.016 inch) (Fig. 23-44).

14. Scraps of medullary bone that have been saved during trimming of the graft are added in the void above the block inlay and in any other spaces not filled or in close contact (Fig. 23-42, *H*, areas marked X).

15. Closure and postoperative care are the same as previously described.

Discussion. There are two objections to this procedure that cannot be circumvented: (1) It is a long operation, requiring 4 to 5 hours. However, with the patient adequately supported during and following the surgery, the course is ordinarily uneventful. (2) Use of the ilium for the donor site is the other objection—patients always complain much more about the hip than the jaw. "Bank" bone is not believed to have the potential for a "take" that autogenous grafts have.

Results in cases of micrognathia treated by this method have been so successful that the principal disadvantages mentioned above can be accepted. By comparison to other methods, the operation has the following advantages:

1. It is adaptable to the usual cases of micrognathia.

2. As much as 1 to 2 cm. of advancement can be secured.

3. The small size and bulk of the body of the mandible are not contraindications.

4. Firm clinical union is rapid, requiring about 8 to 10 weeks.

5. The cosmetic result is excellent because the angle of the mandible is maintained or improved at the same time the body is advanced to provide a good profile.

6. The operation can be done without injury to important nerves (that is, mandibular and facial).

7. Elaborate splints are not needed. Orthodontic appliances or ordinary arch bars will suffice for fixation during the period of immobilization (Figs. 23-44 and 23-45).

A very acceptable substitution for this iliac bone graft procedure is one described by Thoma.[35] A rib graft does not provide quite the bulk of bone substance obtained

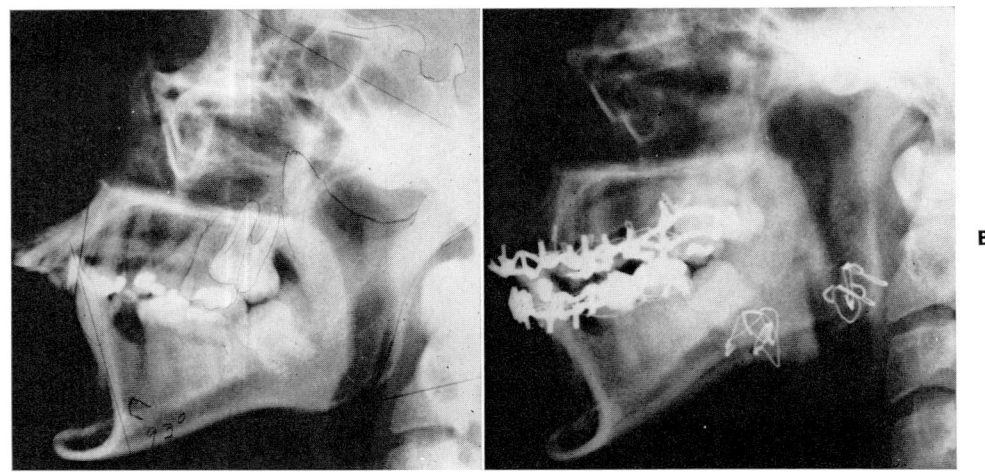

Fig. 23-45. Lateral skull roentgenograms from which tracings (Fig. 23-42) were made. **A**, Preoperative. **B**, Postoperative. (U. S. Army Photographs; Letterman Army Hospital.)

Developmental deformities of the jaws 497

by onlaying with a block from the ilium; however, it is easier to obtain and is less disabling for the patient. The surgical technique is the same as described for placement of iliac bone. Edges of the rib graft are decorticated to afford medullary bone contact when it is interposed between the proximal and distal parts to obliterate the space created as the distal (body portion) is advanced.

Vertical L, L modified, or C sliding osteotomy (without bone grafting)

When there is no need for the addition of bulk in correction of retrognathia (micrognathia is not a factor), but simply an advancement of the mandible to Class I relation is desired, the *vertical L sliding osteotomy* (or modified) is a very excellent procedure and one to be considered.[62] (See Fig. 23-46.)

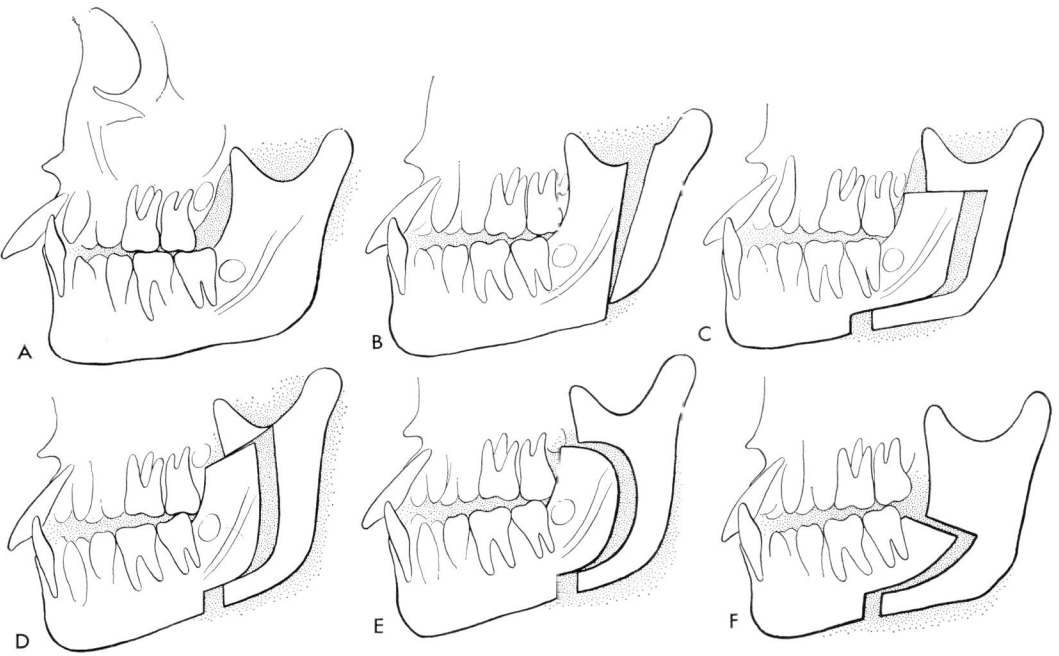

Fig. 23-46. A, Tracing from a lateral cephalogram, which shows the retruded mandible and Class II occlusion of the teeth (note relation of first molars). B, Vertical (or oblique subcondylar) osteotomy in ramus permits advancement of the mandible, but does not allow for much bony contact at site of osteotomy and also reduces prominence of the gonial angle. C, The inverted L of Pichler and Trauner with a horizontal cut made between the base of the coronoid process and the mandibular foramen and then vertically downward parallel to the posterior border of the ramus and rounding anteriorly as in D. D, L osteotomy with line of bone incision made from the mandibular notch "vertically" downward parallel to the posterior border of the ramus and then curved with the angle anteriorly, parallel to the lower border of the mandible for about 3 cm. and then downward through the lower border. Thus a "hockey stick" shape is given to the proximal fragment, and as the mandible is advanced, sliding contact is maintained along the horizontal line of osteotomy at the lower border. Coronoidotomy must be done also. E, Another modification of the cut according to Lister is a circular cut in the form of a C. The effect obtained in C to E is essentially the same. F, Osteotomy suggested by Hayward is paralleled to the arc of movement of the mandibular anterior teeth, resulting in maximum bony contact as the bone is advanced following osteotomy. The operation is done in 2 stages—one intraoral and one extraoral.

1. This operation is accomplished via an extraoral submandibular approach using "curtain draping" to permit access to the oral cavity for intermaxillary immobilization.

2. The incision should be about 5 to 6 cm. in length to ensure adequate access to the whole lateral surface of the ramus and several centimeters of the lower border of the mandible anterior to the angle.

3. The outline of osteotomy should be scribed on the lateral surface of the bone as preplanned from tracings of a lateral cephalogram (Fig. 23-46). This line of osteotomy may be vertical down from the mandibular notch (Fig. 23-46, C) or horizontal from the anterior border of the ramus above the mandibular foramen and then vertically down, to within about 1 or 1.5 cm. of the angle of the mandible (Fig. 23-46, D. The *line of cut is then curved anteriorly* and may be extended in this direction as far as necessary to allow for necessary "sliding" advancement of the jaw and to maintain bone apposition on the horizontal plane at the lower border of the mandible. A third line of osteotomy may be in the shape of a C circling around the mandibular foramen from the anterior border of the ramus to the angle of the mandible and then anteriorly, as already described. Lister used this C cut.[62]

4. If a straight vertical cut from the mandibular notch is planned, coronoidotomy should be accomplished to eliminate interference of the temporalis muscle with the forward placement of the mandible.

5. Osteotomy is accomplished as usual, with much care exercised in the parts of the cut above the mandibular foramen since "guarding" on the medial surface is technically not feasible. We depend on 18,000 rpm, sharp bone drills and the sense of feel to ascertan lack of resistance as penetration of the medial cortex occurs. Points of incomplete osteotomy are severed using short, sharp taps with a broad-bladed, sharp chisel and mallet.

6. From about the height of the mandibular foramen on down parallel to the posterior border of the ramus and anteriorly parallel to the lower border the osteotomy can be accomplished rapidly since medial soft tissue is guarded with a broad, flat Lane periosteotome. A No. 702 or 703 carbide fissure bur in the Jordan Day engine is used to take advantage of the side cutting effect.

7. When osteotomies are completed on both sides, the mouth is entered and the new occlusion relation is fixed by heavy intermaxillary elastics. A clear acrylic "wafer" occlusal guide plate is more routinely used in retrognathic cases.

8. After a change of gloves the "curtain drape" is readjusted and the surgical field is reentered. Freedom of the proximal fragment (posterior, ramus, and condyle part) is ensured from muscle binding. Bone approximation is checked along the horizontal

---

Fig. 23-47. **A,** This 14-year-old girl was a shy introvert, no doubt influenced by her retruded lower jaw. **B,** She had a typical Class II malocclusion. **C,** The overbite and overjet are demonstrated in a profile roentgenogram. The lower incisors related high onto the palatal mucosa. **D,** Bilateral L osteotomies were accomplished—one side according to Fig. 23-46, **C,** and one as seen in Fig. 23-46, **D.** (Photograph after osteotomy, but before advancement of the mandible and wiring.) **E,** A "wafer" was placed to ensure desired occlusion and to prevent extrusion or other injury to these young teeth during the 6 weeks of immobilization. **F,** The intermaxillary space closed almost entirely during the first year postoperative as the permanent teeth erupted to the normal occlusal plane. **G,** Although an overbite still existed 1 year after surgery, her occlusion was orthodontically correctable. **H,** She had a remarkable improvement in personality and appearance.

Developmental deformities of the jaws

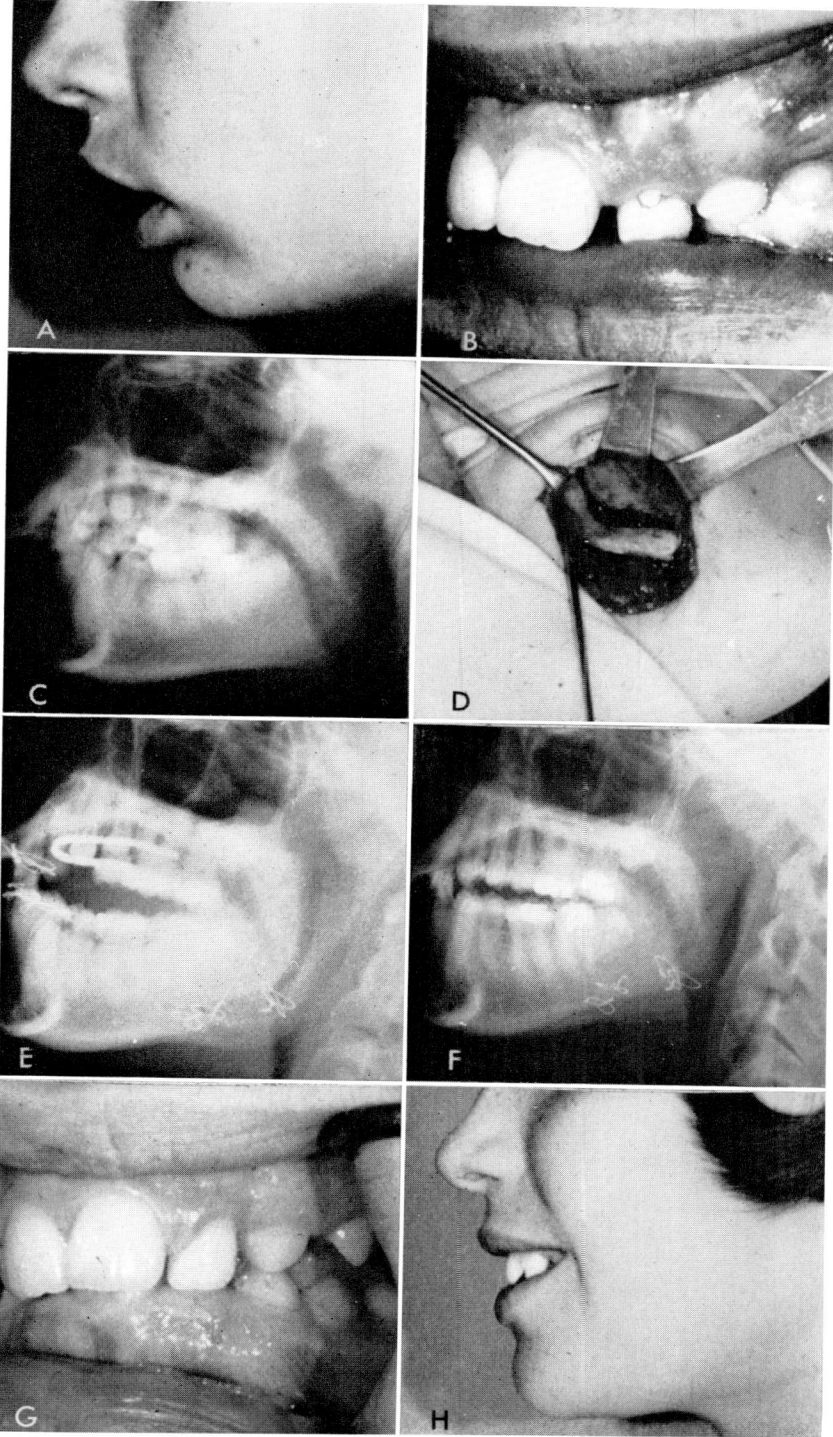

Fig. 23-47. For legend see opposite page.

cut above the lower border. At least one wire suture is placed on each side to ensure proper bone fragment control.

9. Closure of soft tissue follows a standard technique.

Vertical L sliding osteotomy (or one of the modified versions) is a marked improvement over methods heretofore available when bone grafting is not needed. The technique more nearly satisfies all of the criteria set forth at the beginning of this section on micrognathia and is therefore adopted as a standard technique. In Fig. 23-47 an example of the application of the L technique is illustrated.

MICROGENIA AND GENIOPLASTY

Osteotomy and advancement or lengthening the mandible is not always necessary in receding "Andy Gump" facies. Occasionally the occlusion is quite satisfactory and all that is needed to improve appearance is addition of substance to the chin. At the same time much psychological benefit can result. Occasionally, genioplasty is adjunctive to the cosmetic result following one of the previously described osteotomy procedures. Bone, cartilage, tantalum mesh, and alloplastic materials[66-70] are used to build out the mental prominence. Intraoral or extraoral access to the chin is obtained depending on indications and treatment plan.

The least complicated approach to treatment of this problem is by implantation of a contoured-to-measure piece of silicone rubber inserted intraorally. A short, vertical incision is made at the midline, through which a pocket is formed by blunt dissection. The implant is inserted and properly

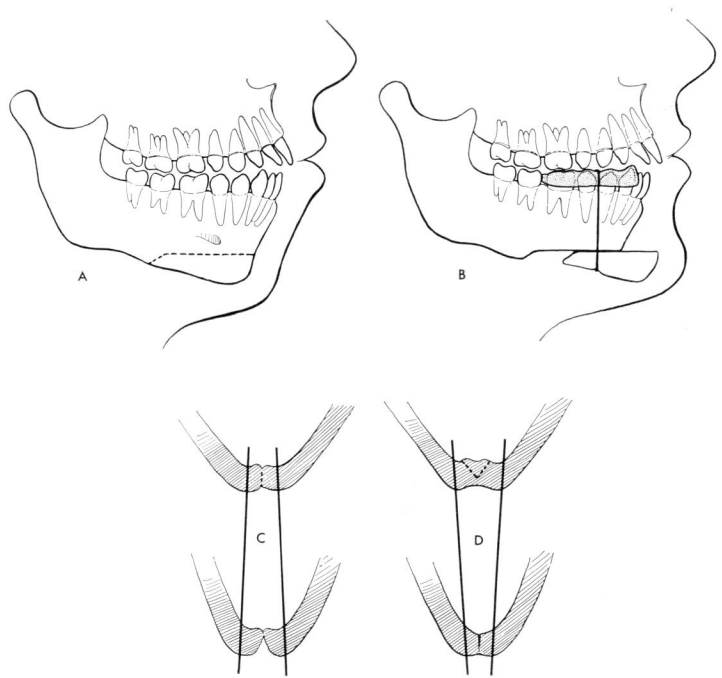

Fig. 23-48. Horizontal sliding genioplasty to afford chin prominence when occlusion is acceptable. Expansion of the chin block is accomplished by a cut in the labial cortex, narrowing by removal of a wedge in the lingual cortex. (Modified from Obwegeser, H.: Oral Surg. **10:**677, 1957.)

positioned, and after closure of the wound a semipressure dressing is carefully placed over the chin and lower jaw to maintain the implant in proper position during the immediate postoperative course. Other foreign materials are also "pocketed" supraperiosteally.

In cases of retrusion of the chin in which occlusion is good but a "long face" is present the horizontal sliding genioplasty of Obwegeser[42] serves ideally to improve the condition (Figs. 23-48 and 23-49). The operation can be done either via intraoral approach (so-called degloving technique) or a submental incision.

Many variations in techniques are used in genioplasty, and a choice of materials to implant is also available; however, autogenous iliac bone remains one of the most reliable of materials, and the latitude of correction is probably greatest when this material is used. Modest corrections can be achieved quite nicely via intraoral incisions. Converse,[71] who favors this approach to genioplasty, places emphasis on the soft tissue dissection to the bone. The incision is made through the mucosa above the labial fold on the inner aspect of the lip, and dissection is carried submucosally in to the periosteum also above the level of the labial vestibule. The periosteum is then incised horizontally and elevated to the extent needed to provide space for the graft. By this "double flap" technique food debris, saliva, etc. are excluded from the depth of the wound after closure. Likewise, less tension is placed on the incision line when closed, and break down of the wound is unlikely.

If large onlays of bone are needed, an extraoral approach is probably safer. The case illustrated in Fig. 23-50, for example, required placement of bone over a large portion of the right lateral surface of the mandible well back of the mental foramen as well as over the symphysis. The incision here was a long one placed well under the shadow of the mandible for two reasons: (1) to place the scar inconspicuously and (2) to have the line of incision well away from the bone graft so that the graft will be well supported. It should be noted in this case that the foreshortened, deformed side was the *left* side, but bone was added to the *right* side and symphysis to develop a symmetrical face. Deformities of this type are ideally corrected in this manner.

APERTOGNATHIA (OPEN BITE DEFORMITY) AND OTHER OCCLUSION AND JAW ABNORMALITIES

Apertognathia, maxillary protrusion and retrusion, and other occlusion and jaw disharmonies and irregularities are correctable surgically or may be improved sufficiently

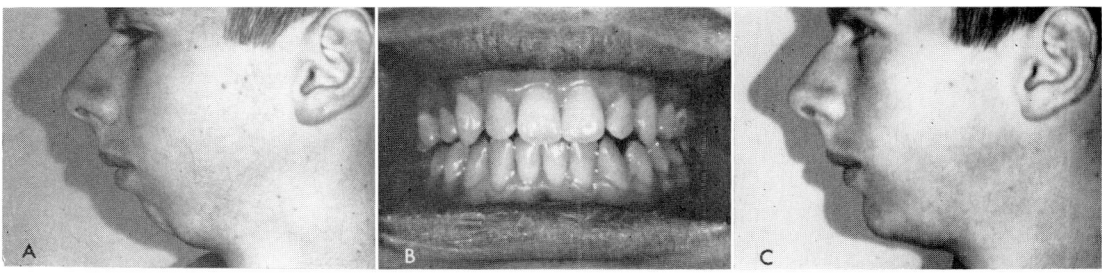

Fig. 23-49. **A,** Microgenia prior to correction in a boy age 17. **B,** He had excellent occlusion, but had been under orthodontic treatment since he was 8 years of age. **C,** Genioplasty by Obwegeser's "sliding" method was used via a submental extraoral approach.

502 *Textbook of oral surgery*

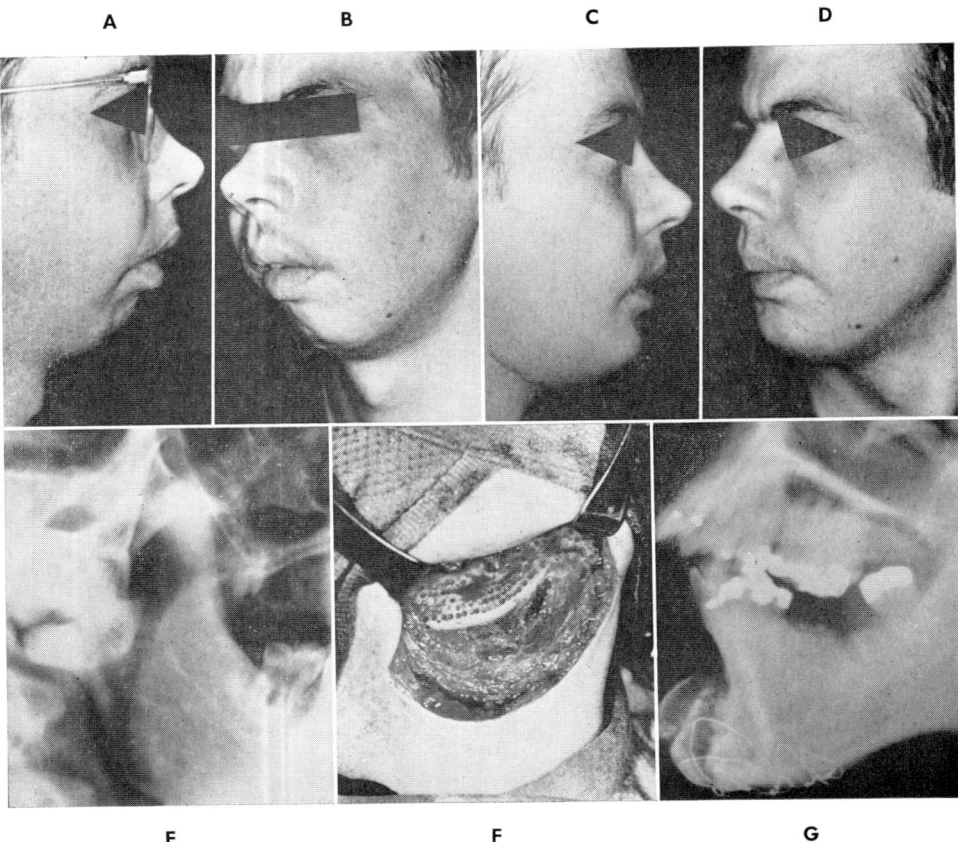

Fig. 23-50. **A** and **B**, Unilateral facial deformity resulting from birth injury of left condyle with underdeveloped *left* mandible. Class II malocclusion could not be improved upon by surgical methods. **C** and **D**, Final cosmetic result. **E**, Deformed *left* condyle. **F**, Bed prepared for correction of deficiency, which will be corrected by addition of a full-thickness bone graft from the ilium to the *right* side of the mandible and symphysis. **G**, Onlay bone graft. (U. S. Army Photographs; Letterman Army Hospital.)

to greatly facilitate subsequent orthodontic or dental restorative care. Selection of a proper operation for correction of a given problem must be based on a critical examination of the patient's appearance, study of models, and cephalometric analysis. The relationship of the upper lip to the upper incisor teeth in resting, speaking, and smiling postions, correlated with the relationship of segments of sectioned study models, provides the most preoperative information. Murphey and Walker[10] emphasize the benefits of combined orthodontic–oral surgery work-up using photographs, study casts, and cephalometric roentgenograms. Depending on the results of these studies, surgery may be accomplished in the anterior maxilla, posterior maxilla, anterior mandible, or mandibular rami, or a combination of more than one site.

A multiplicity of etiological factors exists in this category of deformities and occlusion irregularities. Principle among these causes are interference with the condylar growth center, abnormal tongue habits, and lip and finger sucking. *When the deformity*

Developmental deformities of the jaws **503**

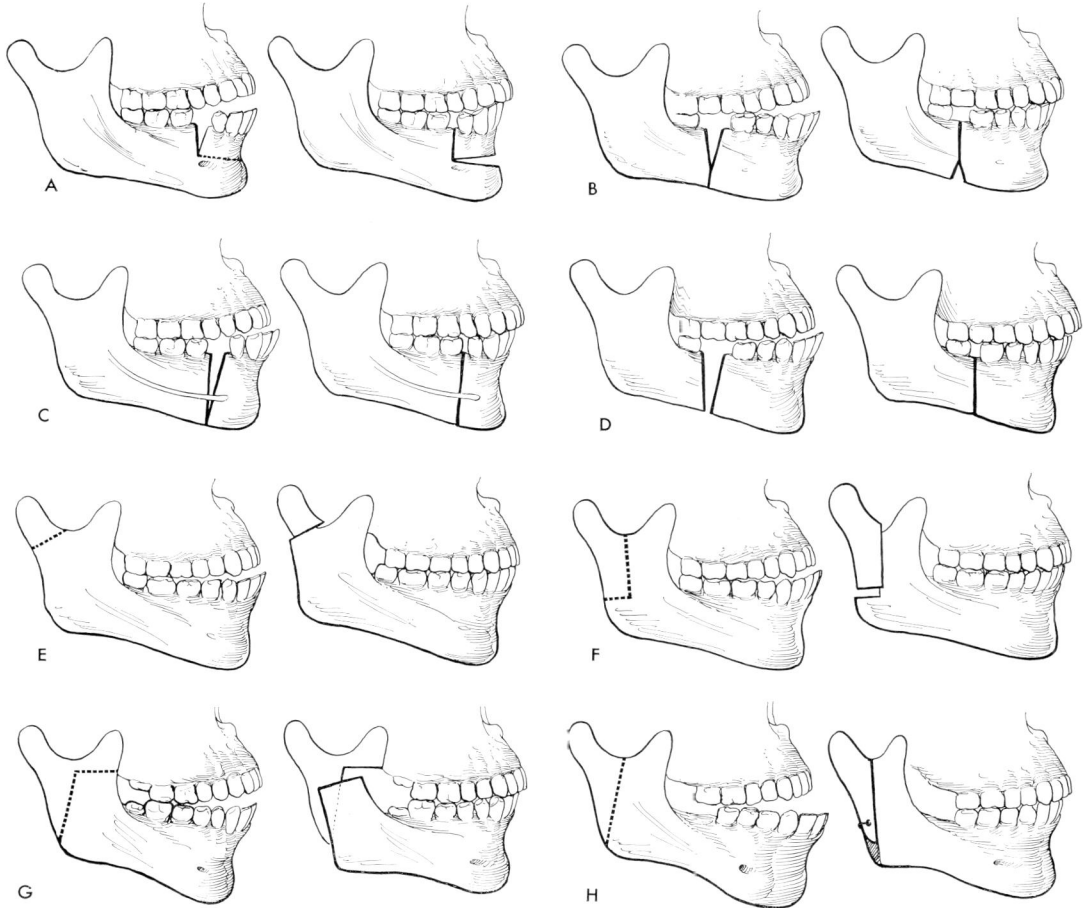

Fig. 23-51. Locations of mandibular osteotomy and ostectomy that have been used to correct anterior open bite deformities. **A**, Hullihen's V-shaped ostectomy. **B**, Lane and Pickerill V ostectomy. **C**, Thoma Y ostectomy. **D**, Thoma's trapezoid ostectomy. **E**, Babcock's osteotomy. **F**, Limberg's osteotomy. **G**, Pichler's and Trauner's osteotomy. **H**, Shira's oblique sliding osteotomy.

is caused by habit, corrective surgery should not be undertaken until the habit has been overcome. This is especially the case in apertognathic conditions caused by tongue thrusting and reverse swallowing.

A number of *basic* operations are available for use in correction of these deformities and occlusal disharmonies, and the surgical techniques will be described later in this section. These basic operations, which are now generally accepted and utilized, have evolved over the years since Hullihen's[1] historical first operation was performed in 1849 (Fig. 23-51, *A*). Blair[2] and many others[35,72,73] since then have recommended the procedure or modifications of *V-shaped ostectomy* for correction of open bite (Fig. 23-51, *B* to *D*). Babcock,[74] Limberg,[61] and Pichler and Trauner[75] suggested operations in the ascending rami of the mandible to allow for repositioning of the mandible anteriorly and closure of the open bite relation (Fig. 23-51, E to G). The principle of vertical sliding osteotomy to lengthen the ramus was suggested in the first edition of this textbook (Figs. 23-53 and 23-54).

When the "open bite" deformity is associated with prognathism, a different problem presents. Thoma[35] suggested a trapezoid ostectomy in the body of the mandible with the amount of bone excision determined by geometric measurement of the degree of open bite (Fig. 23-52, B to D). Shira[30] applied the principles of ramus vertical osteotomy in eight cases of open bite and reported "gratifying results with little tendency for remission" (Fig. 23-51, H). We have also had good success with correction of open bite by *vertical (not oblique) sliding osteotomy* in the rami, but have observed a much greater tendency toward relapse than in ordinary prognathic cases. Since the overall vertical length of the ramus is definitely elongated or extended (by vertical sliding) we are strong in our conviction that *decortication, direct transosseous wiring (over corrected), and coronoidotomy are essential.* Direct transosseous wiring is virtually impossible if subcondylar (oblique)

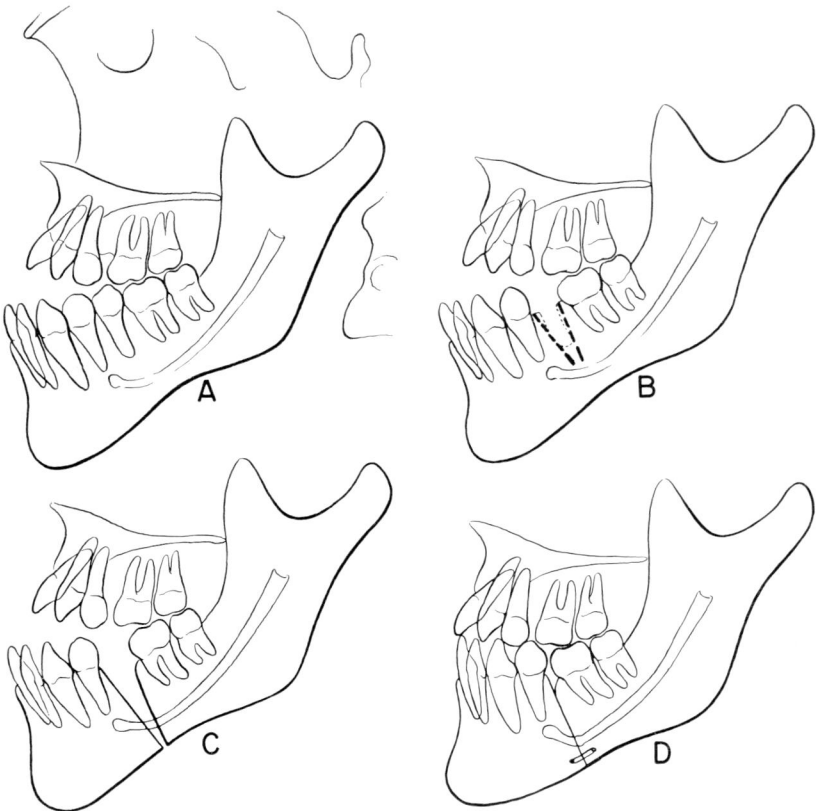

Fig. 23-52. Tracings from cephalograms of a patient with open-bite deformity, or apertognathia. **A,** Preoperative relation. **B,** Intraoral V-shaped bone incisions to a level just above the mandibular canal. **C,** V ostectomy completed via an extraoral submandibular approach. **D,** Transosseous wiring at the lower border of the mandible supplemental to dental splinting and intermaxillary fixation.

osteotomy is used in attempting elongation of the ramus. Mohnac[11] suggests "replacing the musculature at a higher point" when closing the soft tissue in these cases. *Also, one should plan for 5 to 6 weeks of immobilization, but most important of all, the abnormal tongue habits must be corrected preoperatively.* Limberg[61] cut the ramus from the mandibular notch obliquely downward to a point near the lower aspect of the posterior border of the ramus above the angle where a short horizontal extension carried the incision to the posterior border. He did not mention any restraining effect that the attachment of the temporalis muscle might have, but did find it necessary to detach the stylomandibular ligament to permit downward movement of the body of the mandible. According to Pichler and Trauner[75] these difficulties were overcome by altering the bone incision. By sectioning the ramus from its anterior border above the foramen (below the coronoid process) horizontally back and then vertically downward, neither the temporalis muscle nor the stylomandibular ligament impeded movement of the sectioned part. Their vertical bone incision was posterior to the foramen, thus avoiding injury to the nerve.

Technique for V-shaped ostectomy in the body of the mandible

Technique. The principle and technique for V ostectomy are essentially the same as described for ostectomy in the body of the mandible for correction of prognathism. Unless edentulous spaces are present in appropriate locations, a tooth (usually a premolar) must be extracted bilaterally. Two sets of instruments should be set up, one for the intraoral work and the other for the extraoral. The operation is done as a single procedure, the intraoral being accomplished first.

1. The patient is prepared and draped in the customary manner with "curtain" drapes to separate the intraoral operation from the extraoral.

2. Generous mucoperiosteal flaps are elevated bucally and lingually, with care exercised to protect the mental nerve.

3. A long-shanked No. 703 carbide fissure bur is used for all bone incisions in this operation.

4. The posterior vertical or transverse incision is made in the bone through the buccal and lingual cortical plates first, to a depth estimated to be just above the nerve.

5. The predetermined amount of bone

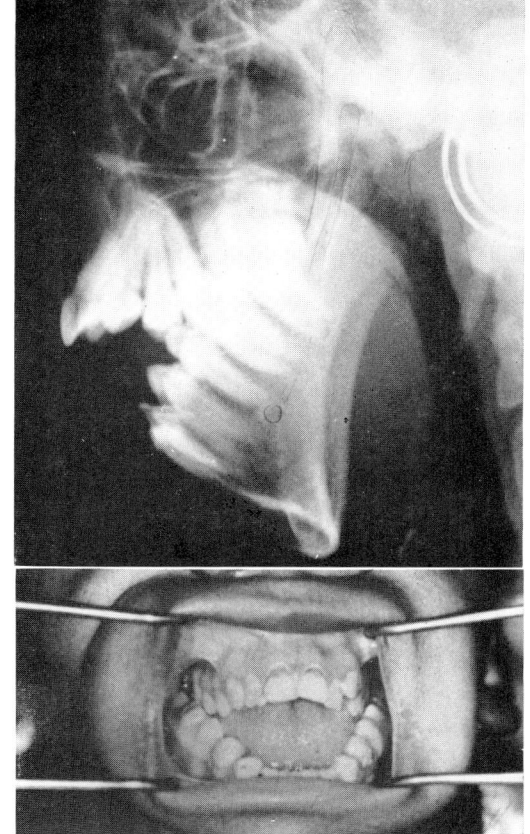

Fig. 23-53. **A**, Lateral cephalogram of a 10-year-old Negro girl with extreme underdevelopment of the mandible and open bite. She was seen on consultation, but nothing was done because of her youth. **B**, Occlusion of same patient. (U. S. Army Photographs; Letterman Army Hospital.)

to be removed is measured with calipers, and the anterior vertical bone incision is made, estimating the degree of angulation necessary to produce the desired V (Figs. 23-52, *B* and *C*, and 23-54, *B*).

6. The intervening bone is then removed with end-cutting rongeurs. Thus, an effort is made to uncover and identify the inferior alveolar nerve and/or its mental and incisive branches. Though this part of the procedure is tedious and painstaking, it is worthwhile to attempt to save the continuity of the nerves.

7. Both sides should be done before the extraoral stage of the operation is begun.

8. The patient is then repositioned, and the operating team prepares for the submental extraoral procedure.

9. The soft tissue dissection does not differ materially from that already described except (a) the mandibular branch of the facial nerve is more superiorly re-

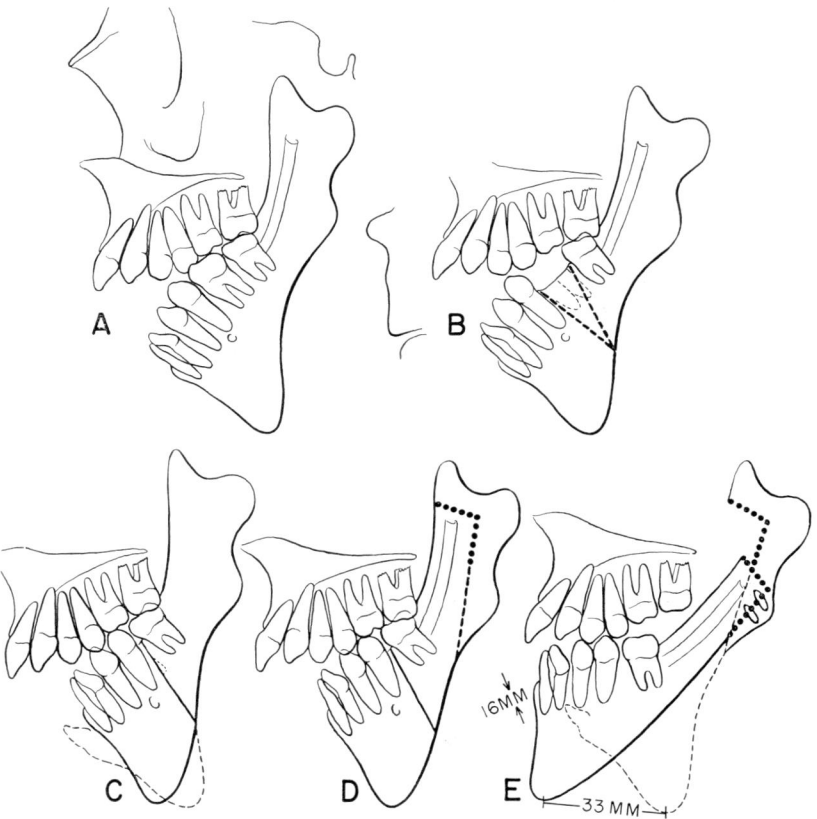

Fig. 23-54. **A**, Initial tracing from the cephalogram of 10-year-old girl shown in Fig. 23-53. A planned series of operations that can be done at the proper age. **B** and **C**, V ostectomy will close the incisal relationship about 12 mm. and move mentum anteriorly about 10 mm. **D** and **E**, L-shaped sliding osteotomy in the ramus (Pichler and Trauner) at a later date will close the incisal relationship about 4 mm. more, and by decortication and overlapping of bone ends, mentum will be extended anteriorly an additional 23 mm., or a total of approximately 33 mm.

lated in this area and usually will not be encountered, (b) considerable vascularity is present deep to the platysma muscle, but none of these vessels has the caliber of the facial vessels, and (c) progress to the bone is therefore easier and more rapidly accomplished.

10. As soon as the periosteum is reached it is elevated widely until communication with the intraoral operation is reached and the intraoral bone cuts are in view.

11. The V excision is completed to the lower border, using a No. 703 bur. Once the anterior part of the mandible is mobilized the segment of bone below the mental foramen can be freed and removed. Trauma to the nerve may result in temporary anesthesia, but even if severed, the nerve usually recovers. Excessive manipulation of the mobilized anterior part of the mandible should be avoided to prevent stretching or tearing the nerve (Fig. 23-52, C).

12. The bone ends are held firmly with larger Kocher forceps clamped to the lower border, as the edges are planed to fit into close approximation. Planing is accomplished with a thin, flat chisel, or with a No. 703 bur principally on the proximal or posterior fragment. Failure of approximation may occur at the lower border because of the sliding up and bending back of the anterior (distal) fragment.[73]

13. The mouth is reentered and the occlusion established anteriorly. Intermaxillary fixation is secured. Although not feasible in every instance, I have had satisfactory results in using a cast lingual splint on the lower teeth in these cases. This splint is cast to fit a study model that has been sectioned and repositioned. The splint can be placed prior to surgery and wired to the teeth posterior to the proposed site of ostectomy. When this stage of the operation is reached and the anterior section of the mandible is moved into position, the teeth in it are wired to the lingual splint or a precast metal labial splint may be used. (Fig. 23-32, B). In any case, positive fixation should be established, by some means, in the dental arch between the anterior and posterior fragments.

14. The bone ends are then wired together inferiorly and the extraoral wounds closed in anatomical layers as described previously (Fig. 23-52, D).

15. Dressings and postoperative care are routine.

16. Healing time is dependent on the accuracy of bone approximation and adequacy of immobilization.

Technique for sliding osteotomy to lengthen the rami (Inverted L, Vertical or Oblique)

Technique. The approach for sliding osteotomy to lengthen the rami is entirely extraoral. It is the same as has been described for other extraoral operations in the ramus. The incisions need not exceed 6 to 8 cm. for adequate access to the lateral aspect of the ramus. The technique of osteotomy is not hazardous and is relatively easy to accomplish.

1. The line of the bone incision is marked with a dye stick. It extends from the anterior border of the ramus at a level above the prominence of the foramen posteriorly to within about 1 cm. of the posterior border. It is then carried vertically downward just posterior to the foramen to the lower border of the mandible.[75] It may be made in the form of an inverted L, in a circular direction, or in a vertical line from the mandibular notch to the angle, depending on indications established by study of templates (Fig. 23-54, D and E).

2. With a No. 15 bone drill in a straight handpiece on a high-speed engine, perforations are made at 2 mm. intervals along the line that has been marked. The engine should be run at high speeds with a light pressure so that the surgeon can feel diminishing resistance as the bur emerges through the medial cortex. Actually a medullary space is imperceptible to touch in the area above and anterior to the foramen.

Both cortices and the medullary space can be felt from about the area where the line changes to a vertical direction. If a sharp, fast-revolving (18,000 rpm) bur is used, no need exists to elevate the medial periosteum and insert a protecting flat elevator. In fact, to do so invites trouble in the form of possible hemorrhage that is difficult to control. Such an instrument may be placed under the lower extent of the bone perforations advantageously, but should not go higher than the region of the foramen.

3. The drill perforations on the lateral cortex may be connected with a No. 703 fissure bur to facilitate the final section. It is done through the medial cortex with short, sharply executed blows with a hand mallet on a thin, sharp, broad-bladed chisel.

4. Once the bone sectioning is completed, the anterior segment and the body of the mandible are distracted downward. Elevation and freeing of medial periosteal attachments may be needed at this time.

5. The mouth is entered, and desired occlusion is established with intermaxillary elastic ligatures applied to previously placed arch bars. Arch bars in this operation are adequate for fixation since immobilization is ordinarily not required for more than 6 to 8 weeks.

6. The surgical team then changes gloves, replaces the "curtain" drape, and returns to the extraoral field.

7. The cut edge of the proximal fragment or posterior portion of the ramus should align itself with the distal (anterior portion of the ramus) fragment on a vertical plane. One or two pairs of drill holes are appropriately placed and the fragments wired into direct approximation. To accomplish this, elevation of the medial periosteum will be necessary, but careful manipulation of fragments makes transosseous wiring easy.

8. Closure of the wound, dressings, and postoperative care follow the routine already described.

The technique of osteotomy just described must never be modified to place the line of incision through the bone in an "oblique" direction from the mandibular notch to the posterior border of the ramus above the angle, but must always be "vertically" to the angle. Decortication is indicated, especially if prognathism coexists with apertognathia. *Direct wiring with overcorrection is always indicated.* Severing the coronoid process (coronoidotomy) to eliminate the pull of the temporalis muscle helps to prevent relapse when a straight vertical cut from the mandibular notch has been made. These extra steps should be routine in correction of apertognathia.

Maxillary osteotomy

Operations performed in the maxilla to correct open bite and maxillary protrusion are not new, although it is only in recent years that this surgery has been undertaken in this country to any extent. In 1935 Wassmund[76] described *anterior maxillary osteotomy* to correct maxillary prognathism (Fig. 23-55). The operation consisted of extracting first premolars bilaterally, performing ostectomy buccally and palatally to a vertical height level with the floor of the nose. Horizontal osteotomy was then accomplished at this level above the apices of the anterior maxillary teeth joining the vertical cuts. When modified and applied to various apertognathic and other anterior malrelations, this operation has much usefulness. Schuchardt[77] recognized the need to reduce the vertical jaw relation posteriorly in cases of anterior open bite in which the lip line would be esthetically too high and closure of the lips difficult if anterior maxillary osteotomy was performed. He recommended *posterior maxillary osteotomy* with impaction of the tooth-bearing alveolar ridges into the maxillary sinuses, bilaterally (Fig. 23-56). In 1959 Köle[65] published a little noticed but beautifully descriptive series of articles dealing principally with "operations on the alveolar ridge

Developmental deformities of the jaws 509

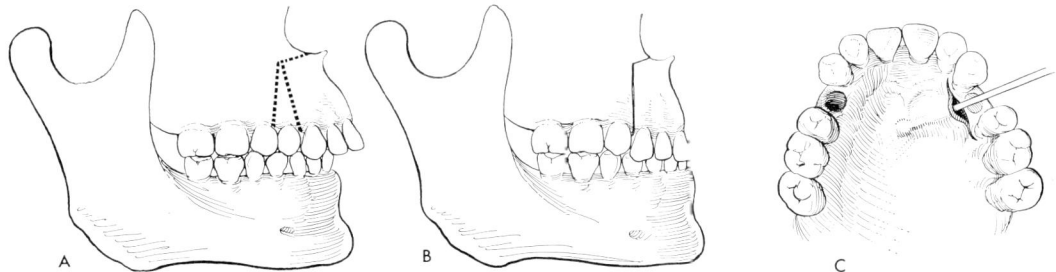

Fig. 23-55. Anterior maxillary osteotomy for correction of maxillary prognathism, retrusion, open bite, and closed bite. **A**, In maxillary protrusion, ostectomy is accomplished in the first premolar area, followed by horizontal osteotomy above the apices of the anterior teeth. **B**, After the palatal osteotomy is completed (**C**) the anterior maxilla is retruded to normal incisal relation. (Modified from Wassmund, M.: Lehrbuch der praktischen Chirurgie des Mundes und der Kiefer, vol. 1, Leipzig, 1935, Johann Ambrosius Barth.)

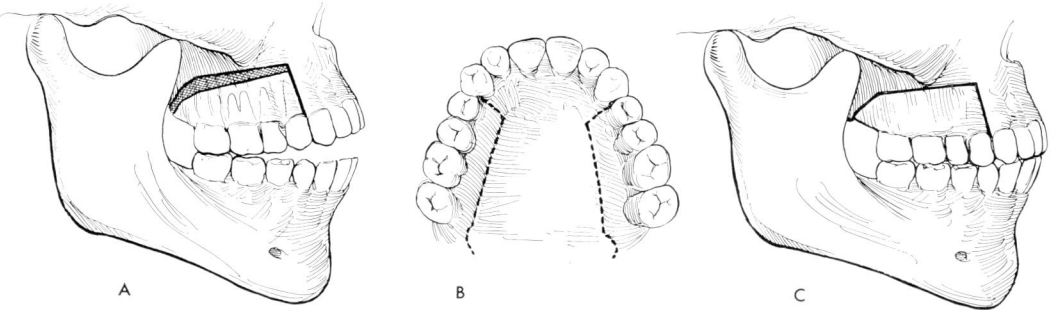

Fig. 23-56. Posterior maxillary osteotomy for correction of anterior open bite or posterior malocclusion. By osteotomy above the apices of the posterior teeth buccally (**A**) and palatally (**B**) in "stage" procedures, the posterior maxillary tooth-bearing alveolar ridges are impacted into the maxillary sinuses bilaterally, thus closing the anterior open bite (**C**). (Modified from Schuchardt, K.: International Society of Plastic Surgeons, Transactions of Second Congress, Edinburgh, Scotland, E. & S. Livingstone, Ltd.)

to correct occlusal abnormalities" that "completely replaces orthodontic treatment" or "facilitates subsequent orthodontic treatment."

More recently in this country considerable notice has been given to this type of surgery. Mohnac[11,78,79] has become very enthusiastic about correction of occlusal irregularities by maxillary osteotomies and has comprehensively outlined indications and descriptions of operative procedures for both anterior and posterior maxillary osteotomies. He states that "surgical corrective procedures can be performed in the maxilla either alone or in combination with procedures performed in the mandible. Specifically, the maxilla or sections of it can be advanced, retracted, raised, lowered, or moved medially or laterally." Parnes, Torres, and Galbreath[80] reported two cases of maxillary protrusion corrected by anterior maxillary osteotomy in a single-stage operation in 1965. They were evidently pleased with results and made no mention of com-

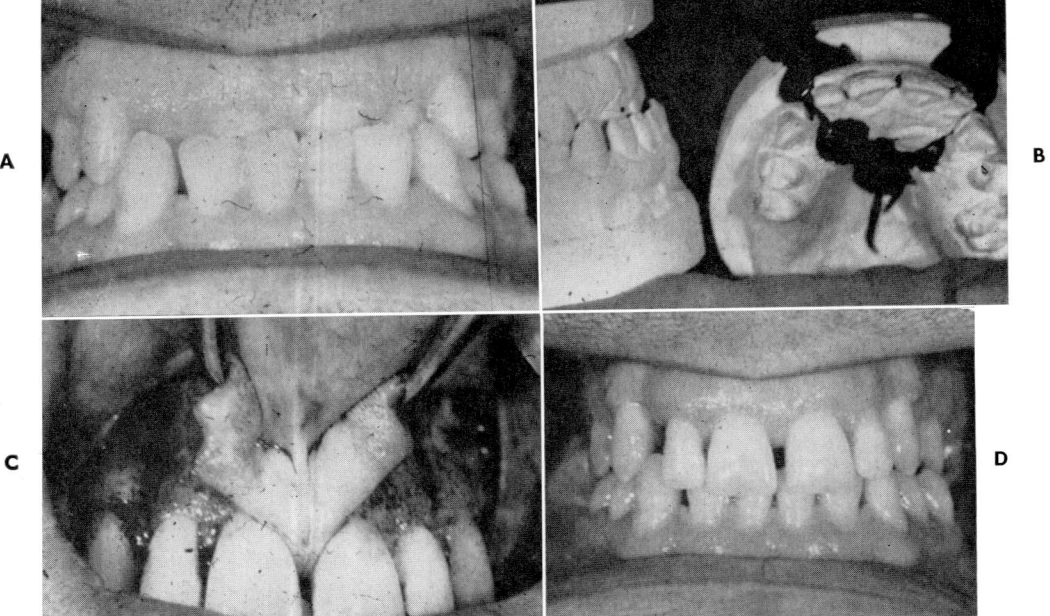

Fig. 23-57. **A**, The patient was a 32-year-old man whose four maxillary incisor teeth were in lingual version. His posterior occlusion was excellent. **B**, The upper study model was sectioned at the suture lines of the premaxilla. **C**, Segmental osteotomy was accomplished in one operation, sectioning free the premaxilla and its four incisor teeth. The surgically fractured anterior maxilla was wired to a cast labial arch splint for immobilization during healing. **D**, An improved incisal relation resulted. Spacing at sites of osteotomy between lateral incisors and cuspids was not objectionable. Thus the anterior maxilla has been moved forward, the reverse of that shown in Figs. 23-55, 23-58, and 23-59.

plications. Reed, Hinds, and Mohnac[81] reported one case of bilateral posterior maxillary osteotomy performed in two stages to correct an anterior open bite. The problem was a complicated one, and included in the planning was bilateral subcondylar osteotomy to correct an associated mandibular deviation and cross bite occlusion. The functional and cosmetic improvement was remarkable. The possibilities offered by "segmental" surgery first came to our attention in 1959,[82-84] and our first anterior maxillary osteotomy was accomplished that same year in August (Fig. 23-57).

Utilization of maxillary osteotomy must be given careful consideration, and definite indications must be present. Anterior facial disharmonies such as incisal line of teeth and related lip line, maxillary protrusion, maxillary open bite, and overbite must be studied carefully. Maxillary osteotomy is not the solution to all of these problems, and indiscriminate use of the operation will produce a percentage of poor results (Fig. 23-58).

Technique for anterior maxillary osteotomy (Figs. 23-58 and 23-59). Whether the anterior part of the maxilla is to be retruded, tipped down, raised, or protruded makes little difference since the surgical approach is essentially the same in each instance.

1. A vertical incision is made at the midline of the maxilla through the periosteum

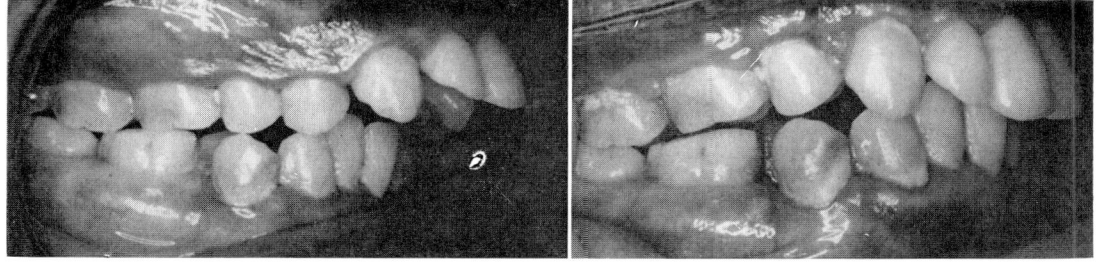

Fig. 23-58. **A**, Preoperative maxillary protrusion. **B**, Postoperative occlusion with correction by removal of first premolars and anterior maxillary osteotomy with set-back of protrusion. (Denver General Hospital with Dr. D. H. Garehime.)

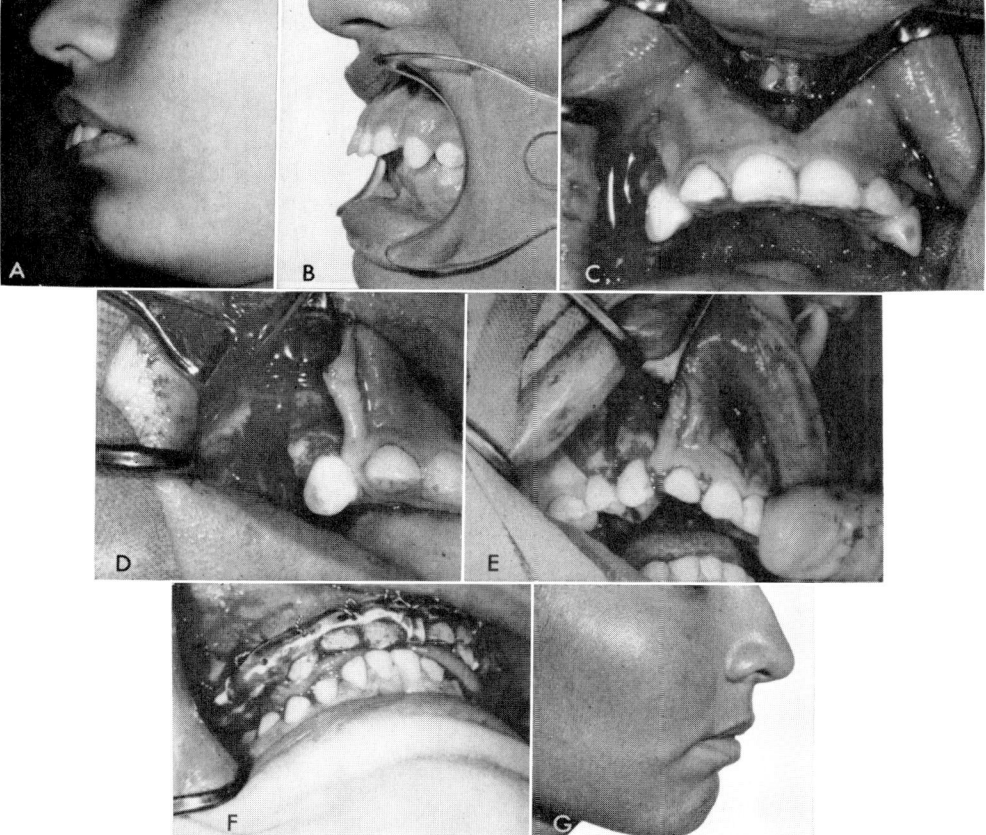

Fig. 23-59. **A**, Profile of 15-year-old girl with maxillary protrusion. **B**, Class II malocclusion. **C**, Through a vertical midline incision horizontal osteotomy was accomplished. Although the bone cut *looks* low in this picture, it is placed just below the anterior nasal spine and floor of nasal fossa, well above the apices of the teeth. **D**, The first premolar is extracted and osteotomy is accomplished in this area from buccal plate right through palate to permit retrusion of the anterior maxilla. **E**, When both horizontal osteotomy and vertical ostectomy are completed, the anterior maxilla is depressed back until space of first premolar is closed or to the pre-established correct relation. **F**, Cast labial splint is fitted, soft tissue wounds are closed, and the splint is wired to the teeth. **G**, Improved incisal relationship and appearance resulted. (Denver General Hospital with Dr. Paul Rowe.)

from just below the anterior nasal spine down almost to the alveolar crest.

2. Periosteum is elevated laterally to the second premolar area.

3. An oblique incision is made on each side upward and posteriorly from the gingiva at the distal buccal aspect of the second premolar into the buccal fold.

4. A large mucoperiosteal flap is elevated from these latter incisions anteriorly, exposing the buccal plate over the first premolar, which is removed.

5. The interdental papilla is incised on the palatal aspect between the teeth adjacent to the first premolar.

6. Soft tissue covering the anterior hard palate is undermined by elevating the periosteum to the midline and creating a connecting "tunnel" from one side to the other (Fig. 23-55, C).

7. The first bone incision is made on the buccal through the socket of the first premolar and extended beyond the apex for several millimeters. The maxillary sinus membrane is usually encountered, but it is of no concern (Fig. 23-59, D).

8. A No. 703 or 702 carbide fissure bur run at 18,000 rpm under copious water irrigation is used for all bone incision and excision.

9. An osteotomy is then accomplished from the midline incision just below the floor of the nasal fossa horizontally back on both sides to join the buccal cut at the premolar location. It may be necessary to angle upward somewhat over the canine area to provide a wide margin at the apex of that tooth (Fig. 23-59, C).

10. Osteotomy is then accomplished across the palate from each side through the "tunnel" to the midline. This is never well visualized and must be done with good retraction protection to the soft tissue and use of a fast-revolving, well irrigated bur. Much dependence is placed on sense of touch and resistance of hard bone to the revolution of the bur.

11. Thin probes are used to seek out incomplete severance of bone, and thin, broad, flat-bladed osteotomes facilitate final osteotomy.

12. Bone is removed as needed to permit placement of the freed anterior maxillary fragment to the desired relation.

13. This relation must be predetermined on study models from which a *cast labial splint* has been made. The splint serves to guide proper positioning of the sectioned part and is then wired to all remaining teeth in the arch. Stability is thus secured during healing, and intermaxillary fixation is usually *not* used (Fig. 23-59, F).

14. Flaps are closed with interrupted sutures, and a pressure dressing is taped to the face across the upper lip to help control the inevitable edema and ecchymosis.

Technique for posterior maxillary osteotomy. Posterior maxillary osteotomy may be used to expand or narrow the maxillary arch unilaterally or bilaterally and to close vertical dimension posteriorly to correct anterior open bite. It is accomplished in two-stage operations, the palatal side being done first.

1. Incisions are made into the interdental papilla from the second molar forward to the central incisor.

2. Palatal mucoperiosteal tissues are elevated from the gingival margin, exposing the greater palatine foramen and contents. It is unnecessary to strip back the entire palatal covering.

3. Using a No. 703 carbide fissure bur, a cut is made anteriorly from the foramen to the first premolar area, where it is angled downward to the alveolar ridge between the premolar and canine teeth. This cut is kept in a vertical plane parallel with the long axis of the teeth and is carried through the palatine process of the maxilla to the maxillary antrum. The cut is then carefully extended posterolaterally to the pterygomaxillary fissure.

4. The palatal flap is replaced and sutured and the second stage is delayed 3 to 4 weeks to ensure nutrition.

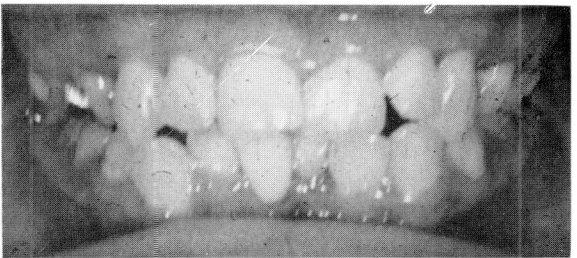

Fig. 23-60. **A**, Preoperative malrelation of the anterior teeth with open bite. **B**, Because of high lip line, posterior osteotomy was performed to close the incisal relationship.

5. After the delay a large buccal flap is raised from the gingival margin, exposing the lateral aspect of the maxilla from the canine prominence posteriorly to the tuberosity.

6. A thin, vertical cut is made between the canine and first premolar using a No. 701 or 702 carbide bur. (Occasionally the first premolar must be removed to permit desired placement of the sectioned part.)

7. A horizontal cut is made with a No. 703 bur from the pterygomaxillary fissure anteriorly under the zygomatic process, above the apices of the teeth, into the maxillary antrum and anteriorly, joining the vertical cut at the canine fossa.

8. If the sectioned part is to be depressed and impacted upward into the sinus, it may be necessary to remove additional bone along the horizontal bone cut.

9. A broad, flat, thin periosteotome is usually needed to complete the surgical fracture.

10. A prefabricated labial cast silver splint is utilized here also to ensure union and resist relapse. Intermaxillary fixation is applied lightly, but only between the anterior teeth.

A case illustrating results of this method for closing open bite deformities is shown in Fig. 23-60.

CONCLUSION

Robinson[85] states that a "standardized outline of surgical technic for prognathism is necessary in teaching residents." We hope this chapter may provide the basis for such outline in surgical technique; however, training must never become stereotyped "by the numbers" process, otherwise variations from normal may not be adequately coped with when encountered. Students (residents) must be stimulated to think independently and individually, while preceptors must teach *all* acceptable methods of corrective jaw surgery, including the more difficult procedures and also those less frequently needed. Imagination and the versatility of many of the operations described herein make possible the correction of almost any conceivable deformity that may be present, but the results will depend largely on how well the operation is planned and the surgical ability of the surgeon. Blair's classical remark 60 years ago that the mandible "is a hoop of bone capable of almost any kind of adjustment" is more realistic in this modern day than ever before.

REFERENCES

1. Hullihen, S. P.: Case of elongation of the underjaw and distortion of the face and neck, caused by burn, successfully treated, Amer. J. Dent. Sci. **9:**157, 1849.
2. Blair, V. P.: Operations on the jaw-bone and face, Surg. Gynec. Obstet. **4:**67, 1907.
3. Sicher, H.: Growth of the mandible, Amer. J. Orthodont. **33:**30, 1947.
4. Engel, M. B., and Brodie, A. G.: Condylar growth and mandibular deformities, Surgery **22:**976, 1947.

5. Sarnat, B. G., and Engel, M. B.: A serial study of mandibular growth after removal of the condyle in the macaca rhesus monkey, Plast. Reconstr. Surg. 7:364, 1951.
6. Sarnat, B. G., and Robinson, I. B.: Surgery of the mandible, some clinical and experimental considerations, Plast. Reconstr. Surg. 17:27, 1956.
7. Pascoe, J. J., Hayward, J. R., and Costich, E. R.: Mandibular prognathism, its etiology and a classification, J. Oral Surg. 18:21, 1960.
8. Graber, T. M.: In Salzmann, J. H., editor: Roentgenographic cephalometrics; proceedings of the workshop conducted by the special committee of the American Association of Orthodontists, Philadelphia, 1961, J. B. Lippincott Co., pp. 21-34.
9. Colle, A. J.: Some clinical applications of cephalometric analysis, J. Canad. Dent. Ass. 20:309, 1954.
10. Murphey, P. J., and Walker, R. V.: Correction of maxillary protrusion by ostectomy and orthodontic therapy, J. Oral Surg. 21:275, 1963.
11. Mohnac, A. M.: Surgical correction of maxillomandibular deformities, J. Oral Surg. 23:393, 1965.
12. Hinds, E. C.: Correction of prognathism by subcondylar osteotomy, J. Oral Surg. 16:209, 1958.
13. Jaboulay, M., and Berard, L.: Traitement chirurgical du prognathisme inferieur, Presse Med., No. 30:173, April 19, 1898.
14. Duformental, L.: Le traitement chirurgical du prognathisme, Presse Med., No. 24:235, March 23, 1921.
15. Pettit, J. A., and Walrath, C. H.: A new surgical procedure for correction of prognathism, J.A.M.A. 99:1917, 1932.
16. Smith, A. E., and Johnson, J. B.: Surgical treatment of mandibular deformations, J. Amer. Dent. Ass. 27:689, 1940.
17. Smith, A. E., and Robinson, M.: Surgical correction of mandibular prognathism by subsigmoid notch ostectomy with sliding condylotomy; a new technic, J. Amer. Dent. Ass. 49:46, 1954.
18. Moose, S. M.: Surgical correction of mandibular prognathism by intraoral subcondylar osteotomy, J. Oral Surg. 22:197, 1964.
19. Reiter, E. R.: Surgical correction of mandibular prognathism, Alpha Omegan 45:104, 1951.
20. Reiter, E. R.: Mandibular prognathism: bilateral osteotomy through the neck of the condyle, lecture course, 36th annual meeting, American Society of Oral Surgeons, Nov. 4, 1954, Hollywood, Fla.
21. Kostecka, F.: A contribution to the surgical treatment of open bite, Int. J. Orthodont. Dent. Child. 20:1082, 1934.
22. Schaefer, J. E.: Correction of malocclusion by surgical interference, Am. J. Orthodont. Oral Surg. (Oral Surg. Sect.) 27:172, 1941.
23. Verne, D., Polachek, R., and Shapiro, D. N.: Osteotomy of condylar neck for correction of prognathism: study of fifty-two cases, J. Oral Surg. 15:183, 1957.
24. Kaplan, H., and Spring, P. N.: Gustatory hyperhidrosis associated with subcondylar osteotomy, J. Oral Surg. 18:50, 1960.
25. Caldwell, J. B., and Letterman, G. S.: Vertical osteotomy in the mandibular rami for correction of prognathism, J. Oral Surg. 12:185, 1954.
26. Letterman, G., Caldwell, J. B., Schurter, M., and Shira, R. B.: Vertical osteotomy in the mandibular rami for correction of prognathism —a ten year follow-up study. Excerpta Medica International Congress, Series #66, Proceedings of the Third International Congress of Plastic Surgery, Washington, D. C., October, 1963.
27. Caldwell, J. B.: Surgical correction of development deformities of the mandible, U. S. Armed Forces Med. J. 3:362, 1954.
28. Shira, R. B. (Major General, Dental Corps; formerly Chief, Dental Service, Walter Reed General Hospital, Washington, D. C.): Personal communication.
29. Caldwell, J. B., and Hughes, K. W.: Prognathism in edentulous and partially edentulous patients, J. Oral Surg. 16:377, 1958.
30. Shira, R. B.: Surgical correction of open bite deformities by sliding osteotomy, J. Oral Surg. 19:275, 1961.
31. Robinson, M.: Prognathism corrected by open vertical condylotomy, J. S. California Dent. Ass. 24:22, 1956.
32. Robinson, M.: Prognathism corrected by open vertical subcondylotomy, J. Oral Surg. 16:215, 1958.
33. Hinds, E. C.: Surgical correction of acquired mandibular deformities, Amer. J. Orthodont. 43:160, 1957.
34. Hinds, E. C.: Correction of prognathism by subcondylar osteotomy, J. Oral Surg. 16:209, 1958.
35. Thoma, K. H.: Oral surgery; ed. 4, St. Louis, 1963, The C. V. Mosby Co., pp. 1162, 1168, 1169, 1141, 1142, 1147.
36. Hensel, G. C.: The surgical correction of mandibular protraction, retraction and fractures of the ascending rami, Int. J. Orthodont. 23:814, 1937.
37. Moose, S. M.: Correction of abnormal man-

dibular protrusion by intraoral operation, J. Oral Surg. 3:304, 1945.
38. Sloan, A. C.: Intraoral osteotomy of ascending rami for correction of prognathism, Texas Dent. J. 69:375, 1951.
39. Skaloud, F.: A new surgical method for correction of prognathism of the mandible, Oral Surg. 4:689, 1951.
40. Kazanjian, V. H.: The inter-relation of dentistry and surgery in the treatment of deformities of the face and jaws. Amer. J. Orthodont. Oral Surg. (Oral Surg. Sect.) 27:10, 1941.
41. Kazanjian, V. H.: The treatment of mandibular prognathism with special reference to edentulous patients, Oral Surg. 4:680, 1951.
42. Obwegeser, H.: The surgical correction of mandibular prognathism and retrognathia with consideration of genioplasty. Part I. Surgical procedures to correct mandibular prognathism and reshaping of the chin, Oral Surg. 10:677, 1957.
43. Dal Pont, G.: Retromolar osteotomy for the correction of prognathism, J. Oral Surg. 19:42, 1961.
44. Harsha, W. M.: Bilateral resection of the jaw for prognathism, Surg. Gynec. Obstet. 15:51, 1912.
45. New, G. B., and Erich, J. B.: The surgical correction of the mandibular prognathism, Amer. J. Surg. 53:2, 1941.
46. Dingman, R. O.: Surgical correction of developmental deformities of the mandible, Plast. Reconstr. Surg. 3:124, 1948.
47. Dingman, R. O.: Surgical correction of mandibular prognathism, an improved method, Amer. J. Orthodont. Oral Surg. (Oral Surg. Sect.) 30:683, 1944.
48. Thoma, K. H.: Oral surgery, ed. 4, St. Louis, 1963, The C. V. Mosby Co., p. 1135.
49. Batson, O. V.: The temporalis muscle, Oral Surg. 6:40, 1953.
50. McCarthy, W. D., and Burns, S. R.: Screw lock sectional splint, J. Oral Surg. 4:343, 1946.
51. Kazanjian, V. J.: Surgical treatment of mandibular prognathism, Int. J. Orthodont. 18:1224, 1932.
52. Van Alstine, R. S., and Dingman, R. O.: Correction of mandibular protrusion in the edentulous patient, J. Oral Surg. 11:273, 1953.
53. Cameron, J. R., and Stetzer, J. J.: Bilateral resection of the mandible to correct prognathism, J. Oral Surg. 6:69, 1948.
54. Caldwell, J. B.: Surgical correction of extreme mandibular prognathism, J. Oral Surg. 26:253, 1968.
55. Blair, V. P.: Underdeveloped lower jaw, with limited excursion, J.A.M.A. 53:178, 1909.
56. Limberg, A. A.: A new method of plastic lengthening of the mandible in unilateral microgenia and asymmetry of the face, J. Amer. Dent. Ass. 15:851, 1928.
57. Kazanjian, V. J.: Surgical correction of deformities of the jaws and its relation to orthodontia, Int. J. Orthodont. 22:259, 1936.
58. Caldwell, J. B., and Amaral, W. J.: Mandibular micrognathia, corrected by vertical osteotomy in the rami and iliac bone graft, J. Oral Surg. 18:3, 1960.
59. Robinson, M.: Micrognathism corrected by vertical osteotomy of ascending ramus and iliac bone graft: a new technique, Oral Surg. 10:1125, 1957.
60. Robinson, M., and Lytle, J. J.: Micrognathism corrected by vertical osteotomies of the rami without bone grafts, Oral Surg. 15:641, 1962.
61. Limberg, A. A.: Treatment of open bite by means of plastic oblique osteotomy of the ascending rami of the mandible, Dent. Cosmos 67:1191, 1925.
62. Caldwell, J. B., Hayward, J. R., and Lister, R. L.: Correction of mandibular retrognathia by vertical-L osteotomy: a new technic, J. Oral Surg. 26:259, 1968.
63. Hofer, O.: Die vertikale Osteotomie zur Verlangerung des einseitig verkurzten aufsteigenden Unterkieferastes, Oest. Z. Stomat. 34:826, 1942.
64. Hofer, O.: Operation der Prognathie und Mikrogenic, Deutsch. Zahn. Mund. Kieferheilk. 9 121, 1942.
65. Köle, H.: Surgical operations on the alveolar ridge to correct occlusal abnormalities, Oral Surg. 12:277, 413, 515, 1959.
66. Kazanjian, V. H., and Converse, J. M.: Surgical treatment of facial injuries, Baltimore, 1949, The Williams & Wilkins Co., p. 433.
67. Barsky, A. J.: Principles and practice of plastic surgery, Baltimore, 1950, The Williams & Wilkins Co., p. 312.
68. Thoma, K. H.: Genioplasty with tantalum gauze, Oral Surg. 2:65, 1949.
69. Millard, D. R.: Adjuncts in augmentation mentoplasty and corrective rhinoplasty, Plast. Reconstr. Surg. 36:48, 1965.
70. Small, I. A., Brown, S., and Kobernick, S. D.: Teflon and Silastic for mandibular replacement: experimental studies and reports of cases, J. Oral Surg. 22:377, 1964.
71. Converse, J. M.: Reconstructive plastic surgery, Philadelphia, 1964, W. B. Saunders Co., p. 901.
72. Pickerill, H. P.: Double resection of the mandible, Dent. Cosmos 54:1114, 1912.
73. Thoma, K. H.: Y shaped osteotomy for cor-

rection of open bite in adults, Surg. Gynec. Obstet. **77**:40, 1943.
74. Babcock, W. W.: Field of osteoplastic operations for the correction of deformities of the jaws, Dent. Items Interest **32**:439, 1910.
75. Pichler, H., and Trauner, R.: Mund und Kieferchirurgie, part 1, vols. 1 and 2, Wien, 1948, Urban & Schwarzenberg, p. 626.
76. Wassmund, M.: Lehrbuch der praktischen Chirurgie des Mundes und der Kiefer, vol. 1, Leipzig, 1935, Johann Ambrosius Barth.
77. Schuchardt, K.: Experiences with the surgical treatment of some deformities of the jaws: prognathia, micrognathia, and open bite, International Society of Plastic Surgeons, Transactions of Second Congress, London, 1959 (Wallace, A. B., editor) Edinburgh, Scotland, 1961, E. & S. Livingstone, Ltd., p. 73.
78. Mohnac, A. M.: Lecture, Rocky Mountain Society of Oral Surgeons, annual meeting, June, 1966.
79. Mohnac, A. M.: Maxillary osteotomy in the management of occlusal deformities, J. Oral Surg. **24**:303, 1966.
80. Parnes, E. I., Torres, I., and Galbreath, J. C.: Surgical correction of maxillary protrusion, J. Oral Surg. **24**:218, 1966.
81. Reid, R., Hinds, E. C., and Mohnac, A. M.: Surgical correction of facial asymmetry associated with open bite, J. Oral Surg. **24**:527, 1966.
82. Obwegeser, H. (Zahnärztliches Institut der Universität, Zürich, Switzerland): Personal communication, Nov., 1959.
83. Köle: Personal communication, International Congress for Maxillo-Facial Surgery, Graz, Austria, May, 1959.
84. Trauner, R.: Personal communication, International Congress for Maxillo-Facial Surgery, Graz, Austria, May, 1959.
85. Robinson, M.: Teaching outline for prognathism surgery at Los Angeles County Hospital, J. Oral Surg. **21**:227, 1963.

Chapter 24

SURGICAL ASPECTS OF ORAL TUMORS

Claude S. LaDow

Tumors, or neoplasms, are new growths of abnormal tissue arising around the oral cavity as in other parts of the body. They may occur in the lips, cheeks, floor of the mouth, palate, tongue, and in the jaw bones. These new growths may be of epithelial, connective tissue, or nerve tissue origin, although neurogenic tumors are extremely rare in the oral cavity.

Tumors may be benign or malignant, depending upon their behavior pattern and cellular structure. A benign tumor grows slowly and is usually encapsulated. It enlarges by peripheral expansion, pushes away adjoining structures, and manifests no metastasis. A malignant tumor, on the other hand, endangers the life of its host by its rapid infiltrating extension into surrounding vital structures and the phenomenon of metastasis, which creates secondary growths in distant parts of the body, usually through the lymphatic system and bloodstream.

Treatment of tumors is essentially the extirpation of the mass, although surgical intervention varies with the nature of the neoplasm. Some benign neoplasms of the mouth possess characteristics rarely encountered elsewhere in the body. These characteristics pertain to tumors of dental origin.

Oral tumors may be classified into those of dental origin and those of nondental origin. Oral tumors of dental origin arise from epithelial inclusions remaining within the jaw bones after tooth formation is completed. This occurs around the teeth and within suture lines of the developing maxillae and mandible. Epithelial tumors may be secreting or nonsecreting, depending upon the presence of secretory epithelium, as occurs in cysts.

TUMORS OF THE HARD TISSUES OF THE ORAL CAVITY
Odontogenic tumors

Odontogenic cysts are discussed in detail in a separate chapter. Dental tumors arising in the jaw bones may be broadly classified into odontomas and ameloblastomas.

Odontoma. *Calcified odontomas, simple enamel pearls,* and *cementomas* usually consist of one or more kinds of tooth elements. Enamel pearls consist of enamel. Odontomas consist of dentine. Cementomas are of cementum. Odontomas may be composite by manifesting two or more tooth tissue elements. These simple tooth tumors arise from some aberration of the tooth germ early in life. Surgical intervention is instituted at an early age to prevent derangement of the permanent dentition. In later years multiple cementomas and ossifying fibromas appear frequently near the roots of teeth. The teeth remain vital with absence of subjective symptoms. Surgical intervention for these innocent tumors is unnecessary since they frequently reach a stage of inactivity and become calcified within the jaw bones without disturbing function and are only apparent in roentgenograms. Composite odontomas are excised since they contain various tooth formations that tend toward destructive cystic change. Some of these masses grow to considerable size in the young, thus interfering with eruption of permanent teeth. They can cause considerable bone destruction. Roentgenographic diagnosis may be the only outstanding evidence of their presence besides a slight aberration of the surrounding structures. Surgical removal of these benign tumors is always conservative. They can be approached by removing the overlying bone (Fig. 24-1). These masses are enucleated from the adjoining bony structures of the jaw with surgical burs or chisels. Controlled sharp dissection is preferred to elevator technique since the surrounding tissue may be damaged when uncontrolled elevator force is applied. Primary closure of the operative site following obliteration of the cavitation with absorbable packs is the treatment of choice. Complications following removal of odontomas may include paresthesia of the lower lip and mandible when the tumor mass contacts the inferior dental nerve, hemorrhage from the cavitation when bleeding areas are not controlled, and secondary infection with breakdown of sutures. Recurrence of these benign tumors has not been reported.

Ameloblastoma. The ameloblastoma is a tumor arising from embryonal cells of developing teeth. Although most forms of this tumor simulate other slow-growing, benign tumors, some can develop malignant tendencies. Degeneration of this tumor into carcinoma has occurred. Patients may have few subjective symptoms during tumor growth. Enlargement of the tumor may expand the buccal, lingual, or palatal bone plates. Teeth may loosen, and pressure symtoms may occur, especially in the region of the maxillary sinuses. Roentgenographic examination may demonstrate unilocular or multilocular types. Unilocular ameloblastomas may be confused with benign cysts. The tumor frequently absorbs the alveolus surrounding the roots of teeth and may absorb root ends (Fig. 24-2). They occur in both jaws. Metastasis is rare, but tumor fragments may find their way into the lungs by aspiration. Ameloblastomas grow by extension into adjacent tissues and may perforate the investing bone. A biopsy should precede treatment since these tu-

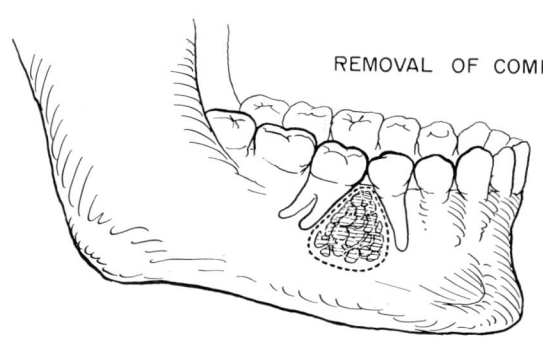

Fig. 24-1. Local excision of benign tumor.

Surgical aspects of oral tumors **519**

mors frequently present individual characteristics. Some are slow-growing, expansive tumors requiring many years to manifest subjective symptoms. Others grow more rapidly and present definite malignant tendencies. Biopsy is satisfactorily performed under local anesthesia. The overlying cortical bone is exposed through a mucoperiosteal incision, and a portion of bone is carefully removed with surgical burs or chisels. A section of the tumor mass is excised sharply without currettage or trauma. The overlying mucoperiosteum is sutured. The extent of the operative procedure will depend upon the histological structure of the tumor and the extent of involvement of the surrounding tissues.

Methods of treatment include extirpation, radical resection of the jaw, chemical cauterization, and electrocauterization. Local excision of a small, accessible tumor is indicated in the young, provided they agree to regular follow-up and a radical resection when recurrence occurs. Recurrences are not unusual following curettage. Incomplete surgical treatment may stimulate

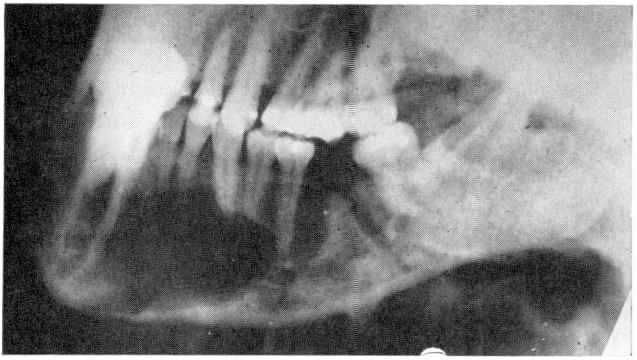

Fig. 24-2. Ameloblastoma. Absorption of alveolus and roots of teeth.

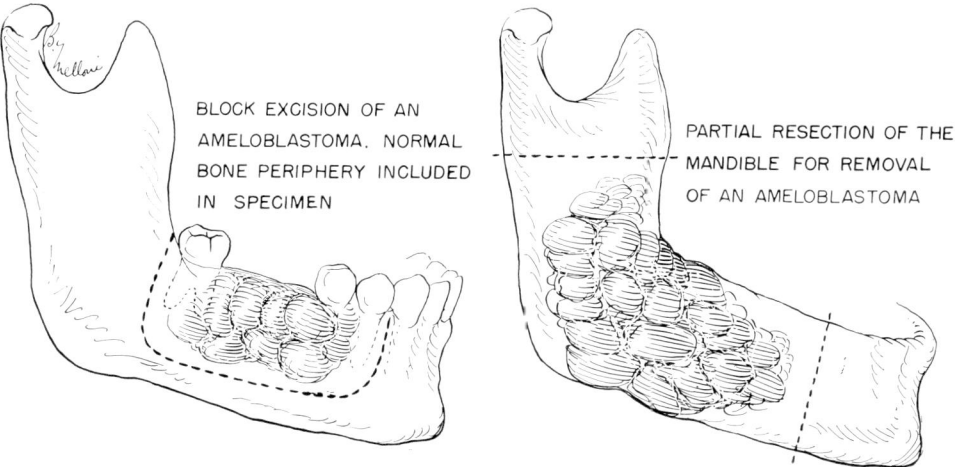

Fig. 24-3. Extension of the tumor through the cortical plate is an indication for partial resection.

tumor cell growth. Ameloblastomas are exposed widely by removing overlying bone, including the buccal plate as far as the base of the tumor. The buccal plate may be very thin because of the expansive enlargement of the underlying tumor. Whenever possible, the inferior border of the mandible is preserved and retained to maintain continuity of the jaw. Block section of the involved bone should extend into and include some normal peripheral bone surrounding the tumor mass (Fig. 24-3). Sharp cutting instruments are used to separate the diseased area from normal osseous structures. The entire base and surrounding margins are then electrocauterized to destroy completely the residual tumor cells. Sedative dressing is placed for drainage, to reduce pain, and allow healing by secondary intention from the bottom of the cavity. The mucoperiosteum is partially approximated, leaving an orifice for removal and renewal of the dressing. The wound dressing is renewed and gradually reduced in size in small amounts each time the packing is changed during the reparative process.

Ameloblastomas that have extended within the maxilla may perforate palatal mucoperiosteum and nasal mucosa. Radical resection of the tumor and the immediate surrounding osseous structures is the accepted treatment of choice. Since these tumors grow by extension into adjoining tissues, adequate surgical resection is accomplished. Frequently a stump of normal bone at one periphery of the resection is retained as in the condylar region of the mandible (Fig. 24-3). This bone may be utilized as a base of attachment for reconstruction of the missing section of the mandible by bone grafts. Bone grafts may be inserted at the time of surgical intervention because of the low incidence of metastasis in this type of new growth. Whenever radical procedures are performed to eradicate the ameloblastoma, conservative efforts are made to maintain function and esthetics.

Osteogenic tumors

Neoplasms arising from the jaw bones are classified as osteomas, fibro-osteomas or fibrous dysplasias, myxomas, chondromas, and sarcomas.

Osteoma. Osteomas of the jaws appear as areas of circumscribed, benign, bony new growths. Osteomas arising from the inner surface of bone cortex are called enostoses or central osteomas. Tumors of this kind consist of dense cortical bone extending into the spongiosa of the jaw. They can be demonstrated in roentgenograms as circumscribed, dense, bony tumors. Treatment may be unnecessary unless symptoms of pain resulting from pressure on nerve fibers are manifest, or superficial ulceration occurs in overlying tissues. All forms of osteoma cast a radiopaque shadow in roentgenograms. Osteomas consisting of spongiosa are much less dense, with outlines more difficult to differentiate from the adjoining bone.

Some forms of osteoma arise from the periosteum proper, from aberrant cartilage cells, and from the cortical plates. These will occasionally assume considerable disfiguring size, in which case surgical removal is indicated to reestablish facial harmony and obviate interference with function. These osteomas are composed of spongy bone with only a thin layer of covering cortex. They cast light shadows on roentgenograms. These tumors may be sharply dissected at their base, where they are contiguous with the bony cortex of the jaws. Osteomas rarely recur following complete excision.

Locally circumscribed bony growths developing outside the cortical plates are called exostoses or peripheral osteomas. These bony outgrowths are benign and slow growing and seem to develop in young adults. They may follow trauma or irritation. Areas of exostosis may occur at sites of muscle insertion or at the junction of two bones. A frequent site of exostoses is the midline region of the hard palate. This is known as a torus palatinus. A torus mandibularis may occur on the lingual aspect of the mandible in the premolar and molar regions.

Fibro-osteoma. The fibro-osteoma, a fibrous dysplasia of bone, is a benign, slow-growing tumor of bone that tends to have its greatest growth in the second decade of life. It is a diffuse, poorly differentiated endosteal tumor replacing the normal spongiosa with fibrous tissue. Increased irregular areas of calcification may occur as new bone formations develop in this tumor. The enlarging neoplasm may displace teeth and expand cortical plates of the jaw bones. A fibro-osteoma tends to occur more frequently in women than in men and is seen more often in the maxilla than in the mandible. This tumor may obliterate the maxillary sinus and may extend into other bone landmarks. It does not invade the nasal structures. This is of diagnostic importance since in both hyperostoses and Paget's disease the nasal meati are obliterated. This tumor is occasionally confused with the fibrosarcoma because of similar histological patterns. The fibro-osteoma grows slowly. The fibrosarcoma, on the other hand, enlarges rapidly. The fibro-osteoma manifests radiopacity following initial development as calcification occurs. Extensive involvement of the mandible will present an enlarged, curved lower border. Treatment of these benign tumors is conservative surgical contouring. The tumor mass can be sectioned from normal bone by local curettage only when it is small. Some growths become large and invade the spongiosa (Fig. 24-4). Excision of a large fibro-osteoma entails resecting the involved segment of the jaw. Enormous fibro-osteomas expanding into the oral cavity, interfering with function, and producing facial deformity are trimmed surgically to reestablish normal facial symmetry and maintain function. X-irradiation may be a useful adjunct to surgical treatment to inhibit the growth potential. These tumors tend to bleed freely following a contouring operation. Pressure packs and electrocoagulation may be necessary to control hemorrhage. The fibro-osteoma frequently recurs when treatment has been instituted at an early age. Cases have been reported in which fibro-osteomas have been reduced several times without any indication of malignant change.

Myxoma and chondroma. The myxoma and chondroma are closely allied tumors of embryonic tissue origin, developing from

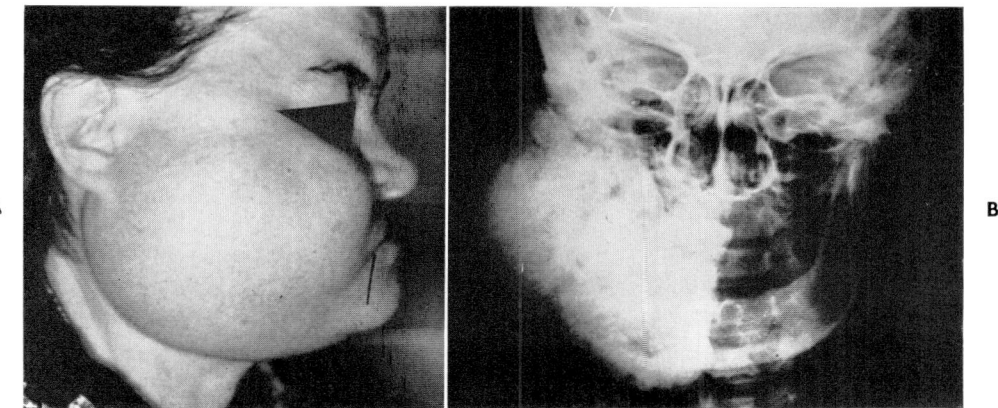

Fig. 24-4. **A,** Ossifying fibroma. The curving lower border of the mandible is the result of the expanding cortical plate of bone. **B,** Radiograph of the same case. Duration of 25 years.

immature primitive bone or cartilage cells. The myxoma may simulate a cystic lesion because of its honeycomb appearance in roentgenograms. Expansion of the bone cortex occurs with the appearance of mucoid material replacing bone architecture. The chondroma arises from aberrant fetal cartilage in specific regions of the mandible, such as the symphysis, coronoid and condyloid processes, as well as the alveolomalar and the paraseptal cartilages of the maxilla. The chondroma may cast a faint shadow outside of the bone in roentgenograms. A chondroma may calcify and cease to enlarge, in which case it is known as an osteochondroma. Both forms of this precocious tumor occur early in life. Myxomas, chondromas, and the osteochondromas may be detected clinically by pain, swelling, and limitation of motion. These tumors grow slowly. They are extirpated surgically.

Some osteochondromas tend to undergo malignant change, thus becoming chondrosarcomas. Chondrosarcomas consist of cartilagenous masses, areas of ossification, and mucoid degeneration. In young individuals they occur between bone and periosteum in areas of active bone growth. Cortex and spongiosa become secondarily invaded. These tumors are extremely difficult to eradicate, hence conservative surgical intervention is never attempted. The absence of early subjective symptoms leads to undetected progression of the disease. The his-

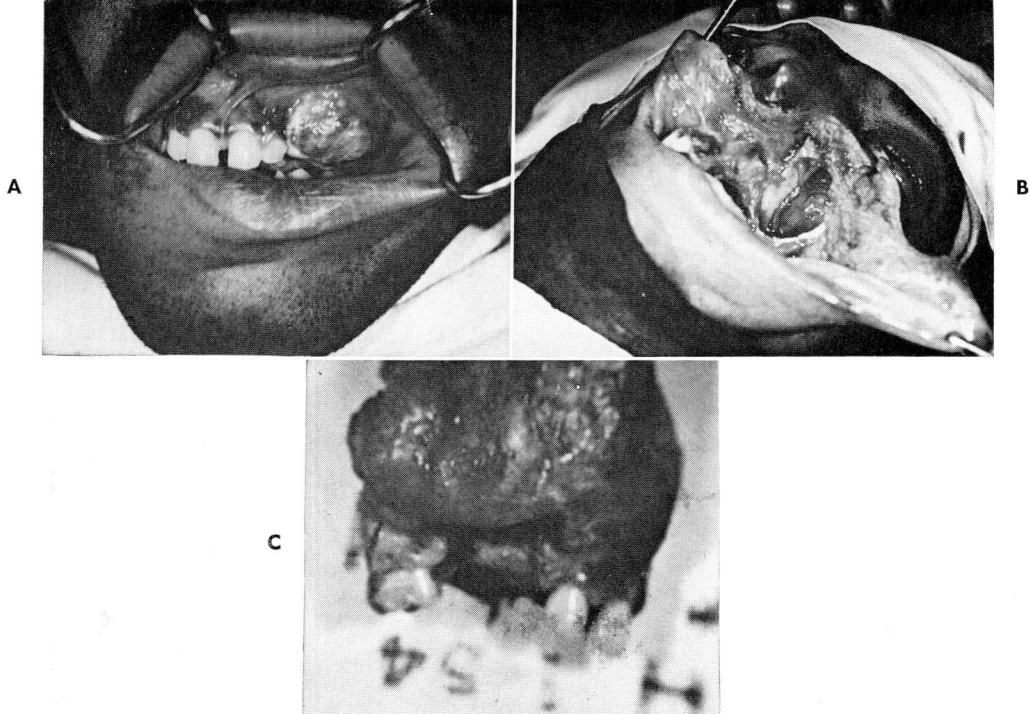

Fig. 24-5. **A,** Chondrosarcoma of maxilla. Early treatment with x-irradiation and radium application did not demonstrate beneficial results. **B,** Excision of tumor area through external approach. Invasion of the nasal fossa and anterior portion of the antrum had occurred. Exposure was sufficient for extirpation of the tumor. **C,** Specimen consisting of excised tumor and the immediate surrounding structures.

topathology of the chondrosarcoma is very obscure, thus making early diagnosis difficult. Surgical intervention with its necessary trauma stimulates cellular activity. Radical resection of chondrosarcoma is performed with thoroughness by including in the excision some of the normal bone surrounding the tumor mass (Fig. 24-5). The resulting cavitation is adequately electrocauterized. Although this tumor spreads principally by local extension, it tends to metastasize elsewhere in the body. Radiation therapy does not seem to have any beneficial effects on chondrosarcomas.

Sarcomas. Osteogenic sarcomas originate from bone-producing cells. These highly malignant tumors are rare and generally occur in children during periods of active growth. Three general types are recognized:

1. *Osteolytic* sarcomas, accompanied with considerable bone destruction and immature tumor cells with little new bone formation
2. *Osteoblastic* sarcomas, producing abundant new bone with manifestations of smaller areas of tumor activity interspersed throughout the bone
3. *Telangiectatic* sarcomas, highly vascular, developing more rapidly, and invading by extension into the surrounding soft tissue

Trauma is considered the main etiological factor in the history of all osteogenic sarcomas. The subjective symptoms include pain, swelling of the jaw bone, interference with jaw function, and loosening and displacement of the teeth. Roentgenograms reveal a poorly demarcated tumor mass with areas of bone destruction and areas of new bone formation giving a sort of mottled appearance. The characteristic "sun-rays" appearance in the osteoblastic sarcoma results from the radiating spicules of bone extending outward from the cortex. The more poorly differentiated forms of osteogenic sarcoma develop rapidly and invade surrounding tissues. The sclerosing and osteoblastic forms seem to grow slowly. All types of sarcomas metastasize to the lungs through the bloodstream. Treatment of osteogenic sarcoma is instituted very early and consists of radical resection of the bone containing the tumor. The adjoining blood supply leading into the tumor mass is included in any attempts of resection. Roentgenograms of the chest are taken early to detect any metastatic lesions. X-irradiation is given to these metastatic areas. Some clinicians believe preliminary x-irradiation of primary sites is helpful in reducing the incidence of metastatic lesions. Bone grafting of the sectioned portion of the jaw bone is not indicated at the time of surgical intervention because of the high incidence of metastasis and exposure of the areas to x-irradiation. A prosthetic appliance is positioned immediately after resection to maintain jaw bone continuity until bone grafting is possible (Fig. 24-6). This maintains facial form and aids jaw function. Prognosis is very poor since much depends upon the accessibility of the tumor, its state of activity, the presence of metastasis, and the thoroughness of operative intervention.

Ewing's tumor. Ewing's tumor is of very obscure etiology. It is believed to arise from the endothelial lining of the blood and/or lymph vessels. Some pathologists regard the tumor as a primary lymphoma of bone. Trauma is the common important factor in its etiology. This neoplasm is seen during the first two decades of life. Subjective symptoms include elevation of body temperature, pain, swelling, and interference with jaw function. The last three subjective symptoms are the usual triad noted with bone sarcomas. Roentgenograms reveal expansion of bone cortex with apparent areas of increased density. The periosteum is thickened and pushed away from the bone. Areas of new bone are formed over areas of bone destruction. Treatment of Ewing's tumor is primarily by x-irradiation

Fig. 24-6. **A,** Defect following excision of osteogenic sarcoma. Metallic appliance placed to maintain mandibular relation. **B,** Intraoral fixed appliance positioned to maintain mandibular relations and function.

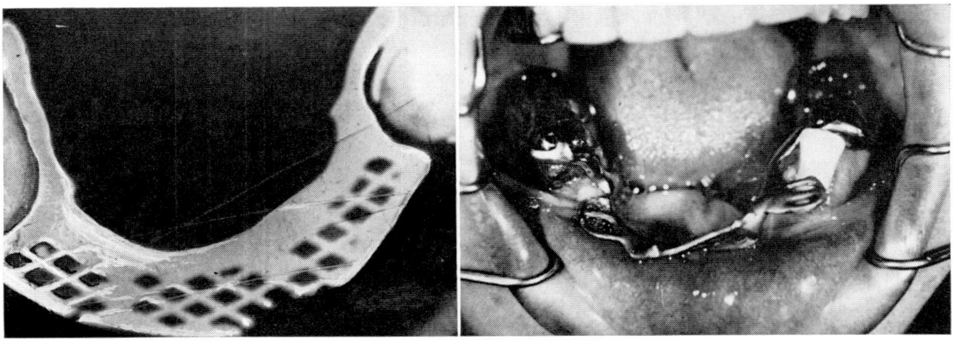

since the growth is extremely radiosensitive. This may be followed by radical surgical treatment after the acute symptoms caused by x-irradiation subside. Metastasis occurs in almost all cases of Ewing's tumor. Favorite sites for metastatic new growths are the lungs, lymph nodes, spine, and ribs. The prognosis in Ewing's tumor is very grave since less than 20% survive once metastasis has occurred.

Multiple myeloma. Multiple myeloma may occur anywhere in the body, although the first indication of its presence may be apparent in the jaw bone (Fig. 24-7). This tumor is of obscure etiology. It is believed to have originated from bone marrow cells. Multiple myelomas are seen in older individuals from the fourth to seventh decades of life. The ribs, sternum, clavicles, and vertebrae reveal, in 90% of cases, small, round lesions that appear radiolucent in roentgenograms. The skull and jaw bone are less often affected, but should be surveyed roentgenographically in all cases of this disease.

Pain of a wandering type is an outstanding symptom. The presence of Bence Jones bodies in the urine is a diagnostic sign. Alkaline phosphatase level is normal in multiple myeloma. Hypercalcemia is frequent. Local biopsy of an accessible lesion con-

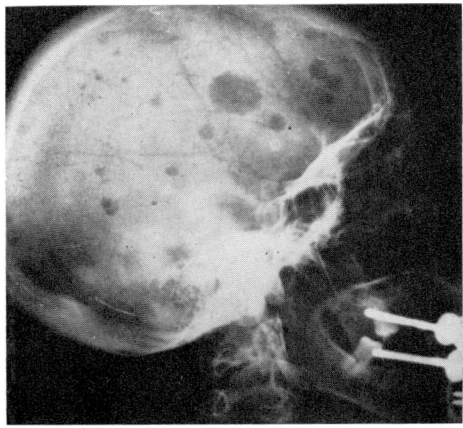

Fig. 24-7. Multiple myeloma with skull involvement in 48-year-old patient. Symptoms of pain and swelling of jaw prior to osteolytic lesions of skull and long bones. Pathologic fractures of lower jaw supported by external pin and screw fixation. Local biopsy of jaw established diagnosis.

firms the diagnosis. Anemia accompanies this disease. Fractures occur when the long bones, ribs, or mandible become involved. Treatment consists of x-irradiation of involved areas to suppress growth of tumor cells and to alleviate pain. Chemotherapy is used to augment treatment. Hormones and nitrogen mustard are employed as adjuncts in therapy. Hormones aid in alleviating pain. Chemotherapy may retard progress of the disease.

Central giant cell tumor. The central giant cell tumor is a benign neoplasm developing in bone of cartilaginous origin. The symphysis and the angles of the mandible and the canine fossa of the maxilla are typical locations. These tumors occur in the second or third decade of life, with trauma as the suspected factor. Pain and swelling of the mandible with occasional fractures occur whenever the tumor reaches a large size. Expansive enlargement of the jaw reduces the vitality of the tissue, thus precipitating fractures. Roentgenograms show no uniform, clear-cut picture of central giant cell tumor since the growth appears as multicystic areas with irregularly outlined, fine trabeculations. The teeth are frequently loosened, with evidence of absorption of their roots. Biopsy is essential to establish adequate diagnosis. These tumors destroy spongy bone and tend to thin out the cortical bone to a frail shell, thus leading to ultimate perforation. The tumor tissue is soft and highly vascular and tends to undergo free hemorrhage when traumatized. This tumor may look yellowish-red because of blood pigment.

Treatment consists of enucleation of the growth following complete exposure. The walls and bed of the resulting cavitation are thoroughly electrocauterized to destroy possible residual areas leading to regrowth. Since this tumor is benign and slow growing, conservative treatment is carried out for ultimate preservation of the bone continuity of the jaw.

TUMORS OF THE SOFT TISSUES OF THE ORAL CAVITY

Papilloma. Papillomas are benign tumors arising from the epithelial tissue of the mucous membranes of the oral cavity. They may be pedunculated or sessile and consist of keratinized epithelium on a connective tissue base. Papillomas are usually small, although they may grow to the size of a grape before the patient seeks treatment. These tumors undergo irritation from the natural dentition or artificial appliances. Malignant changes may occur following trauma. The papilloma is treated by surgical extirpation and electrocauterization of the connective tissue base. Excision is accomplished through a curved incision running around the periphery of the tumor and extending sufficiently into normal tissue to complete removal from the base of attachment (Fig. 24-8). Bleeding may be controlled with electrocautery (Fig. 24-9, A). Closure is accomplished with coaptation by means of nonabsorbable sutures. Recurrences are not common if adequate excision has been accomplished.

Fibroma. Fibromas (Fig. 24-9, B) are benign tumors arising from the submucous and subcutaneous connective tissues of the mouth and face following trauma. They may arise from the periosteum of the jaws. A fibroma is a sessile or pedunculated tumor. It is usually rounded and firm. Fibromas are more vascular than papillomas. They may assume a considerable size and become traumatized from dentures and mastication. Treatment of the fibroma is surgical excision through a curved incision in the normal tissue surrounding the periphery of the growth. The edges of the resulting wound may require freeing and undermining for some distance to permit coaptation of the edges with nonabsorbable sutures. Fibromas will not recur if complete excision, including the base, is accomplished. A fibroma may arise from the jaw periosteum as well as from the connective tissue of the submucosa. These sessile and pedunculated benign tumors are frequently called fibrous epulides.

Fibrous epulis. Fibrous epulides (Fig. 24-9, C) occur around the gingiva quite frequently and seem to arise from chronic irritation of the bone periosteum or dental periodontium attaching to the teeth. Epulides may reach the size of large grapes and may become irritated readily from the

526 Textbook of oral surgery

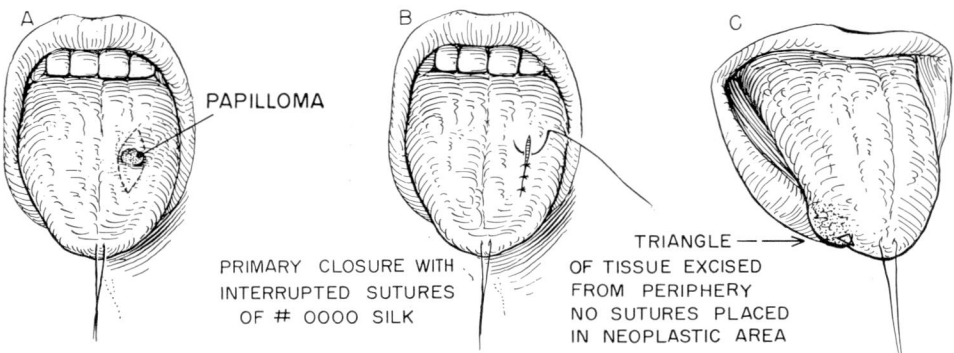

Fig. 24-8. **A** and **B**, Excision biopsy. **C**, Incision biopsy.

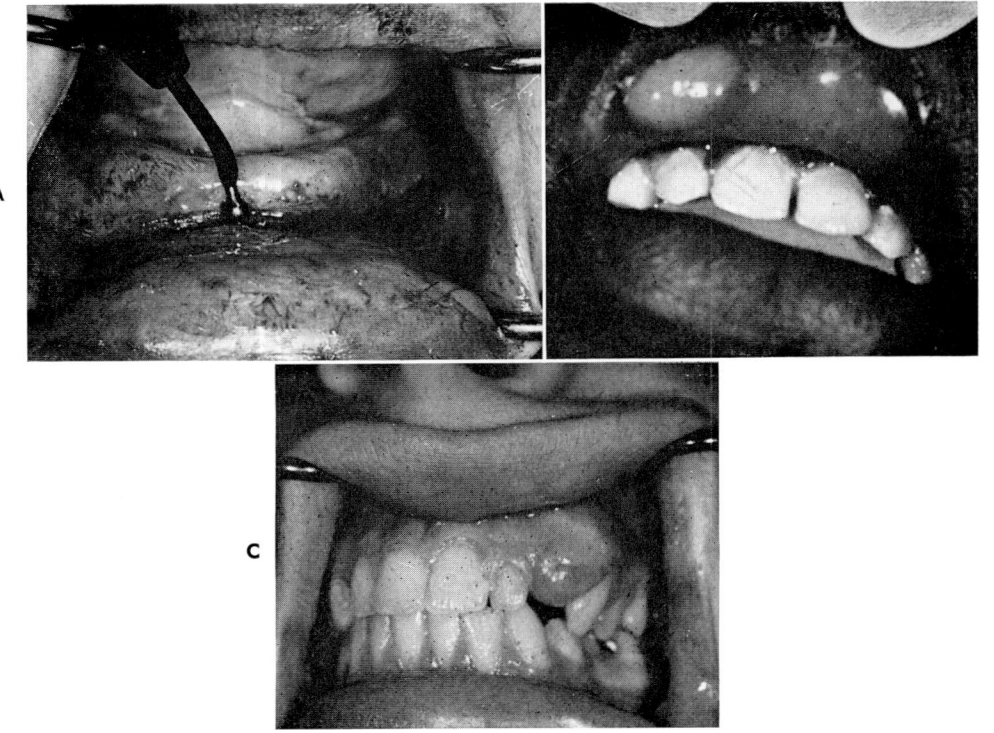

Fig. 24-9. **A**, Electrocoagulation of bleeding area following excision of small tumefaction of gingiva. Bove ballpoint used with 30 ma. **B**, Fibroma of lip. Irritation caused a connective tissue hyperplasia. **C**, Fibrous epulis. Complete excision may involve the adjoining teeth.

act of mastication. The treatment of fibrous epulis demands complete excision of the tumor from the surrounding gingival tissues whenever it is of bone periosteum origin. Epulis of dental periodontium origin calls for removal of the tooth involved in the epulis formation to obviate recurrence and ensure proper healing. Although an epulis is benign, it tends to recur if incompletely removed. The exposed bone, following excision of the epulis, is protected with a covering of surgical cement to permit normal granulation formation and act as a soothing dressing. Surgical cement packing of this type can be left in position for a period of 7 to 10 days.

Peripheral giant cell tumor. The peripheral giant cell tumor is sometimes called a giant cell epulis. It arises from the connective tissues of the dental periodontium that gives the teeth their attachment to the alveolus. This tumor is usually bluish-red because of its highly vascular nature. It may be sessile or pedunculated. Peripheral giant cell tumor occurs at any age and seems to be more common among females. It can assume an extensive size when it pushes the teeth from their normal position. It invades the adjoining bone as enlargement proceeds (Fig. 24-10). Treatment of these tumors is excision. Adjacent teeth should be removed to provide access to the tumor mass. A portion of the sound gingival tissue and bone is included in the excision. The resulting cavitation is electrocauterized to destroy any residual remnants and to con-

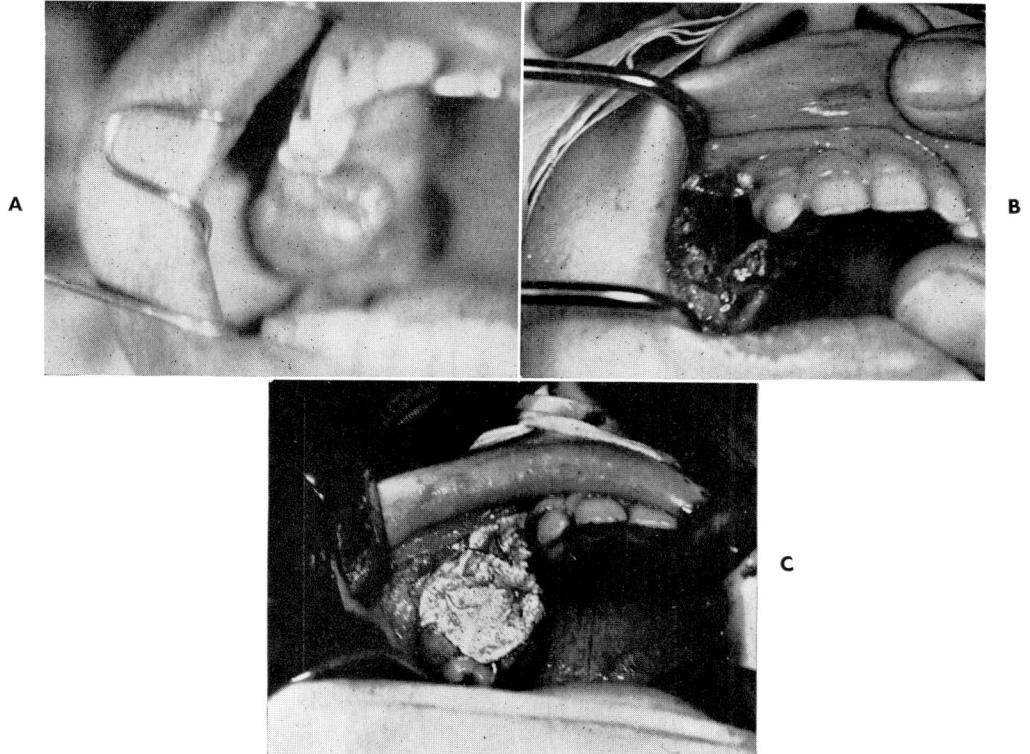

Fig. 24-10. **A,** Peripheral giant cell tumor. The tumor extends superiorly, eroding alveolar bone. **B,** Cavitation following excision and electrocauterization of base. **C,** Medicated packing stimulates healing by secondary intention.

trol bleeding. The cavitation is finally filled with a sedative pack to permit normal granulation and alleviate pain. Peripheral giant cell tumor does not recur after complete excision.

Pregnancy tumor. Pregnancy tumors arise on the gingival tissues of the jaw bones as pedunculated growths during pregnancy as a result of an obscure hormonal reaction. They appear about the second or third month of pregnancy and persist until parturition, when they begin to disappear. A pregnancy epulis consists of highly vascular connective tissue. It is bluish-red, fading slightly on compression, occurring in either dental arch, and bleeding readily on the least trauma. Pregnancy tumors attain considerable size, are unsightly, and may interfere with mastication. Treatment of a pregnancy tumor is local excision followed by electrocoagulation when the tumor is large, to ease the patient's state of mind. Surgical intervention offers better results after parturition whenever they persist since the stimulating hormonal factor is then absent. Pregnancy tumors may be multiple.

Hemangioma and lymphangioma. Hemangiomas and lymphangiomas arise in connection with the blood vessels and lymphatics. They are benign tumors, seem to exhibit a congenital trend, and appear in the young. Their etiology is very obscure, being attributed to aberrant remains of developing blood and lymph tissue elements within areas in which they are not usually found.

Hemangiomas may be classified into capillary and cavernous types. Capillary hemangioma is known as "port-wine stain." It may occur on the face or within the mouth. This tumor fades upon compression and presents a dark, bluish-red hue. The cavernous hemangioma has large blood sinuses and tends to invade the soft tissue or erode the adjoining bony structures by pressure. A pulsation may be detected in the cavernous types. Preliminary biopsies of these bluish, pulsating lesions should never be attempted in the office because of extensive hemorrhage.

Capillary hemangioma has been treated by local excision when the tumor was small. Injection of boiling water into the afferent vessels has been employed to sclerose the vessels. Radium applications and x-irradiation have been used to accomplish the same results. Conservative measures are followed in children. Excision and skin grafting is the treatment of choice in adults whenever surgical intervention is justified. Radium applications and x-irradiation are deferred in infants whenever possible, to obviate injury to developing teeth and jaws.

Cavernous hemangiomas involving soft tissues of the oral cavity may be excised with scalpel or endothermy knife. The incision should extend around the tumor in normal tissue. Feeding vessels are isolated and ligated prior to extirpation of the tumor. Sclerosing solutions have been employed successfully prior to surgical treatment to reduce the size of the hemangioma by fibrosing the feeding vessels. Sotradecol, 3%, 1 to 5 ml., is injected into the afferent vessels. Boiling water may be used in the same fashion. Reduction of tumor size lessens the possibility of injury to adjacent vital structures and enhances esthetic results. Excision with electrocautery may lead to sloughing of wound margins, thus interfering with closure.

Interosseous hemangiomas do not present a clear radiographic appearance and may simulate other osseous lesions such as giant cell tumors, traumatic bone cysts, fibrous dysplasias, or ameloblastomas. Changes in normal bony architecture are poorly defined with lytic areas in the medullary portions. A history of swelling, bleeding from gingival tissue, and mobility of teeth should be an admonition of uncontrollable hemorrhage following a minor surgical procedure in the area. Treatment of the cavernous hemangioma of the jaws is wide local excision under controlled conditions. Hypotensive anesthetic management, ligations of major blood vessels, and adequate blood replacement are necessary adjuncts of the surgical treatment. Dressings of medicated packs are employed and renewed during healing.

The *lymphangioma* is a benign tumor frequently occurring on the lips and cheek, but it may occur in the nasopharynx and tongue. It presents a soft, doughy texture of the tissues. The overlying skin tends to present a wrinkled appearance. Distortion occurs as a result of periods of active growth followed by formation of fibrous tissue. Treatment of the lymphangioma is surgical excision when the tumor has not assumed a large size. Large tumors may be reduced surgically by partial excision in succeeding operations. Sclerosing solutions have been employed with some success for further reduction of drainage channels to these tumors. The lymphangioma is radioresistant. No recurrence follows complete excision.

Lipoma. Lipoma is a benign tumor consisting of adipose tissue, developing anywhere in the oral cavity where fat tissue is present. The lips and cheeks are favorite sites for this tumor. The overlying mucosa may be stretched by the pressure enlargement of the lipoma. A lipoma is a firm and freely movable mass, yellowish in color. It is demonstrable roentgenographically as a hazy mass within soft tissues. Lipoma may be single or multiple and may present extensions into the adjoining soft tissues. This tumor grows slowly.

Treatment of the lipoma is surgical extirpation. The tumor is dissected freely from surrounding soft tissues. Primary closure is accomplished with nonabsorbable sutures in the mucosal tissue and absorbable sutures in the deep layers of tissues, such as muscle.

Myoma. Myomas are benign, well-defined, muscle tissue tumors commonly occurring in the tongue, lips, and soft palate. They appear as firm, sessile masses that may not be encapsulated. A myoma presents few subjective symptoms. The patient may be aware of a painless "lump" in the tongue, cheek, or lips. The tumor is readily traumatized by mastication. Surgical excision is the treatment of choice. The growth is bluntly freed from surrounding structures through an incision in the overlying mucosa or skin. The wound is closed with coaptation sutures. Myomas rarely recur following complete excision.

Pigmented nevus. Pigmented nevi are benign, epithelial tumors seen occasionally in the oral cavity on the buccal mucosa, gingiva, and tongue. They contain melanin pigment. Nevi in the mouth may vary in color from a light blue to black. They may be flat, sessile, or papillary in form. A nevus may simulate pigmented papilloma, hemangioma, or the normal pigmented areas present in people of tropical climes. This tumor can exhibit malignant changes in later life as a result of continued chronic irritation. Symptoms of malignant change are rapid increase in growth rate, darkening in color, superficial ulceration, and bleeding on the least trauma. The nevus usually precedes the malignant melanoma. Incisional biopsy should never be attempted. The malignant melanoma can metastasize very early through the lymphatic channels to the lungs and liver. Treatment consists of very wide excision and complete dissection of the regional and related lymph nodes early in the course of the disease. This tumor is radioresistant. Prognosis is poor despite extensive radical excision.

Mixed tumor. Mixed tumors are new growths arising from salivary gland tissue. They may occur in the lips, cheeks, floor of the mouth, or soft and hard palates within the area of distribution of the major or minor salivary glands. Almost 90% of all mixed tumors occur in the parotid gland. Most clinicians agree that these tumors are of epithelial origin. Lymphoid and mucin-producing cells may be present in these epithelial patterns. The mixed tumor is encapsulated and can be defined from normal structures on palpation. They may be lobulated, firm, slightly movable. The tumor may be attached by stalks to the normal gland tissue or present extensive protrusions of the capsule into surrounding structures. Large mixed tumors of the oral cavity and major salivary glands tend to recur after removal, a result of further growth from remnants of these extensions. The growth rate is slow, but incomplete surgical intervention tends to activate recurrences. Although mixed tumors of the oral cavity are essentially benign, some may become malignant since the occurrence of regrowth is common.

The diagnosis of mixed tumor is accomplished by clinical examination and biopsy. The presence of an encapsulated, firm, lobulated tumor with well-defined borders and a history of slow growth usually indicates mixed tumor. Confirmation of the diagnosis is established by biopsy.

Treatment of mixed tumor is complete surgical removal after adequate exposure of the tumor mass; most of these tumors are radioresistant. Mixed tumors known as papillary cystadenomas (Fig. 24-11) can be easily extirpated, including their capsular extensions. Cylindromas (Fig. 24-12), on the other hand, are difficult to extirpate completely since they tend to recur because of their highly malignant nature. Electrocauterization may be necessary in some cases to destroy all residual tumor cells. Prognosis depends upon the pathological characteristics of the tumor and the success of surgery.

Adenocarcinoma. Adenocarcinoma is a highly malignant tumor usually arising from salivary gland tissue. This tumor can occur in aberrant gland tissues of the lips, cheeks, palate, and oropharynx as well as in the major salivary glands. Primary adenocarcinoma may be differentiated from the

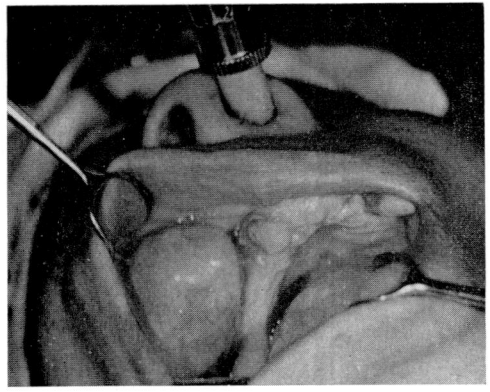

Fig. 24-11. Mixed tumor, papillary cystadenoma type. Local excision with careful dissection of the capsule is the treatment of choice.

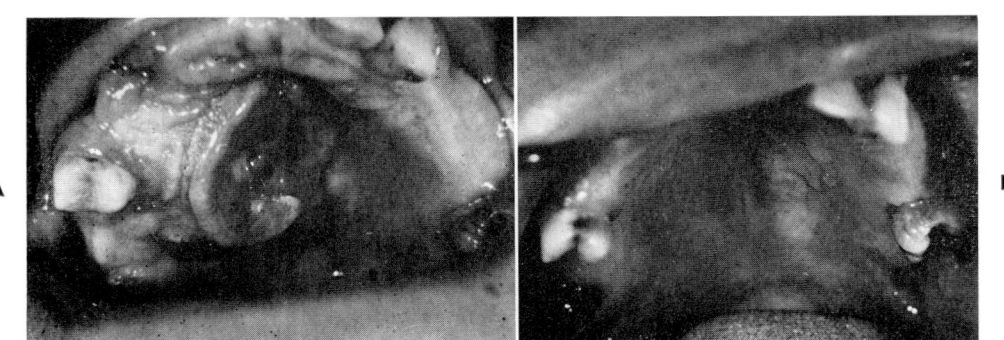

Fig. 24-12. **A,** Mixed tumor, cylindroma type. This tumor is highly malignant. Wide excision followed by electrocauterization is necessary to eradicate the neoplasm. **B,** Postoperative photograph 1 year later.

benign mixed tumor by the rapidity of growth, early pain from sensory nerve pressure, anesthesia of tissue peripheral to neoplasm, and immobility of the tumor mass from extensions into adjacent tissues. Adenocarcinomas metastasize to regional lymph nodes, lungs, and the skeletal system. Diagnosis is established from biopsy. Roentgenograms of the chest are advisable to determine the presence of metastatic lesions. Treatment of adenocarcinoma includes radical excision of the tumor and its accessible extensions. Irradiation therapy may be employed to treat distant metastatic lesions when present. Prognosis is much less favorable when metastasis has occurred.

Neurogenic fibroma. Neurogenic fibroma is a very rare tumor arising from nerve tissue. This tumor grows slowly by expansion and is therefore osteolytic in character. This benign tumor can develop into malignant fibrosarcoma and is therefore excised widely. Fibrosarcoma occurring in bone from neurogenic elements is surgically treated by extensive resection of the involved jaw.

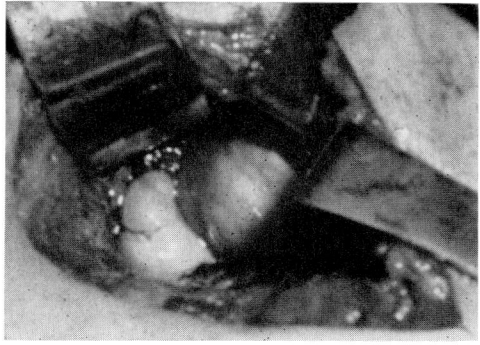

Fig. 24-13. Submandibular surgical approach to fibrosarcoma of the right pterygoid fossa. Lower jaw sectioned at angle. Dissection through medial pterygoid muscle. Patient presented with anesthesia of lower lip and temporomandibular pain of 3-year duration. Previous treatment consisted of equilibration of teeth and psychotherapy.

Fibrosarcoma. Fibrosarcoma rarely develops in the soft tissues of the oral cavity. These tumors are found occasionally in the pharyngeal region (Fig. 24-13). Ulceration of these smooth, firm tumors is rare and, according to Padgett, the point of origin is obscure.

Neurinoma and ganglioneuroma. Neurinoma and ganglioneuroma are very rare nerve tumors. A few cases of these benign neoplasms have been reported by Thoma and have been treated conservatively without recurrence.

CARCINOMA OF THE ORAL CAVITY

Carcinoma arises in connection with the cutaneous surface of the face and mucous membrane of the mouth. The *basal cell* form of carcinoma develops on the skin of the lips and face. *Squamous cell* carcinoma occurs on the vermilion borders and mucosa of the mouth. Carcinoma of the mouth accounts for approximately 5% of all carcinomas occurring in man. Carcinoma of the oral cavity develops as a result of invasion of malignant epithelial cells through the normally intact basal cell layer into subcutaneous and submucosal tissues. The etiology is obscure, although certain contributing factors may be present. *Chronic irritation* from overexposure of the lips to sunlight and traumatism by jagged teeth and ill-fitting dentures are among the predisposing factors in some individuals. The use of *tobacco* is considered as an etiological factor. Areas of leukoplakia are frequently present as premonitory lesions in the history of squamous cell carcinoma. Leukoplakia is a lesion of the mucous membranes, appearing as a painless, hard bluish-white, shiny patch. It occurs in older patients following continued, chronic irritation. Patches of leukoplakia may undergo malignant change by malignant cells in the mucosa invading the underlying tissue (Fig. 24-14, A).

Plummer-Vinson syndrome is considered a precancerous manifestation. This syn-

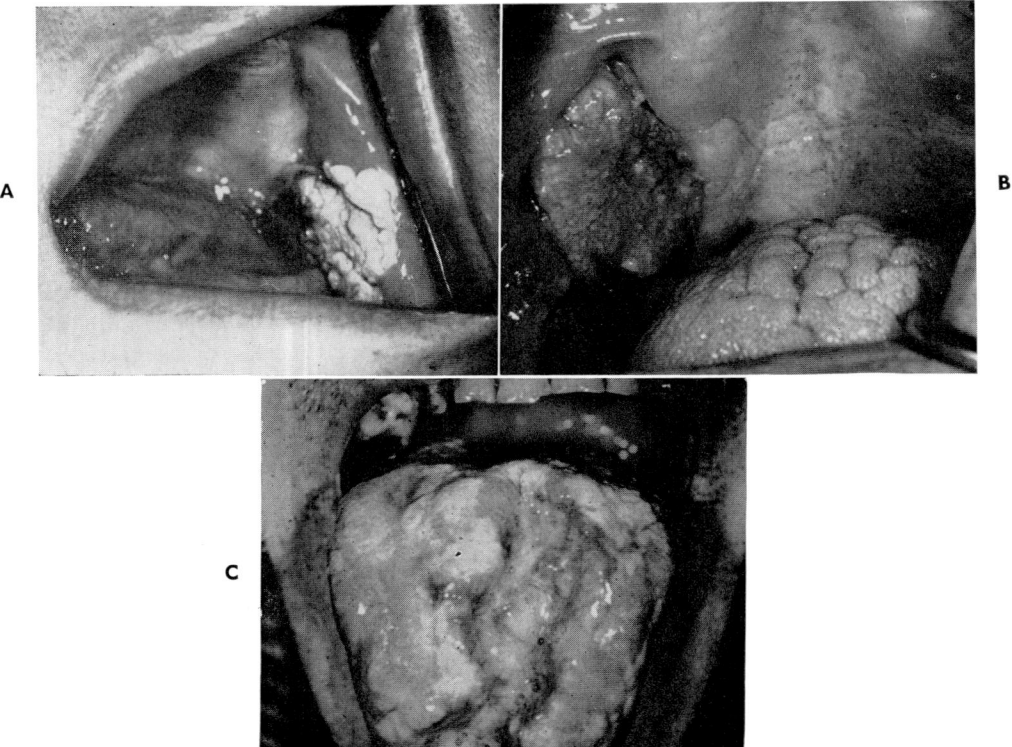

Fig. 24-14. **A**, Leukoplakia of the cheek beginning to show malignant change as demonstrated by the indurated, leathery appearance and fissuring of the surface. **B**, Squamous cell carcinoma, verrucous type, of buccal mucosa. X-irradiation and interstitial radium implantations constitute the treatment. **C**, Carcinoma of dorsum of tongue and overlying syphilitic lesion.

drome is characterized by dysphagia, glossitis, and a hypochromic, microcytic anemia. It occurs principally among females with dietary deficiency.

Carcinoma may present an ulcerative or verrucous lesion (Fig. 24-14, B). Squamous and basal cell carcinomas invade submucosa and subcutaneous tissues, including bone. They may arise insidiously with little pain in their early growth. The patient may be aware of a "blister" on the lip or an ulcer or "lump" in the mouth, which persists. Clinical examination may demonstrate an ulcerated area presenting raised or rolled borders with infiltration and induration about the margins. Induration of the surrounding tissue may not be present in early stages. Superficial ulceration or areas of leukoplakia may precede the neoplasm. Syphilitic lesions may complicate carcinoma of the tongue (Fig. 24-14, C). Carcinoma of the mouth metastasizes to regional lymph nodes during its extension. Metastasis to the cervical nodes may be detected by bimanual palpation of the local sites of lymphatic drainage. Metastatic nodes may be discrete and difficult to palpate, but lymphatic dissemination of the neoplasm has progressed. Large, extensive, fixed metastatic nodes indicate an advanced primary tumor.

Diagnosis is established from a biopsy, which is taken as early as possible with little trauma. Local anesthesia is indicated for biopsy, provided the injection is not delivered into the tumor area. Excision biopsy is done if the lesion is very small. When the lesion is large, an incision biopsy is performed prior to surgical intervention. This is accomplished by removing a wedge-shaped segment of the tumor, using the scalpel or the electrocautery (Fig. 24-8, C). The electrocautery is advantageous for controlling hemorrhage since it seals off the bleeding vessels and prevents passage of tumor cells into the circulation. Sutures are avoided to prevent extension of the neoplasm. Aspiration biopsy is useful in cases of deep, inaccessible sites of metastasis. Aspiration biopsy is performed by employing a specially constructed, large-caliber needle and glass syringe. Some tumor cells are drawn or aspirated into the syringe after the tip of the needle is introduced into the tumor bed. This technique is very difficult, even in the hands of an experienced clinician.

Biopsy material may be obtained by rubbing the tumor site gently with a sponge material, thus transferring some of the tumor cells to the sponge for histological examination. This is an adequate method when screening large numbers of patients with suspicious oral lesions. It has been employed with satisfactory results in gynecology and is known as the Papanicolaou test. A negative pathological report could be misleading because the tumor surface may contain only inflammatory exudate or necrotic tissue. A positive report would still require an incision or excision biopsy for confirmation of the diagnosis.

Treatment

Treatment planning for malignant tumors will depend upon the histology of biopsy, location of the neoplasm, its radiosensitivity, the degree of metastasis, and the age and physical condition of the patient.

The location of the tumor in the oral cavity may complicate treatment. Neoplasms in the posterior part of the mouth are less accessible and frequently encroach on vital structures. Adjunctive irradiation therapy may be indicated in certain cases. Eighty percent of cancers of the lip may be successfully treated by prompt therapy, but carcinoma of the floor of the mouth, tongue, and gingiva presents a poorer prognosis. Carcinoma arising in the posterior part of the mouth is not always diagnosed and treated early in the course of the disease. These carcinomas infiltrate rapidly into adjacent structures and metastasize early to cervical lymph nodes. Less than 25% of these neoplasms may be successfully treated following extensive metastasis.

The age and physical condition of the patient are important in the treatment plan. Aged, debilitated patients can withstand extensive surgical procedures only after careful preoperative preparation. This may delay treatment and permit progression of the disease.

Irradiation therapy. Sensitivity of the tumor to irradiation therapy influences treatment. Radiosensitive tumors may be advantageously treated with x-ray or radium emanations alone or in combination with surgery.

Treatment of carcinoma is the responsibility of a team consisting of the pathologist, radiologist, internist, oncologist, and oral surgeon. Irradiation therapy for treatment of malignant neoplasms is based upon the fact that tumor cells in stages of active growth are more susceptible to radiation than adult tissue. The more undifferentiated these cells appear histologically, the more radiosensitive the tumor is likely to be. The more the cells appear like normal adult cells, the less reaction to irradiation. Mode of action upon the active, growing neoplasm by irradiation is the immediate or delayed death of the tumor cells and a suppression of reproduction. Agents employed for irradiation are the short-wavelength roentgen rays or the gamma rays of radium. Although these agents have a selective effect upon active neoplastic tissues, normal tissue must be protected.

Three methods are generally used for application of irradiation. The emanations are delivered to the tumor area from a distance, the radioactive agents are implanted into the tumor bed, or a combination of both methods may be used with or without surgery.

X-irradiation is frequently used to sterilize the tumor from a distance outside the oral cavity. Filters of aluminum and copper may be employed to protect tissues. Intraoral cones have been devised to increase tumor dosage and reduce exposure of normal tissues. Radium can also be applied by means of an extraoral bomb. This is not always practical because of cost of large quantities of radium needed for this method. Newer methods of treatment include other radioactive metals. Radioactive cobalt is used extensively to irradiate tumor sites. Increased kilovoltage of roentgen equipment is now employed so that undesirable side effects of irradiation are reduced.

Radioactive agents such as radium, radon gas, or activated iridium can be implanted directly into the neoplasm (Fig. 24-15, A). Radium and radon gas are enclosed in gold or platinum to reduce immediate tissue necrosis and permit even distribution of the emanations. Careful irradiation treatment planning is essential so that proper distribution of the radioactive agents is accomplished to sterilize the tumor. Consid-

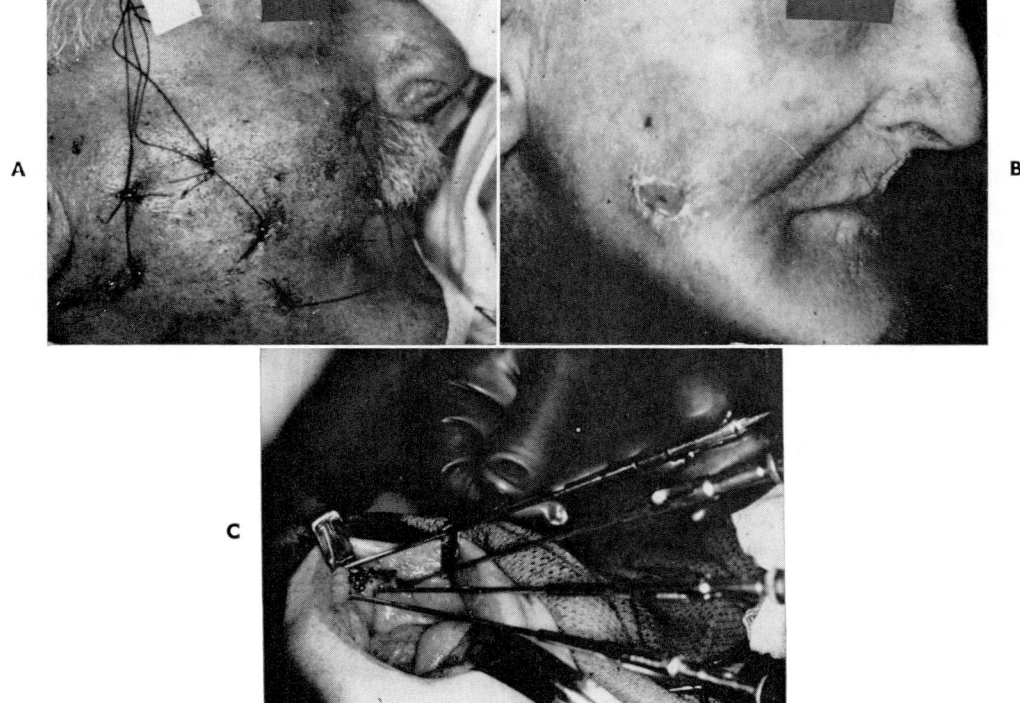

Fig. 24-15. **A,** Interstitial implantation of radium needles for squamous cell carcinoma of the buccal mucosa. **B,** Erythema of the skin 4 weeks following use of interstitial radium implant. **C,** Radon seed implantation by means of applicators to neoplasm on mucosa of cheek. Insertion is made to a predetermined depth and at calculated distances from the center of the neoplasm.

eration of the surrounding normal tissue is given since it receives some of the emanations. Areas of irradiation develop erythema (Fig. 24-15, B), and normal tissue function is impaired. Skin tolerance to irradiation must be determined to avoid severe injury. Necrosis of bone also occurs following intensive treatment. Osteoradionecrosis may follow irradiation therapy because of the interference with normal bone nutrition by the radioactive agents in the presence of infection (Fig. 24-16). Progressive necrosis can involve the entire jaw, necessitating sequestration or resection. Teeth in the irradiated area should be removed prior to therapy so that this retrograde process is avoided.

Surgical treatment. Surgical treatment of malignant tumors of the oral cavity requires wide excision. Squamous cell carcinoma of the oral mucosa invades adjacent tissues and metastasizes more readily than cutaneous carcinoma. Prompt, adequate treatment is essential to eradicate the growth. Wide excision is important since growth of the tumor extends into surrounding normal tissues with considerable invasion, which may not be visible clinically. Scalpel and electrocautery are employed to excise the tumor. Primary healing does not always occur following excision with the electrocautery since scar tissue formation is extensive in this case. Scar tissue is removed following successful treatment of malignant disease because extensive scar formation interferes with function.

Extension of the neoplasm into the periosteum and bone requires complete or partial resection of the jaw. Resection can be extensive when the bony cortex is invaded. Partial resection may be indicated whenever the periosteum alone is involved. Malignant tumors can involve the medulla of bone, thus revealing osteolytic areas in roentgenograms. Infiltrating carcinoma of the jaw may cause paresthesia by invading branches of the trigeminal nerve. Extensive resections of the jaws for squamous cell carcinoma should include an adequate resection of blood vessels of the affected side. The adjoining soft tissue should be supported whenever possible by prosthetic appliances attached to the bone stumps (Fig. 24-17). Immediate bone grafting is not advisable following radical resection for carcinoma. A period of observation is necessary to ensure no recurrence.

Squamous cell carcinoma may metastasize to the cervical lymph nodes early in the progress of the disease. Regional lymph nodes become enlarged and can be detected by palpation. These lymph nodes are

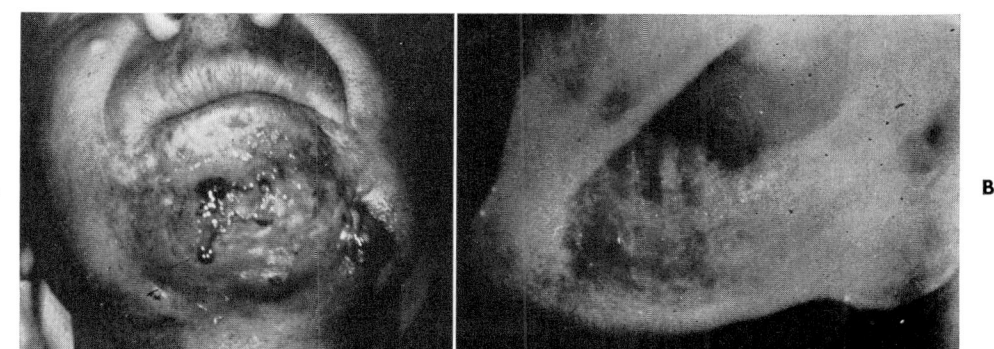

Fig. 24-16. A, Osteoradionecrosis of the mandible with draining sinuses in the overlying soft tissues. B, Early osteoradionecrosis 5 years following x-irradiation of the tonsillar region. No protection was given to the osseous structures during therapy.

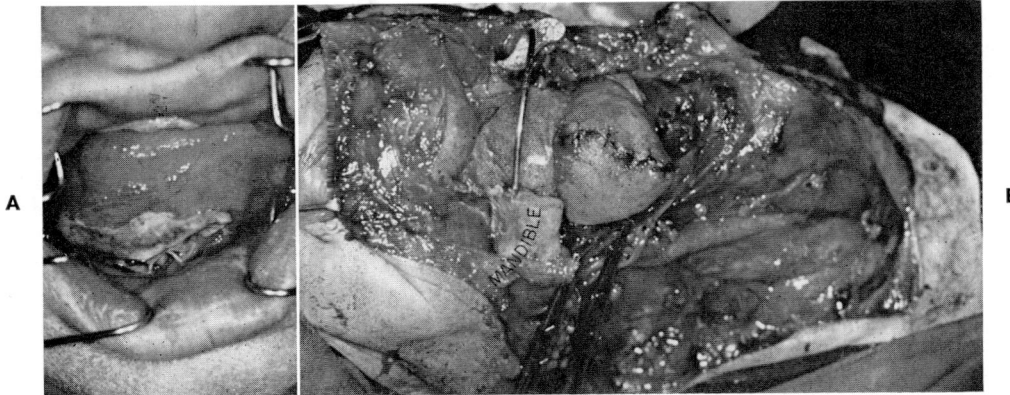

Fig. 24-17. **A,** Ulcerative carcinoma with infiltration of intrinsic and extrinsic tongue muscles. Metastasis to the cervical lymph nodes occurred on both sides. **B,** Resection of anterior third of tongue and floor of mouth and partial resection of mandible in continuity with bilateral neck dissection. Zimmer pin placed for stability of mandible.

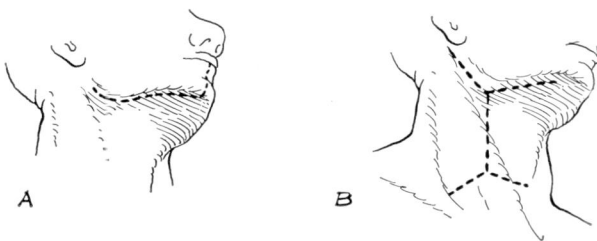

Fig. 24-18. **A,** Incision line for hemisection of mandible. Extension through lip is optional when an anterior segment of bone is resected at the symphysis. **B,** Incision lines for skin flaps for radical dissection of the cervical lymph nodes. The superior incision exposes the entire lower border of the mandible and its associated structures.

excised widely before further extension occurs. Skin flaps are reflected widely to expose underlying, involved tissues (Fig. 24-18). Although some lymph nodes within the operative field may appear normal, their removal in continuity with fascial attachments is imperative. Some normal structures are sacrificed in this procedure. Ligations and excisions of some blood vessels are necessary to control hemorrhage and completely extirpate contiguous lymph tissues. Closure is accomplished with nonabsorbable coaptation sutures after drains have been positioned to reduce hematoma formation. Pressure bandages are useful to aid healing.

Chemotherapy. New advances in therapy, better patient management, and advanced anesthetic techniques, have improved the prognosis of oral carcinoma. Infusion of chemotherapeutic agents into major blood vessels supplying tumor areas around the oral cavity has been successful in some cases. These agents seem to have a predilection for anaplastic tissues and destroy the tumor. A promising group of synthetic chemical agents used for treatment of oral cancers are the antimetabolites.

These chemicals interfere with the metabolism of the rapidly growing and dividing cancer cells. Agents such as methotrexate and 5-fluoro-uracil are infused under controlled pressure into the arterial stream nourishing the tumor site. The quantity of the chemical compound necessary for consistent cancericidal effect may have to be reduced in concentration because of depressant effects on the hemopoietic system of the patient. Nausea, vomiting, and general malaise are anticipated subjective symptoms. Remission of tumor activity occurs, and the local site usually sloughs. Follow-up treatment may be threefold and consist of additional chemotherapeutic agents, x-irradiation, and surgical extirpation of a smaller and less aggressive tumor.

Cryosurgery. Recent improvements in freezing of selected tissues have given new impetus to the treatment of benign and malignant neoplasms, and cryosurgery has recently been successfully attempted in treatment of tumors. The technique of freezing selected areas in the oral cavity is accomplished by a probe tip contacting neoplastic tissue after liquid nitrogen has entered the tip in controlled amounts. The temperature of the contacted tissues is lowered to around $-180°$ C. Cell injury and death occur as a result of this brief contact. Usual sequelae of swelling, necrosis, and slough of affected tissues follow this treatment.

The advantages with chemotherapeutic infusion agents and selective cryosurgery are inclusion of the poor-risk patient with advanced neoplastic disease, conservation of bony support to contiguous soft tissues involved with tumor tissue, minimal blood loss through a more conservative treatment, and less postoperative pain and cosmetic deformity.

Comment

The dentist has the opportunity to regularly examine patients for all aspects of oral diseases. He should maintain a high index of suspicion regarding any changes in the character of the oral mucosa. Recognition of early malignant changes in oral tissues should be a challenge and stimulate continued study to improve diagnostic ability. Prompt referral of patients for definitive treatment is most important for satisfactory results.

REFERENCES

1. Ackerman, L. V., and Del Regato, J. A.: Cancer: diagnosis, treatment and prognosis, ed. 3, St. Louis, 1962, The C. V. Mosby Co., pp. 100, 109, 111, 218, 282.
2. Anderson, W. A. D.: Pathology, ed. 4, St. Louis, 1961, The C. V. Mosby Co., p. 1319.
3. Blair, V. P., Moore, S., and Byars, L. T.: Cancer of the face and mouth, St. Louis, 1941, The C. V. Mosby Co., pp. 174, 180.
4. Blair, V. P., and Ivy, R. H.: Essentials of oral surgery, ed. 4, St. Louis, 1951, The C. V. Mosby Co., pp. 342, 507, 533.
5. Bland, S. J.: Tumors, innocent and malignant, London, 1922, Cussell & Co., Ltd., p. 236, 241.
6. Brown, J. B., and Byars, L. T.: Malignant melanomas, Surg. Gynec. Obstet. 71:409, 1940.
7. Cade, S.: Malignant disease and its treatment by radium, vol. 1, Baltimore, 1948, The Williams & Wilkins Co., p. 167.
8. Cahn, W. G.: Cryosurgery of malignant and benign tumors, Fed. Proc. 24:S 241, 1965.
9. Catlin, D., Das Gupta, T., McNeer, G., et al.: Noncutaneous melanoma, CA 16:75, 1966.
10. Crowe, W. W., and Harper, J. C.: Ewing's sarcoma with primary lesion in mandible, report of a case, J. Oral Surg. 23:156, 1964.
11. Curreri, A. R.: Current concepts and practices in cancer chemotherapy, Cancer 16:5, 1966.
12. Doner, J. M., Granite, E. L., Laboda, G., and Finkelman, A.: Primary oral carcinoma with pulmonary metastasis, report of a case, J. Oral Surg. 25:173, 1967.
13. Emmings, F. G., Koepf, S. W., and Gage, A. A.: Cryotherapy for benign lesions of the oral cavity, J. Oral Surg. 25:321, 326, 1967.
14. Emmings, F. G., Neiders, M. E., Greene, G. W., Koepf, S. W., and Gage, A. A.: Freezing the mandible without excision, J. Oral Surg. 24:145, 1966.
15. Freeman, F. J., Beahrs, O. H., and Woolner, L. B.: Surgical treatment of malignant tumors of the parotid gland, Amer. J. Surg. 110:532, 1965.
16. Geschickter, C. F., and Copeland, M. M.:

Tumors of bone, ed. 3, Philadelphia, 1949, J. B. Lippincott Co., pp. 194, 415.
17. Ivy, R. H., and Curtis, L.: Adamantinoma of the jaw, Ann. Surg. **105:**125, 1937.
18. LaDow, C. S., Henefer, E. P., and McFall, T.: Central hemangioma of the maxilla with Von Hipple's disease, a case report, J. Oral Surg. **22:**252, 1964.
19. Lewin, R. W., and Cataldo, E. Multiple myeloma discovered from oral manifestations, report of a case, J. Oral Surg. **25:**72, 1967.
20. Lichtenstein, L., and Jaffe, H. L.: Fibrous dysplasia of bone, Arch. Path. **33:**783, 1942.
21. Loré, J. M., Jr.: Head and neck surgery, Philadelphia, 1962, W. B. Saunders Co., 316, 317.
22. Marchetta, F. C., Sako, K., and Camp, F.: Multiple malignancies in patients with head and neck cancer, Amer. J. Surg. **110:**538, 1965.
23. Martin, H., Del Valle, B., Ehrlich, H., and Cahan, W. G.: Neck dissection, Cancer **4:**441, 1951.
24. Martin, H.: Surgery of head and neck tumors, New York, 1957, Hoeber-Harper, pp. 246, 248.
25. Pack, G. T., and Boyki, G. V.: Resection of mandible for medullary osteosarcoma, Amer. J. Surg. **43:**754, 1939.
26. Padgett, E. C.: Diseases of the mouth and jaws, Philadelphia, 1938, W. B. Saunders Co., pp. 507, 513, 569, 571.
27. Robinson, H. B. G.: Ameloblastomas—survey of 379 cases from the literature, Arch. Path. **23:**831, 1937.
28. Rush, B. F., Jr., and Klein, N. W.: Intraarterial infusion of the head and neck. Anatomic and distributional problems, Amer. J. Surg. **110:**513, 1965.
29. Scudder, C. L.: Tumors of the jaws, Philadelphia, 1912, W. B. Saunders Co., p. 246.
30. Seldin, H. M., Seldin, D. S., Rakower, W., and Jarret, W. J.: Lipomas of the oral cavity, report of 26 cases, J. Oral Surg. **25:**271, 1967.
31. Sherman, R. S., and Sternbergh, W. C.: The roentgen appearance of ossifying fibroma of bone, Radiology **50:**595, 1948.
32. Sullivan, R. D., and McPeak, G. J.: A favorable response in tongue cancer to arterial infusion chemotherapy, J.A.M.A. **179:**294, 1962.
33. Sullivan, R. D.: Continuous intra-arterial infusion chemotherapy for head and neck cancer, Trans. Amer. Acad. Ophthal. Otoloryng. **66:**111, 1962.
34. Thoma, K.: Oral surgery, ed. 3, St. Louis, 1958, The C. V. Mosby Co., pp. 1096, 1197, 1207, 1228.
35. Thoma, K.: Oral pathology, ed. 4, St. Louis, 1954, The C. V. Mosby Co., p. 1306.
36. Ward, G. E., and Hendrick, J. W.: Diagnosis and treatment of tumors of the head and neck, Baltimore, 1950, The Williams & Wilkins Co. pp. 315, 324, 325, 326, 351, 738, 747.
37. Ward, G. E., Williamson, R. S., and Robben, J. O.: The use of removable acrylic prostheses to retain mandibular fragments and adjacent soft tissues in normal positions after surgical resection, Plast. Reconstr. Surg. **4:**537, 1949.
38. Ward, T. G., and Cohen, B.: Squamous carcinoma in a mandibular cyst, Brit. J. Oral Surg. **1:**12, 1963.
39. Weinmann, J. P., and Sicher, H.: Bone and bones, ed. 2, St. Louis, 1955, The C. V. Mosby Co., p. 408.
40. Wilde, N. J., Tur, J. J., and Call, D. E.: Hemangioma of the mandible, report of a case, J. Oral Surg. **24:**549, 1966.
41. Willis, R. A.: The spread of tumors in the human body, St. Louis, 1952, The C. V. Mosby Co., p. 3.

Chapter 25

SALIVARY GLANDS AND DUCTS

Donald E. Cooksey

STRUCTURE OF THE SALIVARY GLANDS

Salivary glands may be divided for purposes of description into major and minor glands. The major salivary glands are the parotid, submandibular, and sublingual glands. The minor salivary glands are those smaller glands and groups of glands in the palate, buccal mucosa, and floor of the mouth that secrete primarily mucus. Since the salivary glands have frequently been described in detail in various texts on anatomy, histology, and surgery, this discussion is limited to such descriptions as are pertinent to oral surgical problems.

Gross anatomy

Parotid gland. The parotid gland (Fig. 25-1, *A*) is a paired, bilobular serous gland overlying the masseter muscle. It extends upward to the level of the auditory canal and downward to, and frequently below, the lower border of the mandible. Posteriorly it wraps itself around the posterior border of the mandible, and anteriorly it extends into the buccal fat pad, where it gives off its excretory duct. In the fat substance a small lobule of gland usually attaches itself to the duct. The superficial lobe and the deep lobe are connected by an isthmus at the posterior border of the gland.

The motor portion of the seventh cranial, or facial, nerve emerges from the stylomastoid foramen and passes laterally and anteriorly to the isthmus, where it divides into two main branches. These branches pass above and below the isthmus between the lobes, branching and rejoining along their course. Thus, the seventh cranial nerve is deep to the superficial lobe of the parotid gland and passes between the lobes rather than within the parotid substance. As a result, it is possible to remove the superficial lobe without sectioning the nerve.

The parotid duct passes anteriorly and medially from the gland along the lateral border of the masseter muscle and turns at a right angle around the anterior border of the masseter muscle. It then penetrates the buccinator muscle and the oral mucosa and opens, at the level of the neck of the maxillary second molar, into a small caruncle. Thus, from 1.5 to 3 cm. of the duct is accessible from the mouth. Dissection through the mouth past the right angle turn at the anterior border of the masseter muscle is most difficult; and an element of risk is present since portions of the seventh cranial nerve may be encountered at this level.

Submandibular gland. The submandibular gland (Fig. 25-1, *B*) is a paired mucoserous gland lying in the submandibular space. It extends inferiorly to the digastric muscle, superiorly to the mylohyoid muscle, anteriorly to the midbody of the mandible,

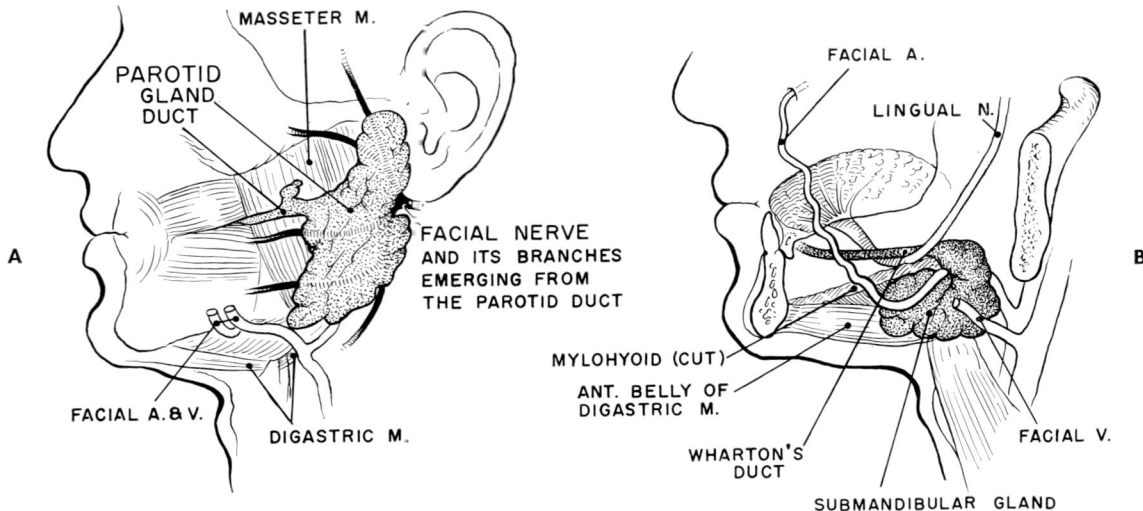

Fig. 25-1. **A**, Anatomical relations of parotid gland and duct. **B**, Anatomical relations of submandibular gland and duct.

and posteriorly to the angle of the mandible. It is bordered laterally by the medial border of the mandible and medially by the hyoglossus muscle. Inferolaterally it is covered by the skin and platysma muscle.

At the posterior border of the mylohyoid muscle the submandibular gland turns up and forward, entering the sublingual space and giving off its excretory duct. The duct passes anterosuperiorly in the sublingual space and opens into the mouth beneath the anterior portion of the tongue at a caruncle lateral to the lingual frenum. In its course the duct travels from lateral to medial and from below upward, crossing beneath the lingual nerve at the level of the third molar and then above the lingual nerve at about the level of the second molar. Thus, in a transoral procedure for removal of a stone, the lingual nerve would be encountered above the duct posteriorly, but beneath the duct or not at all from the second molar forward.

The facial artery passes from behind and medial to the gland up and over the gland to emerge from the submandibular space laterally and proceeds into the face at the level of the anterior border of the masseter muscle. Thus, the facial artery would not be encountered in the incision for removal of the gland, but would have to be located by dissection. Its location is usually indicated by the presence of two lymph nodes, the prevascular and retrovascular nodes, which overlie it at the level of the inferior border of the mandible. Superior and deep to these nodes is the marginal mandibular branch of the seventh cranial nerve, and posterior to the nodes is the facial vein. Since the facial vein is lateral to the gland, this vein may be cut in the incision and cannot be depended upon as a landmark once it has been disturbed.

Just medial to the course of the facial artery, at the superior pole of the gland and at the posterior border of the mylohyoid muscle, are several ganglionic connections from the lingual nerve. The submandibular ganglion is included in this plexus, but is seldom identified at surgery. The lingual nerve may be identified above these connections and follows an anterior and medial course into the sublingual space in proximity to the submandibular duct.

The hypoglossal nerve and sublingual vein cross the lateral surface of the hyoglossus muscle in the medial wall of the submandibular niche. They are separated from the gland capsule by a thin layer of fascia, through which they may be identified, and therefore need not be disturbed. The hypoglossal nerve and sublingual vein, together with the posterior border of the mylohyoid muscle and the pulley of the digastric muscle, form a triangle having the hyoglossus muscle as its floor. By spreading the fibers of the hyoglossus muscle at this point the lingual artery may be exposed.

Sublingual gland. The sublingual gland is a paired mucous gland lying in the sublingual space, above the mylohyoid muscle, in a line parallel to the course of Wharton's duct. Its landmark is a ridge, called the plica sublingualis, which runs anteroposteriorly in the floor of the mouth. It secretes principally mucus from a series of small short ducts, which vary in number from person to person, and seldom becomes involved in the problems of its fellows, the submandibular and parotid glands. Occasionally, glands normally occupying the anatomical position of the sublingual gland attach to the submandibular duct and open into it rather than into the mouth.

Minor salivary glands. The minor salivary glands are scattered throughout the oral mucous membrane and are simply clusters of mucous acini attached to short ducts that open into the mouth. They are sometimes clustered in groups, as are those beneath the tongue, and their ducts emerge in large numbers in relatively small areas. These glands are very superficial, lying just beneath the mucosa.

Microscopic anatomy

Microscopically these glands are all very similar in construction, being composed of mucous or serous acini or combinations of both. The primary differentiating characteristic in any given fragment of tissue is the relative number of mucous or serous forms, the parotid gland being almost entirely serous.

Since the minor glands and the sublingual glands are very simple systems, their epithelium-lined excretory ducts are small and short. The parotid and submandibular duct systems are composed of a series of very small ducts that drain a single acinus and join to make larger ducts. These larger ducts drain lobes and in turn join the principal excretory duct to the mouth. Thus, if the ductal pattern were seen in its entirety, it would resemble a leafless tree with the termination of each twig an in-

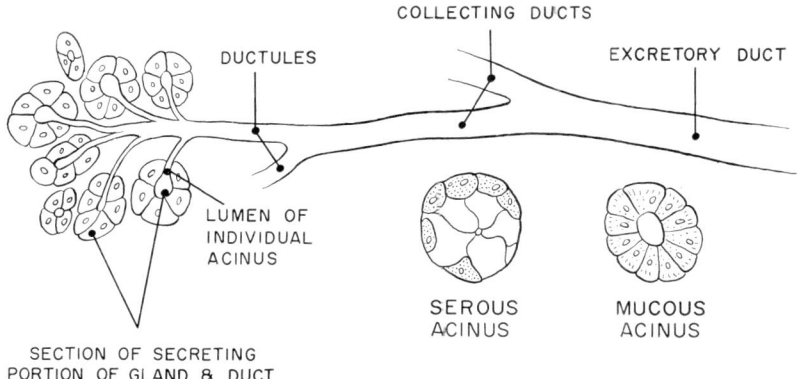

Fig. 25-2. Microscopic anatomy of salivary glands.

dividual acinus, the branches the lobular ducts, and the trunk the main excretory duct (Fig. 25-2).

The principal tissue elements seen microscopically are glandular epithelium representative of the secretory portion of the gland, cuboidal epithelium lining the ducts, connective tissue compartments dividing the individual lobes, and a capsule of connective tissue.

Anatomical weaknesses

Study of the salivary glands reveals several distinct anatomical weaknesses. The minor glands and the sublingual glands, having short, straight, simple duct systems, are seldom affected by inflammatory conditions, but may react to anything causing partial closure or rupture of the duct. A mucocele is the usual result. Complete closure produces atrophy of the gland.

The other systems have more serious weaknesses. First, the entire submandibular gland and duct system lies in a dependent position, which predisposes it to retrograde invasion by oral flora. Second, both the submandibular duct and the parotid duct are slightly larger along their course than at their caruncle. This permits storage of secretions so that a ready flow may be available on stimulation without waiting for the secretory process. This relatively static reservoir, however, permits settling out of epithelial cells and inspissation of salivary fluids, which tend to form obstructions and are a ready nidus for bacterial activity. Third, both the submandibular and the parotid ducts make a radical turn along their course. The submandibular duct turns sharply at the posterior border of the mylohyoid muscle, just anterior to the hilus of the gland. The parotid duct turns sharply at the anterior border of the masseter muscle, fairly close to the caruncle. These two areas are favorite points of lodgment of obstructions, just as the mechanical aspects of the arrangement would suggest. Finally, since both glands are dependent on one mode of disposal of secreted fluids, anything tending to reduce the flow tends also to alter the composition and function of the glands.

DISEASES OF THE SALIVARY GLANDS
Inflammatory diseases
Acute sialadenitis

Any acute inflammation of the salivary glands may be termed acute sialadenitis. What is discussed in this instance, however, is the nonspecific acute adenopathies not related to any other condition.

Symptoms. These swellings are usually sudden in onset, although they may be the acute phase of some chronic condition. The gland becomes sore and tense, usually on one side only, and pus may be seen at the orifice of the duct or may be milked from the duct system. The patient's temperature may rise, and the blood picture will reflect the relative toxicity of the infection. If uncontrolled, these infections will sometimes localize beneath the skin and require incision and drainage.

Etiology. Smears and cultures to determine the predominant organism reveal a wide range of bacteria, most of which are normally found in the oral cavity. These include *Streptococcus salivarius* and *Streptococcus viridans, Diplococcus pneumoniae,* and *Staphylococcus pyogenes* var. *aureus* and *Staphylococcus pyogenes* var. *albus.* Occasionally yeast forms are found. Thus, evidence does not indicate any specific cause or predominant pathogen. Acute stomatitis seldom plays an appreciable role in the onset of such conditions.

Treatment. Treatment of these infections is by medicinal means. Use of antibiotics or sulfonamides to control the acute infection is indicated. If a sample of pus is obtainable, tests for specific antibiotic sensitivity are of great help. Care should be taken when making the culture to obtain the secretions of the duct rather than samples of the oral flora.

After the acute phases of the infection subside, or the patient is under adequate antibiotic control, the duct may be dilated with a blunt probe to assist drainage. Sialograms aid in assessing the cause or amount of damage and frequently are of great assistance in treatment because of the antimicrobial effect of the iodized solution used to make them. Adequate hydration of the patient is important, and the use of sialogogues to increase the salivary flow and produce a washing action may be beneficial.

Prognosis. Once established, this condition tends to recur. Frequently the recurrent disease takes the form of a chronic or subacute type, and later in the course of the disease, obstructions may appear in the duct, or cavitations may appear in the gland structure.

Differential diagnosis. Occasionally one sees conditions that may be confused with acute sialadenitis, and vice versa. Unilateral epidemic parotitis, for example, is always a consideration in differential diagnosis. Often one sees cases of what has been termed idiopathic parotitis or submandibular adenitis for want of a better understanding of the condition. In these instances the gland has become hard and tender. No increase in temperature and no pus formation occurs. Sialograms reveal no evidence of disease, and the gland and duct substances appear normal. This condition is recurrent and subsides variously after administration of antibiotics, antihistaminics, or lemon drops, after massage, or upon neglect. Two possible explanations have been advanced for this phenomenon: (1) that it is caused by the presence of small mucous plugs, which eventually pass out of the salivary caruncle when placed under enough pressure, and (2) that it is caused by the transmission of noxious stimuli to the sympathetic nerves supplying the mucous acini, which produces hypersecretion of mucus and relative stasis as a result of increased viscosity.

Not infrequently the lymph nodes within the submandibular gland substance become enlarged. This enlargement may be accompanied by adenopathy of the adjacent prevascular and retrovascular nodes and is usually the result of infection higher in the head or jaws; but it simulates inflammation of the submandibular gland. Upon palpation the vascular nodes can be separated from the gland and trapped against the mandible; however, the intraglandular node stays with the gland and is difficult to differentiate from glandular adenopathy except by the size and texture of the remainder of the gland. A similar situation obtains with the parotid gland, a frequent cause being minor infections of the eye.

Chronic sialadenitis

Any of the acute salivary gland infections just described may become chronic. The chronic disease, however, is most frequently found behind an obstruction that has produced long periods of stasis. In this condition, the duct system dilates and exerts pressure against the adjacent gland. Obstruction and stasis increase the pressure, and atrophy and fibrosis of the gland occur. The gland becomes firm and hard, and may or may not be tender, depending upon the phase of the inflammatory change and the degree of chronicity. Abscesses and cysts may occur in the gland substance that require drainage, or they may smolder for years in a series of remissions and recurrences. Conservative treatment in the form of removal of the obstruction, dilatation of the duct, and diagnostic and therapeutic sialography may abate the condition. Unfortunately, recurrence is not unusual, and surgical removal of the gland may be necessary.

Chronic sialadenitis may also follow long periods of general anesthesia, general debilitation, pneumonia, or other diseases involving high febrile courses, or any factor possibly tending to produce long periods

544 *Textbook of oral surgery*

of dehydration, all of which permit bacteria to retrograde and incubate in the duct system. The resultant sialodochitis produces strictures of the duct, stasis, dilatation, and chronic infection that resists permanent cure.

Diseases due to obstruction
Sialolithiasis

The series of events leading to both gross and microscopic chronic inflammatory changes in salivary glands is somewhat obscure. It is well known, however, that one of the most prominent signs is the production of a salivary stone, or sialolith. The most popular theory of sialolith formation is that an accretion of mineral salts forms in and around a soft plug of mucus, bacteria, or desquamated epithelial cells. This theory seems to be well founded, in that some sialoliths are quite radiopaque and well calcified, whereas others are soft and rubbery and are not demonstrable radiographically. Sialoliths occur in a wide variety of sizes and shapes, a fact indicating that their development is progressive once they become lodged in the duct. The development of a sialolith inevitably leads to stasis and infection of the duct system and produces the changes described under chronic sialadenitis.

Symptoms. Symptomatically, the gland involved may swell, especially at mealtimes, and may become tense and sore. This swelling and tenderness may subside, only to recur later. Pus may be seen at the orifice of the caruncle, which may be inflamed, and pus or cloudy saliva may be obtained by milking the gland. The stone may be palpable by bimanual manipulation and may be movable up and down the duct. The stone may be visualized in radiographs, and dilatation at the site of the stone and of the ducts of the gland will be evident in a sialogram.

Management. Management of these stones is surgical. Generally the stone can be removed transorally; however, extreme damage to the gland or recurrence of the disease after transoral removal of the stone may indicate removal of the gland (Fig. 25-3).

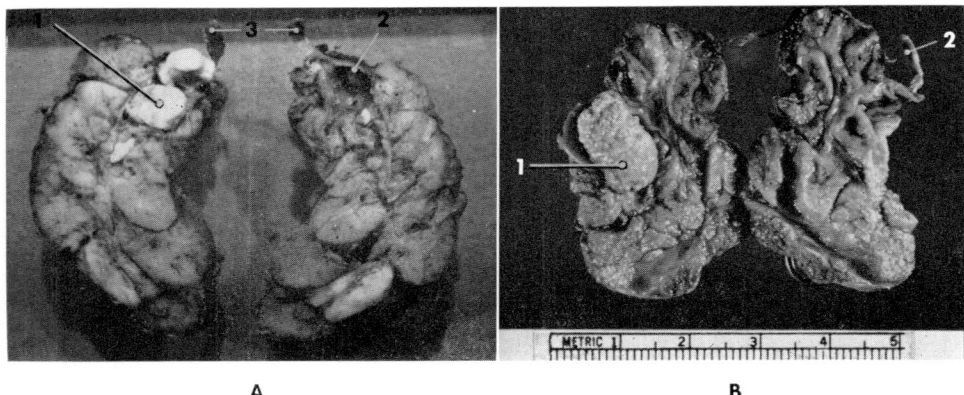

Fig. 25-3. **A,** Surgical specimen of a submandibular salivary gland containing several large stones. 1, Clump of four stones in the pelvis of the gland; 2, gland pelvis showing dilation of the pelvis from the stones; 3, submandibular duct, demonstrating the relative size of the stones compared to the duct. **B,** Surgical specimen of submandibular salivary gland containing one large stone. 1, Solitary stone in the pelvis of the gland; 2, duct of the gland demonstrating difference in size of duct and stone. Stones such as shown in **A** and **B** are difficult to remove transorally and not infrequently do sufficient damage to the gland during their tenure to require their ultimate removal.

Sialoangiectasis

This term is employed to describe a gland and duct system vastly dilated by stasis of salivary secretion resulting from obstruction. The most frequent cause is a sialolith, although a simple stricture may be the cause. It is not unusual to observe glands with a long history of chronic infection from no obvious cause that demonstrate this extensive dilatation.

The prognosis for such glands is poor since their natural history is one of repeated acute attacks ultimately resulting in removal of the gland.

Retention cysts

Retention cysts result from rupture of a duct into the gland parenchyma. This rupture fills with salivary secretion and is eventually encapsulated with fibrous connective tissue. A complete or partial epithelial lining may or may not be present.

Since these cysts seal themselves off from the duct system, they do not fill with radiopaque contrast medium in sialography; instead, they demonstrate themselves radiographically as nonfilling, space-occupying defects in the gland substance. They may have an obscure opening into a duct, which permits them to drain and refill periodically, but which does not admit the radiopaque oil. For this reason, they are prone to enlarge and subside (a characteristic that readily differentiates them from mixed tumors, which do not subside). To palpation they are usually soft and may be doughy or fluctuant; and they are sometimes tender. (Mixed tumors are hard and seldom tender.)

Treatment. Surgical removal is the treatment of choice. This is necessary not only to eliminate the lesion, but to establish the diagnosis as well. Incision and drainage usually result in eventual recurrence. Exteriorization should not be considered.

Atrophy

Degree plays an important part in the effect of obstruction on glandular tissue. Partial obstruction results in sialoangiectasis; obstruction with rupture of the duct produces retention cysts; partial obstructions are usually accompanied by infection; complete obstruction produces atrophy. Complete obstruction productive of atrophy is rare and is usually the result of surgical accident in which the main excretory duct is tied and all avenues for the escape of fluid are obliterated. Another prominent cause of salivary gland atrophy is heavy doses of irradiation, usually in the treatment of malignant tumors.

The loss of one salivary gland because of atrophy or excision is of little importance. The loss of several of the major glands, however, produces xerostomia and atypical caries.

Lack of salivary secretion, collapse of the duct, and inability to receive iodized oil for sialography are typical of this condition. No treatment is available once the atrophy has occurred.

Tumors of the salivary glands

Like tumors in most locations, tumors primary in the major and minor salivary glands can be roughly classified as benign and malignant. Even this classification will be disputed, since at least two tumors, the mixed tumor and the mucoepidermoid tumor, though benign in biological behavior at the outset, are well known to undergo malignant changes. In addition, at least one developmental defect, the branchial cleft cyst, so simulates a tumor clinically as to defy differential diagnosis short of formal biopsy. For this reason these tumors will be discussed according to their biological behavior when observed clinically. For a better understanding of these lesions, further study of the extensive pathological literature on the subject should be carried out.

Benign tumors

Salivary adenoma. This tumor is a benign neoplastic proliferation of secretory cells in a salivary gland. It is usually confined to the substance of the parotid gland.

It is firm, painless, usually well encapsulated, and slow growing, and it is readily moved from its growth site on pressure and returns to its original position on release. This is an important sign since most malignant growths are indurated and cannot be so displaced. Few, if any, visible changes appear in the sialogram, and differential diagnosis is not positive without biopsy. This tumor is regarded as biologically benign. Management is surgical.

Papillary cystadenoma lymphomatosum (Warthin's tumor). This benign and slow-growing tumor may occur anywhere in or near the parotid gland, usually in the region of the angle or ramus of the mandible or beneath the ear lobe. It is firm and nontender and may be sufficiently circumscribed to be readily moveable. Changes in the sialogram are minimal until the tumor has attained sufficient size to display nonfilling, space-occupying, tissue-displacing tumor substance. Even then, differential diagnosis is questionable without biopsy. Warthin's tumor occurs most frequently in males in their fifth decade, but it may occur in either sex and somwhat earlier or later. Management is surgical.

Branchial cleft cyst. A branchial cleft cyst is a nonneoplastic and nonmalignant developmental anomaly originating from epithelium that is enclaved between branchial arches at the time they fuse. It usually manifests itself as a swelling on the lateral aspect of the neck or in the floor of the mouth; but it is known to develop in sites adjacent to or within the major salivary glands, in such fashion as to defy differentiation from tumors of the gland by clinical means. A branchial cleft cyst is firm, but softer, as a general rule, than any of the true neoplasms. It may undergo periodic recessions, a sign that is never present in a true neoplasm. Movement may be possible, but this is not always a characteristic since the cyst may be attached to structures that move with difficulty, or it may have had a previous inflammatory episode that has produced circumferential fibrosis. During its tenure it may become tender to palpation, at which time it is usually tense and firm.

A branchial cleft cyst appears in the sialogram as a space-occupying, nonfilling defect, similar in many respects to other solid or cystic lesions of the salivary glands. Usually, however, it does not exhibit the typical "ball-in-hand" deformity common to mixed tumors.

Mixed tumors. Wide disagreement is present among pathologists as to the essential nature of mixed tumors and among surgeons as to the proper method of treating them. For clinical purposes, the most arguable question is: Are they malignant or benign? Perhaps the best way to answer this question for the clinician is to point out that since mixed tumors do not generally metastasize, or, when untouched, do not invade until late in their development, they may be regarded as benign. Unfortunately, they have a strong propensity to recur. The recurrences are probably the result of either incomplete excision at operation or multicentric origin of the lesion; they are frequently more serious than the primary lesion because pathways of invasion are opened. Some say that a mixed tumor may undergo metaplasia after surgical intervention and recur as a true malignant neoplasm. This theory leads to the differences among surgeons, who variously recommend enucleation, wide excision, or radical resection of the gland, seventh cranial nerve, integuments, and lymph node-bearing tissues that furnish drainage to the area. The best solution probably lies in the middle course, in which the lesion together with a portion of the gland supporting it is widely excised. It is seldom necessary to sacrifice the seventh cranial nerve in this procedure, and cure is the rule rather than the exception. When reoperation becomes necessary on account of recurrence, seventh cranial nerve damage is more common and the incidence of cure is reduced. This fact emphasizes the need for adequate management at the original operation.

Clinically, mixed tumors are very hard, probably, in part, because they are composed variously of epithelial and connective tissue elements. They are usually loosely encapsulated in fibrous tissue and are readily moveable, although as they advance in size, involving more tissue, they may become firmly fixed and even give the impression of induration. Recurrences, on the other hand, almost without exception are firmly fixed. Mixed tumors are generally nodular to palpation and give the impression of being composed of one or more globular masses.

Mixed tumors occur most frequently in the parotid gland, usually at the angle of the mandible or beneath the ear lobe. They occur less frequently in the submandibular gland and in the minor salivary glands of the palate and lips. (The author has not encountered this tumor in the sublingual glands, although no reason is known why these should not be affected.)

Mixed tumors are painless and slow growing and are usually brought to the patient's attention by touch while shaving or applying make-up, etc. Frequently they are thought to be wens by the patient because of their proximity to a common epidermoidal cyst-bearing area. For this reason some mixed tumors are large when first seen, whereas others are relatively small.

It is difficult to differentiate mixed tumors from the several other benign tumors of the area or from hyperplastic lymph nodes. Tissue examination is the most reliable method, and diagnosis can usually be rendered by means of frozen section with sufficient accuracy to guide the surgeon in completing the procedure. Sialograms may show displacement of the glandular structure, particularly of the superficial lobe of the parotid gland. As a result of this displacement the collecting ducts curve around the lesion, giving the appearance of a hand carrying a ball. Unfortunately this characteristic is not limited to mixed tumors, and to be present it requires that the tumor be of sufficient size to produce the deformity. For this reason, as with most tumors extrinsic to the duct system, sialograms are of limited benefit in the diagnosis of mixed tumors.

Treatment is always surgical. Since these lesions do not metastasize unless they have undergone metaplasia and are behaving like a true malignant tumor, dissection of the lymph node–bearing area appears to be excessively radical. On the other hand, in view of the well-known tendency toward recurrence, an original attempt at enucleation seems dangerously conservative. Thus, wide, adequate excision of the area, with efforts toward preservation of vital structures, seems the technique of choice. Mixed tumors do not respond to irradiation.

Neurilemoma (schwannoma). Neurilemoma is included in this discussion, not because it occurs in salivary gland tissue, but because it occasionally affects branches of the seventh cranial nerve, and because it bears such a similarity to mixed tumors clinically that differentiation is almost impossible.

This tumor is benign, slow growing, and asymptomatic. It is encapsulated and readily moveable.

No sialographic findings appear until the tumor reaches a large size; then the sialogram shows displacement of gland substance, similar in all respects to that of the mixed tumor.

The primary problem inherent in a tumor of this type is its removal. A neurilemoma is firmly attached to the sheath of the nerve that it involves, and although the tumor has no special effect on the function of the nerve, its removal usually results in damage or section of the nerve at the point of attachment. Since this lesion does not ordinarily undergo malignant transformation, it would be better left alone if the diagnosis of neurilemoma were established. All too often, however, the damage to the nerve occurs at the time of investigation, and the diagnosis arrives too late. A neurilemoma does not respond to irradiation.

Malignant tumors

Mucoepidermoid tumors. Mucoepidermoid tumors have been variously subdivided in the past into two groups, malignant and benign. Even now reasons seem adequate to believe that some are of a higher degree of biological activity than others and therefore more malignant than others. The class in general, however, is malignant and should be regarded and treated as such.

Mucoepidermoid tumors may grow either rapidly or slowly. They seldom exhibit pain unless infection or invasion of vital structures occurs. They occur most frequently in the parotid gland, but may occur anywhere salivary gland tissue exists. On palpation they feel firm, indurated, and bound down to the surrounding structures; they do not move readily.

Since mucoepidermoid tumors involve the ductal and acinar structures of the gland, changes may be observed in the sialogram. Evidence of cavitations may appear where necrosis has occurred, or of hyperplastic glandular activity with new duct formation, or of a stricture caused by the filling of a duct with neoplastic tissue. Because any of these findings may also be typical of inflammatory disease, care should be taken to coordinate the clinical and sialographic findings carefully before risking a diagnosis. In the final analysis, tissue examination is the only method by which an accurate diagnosis may be reached.

Treatment of these tumors is surgical. Resection may of necessity be more radical than in the mixed tumors, depending upon the extent of the tumor. Conservative management of the seventh cranial nerve must not be considered important; instead, the surgeon should be governed by the extent to which the lesion has invaded adjacent tissue. This is not to imply that the nerve must always be sacrificed. If conservation of the nerve jeopardizes a surgical cure, however, sacrificing the nerve is indicated. Radical neck dissections are not generally indicated unless evidence exists of regional node metastasis, although some schools of thought regard prophylactic neck dissection at the original operation as the mode of choice.

Irradiation may be of benefit in controlling metastasis or in palliative therapy, but it is not thought by most to afford a cure or to be indicated as a postsurgical prophylaxis.

Squamous cell carcinoma. Like the mucoepidermoid tumors, squamous cell carcinomas originate from the epithelium lining the salivary glands and ducts, As is not the case with mucoepidermoid tumors, however, no doubt exists about the malignancy of carcinomas, only about the relative degree of this malignancy. Although it is thought that these tumors probably originate within the ducts, invasion of the surrounding glandular tissue occurs promptly. Metastasis to the regional lymph nodes may occur early or late, depending on the individual behavior of the tumor.

The symptoms, signs, and sialographic evidence of these tumors are similar to those of mucoepidermoid tumors, and no clear-cut clinical differentiation may be made.

Treatment is also similar in all respects, with radical neck dissection figuring more prominently in the treatment by most surgeons.

Irradiation has a noticeable effect in the control of these lesions and their metastasis, particularly in the control of the more anaplastic types. However, control and palliation, rather that cure, are the usual goals of irradiation.

Adenocarcinoma. A large number of lesions, bearing an even larger number of names and subclassifications, may be grouped under the general heading of adenocarcinoma. Included in these are the pseudoadenomatous basal cell carcinoma (adenocystic basaloid mixed tumor, or cylindroma), papillary adenocarcinoma, serous cell adenocarcinoma, mucous cell adenocarcinoma, malignant oncocytoma, and malignant mixed tumor. These and many other terms serve largely to confuse the clinician. For the sake of clarity in thinking of these lesions it should be understood that all are malignant, all are potential killers, and all require some form of radical surgery or cancericidal irradiation if they are to be cured.

The symptoms of these lesions, with the notable exception of cylindroma, are generally those seen in mucoepidermoid tumor and squamous cell carcinoma. A cylindroma is usually a very slow-growing lesion, and its mild-appearing histological characteristics and growth history may lead the surgeon to believe that it is not an aggressive lesion. Actually, it has a powerful propensity for recurrence and extensive invasion with local destruction, frequently leading to successive, disfiguring operations and ultimately metastasizing to distant sites late in the disease.

Other adenocarcinomas may grow with great rapidity and may be so anaplastic in their microscopic characteristics as to defy subclassification.

Sialographic identification of an adenocarcinoma is questionable since the appearance of its internal structure may be very similar to that of any other lesion that produces spaces resulting from central necrosis. In some of the more slowly growing tumors, however, attempts by the tumor to form tissue morphologically similar to the parent tissue produce abnormal acinar structures that are capable of receiving the iodized oil and simulate hypertrophic glandular substance.

The treatment of choice is usually radical surgery. Radical neck dissection may be performed when indicated.

Irradiation is effective in individual cases, but by no means effective in all cases. Cylindroma in particular is very radioresistant. If the tumor is accessible to effective irradiation, it is usually accessible to surgery. For this reason, irradiation is usually reserved for control, palliation, and, in some cases, prophylaxis rather than for primary treatment—the condition and life expectancy of the patient and the size, grade, and location of the lesion all being factors for consideration.

DIFFERENTIAL DIAGNOSIS OF SALIVARY GLAND LESIONS

One of the principal problems associated with the treatment of salivary gland lesions is the decision of the clinician regarding the type of lesion being treated and its anatomical location in relation to the various associated structures. Cytological examination is becoming increasingly important in diagnosis because of improvements in technique and understanding of the specimens obtained. The validity of this examination and of needle biopsy depends largely upon the accuracy of the technique by which the tissues were obtained, and upon the training and ability of the pathologist responsible for analyzing the tissues. Formal biopsies are dependable, but they involve openings on the face and are contraindicated in inflammatory diseases. It rests with the clinician to decide with the nonsurgical means at hand what, if any, further steps are required to secure an accurate diagnosis. The means available are principally the history, the physical examination, and the radiographic examination. From these a rational course of treatment or further diagnostic needs can be determined. Occasionally, clinical laboratory examinations may aid in making the decision.

History

A history of the lesion concerned frequently aids in the determination of its nature.

Duration. The duration of a lesion is an important factor. If a lesion is old and has a history of remission and exacerbation, it is probably of an inflammatory nature. If it is old and has a history of slow, steady growth, it is usually a benign or very low-grade malignant tumor. If it is a new lesion with acute symptoms, inflammation is suggested. A new lesion with a painless swelling, however, is suggestive of early malignancy.

Nature of onset. The nature of the onset may offer some clue. If the onset is gradual and painless, but continuous, tumor is suggested. If it is sudden and painful, the diagnosis of inflammation is more proper, although rapidly growing tumor with overlying infection cannot be discounted.

Rapidity of growth. The rapidity of growth is a very important diagnostic point and indicative of the degree of malignancy. A slow but continuously growing lesion is seldom inflammatory or of a high grade of malignancy. A rapidly growing lesion may be either; but pain, exudate, inflammation, fever, or alterations in the differential blood count toward immaturity usually accompany inflammations. (It is to be remembered that tumors as such are not painful until they either invade surrounding sensitive structures or become infected.) Rapidly growing lesions with a history of resolution and remission are odds-on favorites to be inflammations. Slowly growing lesions with a history of remissions are usually cysts or other retention phenomena. It is not typical of any true neoplasm to remit or regress, although some will have periods of biological inactivity.

Coincidental conditions. A history of other conditions coincidental to the present complaint frequently offers a clue or an explanation of the problem. A history of juvenile tuberculosis or tuberculosis in the family may explain the presence of a calcified body in the region of a salivary gland when no connection with the gland is demonstrable. A history of pneumococcal pneumonia or other acute febrile disease may mark the beginning of chronic sialadenitis, particularly of the parotid gland. Long general anesthesias, usually with the employment of antisialogogues, are pertinent to the observation, as would be the coincidental presence of any cachectic or dehydrating condition.

Physical examination

A proper physical examination is the most important single factor in the differential diagnosis of any given condition. In addition to a general physical survey to detect systemic factors that might be contributory, a careful appraisal of the adnexa of the glands should be carried out. It is important to remember that both the submandibular and the parotid glands have adjacent lymph nodes and nodes within the glandular structure itself. Adjacent infections or tumors in the drainage areas of these nodes frequently cause swellings that only appear to be primary in the glands. Typical of such infections are those of the eye that produce enlargement of the parotid nodes, or those of the teeth that cause enlargement of the submandibular nodes. Tumors of the facial skin such as melanoma, of the oral cavity, and of the facial structures may all produce enlargements of the lymph nodes of the head and neck. Metastasis from more distant parts is relatively rare, although involvement of these nodes by the malignant lymphomas is common.

Bimanual appraisal of these lesions is a necessity, and much information can be transmitted to the examining finger. Manual examination is correctly done by placing one finger into the mouth and the opposite hand over the lesion. Careful manipulation of both hands is calculated to estimate the following circumstances.

Location of the lesion. Ductal lesions are best palpated from within the mouth when the lesion is in the submandibular duct or in the anterior third of the parotid duct. Lesions in the hilus of the submandibular gland just superior to where it passes beneath the mylohyoid muscle are also best palpated from within the mouth. Most salivary stones fall into this category.

Lesions lateral to the musculature of the

mouth can be displaced laterally by the intraoral finger and more readily felt by the extraoral hand. Portions of the gland itself can be displaced and its texture more readily felt. Nodes and swellings can be fixed and identified. Lesions not palpable or movable from within the mouth are then better related as to the relative position they bear.

Milking the gland and duct bimanually offers an estimate of the nature of the secretion and hence of the location of the lesion. Extraductal lesions seldom produce pus within the duct system unless they are so far advanced as to occlude the ducts by pressure.

Consistency of the lesion. Circumscribed lesions such as mixed tumors, enlarged inflammatory nodes, and schwannomas are readily moveable. The inference from this phenomenon is that the lesion has not invaded the surrounding tissues and is not surrounded by diffuse inflammatory exudate. Acutely inflamed areas, abscesses, invasive malignant tumors, or their lymphatic spread are not readily moveable, a result of the infiltration of the surrounding tissues by the disease. An exception is the lymph node involved in early metastasis that has not yet lost its capsular integrity.

Indurated lesions bear a graver prognosis. Although the primary differential sign between a malignant lesion and an indurated inflammatory lesion is the presence or absence of pain, this sign is not always dependable since overlying infection may be involved in any advanced malignant growth. In general, however, induration and boardlike hardness of the area in question is a grave sign, particularly if the cardinal signs of infection are absent or not in proportion to the extent and history of the change. Induration is typical of invasive malignant lesions, and this sign must be considered diagnostic until proved otherwise.

Consistency of the remainder of the gland is very important. Malignant lesions rarely involve the entire gland unless they are infected or far advanced. Thus, a portion of the gland should feel normal to the examining hand. Infections, conversely, usually produce tenseness throughout the entire gland, as does ductal obstruction.

Separation of the gland from lesions not actually involving the gland is also very important. In many cases swellings may seem to involve the gland, but palpation and fixation by finger pressure of either the gland or the lesion demonstrate that the lesion bears only an anatomical rather than a histological relation to the gland. This characteristic is particularly true of branchial cleft cysts, dermoid cysts, nodes, and inflammatory swelling primary in the teeth. In these cases the consistency of the uninvolved gland will be normal.

Many conditions have a typical consistency. Abscesses are usually fluctuant; dermoids and other thick-walled cysts are usually doughy; stones are dense and may be stellate; infected or obstructed glands are usually firm and tense. It becomes obvious that the consistency of the lesion is an important differential sign.

Subjective response. The subjective response of the patient to the bimanual examination frequently varies in accordance with the nature of the disease. Inflammatory conditions are usually accompanied by pain. This pain is increased with manipulation and is quite reliable. At the risk of repetition, it should be remembered that tumors that have become infected or have invaded sensory nerve-bearing structures may also be painful, but that pain is usually a late rather than an early sign of malignancy.

Benign tumors, low-grade malignant tumors, and early malignant tumors are seldom painful. Manipulation may be carried out without complaint from the patient until it has continued long enough to become nettlesome.

The tissues overlying a salivary stone, on the other hand, are almost always tender because of the incompressibility of the

552 *Textbook of oral surgery*

stone, the sharp processes sometimes present, and the inflammation occurring in the ducts surrounding it.

Radiographic evaluation

Ordinary radiographs are of little value except in the presence of a calcified stone or advanced invasion of nearby bony structures. For this reason routine radiography may be omitted unless the examiner has reason to suspect one of these conditions. When a salivary stone is suspected, the mandibular occlusal and the lateral oblique jaw views are of the most value in locating submandibular stones (Fig. 25-4). The posteroanterior and lateral views of the face, coupled with an occlusal film placed in the buccal parietes and shot with a very short (½ to ¾ second) exposure, may be of value in locating parotid stones. A submentovertex view outlining the zygomatic arch may also be useful.

The sialogram offers more diagnostic information. This special study is carried out by instilling radiopaque oil into the duct system of the gland and taking such views as are indicated. Many techniques and forms of equipment to accomplish this study have been described. One that has been successful in the author's hands is illustrated (Fig. 25-5).

Materials. The following materials are required:
1. Several sizes of polyethylene tubing about 18 inches in length, one end of which has been sharply and smoothly beveled
2. A Luer-Lok connector of the type employed in continuous spinal anesthesia
3. A ring-handle 3 ml. Luer-Lok syringe
4. A broken explorer, the end of which has been rounded and polished, to be used as a dilator
5. Any radiopaque oil contrast medium

Method. A length of polyethylene tubing of suitable caliber is selected and fitted into the connector. The syringe is filled with contrast medium and attached to the connector. All air is removed from the system. Extra oil will serve as a lubricant.

The syringe is detached, and the duct in question is cannulated. If pain is encountered, a few drops of local anesthetic around the caruncle may be used. If cannulation proves difficult, the explorer may be introduced to dilate the duct opening.

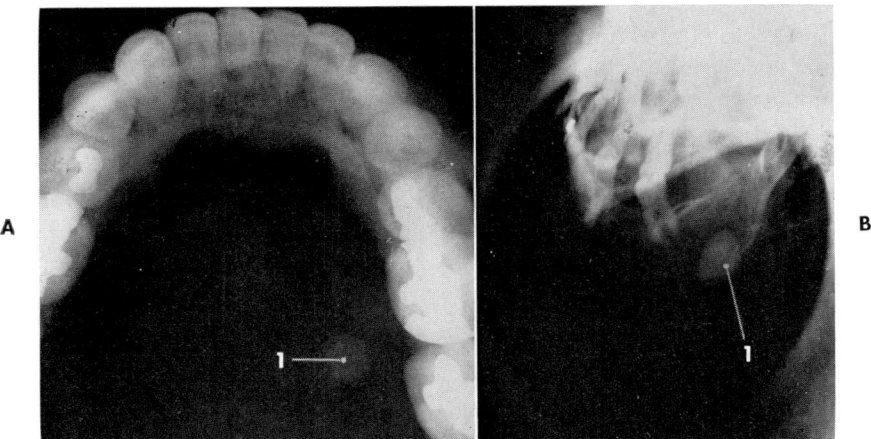

Fig. 25-4. **A,** Submandibular stone (sialolith) in the posterior portion of the duct demonstrated in the occlusal view. **B,** Submandibular sialolith in the gland pelvis demonstrated by a lateral oblique jaw radiograph.

Factors leading to difficulties in cannulation are as follows:
1. Too large caliber tubing
2. Rough bevel on tubing
3. Short or blunt bevel on tubing
4. Lack of lubrication on tubing

The tubing is inserted well into the duct. In the parotid duct an anatomical block is usually encountered where the duct turns posteriorly around the anterior border of the masseter muscle. In the submandibular duct a distance of 3 to 4 cm. is usually sufficient.

The patient is then asked to close his mouth, and the tubing may be held in place through any convenient embrasure without being crushed. The syringe is reconnected, and the patient is instructed to hold it against his chest. In this way, the patient may be moved and positioned at the convenience of the radiologist. When the radiologist has positioned the patient satisfactorily, injection of the contrast medium is started. The patient is instructed to raise his hand when pressure is felt and again when definite pain is felt. The amounts of solution used are subject to individual variation, and symptomatic filling is usually more reliable than the use of predetermined amounts.

Pressure is maintained for 10 seconds after pain is elicited, and then the sialogram is taken. Light pressure is maintained during repositioning for additional views. Posteroanterior and lateral skull views may be taken at the discretion of the operator.

After all views are taken the tubing may be removed, and the patient is instructed to assist in emptying the gland by massage. Residual oil in the gland and duct system is not harmful and may be beneficial in some low-grade inflammatory conditions.

A great deal may be learned from the sialogram, especially if the information is accurately integrated with the clinical findings. Not all lesions have typical sialographic findings, however, and in many cases the final diagnosis depends on formal biopsy techniques. Fortunately, most inflammatory conditions display fairly typical findings when these are coupled with the clinical course, while tumors are frequently characterized by the singular absence of sialographic evidence. An example of mis-

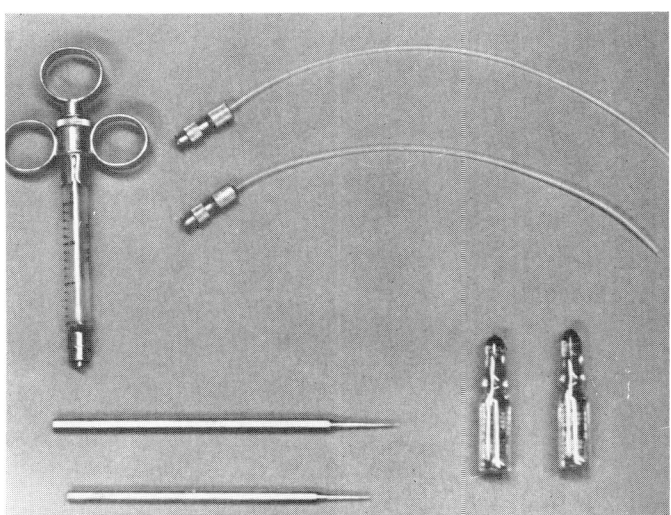

Fig. 25-5. Setup for sialography.

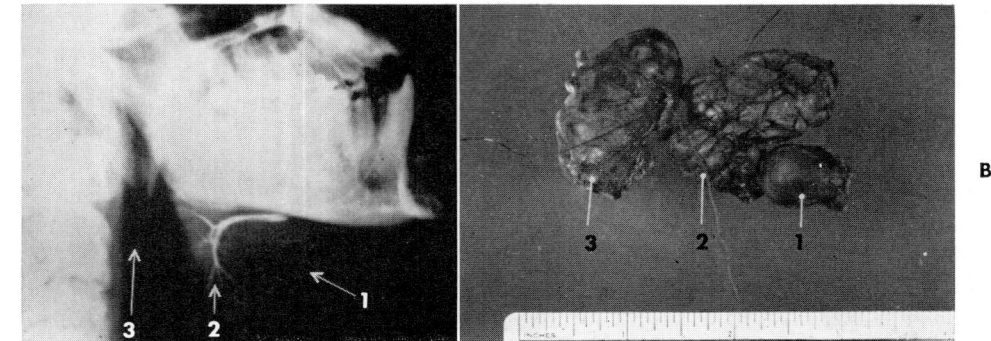

Fig. 25-6. This patient had a very marked swelling of the submandibular region. There were no laboratory findings or other physical findings of note. **A**, Preoperative sialogram demonstrated marked displacement of the gland architecture (1) by some tumefaction. The gland was otherwise normal. Major swelling (2) posterior to this area is not noted in the sialogram. The lesion (3) proved to be marked lymphoid hyperplasia when investigated surgically. **B**, Surgical specimen of the submandibular gland and two associated lymph nodes. The preglandular node (1) is the same as 1 in A. The salivary gland (2) is slightly deformed anteriorly by the hypertrophy of the preglandular node. The retroglandular node (3), since it was not tightly confined, did not distort the gland.

interpretation of equivocal findings is seen in Fig. 25-6.

Sialographic interpretation is best studied by integrating sialographic findings with clinical and historical findings and a knowledge of the basic anatomy and pathoses of the region. For this purpose a group of typical cases are presented, in which the sialographic findings and the clinical and historical findings were sufficiently clear to reach an accurate diagnosis (Figs. 25-7 to 25-23).

Laboratory procedures

Several laboratory procedures are useful in the differential diagnosis of salivary gland lesions. Mumps, infectious mononucleosis, and acute sialadenitis, which tend to resemble one another in the early stages, may be differentiated by an examination of the blood and blood serum. Infectious mononucleosis usually displays a very high percentage of atypical lymphocytes, as well as an increased over-all lymphocyte count, in the blood examination. Sialadenitis, if acute, may show an increase in the number of immature polymorphonuclear leukocytes in the blood examination. A heterophil agglutination test of the blood serum is of benefit in distinguishing infectious mononucleosis.

Most laboratories regard cytological smears as undependable in the differentiation of extraductal salivary gland lesions. Aspiration or needle biopsies are difficult to read because of the small amounts of tissue they offer. Frozen sections and formal biopsies, however, are highly dependable and complete the generally used clinical laboratory examinations.

A complete blood count and a differential blood count may offer some clue as to the relative toxicity of the disease, but they are in no way specific since they demonstrate only the blood's response to an infectious process.

Cytological examination may be carried out if malignant involvement of the duct system is suspected. It is to be remembered, however, that simple saliva from the mouth is not a useful sample, and material for this examination should be obtained from

Text continued on p. 560.

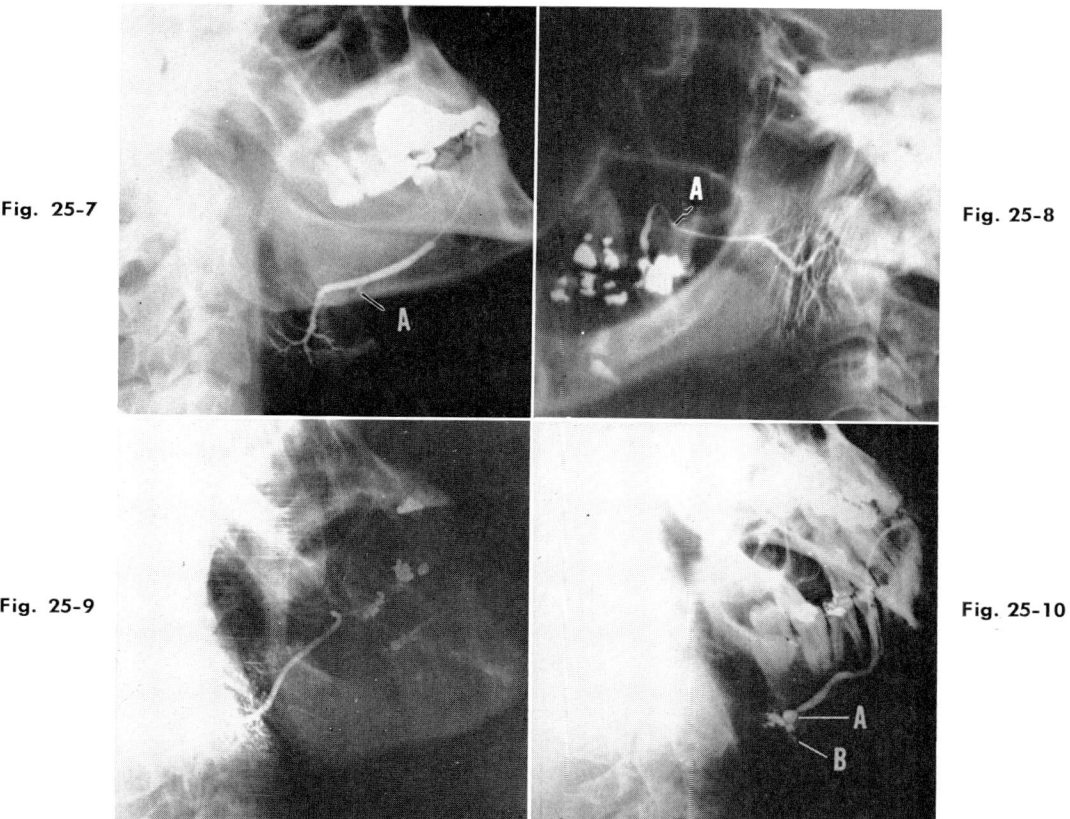

Fig. 25-7.

Fig. 25-8.

Fig. 25-9.

Fig. 25-10.

Fig. 25-7. Normal submandibular gland. In the normal film it is noted that the principal duct is of greater caliber than any of the smaller collecting ducts. The presence of ancillary connections (**A**) with small glands in the sublingual area is not unusual. The collecting ducts are noted to be of comparatively small size, and the terminal acini fill without dilatation. A follow-up film in 20 minutes would reveal little, if any, residual oil in the gland if proper secretory function is present.

Fig. 25-8. Normal parotid gland. The course of the excretory duct around the anterior edge of the masseter muscle is well demonstrated (**A**). The parotid duct is usually somewhat smaller in caliber than the submandibular duct, and its volume may not appear to be equal to the total volume of the collecting ducts. The acinar structure looks much like a leafless tree, and the collecting ducts are fine. (Accessory gland tissue frequently present in the buccal fat pad is not demonstrated in this figure, but can be readily demonstrated in Fig. 25-17.)

Fig. 25-9. Sialadenitis. This sialogram demonstrates the typical "leafy tree" appearance in which the terminal acini of the parotid gland are dilated. This is the early manifestation of inflammation as seen in the sialogram and is usually reversible under proper therapy.

Fig. 25-10. Sialolith. This sialogram demonstrates a small submandibular salivary stone (**A**) at the hilus of the gland effectively blocking the glandular secretions and producing a "link sausage" dilatation (**B**) of the collecting ducts behind the stone.

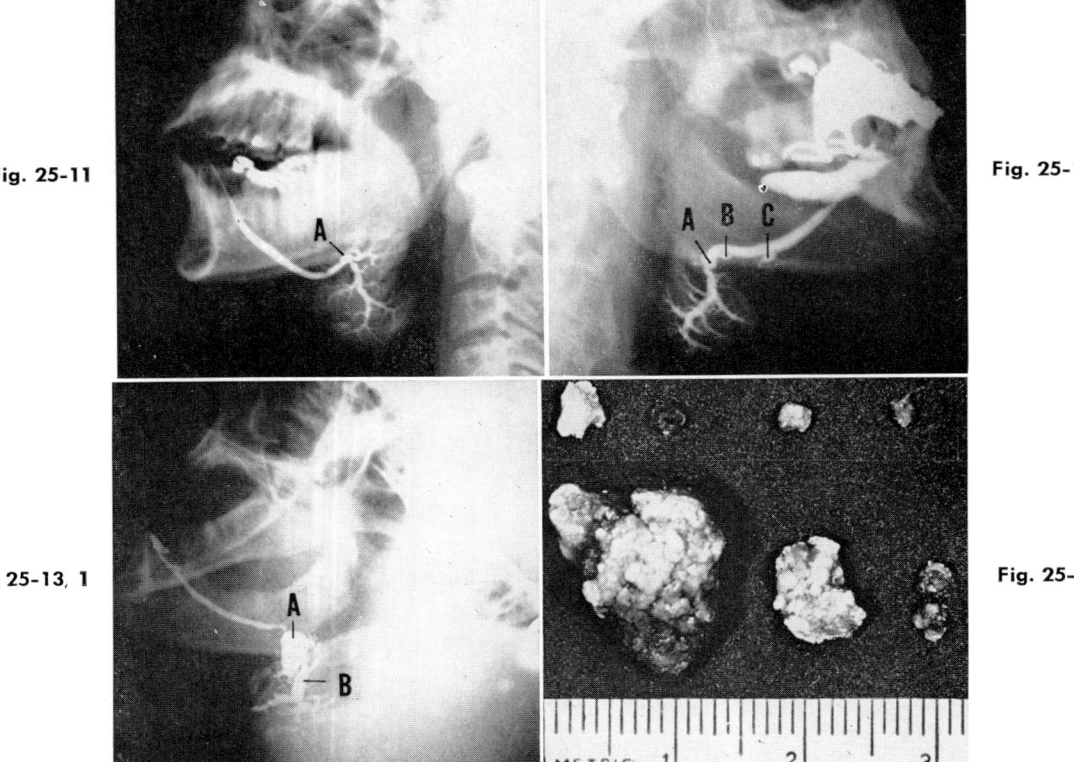

Fig. 25-11.
Fig. 25-12.
Fig. 25-13, 1
Fig. 25-13, 2

Fig. 25-11. Sialolithiasis of submandibular gland. The dilated space (**A**) at the hilus of the gland represents a small, poorly calcified stone that impairs but does not prevent excretion. There is slight dilatation of the duct system behind the obstruction. Transoral sialolithotomy is the treatment of choice in such cases. Access to stones this far distal is frequently technically difficult.

Fig. 25-12. Sialolithiasis, multiple, of submandibular gland and duct. This patient had several stones in the duct and gland and had undergone repeated probings and surgical procedures for their removal. Dilatation **A** at the hilus of the gland represents the principal salivary stone. Dilatations **B** and **C** of the ancillary sublingual ducts are typical of obstruction further forward and represent residual defects resulting from previous stones. Considerable sialoangiectasis is noted in the collecting ducts. This gland continued to be suppurative and symptomatic following the removal of the principal stone and eventually had to be extirpated.

Fig. 25-13. **1**, Sialolithiasis; an example of an extremely large submandibular salivary stone (**A**) occupying the hilus of the gland; marked dilatation of the ducts (**B**) noted behind the obstruction. This patient was successfully treated by transoral sialolithotomy. **2**, Some of the larger stones removed from the gland shown in **1**. Note the marked stellate formation of these calcified foreign bodies. Such a rough configuration prohibits the movement of stones within the duct.

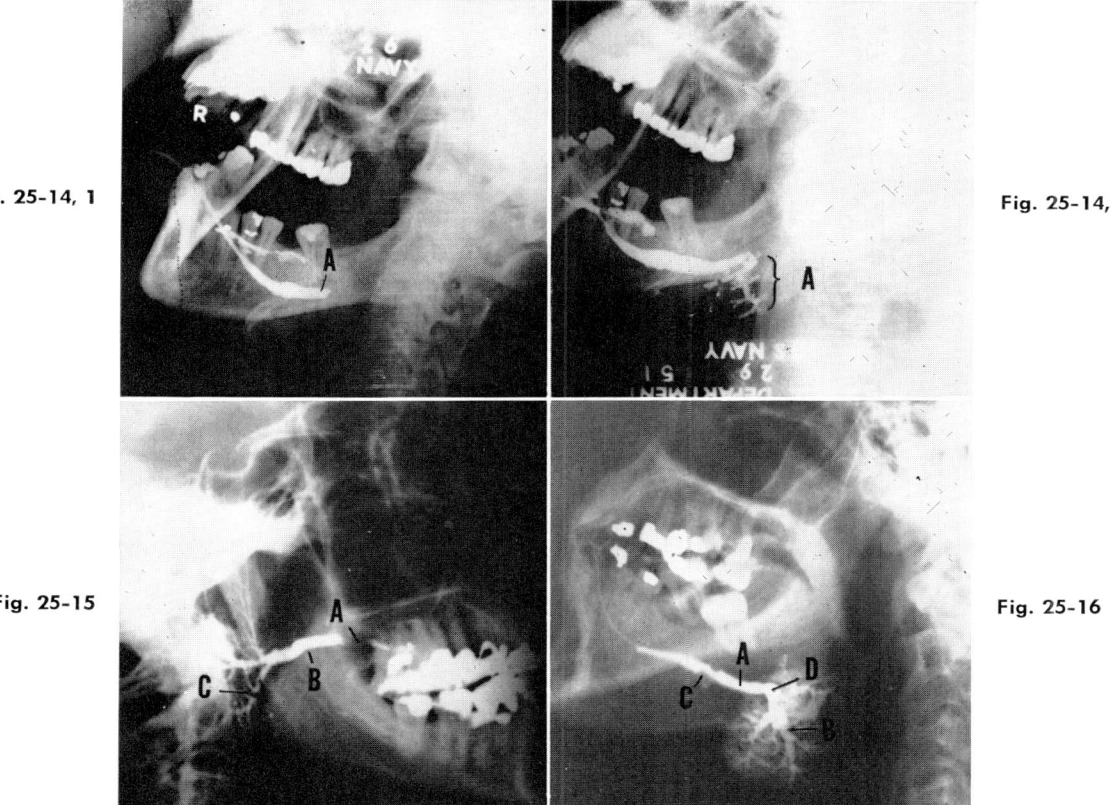

Fig. 25-14, 1
Fig. 25-14, 2
Fig. 25-15
Fig. 25-16

Fig. 25-14. 1, Sialolith. This patient had symptoms of submandibular gland obstruction. The sialogram failed to disclose the gland because of the inability to force the contrast medium past the obstruction (A). Seven salivary stones were removed transorally. 2, Postoperative sialogram of same case illustrated in 1. Note the vastly dilated duct, as well as the clubbing and dilatation of the collecting ducts (A). In spite of the extreme damage to this gland, it was not necessary to remove it.

Fig. 25-15. Obstructive parotitis with sialolith and sialoangiectasis. The interruption (A) in the main excretory duct, just behind the second molar, represents a poorly calcified sialolith that totally occupies the lumen of the duct. Extreme dilatation of the duct (B) is noted behind the defect. The interruptions (C) in the collecting ducts represent inspissated salivary fluid, which, it is believed, may well form the nidus for additional stones. This obstruction was accessible to the surgical procedure described later.

Fig. 25-16. Sialoangiectasis resulting from sialolith and stricture. Large dilatation of the excretory duct (A) is noted, with concomitant dilatation of the collecting ducts (B). The nonfilling defect (C) in the midportion of the excretory duct represents a stricture, whereas the large dilatation (D) in the hilus of the gland represents a smooth sialolith. This stone could be moved by bimanual manipulation from its posterior position forward to the stricture. It was removed transorally from the anterior position after first being fixed by means of a suture passed posterior to it. The patient has remained asymptomatic, in spite of the fact that there appears to be greater structural change in this gland than in the gland shown in Fig. 25-12. Such differences in individual response are difficult to explain, and a decision to remove a gland must be based on the presence of symptoms.

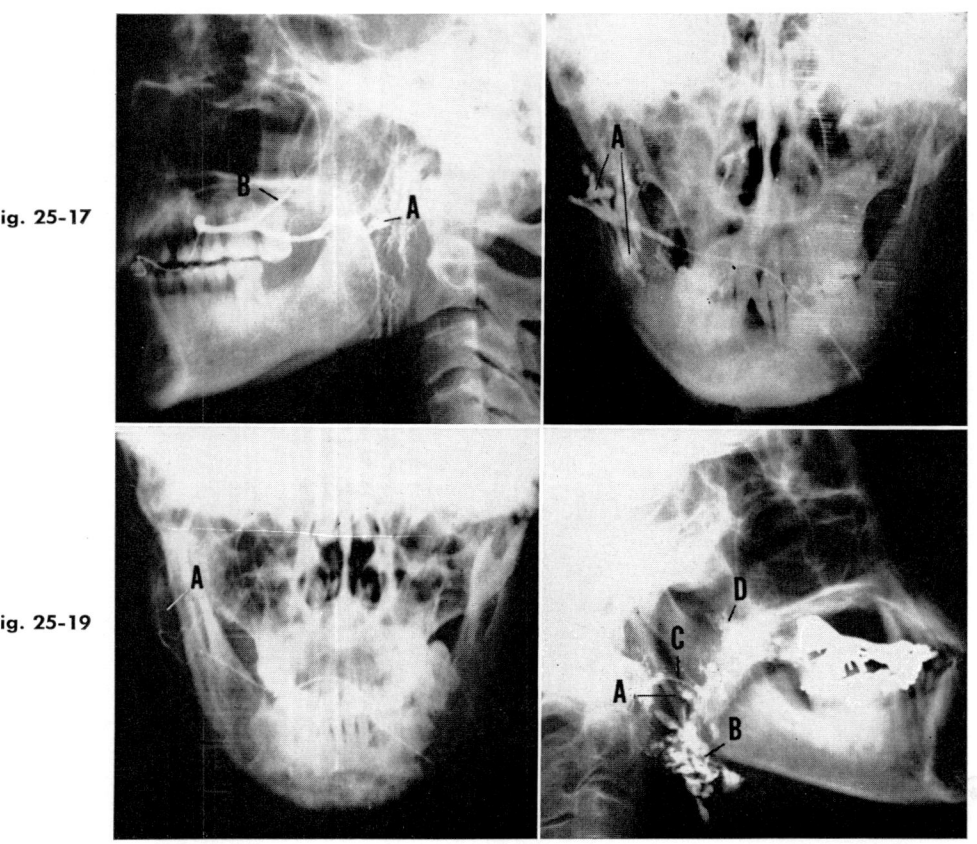

Fig. 25-17.
Fig. 25-18.
Fig. 25-19.
Fig. 25-20.

Fig. 25-17. Sialoangiectasis of parotid gland. This glandular pattern is typical of a chronic sialadenitis with areas of sialoangiectasis in the duct system. The rather large filling defect (**A**) represents destruction of the gland parenchyma by abscess formation. These areas of destruction may be much larger or smaller, depending on the severity of the disease. Dilatation and clubbing of the terminal acini gives the collecting ducts the overall appearance of coarseness typical of salivary stasis. An incidental finding in this sialogram is the presence of the accessory gland structure (**B**) in the buccal fat pad. This is a fairly common anatomical variation and is in no way abnormal.

Fig. 25-18. Sialoangiectasis with chronic sialadenitis. Marked destruction caused by abscess formation (**A**) is noted in this parotid gland. This was a chronic, recurrent condition, which eventually required removal of the gland. The condition was bilateral and followed a severe bout of pneumonia with dehydration and a high febrile course.

Fig. 25-19. Retention cyst of parotid gland. The small nonfilling defect (**A**) in the parenchyma of the parotid gland has displaced the normal architecture. At operation this defect proved to be a retention cyst filled with salivary fluid.

Fig. 25-20. Developmental cyst of parotid gland. This patient had a soft mass in the parotid gland that varied in size and was tender when it became enlarged. A large nonfilling defect (**A**) has pushed aside a part of the gland parenchyma. The remainder of the gland, particularly the inferior pole (**B**), is greatly dilated, suggesting that the mass obstructs the drainage ducts and prevents excretion. The superior pole is more nearly normal in appearance, and the duct course can be seen passing around the superior pole of the cyst (**C**). Accessory glands (**D**) are noted along the entire course of the duct. On removal this lesion was noted to have all the histopathological characteristics of a branchial cleft cyst. The sialoangiectasis was incident to the blocking action caused by the enlargement of this cyst. Retrograde infection followed the blocking.

Salivary glands and ducts **559**

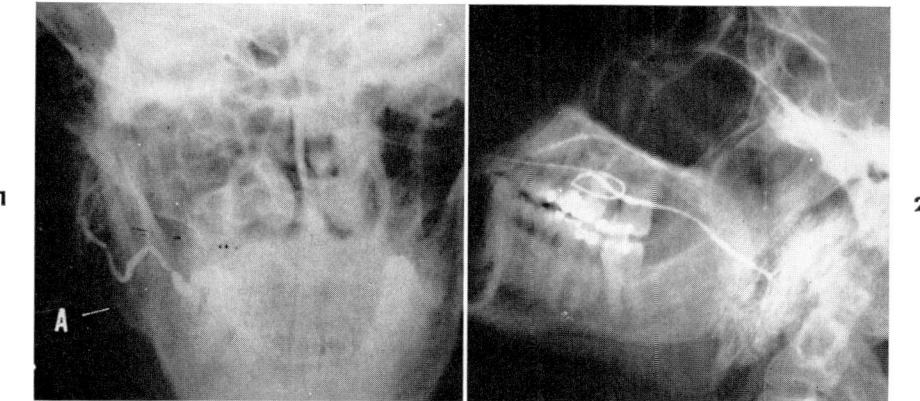

Fig. 25-21. **1,** Mixed tumor, parotid gland. The parotid gland in this case is normal insofar as the sialogram is concerned. The stricture seen in the anterior third of the duct is technical rather than anatomical. The only noticeable feature is that the gland appears to be separated from the angle of the mandible (**A**) by some nonfilling mass that has displaced the superficial lobe of the gland. The inference from such a picture is that of extraductal involvement, which may result from a swollen lymph node, a developmental cyst, a mixed tumor, or any other tumefaction that tends to displace parotid structures. **2,** This lateral view of the patient shown in **1** offers no clue to the presence or identity of the lesion, which in this case was a mixed tumor of the parotid gland, but could have been any one of several extrinsic tumefactions. Sialography in such cases does not offer diagnostic evidence, as it may in conditions that invade the gland or duct system, but there is always some clinical manifestation that can be seen or palpated. Sialograms may or may not tend to support clinical impressions, yet the absence of sialographic findings is of value in determining that the disease is extraductal or extraglandular in nature

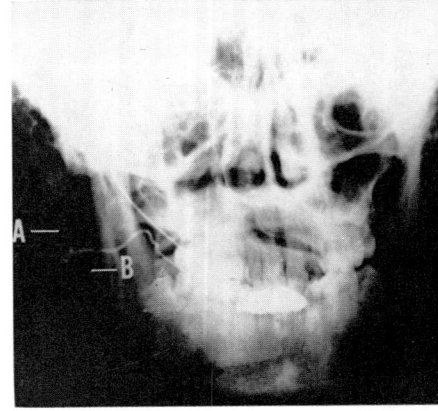 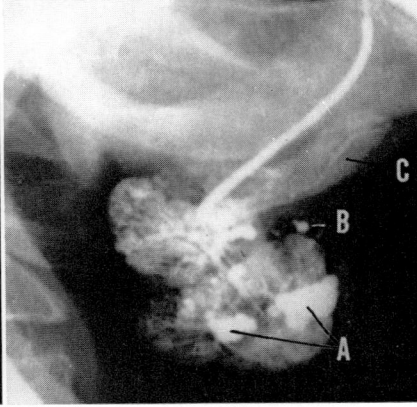

Fig. 25-22. Mixed tumor of parotid gland. This sialogram shows the typical ball-in-hand deformity (**A**). There is considerable displacement of the superficial lobe of the parotid gland, causing it to stand away (**B**) from the body of the mandible and curve around the tumor mass.

Fig. 25-23. Squamous cell carcinoma, primary in the submandibular gland, which is obviously involved with neoplastic disease, has invaded the gland parenchyma. The duct is normal, but the gland substance displays an unusual network pattern suggesting complete arborization of the gland parenchyma. The numerous spaces filled with radiopaque fluid (**A**) are typical of necrotic areas destroyed by tumor. In one area the gland capsule has ruptured sufficiently to permit radiopaque fluid (**B**) to enter the surrounding space. Of interest is the large sublingual extension of glandular tissue (**C**) (which represents hypertrophic extension) that was also invaded by tumor, as were the mandible and the contiguous lymph nodes of the neck. It is impossible to predict the cell type in such tumors; but this sialographic picture, coupled with the clinical findings of a firm, indurated, nonpainful submandibular mass of several years' duration, makes the diagnosis of malignant lesion of the submandibular gland reasonably obvious. Before biopsy it was thought that this might well be either an adenocarcinoma or a mucoepidermoid carcinoma, either of which might well display this clinical and sialographic picture. Accurate diagnosis can be established only by formal biopsy.

the duct of the suspected gland by cannulation. The uses of this examination are limited, and if the results are negative, they are by no means conclusive.

Smears, cultures, and antibiotic sensitivity tests are valuable when the type of organism and the specific antibiotic to be employed are at issue. Again, the sample must be taken from the cannulated duct to avoid oral contamination.

SURGICAL PROCEDURES

With the possible exception of the surgical management of retention cysts such as mucoceles and ranulas, the transoral sialolithotomy is the most frequent operation performed on the salivary system (Fig. 25-24). It is a simple operation, frequently overlooked by medical practitioners untrained in oral surgery in favor of enucleation of the gland. If the stone is favorably located, its removal through the mouth preserves the gland and hence the function of the gland. Although sialoliths are known to recur and glands may be so badly damaged by infection as to require subsequent or eventual enucleation, the more conservative course is usually indicated at the original operation because of its widespread success in the hands of most operators.

The submandibular gland can be enucleated without sequelae if the operation is

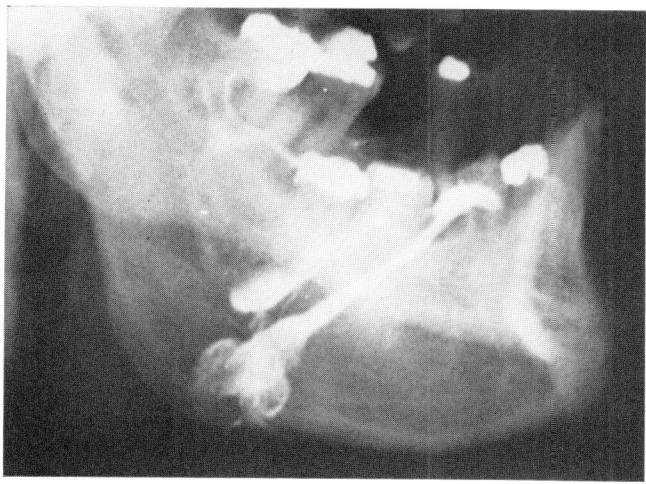

Fig. 25-24. Retained sialolith following incomplete surgery. This patient's submandibular gland was removed by a general surgeon before any effort was made to remove the stone transorally. Symptoms persisted and pus was constantly discharged from the salivary caruncle. The sialogram shows why. The patient still has the salivary stone and part of the gland that lies above the mylohyoid muscle. It is apparent that the underlying condition that produced the glandular dysfunction has not been dealt with. It is usually prudent to attempt the removal of stones transorally before condemning the gland. If it becomes necessary to remove the gland, the operator must assure himself of adequate operative procedure to section the duct above the area occupied by the stone.

properly accomplished. Before removing this gland, however, thought should be given to the results of the loss of its function, although in most patients with normal salivary secretion in the remaining glands its removal is of no consequence.

Removal of the parotid gland is of greater consequence. Danger to the seventh cranial nerve is always present, although careful surgery permits the removal of this gland with only transient weakness in most instances.

The removal of either gland results in slight facial deformity. In the case of the submandibular gland a scar plus a depression or, more accurately, a lack of fullness in the submandibular region results. When the parotid gland is involved, a retromandibular scar plus a loss of some facial contour is experienced. These factors are not significant if the operation is necessary, but contraindicate such procedures when conservative methods would suffice.

Transoral sialolithotomy of submandibular duct

Transoral sialolithotomy is best done with the patient under local anesthesia and in a sitting position.

The stone is first located accurately by radiography and palpation. If possible, and especially if the stone is small and smooth, a suture is passed through the floor of the mouth, below the duct and behind the stone, and tied to prevent the stone from sliding backward. A towel clamp is placed through the tip and, if necessary, the side of the tongue to obtain retraction and control of this member. This step is especially important in obese persons or in those who are unable to control their tongue voluntarily. In slim or especially cooperative persons the tongue can be held in a gauze sponge. How the tongue will be retracted and controlled should be determined at the time of examination, but towel clips should be included in the armamentarium in any case.

The gland is then palpated extraorally and pushed upward toward the floor of the mouth to fix the intraoral tissues under tension and make the stone easier to palpate.

When the incision is made, consideration is given to two structures, the lingual nerve and the sublingual gland. Posteriorly the lingual nerve is superior and lateral to the duct, crossing beneath it at the posterior end of the mylohyoid ridge and passing medially and deep. Thus, if the stone is posterior, the incision is shallow, and blunt dissection is employed immediately to prevent injury to the lingual nerve. If the stone is more anterior, the incision must be made medial to the plica sublingualis (Fig. 25-25) or the operator will find the sublingual gland between his instrument and the stone and a portion of the gland will be transected. Thus the incision for an anterior stone is designed to be over the stone and medial to the plica.

As soon as the operator progresses through the mucosa, blunt dissection is used. Both the incision and the opening obtained by spreading the tissues should be large enough to permit the entrance of the examining finger since reorientation is frequently necessary. Dissection is continued bluntly through the loose tissues of the space until the duct is encountered. If the lingual nerve is encountered in the incision, it must be retracted gently, but never cut. Bleeding is seldom a problem, but, if it occurs, it should be controlled by ligation before proceeding.

The duct is best identified at the point where the stone is lodged. If difficulty arises at this stage, a probe may be passed into the duct to aid in its location. When the duct is located, a longitudinal slit is made directly over the stone. The duct should not be cut transversely because retraction may complete the division and a fistula may result. The opening should reveal the stone and should be of sufficient length to

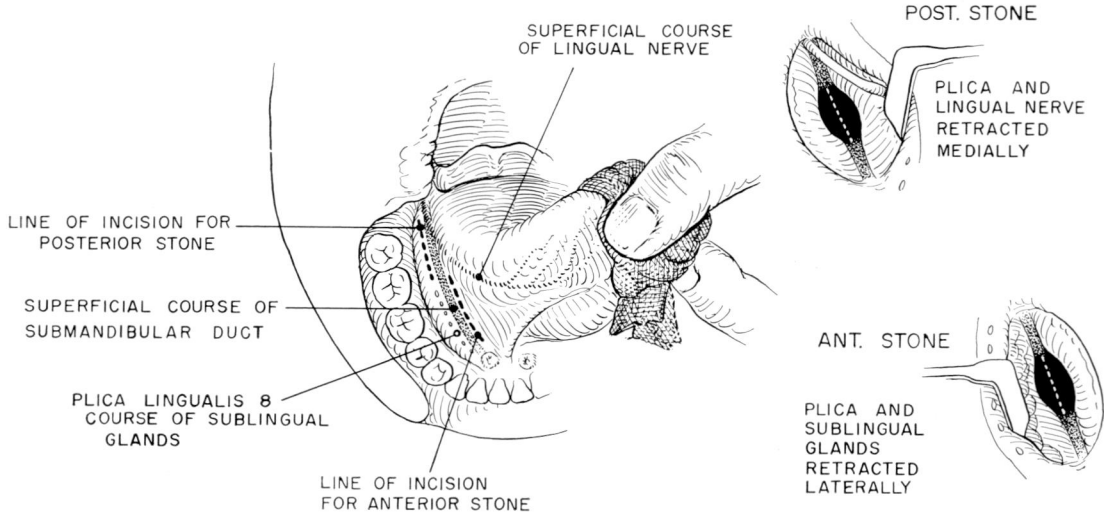

Fig. 25-25. Intraoral landmarks and lines of incision for transoral sialolithotomy of the submandibular duct

permit its removal. The stone can usually be carefully removed with small forceps, but large stellate stones may have to be broken by crushing them with a forceps. After the stone is removed a small aspirating cannula may be passed toward the gland to remove any pus, mucous plugs, or satellite stones that remain. A probe is then passed from the caruncle to the surgical opening to ensure patency of the anterior end of the duct.

No effort is made to close the duct proper. The wound edges are sutured at the level of the mucosa only, and recanalization occurs without further intervention.

Transoral sialolithotomy of parotid duct

The approach to calcifications in the parotid duct may be more difficult than to similar lesions in the submandibular duct. The reason for this is the anatomical peculiarity of the parotid duct. After following a short, superficial course from its caruncle the parotid duct turns laterally and rounds the anterior border of the masseter muscle, proceeding posteriorly to join the gland. A direct cut-down on stones in this duct, therefore, is possible only when the stone is anterior to the anterior border of the masseter muscle. Since most parotid duct stones lodge at or posterior to this point, a direct cut-down is seldom effective. Splitting the duct to follow the channel posteriorly frequently so damages the duct and caruncle that strictures are produced, which lead to new stasis and stone formation.

The suggested procedure, therefore, involves making a semilunar incision running from above downward in front of the caruncle (Fig. 25-26, A and B). The caruncle, mucosal flap, and duct are then retracted medially, the cheek is retracted laterally, and free access is gained to the more posterior segments of the duct by simply following the duct with blunt dissection. This procedure also permits the duct to be retracted anteriorly so that the stone can be delivered into the wound. When the stone becomes accessible, a longitudinal incision

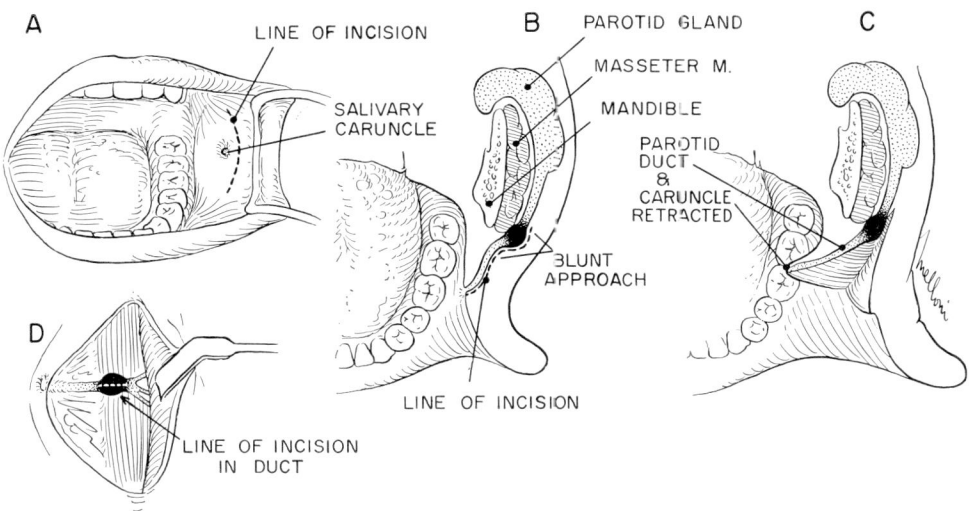

Fig. 25-26. **A**, Intraoral view of line of incision for transoral sialolithotomy of the parotid duct. **B**, Sectional view of line of incision and blunt approach for transoral sialolithotomy of the parotid duct. **C**, Retraction for removal of parotid duct stone, sectional view. **D**, Retraction and duct incision for removal of parotid duct stone, intraoral view.

564 *Textbook of oral surgery*

is made in the lateral side of the duct, and the stone is deliverd (Fig. 25-26, *C* and *D*). The duct need not be sutured since simply closing the mucosal flap with deep mattress sutures will serve to produce recanalization of the duct.

Removal of submandibular gland

Occasionally, because of previous damage from stasis and chronic infection, removal of the submandibular gland is necessary. Usually this is not done until conservative means have been exhausted.

The extraoral incision parallels the course of the digastric muscle. To determine this course the mastoid eminence, the lateral surface of the hyoid bone, and the genial tubercle are palpated. A curving line connecting these three landmarks represents the course of the anterior and posterior bellies of the digastric muscle. A 2-inch incision is made along this curving line (Fig. 25-27) directly over the inferior pole of the gland, and the platysma muscle is sectioned.

The first structure encountered is the facial vein, which is ligated and cut. At the level of the deep fascia the cervical ramus of the seventh cranial nerve is encountered where it communicates with superficial cervical nerves from the cervical plexus. This ramus can usually be retracted posteriorly by passing a hernia tape around it, although cutting it represents no serious loss since it provides only partial innervation to the platysma muscle on one side only.

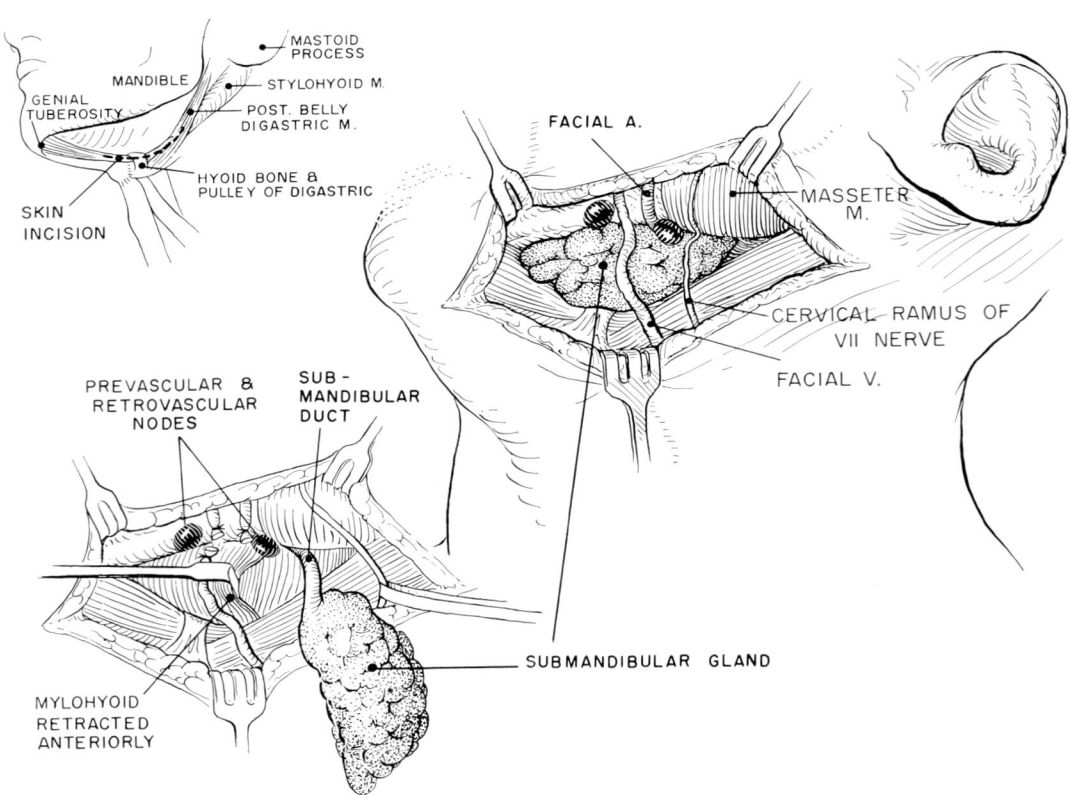

Fig. 25-27. Landmarks and line of incision for removal of submandibular gland.

Beneath the fascia lies the submandibular niche. Blunt dissection between the pulley of the digastric muscle and the gland will free the anterior and inferior portions of the gland. The dissection is continued around the posteroinferior pole, leaving the superior and medial portions of the gland attached.

Vital structures to be considered at this point are the facial artery, the lingual nerve, and the submandibular duct. The facial artery curves up and over the superior aspect of the gland and emerges on the lateral side of the mandible at the anterior border of the masseter muscle. This artery can usually be located by the presence of the prevascular and retrovascular lymph nodes that lie on either side of the vessel. In most instances it is wise to identify and double ligate the facial artery below the gland and to separate it before proceeding with the dissection because its connections with the gland are usually short and difficult to tie and the vessel is frequently buried within the gland.

The gland may then be retracted posteriorly and detached from its ganglionic connections with the submandibular ganglion. The lingual nerve can be identified at this point, but the ganglion is seldom seen at surgery.

As the dissection proceeds bluntly, the submandibular duct may be noted passing superiorly and anteriorly over the roof of the submandibular niche, which is formed by the mylohyoid muscle. This muscle should be retracted anteriorly, the duct retracted posteriorly, and a ligature placed anterior to the ductal pathosis if such exists. A second ligature is placed posterior to the first, but still anterior to the ductal pathosis, and the duct is sectioned between the ligatures. This procedure prevents seepage of infected material into the wound from either the residual duct or the gland. The gland may then be removed and consideration given to the closing of the wound.

Dead space resulting from removal of the gland must be closed or drained. Closure can usually be accomplished by approximating the fasciae of the digastric, stylohyoid, hyoglossus, and mylohyoid muscles with absorbable catgut sutures. If this cannot be done and a dead space remains, or if it is believed that the crypt has become contaminated or is infected, a Penrose drain should be inserted into this area. A second layer of absorbable sutures should be used to close the deep fascia and platysma muscle. A third layer of subcutaneous or subcuticular absorbable sutures is used to close the skin, and the skin edges are then carefully approximated with interrupted silk sutures, size 4-0 or smaller.

The wound should always be covered with a pressure dressing. The drain, if one is placed, should emerge from the wound at the most dependent point, which is usually at the posterior aspect of the wound. This drain may be removed after 24 to 48 hours if no suppuration is present. After 4 days the pressure dressing may be discontinued and half of the sutures may be removed. The incision should be bridged with adhesive butterflies or with a firm collodion dressing. The remaining sutures may be removed on the fifth to seventh day, but the wound should continue to have bridging support for at least 2 weeks.

Removal of parotid gland

In general, removal of the parotid gland is not considered to be within the purview of the oral surgeon. By virtue of special training or because of local circumstances, however, he may include this operation in his repertoire. In any case he should have some knowledge of the problems involved so that he can make decisions regarding treatment.

Because of certain inherent risks of permanent damage to the seventh cranial nerve, this operation is not usually done without strong indications. The presence of a tumor or suspected tumor or of chronic inflammatory disease resistant to conservative treatment is the primary reason for such an undertaking. Most surgeons make every attempt to conserve the seventh cranial nerve by careful dissection or partial removal of the gland. A malignant lesion, however, suffers no compromise, and when attacked surgically, it must be extirpated without regard for the possible resultant deformity.

The incision runs from the superior attachment of the pinna downward, turns anteriorly at the angle of the mandible, and stops at the hyoid bone. A second incision, which may be made posterior to the pinna, joins the first at the inferior margin of the pinna (Fig. 25-28). The ear is retracted from the operative field, and the skin flap is developed on the cheek side of the incision.

The facial nerve may be located in either of two ways: (1) by finding the peripheral portion where it emerges from the anterior edge of the gland and then dissecting backward or (2) by dissecting directly down the posterior aspect of the gland and identifying the main trunk between its entrance into the gland substance and the stylomastoid foramen (Fig. 25-1, A). An electric stimulator is of great assistance in this maneuver. After the nerve has been identified the course of the trunks is followed and the superficial lobe is freed from its attachments. The duct is ligated and cut. Some of the smaller connections between the main trunks may be destroyed in this process, with resultant postoperative facial weakness. Preservation of the main branches of the nerve, however, ensures eventual return to full function.

After the superficial lobe of the gland has been freed and the main branches of the facial nerve have been identified, the deep lobe may be approached. This lobe wraps around the posterior border of the mandible, and dissection in this confined space is facilitated by posterosuperior retraction of the ear. Care should be taken to protect the external carotid artery and the retromandibular vein during this operation. Ligation of these vessels may be prudent because either or both of them may be embedded in the gland substance in a part of their course, and because hemorrhage from the rather large maxillary branch of the external carotid artery may be very difficult to control because of its relative inaccessibility.

The parotid capsule is very tough along its posterior attachment, particularly where the gland encounters the sternocleidomastoid muscle and the acoustic meatus. Care must be exercised, while the pinna is retracted, not to incise the acoustic meatus during separation of the gland.

Most dead space may be closed by careful suturing after removal of the gland. A drain may be indicated in the wound, especially if a portion of the gland is removed and salivary accumulation is expected.

CONCLUSION

A very important part of the mission of oral surgery is the diagnosis and treatment of certain diseases of the salivary glands. Careful diagnosis is the key to success and usually indicates the method of treatment. The ability to distinguish between those

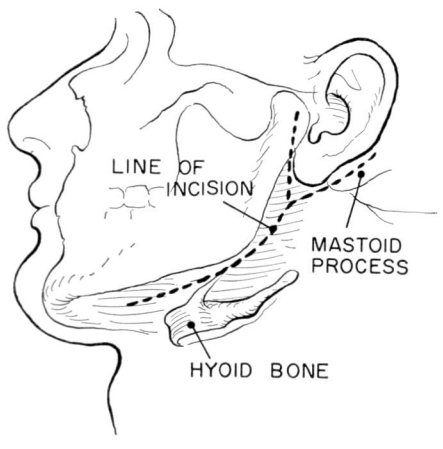

Fig. 25-28. Landmarks and line of incision for removal of parotid gland.

diseases and conditions the treatment of which is a part of oral surgical training and those the treatment of which is within the province of one of the medical specialties is paramount. A knowledge of the anatomy of the salivary glands, an adequate examination, a thorough history, and diagnostic radiographs are a necessity. Clinical laboratory procedures may be of some assistance. Formal biopsy is the only sure method of establishing a firm diagnosis when a malignant condition cannot otherwise be ruled out.

REFERENCES

1. Abaza, N. A., El-Khashab, M. M., and Fahim, M. S.: Adenoid cystic carcinoma (cylindroma) of the palate, Oral Surg. 22:429, 1966.
2. Alaniz, F., and Fletcher, G. H.: Place and technics of radiation therapy in the management of malignant tumors of the major salivary glands, Radiology 84:412, 1965.
3. Blatt, I. M.: Systemic diseases and their relation to the major salivary glands, Trans. Amer. Acad. Ophthal. Otolaryng. 69:1115, 1965.
4. De la Pava, S., Karjoo, R., Mukhtar, F., and Pickren, J. W.: Multifocal carcinoma of accessory salivary gland. A case report, Cancer 19:1308, 1966.
5. Eisenbud, L., and Cranin, N.: The role of sialography in the diagnosis and therapy of chronic obstructive sialadenitis, Oral Surg. 16:1181, 1963.
6. Frank, R. M., Herdly, J., and Philippe, E.: Acquired dental defects and salivary gland lesions after irradiation for carcinoma, J. Amer. Dent. Ass. 70:868, 1965.
7. Frazell, E. L., Strong, E. W., and Newcombe, B.: Tumors of the parotid, Amer. J. Nurs. 66:2702, 1966.
8. Garusi, G. F.: The salivary glands in radiological diagnosis, Bibl. Radiol. 4:1, 1964.
9. Huebsch, R F.: Acute lesions of the oral cavity, Dent. Clin. N. Amer. p. 577, Nov., 1965.
10. Kashima, H. K., Kirkham, W. R., and Andrews, J. R.: Postirradiation sialadenitis; a study of the clinical features, histopathologic changes and serum enzyme variations following irradiation of human salivary glands, Amer. J. Roentgen. 94:271, 1965.
11. Morel, A. S., and Firestein, A.: Repair of traumatic fistulas of the parotid duct, Arch. Surg. 87:623, 1963.
12. Moskow, R., Moskow, B. S., and Robinson, H. L.: Minor salivary gland sialolithiasis. Report of a case, Oral Surg. 17:225, 1964.
13. Prowler, J. R., Bjork, H., and Armstrong, G. F.: Major gland sialectasis, J. Oral Surg. 23:421, 1965.
14. Rosenfeld, L., Sessions, D. E., McSwain, B., and Graves, H., Jr.: Malignant tumors of salivary gland origin; 37 year review of 184 cases, Ann. Surg. 163:726, 1966.
15. Ross, D. E., and Castro, E. C.: Recurrent inflammatory swellings of the salivary glands: emphasis of sialangiectasis, Amer. Surg. 30:434, 1964.
16. Simons, J. N., Beahrs, O. H., and Wollner, L. B.: Tumors of the submaxillary gland, Amer. J. Surg. 108:485, 1964.
17. Wallenborn, W. M., Sydnor, T. A., Hsu, Y. T., and Fitz-Hugh, G. S.: Experimental production of parotid gland atrophy by ligation of Stensen's duct and by irradiation, Laryngoscope 74:644, 1964.
18. Waterhouse, J.: Inflammation of the salivary glands, Brit. J. Oral Surg. 3:161, 1966.
19. White, N. S.: Sjögren's syndrome, J. Oral Surg. 22:163, 1966.

Chapter 26

NEUROLOGICAL ASPECTS OF DENTAL PAIN

Athol L. Frew, Jr., and Don M. Ishmael

Whenever the symptoms of pain present themselves, the whole spectrum of neurological surveys may have to be called upon to properly diagnose the cause. Pain-producing entities may be grossly apparent, as in the case of a simple pulpitis initiated by a deep carious lesion affecting a single tooth; on the other hand, pain may present a vastly complicated picture requiring the utmost care in diagnostic studies. Formerly the dentist was concerned with pain only as it affects the teeth and their surrounding structures, but the field of dentistry has had to broaden its horizon to include those areas that may refer pain to the dental structure. Consequently, the requirement today is that the dentist must be a specialist in dental and facial pain, a requirement that necessarily requires utilizing his basic knowledge of physiology, anatomy, neurology, and pathology of the facial areas.

CLINICAL EXAMINATON FOR LOCALIZATION OF DENTAL FOCUS

Pain may be defined as a subjective response to an unpleasant stimulus that is perceived by the conscious mind as such. The perception of pain begins upon a process of electrochemical conductivity along known neuropathways from the end organ of nerves or pain receptors up to the thalamus of the brain. The act of conduction must be initiated by a sensation that depends upon impulse excited by an adequate stimulation of the receptors and conveyed by the afferent or sensory fibers of nerves to the central nervous system. This process is known as pain perception. Pain perception is dependent upon two main types of sensory receptors: (1) the *exteroceptors*—those receptors capable of transmitting external stimuli from the world about, and (2) the *proprioceptors*—those receptors that take the internal stimuli from the world within.

Pain perception depends upon the proper functioning of the total nerve mechanisms up to but not including the thalamus. Impairment of function in perceptors can often be a valuable diagnostic tool in a neurological survey; that is, an electrical current sufficient to elicit a response when passing through a normal tooth will not produce a sensation in a devitalized one. Hence, the knowledge of impaired perception will enable one to pinpoint a defective dental organ. Pain response or pain reaction begins where the pain perception leaves off, that is, with the thalamus and cerebral cortex. The integrity of the sensory cortex is mandatory in determining an accurate localization of painful stimuli. Reaction to pain that is dependent upon the proper functioning of the thalamus and cortex involves complex psychology, physiology, and neurological anatomical processes. A patient's reaction to pain depends greatly upon his individual tolerance (pain threshold) and his psychological make-up (emotional status), that is, his reaction by reason of fear, past experiences, age, fatigue, even sex, etc.

One must take these factors into consideration when making a neurological survey of the facial areas where dental pain is involved. For instance, a hyperreactive patient might react so violently in the course of examination that he will lead one to suspect a major neuralgia when only a pulpal neuritis may exist.

The process of nerve conduction is done along the main sensory nerve of the head—the fifth cranial nerve. The seventh, ninth, and tenth cranial nerves along with the second and third cervical nerves may be utilized for the mediation of pain. Occasionally one finds that referred pain along the minor sensory areas elicits a pain either concomitantly or exclusively in the fifth nerve region, as in the case of a glossopharyngeal neuralgia or a cervical radicular tension syndrome.

It is equally important that one learn to interpret loss or lack of sensation as well as pain sensation. The examination for determining sensation is a very difficult procedure because it depends totally on subjective measures. Psychological and physical factors must be taken into consideration. These would include age, education, sex, intelligence, fatigability, and suggestibility. Areas to be tested are those that follow known neural distribution. These areas may be specifically evaluated by the use of sweet and sour substances, a pin, or a wisp of cotton. For more details in conducting a neurological examination a textbook on neurology should be consulted.

A cursory examination of this type is valuable in the sense that it may detect sensory defects that the patient is not aware of, and it may indicate that a more thorough examination is in order.

The principal manner in which nerves of the face may be affected are (1) through paralysis and spasm, as in the case of the motor nerves, and (2) through the manifestation of pain, in the case of the sensory nerves. This may be symptomatic (presenting a definite organic origin) or idiopathic (based on a nonorganic origin).

Motor nerves

The motor nerves of the face are principally supplied by the facial or seventh cranial nerve. For instance, the lower lip is supplied by the mandibular branch of the seventh nerve, and the upper lip is supplied by the buccal branches of the seventh nerve. The ninth and eleventh cranial nerves, however supply the pharynx and the soft palate, respectively. The fifth cranial nerve carries motor fibers to the muscles of mastication and sensory fibers to the face.

Paralysis of the face, which is an involvement of the motor nerves, may be brought on by interference with proper functions of the nerve by pressure, severance, or invasion of microorganisms. This may be done centrally within the neuropathways of the brain or peripherally at some distal point.

Intracranial pressure diseases commonly affecting the motor nerve to the face are brain tumors. These tumors present some difficulty in removal because of their infiltrating ability, either by self-perpetuation or by cyst formation. Other types of brain tumors are the meningiomas (which arise from the coverings of the brain), pituitary tumors (endocrine in nature), the angioblastomas and hemangioblastomas (congenital vascular malformations), and true vascular tumors. Other brain tumors are the metastatic tumors (tumors of any of the organs of the body) that may metastasize to the brain. Metastases from the lungs and the breast are the most common. The neurofibromas are tumors arising from the sheath of any of the cranial nerves. These tumors are most often found on the vestibular portion of the eighth cranial nerve. They present symptoms of tinnitus and loss of hearing. With continued growth these tumors may compress the fifth, seventh, and other cranial nerves.

One should observe the fact that from a motor standpoint our brains are upside down; that is, the motor centers controlling the muscles of the face are situated in the lowest portion of the motor area, whereas the centers affecting the foot muscles are situated high on the brain. Also, in some areas the neuropathways of the brain are crossed. For instance, a right frontal lobe tumor will result in a left facial palsy. In general, lesions located within the cortex at the site of the nucleus of the facial nerve will produce a paralysis of the opposite side of the face. Should the lesion occur below the point where the nerve tracts cross, paralysis of the face on the same side of the lesion will occur.

Regardless of the type, certain symptoms are common to most brain tumors: headache, occasionally unilateral, usually limited to the side of the neoplasm; difficulty in vision; sensory symptoms; vomiting (often projectile); convulsions; personality changes; and Cheyne-Strokes respiration.

Extracranial pressures that paralyze the nerves of the face result from neoplasms, accidental injury resulting in pressure of bone or foreign objects, or microorganisms. Paralysis of the face may result from an affection of the motor nerve through traumatic experiences caused by pressures upon the nerve or severing of the nerve. For instance, if the posterior root of the gasserian ganglion of the fifth cranial nerve is sectioned or if the seventh (facial nerve) is injured by severance, facial paralysis ensues. If the paralysis is produced by pressure in a localized neuropathy, then simple removal of the pressure will result in spontaneous and usually instant recovery of function. But if a complete division has occurred, as in severing, then recovery of function can take place only when the divided ends lie in apposition or have been sutured. Growth of nerve fibers from the central ends proceeds at a rate of about 1 mm. a day, and the time of recovery can be estimated by the distance between the site of the injury and the destination of the nerve. Occasionally one finds that the peripheral nerves may be compressed or invaded by primary or metastasizing tumors arising in other tissues.

A classic example of paralysis of the seventh nerve of the face, which is caused by compression of the facial nerve in the fallopian canal as a result of an acute inflammatory process involving the nerve, is Bell's palsy. In this instance, edema leads to compression of nerve fibers, with resulting unilateral paralysis of the facial muscles. This condition is sometimes called peripheral facial palsy. It may result from exposure to cold, or it may occur in the course of an acute infectious disease, or it may result from injury to the nerve in operations in the regions of the mastoid. Tightening of the face and drooping of the angle of the mouth are characteristic changes. In this type of paralysis the face usually shows characteristic changes that vary with the extent of the paralysis. Actually a one-sided paralysis is much more noticeable. One eye seems to stay open while the other eye is able to function normally. When an individual has Bell's palsy for any length of time, considerable irritation of the eye may result from the inability to close it. The mouth appears to be drawn to one side, and actually one side of the face is expressionless. In a complete facial paralysis a masklike, expressionless face is seen that gives the patient a vacant, dumb appearance.

The prognosis in peripheral facial palsy, when it is nontraumatic in origin, is usually good. Patients with milder cases may recover in a month to 6 weeks, and the usual duration does not exceed 5 months. In the traumatic form the prognosis necessarily depends upon the character and the extent of the injury. In some patients whose facial nerve has been injured in operation or accident, anastomosis of the central end of the hypoglossal or the spinal accessory nerve with the distal end of the facial nerve has been reported to be successful. More recently a method of free transplantation of a section of nerve between the proximal and distal ends of the seventh nerve by a method attributed to Ballance and Dual has been reported. Fortunately, even for the most stubborn cases, there is now hope in the future.

Besides the paralysis of the motor nerves of the face and other affections of motor nerves, there are the spasmodic attacks that one occasionally sees. These may be termed fascicular twitchings. The most common seen in dental practice is the hemifacial spasm, which is a very curious condition indeed in that all or part of the muscles supplied by the facial nerve on one side contract intermittently or spasmodically. On occasion it follows Bell's palsy; it may occur without previous involvement of the facial nerve. The current view of this condition is that it is caused by a constriction of the facial nerve in the fallopian canal. Many of the facial tics seem to have no pathological or organic basis and are necessarily looked upon as habit spasms. No doubt these facial tics are largely based upon psychological phenomena, and sometimes, if repeatedly brought to the attention of the patient, voluntary control may be induced and thus the tic eliminated.

Sensory nerves

Motor nerve disturbances of the face can be diagnosed objectively since they are visable. Sensory nerve disturbances, however, must be diagnosed not only from objective tests, but also largely from subjective symptoms and history. In most cases definite neuropathways are followed by the disturbance, but in some instances no clear-cut pathway is followed. In dealing with facial pain few objective signs are apparent, and the absence of organic changes makes diagnosis in this realm much more difficult.

According to Chor,[4] there are perhaps five different facial pains. Brief descriptions of these follow:

Neuralgia. Paroxysmal, sharp, severe, lancinating pain, last only a few seconds, intensely painful, follows course of nerve distribution, has a definite trigger zone (area on the skin or mucous membrane, from which, if touched, pain may be elicited). Presence of sore spots, essentially unilateral (trigeminal neuralgia, etc.). If pain lasts longer than a few seconds, in general, it cannot be diagnosed as neuralgia. Cause is unknown. Frazier[5] suggests neuralgia may be caused by peripheral stimulation of affected nerve in the presence of thalamic lesions. Example: trifacial neuralgia, or tic douloureux.

Neuritis. Nerve inflammation, pain, and paresthesia (tingling, numb, or prickling sensation). May be dull ache or may be sharp and radiating. Nerve involved may be exquisitely tender, swollen, and indurated. Pain usually gradual with increasing intensity; not paroxysmal but constant, not letting up; cause is bacteria invasion, pressure, trauma, etc. Examples: dental infection, inflammation of dental pulp, or infection of impacted teeth.

Referred pain. Transmission of painful stimuli along a course far distant from the original source of its production by virtue of the complex anastomotic connections of the sensory nerves within the cerebral spinal and the sympathetic nervous system. Examples: heart disease, pain down the arm, and angina pectoris.

Central pain. Spontaneous pains and dyesthesias. Probable cause: chronic lesions of the thalamus (DéJerine and Roussy), which result in loss of inhibitory control of subcortical centers. Concerned in perception of sensations. Loss through lesions in the thalamus.

Psychalgia. Emotional stress and worry most prominent cause; does not follow in anatomical boundaries. Varies in intensities and character. Patient usually has a nervous background. Example: neurosis (anxiety or hysteria).

The neuralgias, neuritis, referred pain, central pain, and psychalgia (or mental pain) are in turn separated by whether they are symptomatic (organic) or idiopathic (nonorganic) in origin. Those of idiopathic origin are the neuralgias, central pain, and psychalgia. Those of symptomatic origin are the neuritic pain and the referred pain.

Peripheral organic pain

Under the heading of neuritis is found the odontalgias, the sinus pains, the otalgias, inflammatory lesions of the eye, and local lesions of the jaw. This type of pain is based upon nerve inflammation and is accompanied by pain and paresthesia (tingling, numb, or prickling sensations). Pain may be a dull ache, or it may be sharp and radiating. The nerve involved may be exquisitely tender, swollen, and indurated. The pain usually is gradual with increasing intensity, not paroxysmal but constant, not letting up. The cause is bacterial invasion, pressure, trauma, etc.

In the referred or reflex pain group is found pain resulting from temporomandibular joint affections, impacted or unerupted teeth, or pulp stones. Reflex pain is a type of pain resulting from the transmission of painful stimuli along a course far distant from the original source of its production, such as the pain which radiates down the left arm in a coronary occlusion patient, when the pain is actually within the heart.

Neuritis. In a consideration of the symptomatic pain or pain that presents a definite organic origin, pain originating from dental conditions or odontalgias, including pulpitis, inflammation of the periodontal membrane (periodontitis, or pericementitis), and pericoronal infection, may be brought under the general heading of a neuritis or a neuritic-like pain.

Odontalgia. Primary is pain of dental origin, arising in the pulp. Pain of this type is referred to as a pulpitis; it may be termed acute, subacute, or chronic (the stages of hyperemia and suppuration). A pulpitis is a painful inflammation of the neural substance and blood-vascular supply of the pulp of the tooth. This occurs when the pulp is exposed or nearly exposed to various thermal, mechanical, chemical, or bacterial irritants. Necessary changes evolve in the dental pulp brought on by any of these irritants. Examples include trauma from an external source such as a severe blow, microtrauma from malocclusion or traumatic occlusion, pulpal exposures from bacterial invasions or the close proximity of a large restoration, or overheating during operative procedures.

Some pulpal pain may also be associated with various systemic disturbances that affect the nutrition. Pain associated with the pulp is often difficult to localize because no proprioceptive fibers are present in the chamber of the pulp, the nerves merely emanating from the branches of the trigeminal nerve. If and when the inflammation extends beyond the apices of the tooth and involves the periodontium, then localization and pain associated with percussion can be ascertained. Diseases of the pulp often manifest themselves in both the neuritic type of pain and the reflex pain because the pulp is not supplied with a localizing sensation by means of proprioceptive fibers. As has been noted, reflex pain also occurs from pulp stones or denticles growing within the pulp as well as from pulpal exposures, and sometimes even impacted and unerupted teeth may be a cause of reflex pain. To make a diagnosis in this realm it is highly important that a careful examination and analysis be made of all the signs and symptoms.

Pain arising in the pulp may also result from a hypersensitive dentin or cementum. A knowledge is necessary of the sequelae of pulpal irritation and the changes that occur within the pulp, which manifest themselves in distinct clinical signs. It is not always easy to make a diagnosis quickly and accurately. An orderly, definite, and precise approach must be kept in mind in making any differential type of diagnosis. Often a diagnosis must be made from symptoms that are common to two or more conditions. For instance, an acute apical alveolar abscess and a pericemental abscess may simulate each other and may present the same clinical symptoms although the two are not the same, and one could be successfully treated by one method, which could be totally different than the treatment applied to the other. Naturally, any successful treatment must depend upon a correct diagnosis.

Often, pain of dental origin can be easily localized by careful clinical examination, the use of dental roentgenograms, a careful history, and analysis of the symptoms. If a cavity is present in the tooth or an extremely large restoration, then a strong possibility usually exists of some pulpal disturbance. On the other hand, in the presence of gingival recession, looseness of the tooth, pocket formation, or loss of bone, a periodontal origin is naturally assumed.

If a graphic form of classification is used, it is easier to distinguish between an infected pulpal disease and a disease of the periodontal structures. In general, a good differential diagnosis of inflammatory diseases is given in Table 26-1.

Sinus pain. Other types of pain, neuritic in origin and symptomatic or organic, that confront the dentist are pains of paranasal sinus origin. These are not always easily differentiated by the dentist (particularly since they simulate pain of an odontalgic origin) because of the close proximity of the various sinuses in relation to roots of teeth. However, a few simple diagnostic tests that are easily at the disposal of the dentist may be employed to clarify the picture. It is important in dealing with this type of pain to obtain a good history from the patient; for instance, is there a history of a recent cold, influenza, or other upper respiratory tract infection? Often a few simple questions will help the dentist to determine whether or not pain is of a sinus origin and, if so, which sinus in particular might be involved. For instance, the patient may be asked if the pain is bilateral or unilateral. If the pain is bilateral, then it is more likely to be a frontal sinus involvement, particularly if the patient feels better when sitting in an upright position. If the pain is unilateral and the patient is relieved by a recumbent position, then one may assume that the pain is more probably

Table 26-1. Differential diagnosis of inflammatory diseases*

Pulp	Periodontal membrane
1. The pain is not always localized; often difficult to locate.	1. The pain is always localized; easily located.
2. The pain is sharp, lancinating, intermittent, and throbbing. Usually worse during fatigue and at night when in reclining position.	2. Pain is dull, steady, and continuous. Is not affected by position of body or time of day.
3. The pulp is very sensitive to thermal changes and other irritants.	3. The tooth is not affected by thermal changes or chemical irritants.
4. The tooth is not tender to percussion.	4. In early stages, pressure relieves and later intensifies the pain.
5. The tooth does not seem elongated. Does not interfere in occlusion.	5. The tooth is raised in its socket and strikes first in occlusion.
6. The tooth usually shows extensive caries or a large restoration.	6. A sound unfilled tooth often develops periodontal pain.
7. The regional lymph nodes in the submaxillary area are not affected.	7. The regional lymph nodes are usually enlarged and tender to palpation.
8. Body temperature is not affected.	8. Body temperature is usually increased.

*From Prinz, H.: Diseases of the soft structures of the teeth and their treatment, Philadelphia, 1947, Lea & Febiger, p. 84.

of a maxillary sinus origin. Usually tenderness is present over the affected sinus. This examination may be made by pressing the fingers against the outline of bone overlying the wall of either sinus. If a marked tenderness is found, then it may be assumed that a sinus infection is present. It is not to be confused with the periapical tenderness, which is also felt upon palpation. This can be differentiated by tapping of the teeth in this area. When tenderness of more than one tooth to percussion is the situation, then it is likely that the cause is related to the sinuses rather than to the teeth.

Also, those who are suffering from sinus pain often complain that it hurts to walk or bend over. Transillumination may be used by darkening the room and using the transilluminating light to note if a sinus is cloudy. If doubt is still present, it is good procedure to make radiographs of the sinus area. The roentgenographic examination must be made by the use of large roentgenograms to be used in a cassette. The most effective technique available is the Waters view, which provides an excellent diagnostic field in which both sides are readily made available for study. The typical dental films routinely used in a dental office do not offer enough area to make a diagnosis of sinusitis. It is obvious that the importance of finding pain of a sinus origin is in differentiating it from pain of a dental origin and also in helping the patient to find the proper medical assistance. Never be hasty in extracting teeth in the presence of an existing allergy or cold.

Otalgia. Often an otalgia is also a neuritic type of pain, symptomatic in origin, that produces facial pain at the onset by referring pain along one or more of the branches of the trigeminal nerve. This sometimes is confusing when determining whether or not a tooth or teeth are involved. But usually the pain localizes in the aural region in a relatively short time if the ear is inflamed.

Inflammatory lesions of the eye. Other neuritic-like pains occurring in the face may be the inflammatory lesions of the eye: (1) acute iritis, (2) herpes zoster ophthalmicus, (3) acute retrobulbar neuritis, (4) heterophoria, (5) acute glaucoma. It is seldom that pain originating in the eye will reflect into the area of the teeth, but sometimes acute pain is referred to the area of the nose or the periorbital tissues, and, in such instances, disease of the eye should always be suspected.

Local lesions of the jaw. In a consideration of the local lesions of the jaw such entities as alveolitis, dry socket, and osteomyelitis present neuritic pains that are easily discernible by careful history-taking, good local examination, and the use of radiographs.

All of the aforementioned types of neuritic pain definitely have an established causal phenomenon and are said to be of organic origin, that is, produced by a known cause such as bacterial invasion, pressure, trauma, or other causative mechanism that is definable. This type of pain is strictly inflammatory. It is not to be confused with the neuralgias, which are idiopathic in origin, that is, of unknown cause.

Referred pain. Referred or reflex pain that occurs in the face is usually symptomatic, based upon some definite organic cause, and is referred to as a neuritic-like pain.

Temporomandibular joint affections. Temporomandibular joint affections include conditions such as temporomandibular joint arthritis, temporomandibular joint neurosis, temporomandibular joint neuritis, or Costens' syndrome, all nondescript but applicable terms of the same ailment; this is a condition first observed by Costen as a syndrome arising from malocclusion of natural teeth, or artificial teeth in edentulous mouths, which resulted in a specific affection of the temporomandibular joint. Many symptoms were noted in this disease, mainly pain in or about the temporomandibular joint that radiated up the side of the head and into the face and sometimes even into the neck. A conjoining snapping or cracking noise in the ear upon opening and closing the mouth, severe headaches (particularly the occipital or posturicular type), stuffiness or feeling of fullness in the external auditory meatus, referred pain in the ears, and, on occasion, dizziness or a deafness was attributed to this condition.

Diseases of the temporomandibular joint are usually unilateral, but occasionally may be bilateral. More recent studies have revealed that this condition usually occurs in patients who exceed the limit of load tolerance upon the temporomandibular joint, either by bruxism (night grinding), constant clenching of the teeth while under stress and strain, or other manifestations of nervous origin in the presence of an occlusal disharmony. The symptoms of temporomandibular joint diseases have been attributed to the erosion of the bone of the glenoid fossa by the head of the condyle in instances of distal displacement of the condyle of the mandible caused by the occlusal relationship of the teeth. Costen erroneously attributed this condition to impingement of the auriculotemporal nerve through direct irritation and reflex pain and sensory disturbances in the chorda tympani nerve. It is more probable that this condition is of an osteoarthritic nature (degenerative arthritis) rather than a nerve impingement.

The symptoms often can be relieved by proper treatment, which consists of repositioning the jaws by the use of an acrylic splinting mechanism, metal splints, or other prosthetic appliances that tend to reposition the jaws into a normal occlusion for that individual and thereby rest the joint. Selective grinding (occlusal equilibration) results in occlusal rehabilitation.

A condition that may simulate a temporomandibular joint distubance is one of referred pain from a temporary strain involving the ligaments or muscles of mastication. A painful episode may follow an accident in which the chin has received a blow or a condition in which the jaw has been opened too wide while sneezing or yawning. These temporary disturbances resulting from a traumatic experience will usually alleviate of their own accord and require no treatment beyond heat application and rest.

Differentiation between a muscle strain and a joint disturbance depends upon taking an accurate history before attempting to diagnose from the symptom of pain only. In the process of administering a local anesthetic an inadvertent injection through a muscle may bring on pain and trismus as a sequel. The mandibular block involving the medial pterygoid muscle is the most common example.

Keep in mind that pain referred to the temporomandibular joint might be malignant in origin, as in the case of a parotid gland tumor that causes pain and trismus before it is manifest through the motor nerve disturbance. Another problem to consider when pain is a complaint involving the angle of the mandible is coronary artery occlusion.

Idiopathic pain

Neuralgia. The underlying difference between a neuritic and a neuralgic pain is that though both are of an inflammatory nature, the neuritic pain is produced by a known cause and the neuralgic pain is one of an unknown origin. A neuralgia is distinctive in that the pain is paroxysmal, sharp, severe, and lancinating, lasting, however, only a few seconds. It is intensely painful and follows the course of a known nerve distribution. It is also distinctive in that it has a definite trigger zone (an area on the skin or mucous membrane from which, if touched, pain over the course of the affected nerve may be elicited). Sore spots are present. It is essentially unilateral. If pain lasts longer than a few seconds, generally it cannot be diagnosed as neuralgia. The pain of a neuralgia is much more severe than the pain of a neuritis, but, since it lasts such a short time, it is bearable. The intensity of the pain is such that, when it is seen in a patient, the practitioner is highly impressed by the terrible suffering that the patient must endure during an attack. The etiology and pathology of the neuralgias remain undetermined. However, some conditions seem attributable, such as tumors involving the sensory nerves, multiple sclerosis, syringobulbia, chronic syphilitic basilar meningitis, thrombosis of the posteroinferior cerebellar artery, and chronic intracranial lesions.

The more common types of neuralgias of the face are trigeminal, sphenopalatine, and glossopharyngeal.

Trigeminal neuralgia (tic douloureux). This is an involvement of the fifth cranial nerve and more specifically within the gasserian ganglion. The second and third divisions, separately or together, are most often involved. On occasion, an involvement of the first division is found, but this is more rare. Frazier[5] suggests that this type of neuralgia may result from peripheral stimulation of the affected nerve in the presence of thalamic lesions.

Treatment consists of inhalation from 20 to 30 drops of trichlorethylene on a bit of cotton, which gives a temporary measure of relief, and the administration of large doses of vitamin B with concentrated liver extracts rich in the antianemia factors of vitamin B_{12}; more recently, Tolseram plus Dilantin sodium has been utilized. Alcoholic injection of the trigeminal branches may be performed to give relief for a period of a year or slightly longer. The most permanent results are obtained by surgical resection of the posterior sensory root of the gasserian ganglion, which is the definitive treatment.

Sphenopalatine neuralgia. Another neuralgia producing pain in the face is known as sphenopalatine neuralgia (Sluder's syndrome). In this type of neuralgia the sphenopalatine (Meckel's) ganglion is believed to become irritated by infection or hyperplasia of the sphenoid or posterior ethmoid sinuses. Anemia, fatigue, emotional upsets, toxemia, etc. are factors to be considered in the etiology at times. It has also been attributed to an intumescence of the nasal mucosa when enlarged turbinates, abnormal growths, deviated septa, etc. are present. Some have stated that this type of neuralgia is a result of allergic manifestation or of vasomotor imbalance.

The clinical picture is one of pain around the eye, the upper teeth, and the upper jaw, extending sometimes to the zygoma, and to the temple and, occasionally, producing earache and pain in or around the ear or mastoid process. One sometimes finds a photophobia, lacrimation, rhinorrhea, or some sympathetic syndrome involving a sneezing mechanism. Often symptoms within the tongue occur such as a glossodynia and a peculiar sensation of diminished taste on the anterior half of the tongue. The pain of a sphenopalatine neuralgia differs from that of a trigeminal neuralgia in that it is more constant, lacking the severe paroxysmal attack. The best diagnostic technique available is to cocainize Meckel's ganglion. This also happens to be the best form of treatment. The most permanent results are obtained with alcohol-phenol injections of the ganglion.

Glossopharyngeal neuralgia. Glossopharyngeal neuralgia closely resembles trigeminal neuralgia except for the location of the pain, which follows the distribution of the ninth nerve as well as the fifth nerve. The pain radiates from the lateral wall of the pharynx to the side of the neck and ear. This is a paroxysmal, lancinating type of pain, with a trigger zone present at some point on the pharyngeal mucous membrane. Glossopharyngeal neuralgia can usually be differentiated by painting the throat with cocaine or lidocaine ointment in the region of the tonsillar fossa and lateral pharyngeal walls. The glossopharyngeal nerve lies in close proximity to the vagus, the hypoglossal, and the spinal accessory nerves, and because it lies deep it is unwise to attempt alcohol injections. The best treatment here is surgical section of the sensory pathway.

In general, in making a diagnosis of idiopathic neuralgia the following points must be satisfied: the age of onset is usually more than 35 years of age; the general character of the pain is severely intense and paroxysmal (not more than 30 seconds' duration); it has a definite trigger point that does not change its location; it follows the anatomical distribution of one or more of the affected nerves or their endings; it is unilateral; and it is accompanied by various reflex, vasomotor, sensory, and trophic phenomena such as cutaneous flushing, photophobia, lacrimation, and salivation, as well as a subjective sensation of swelling in the affected tissue and the excitability of the attacks by peripheral stimuli.

The dentist has available an invaluable diagnostic aid when it comes to all types of facial pain, and that is the skillful use of regional anesthesia and analgesia. It is vitally necessary that he master an excellent technique based on a thorough knowledge of anatomy, and, more specifically, neuroanatomy, so that he may pinpoint deposition of an anesthetic solution into an anatomical area and thus by the knowledge of the relief obtained be given a clue to the exact locality of an impending pain and further be able to discriminate the various probable causes of pain.

In making any survey of the neuralgic problems the dentist should constantly keep in mind the fact that any major neuralgia may be caused by an organic lesion of the affected nerve or its roots, tumors at the base of the brain and the middle fossa, tumors growing from the base of the skull in the neighborhood of the foramen ovale or foramen rotundum or on some specific peripheral nerve itself; hence, the dentist should inquire always if vomiting has occurred, with headaches, and if any impairment of sensibility existing in the cutaneous territory of the affected nerve or any evidence of impairment in the motor power or the muscles of mastication is present, since these are all a part of the clinical picture of a more serious brain tumor involvement.

Central pain. Other idiopathic phenomena with which the dentist must concern himself are the headaches that produce facial pain.

Migraine headache. The migraine type of headache is most often unilateral in onset and is a steady ache with spasmodic throbbing. It is very severe, requiring the patient to cease from all activity and go to bed until the pain ceases. It often lasts a few hours, but more frequently lasts 24 to 48 hours. These headaches are ushered in by a feeling of nausea and irritability, and often vomiting occurs. Occasionally present are paresthesia, hemianopia, and scotomas. It is believed that the etiology of this type of headache, though not known, is probably related to allergy and some hereditary factors. Wolff[10] states that certain individuals have a predisposition and psychobiological equipment that makes them prone to sustained and pernicious emotional states. During such states, liable, physiological mechanisms set off a chain of events constituting the attack of migraine. These persons are more often perfectionistic, rigid individuals who become more and more tense and fatigued because of their driving, order-loving routine, and the headache occurs particularly during periods of stress.

Evidence has been presented that tends to place the pathology of migraine headaches in the realm of derangements of cranial vascular function, primarily concerning the branches of the external carotid or any other pain-sensitive artery in the head. The pain is the result of vasodilation and distention of the relaxed cranial arteries. Because the pain is caused by excessive vasodilation, vasoconstricting agents have been used in the treatment of this disorder. These include ephedrine, epinephrine, and caffeine.

Temporal arteritis. Temporal arteritis is temporal in origin, with malaise, fever, sweats, and leukocytosis, and in from 2 to 6 weeks a prominent, reddened, swollen temporal artery exists. This phenomenon is thought to be caused by some focus of infection and has been attributed to bad teeth on occasion. It has also followed in the wake of extracting infected teeth. The only treatment suggested has been resection of a segment of temporal artery. Sometimes a little pressure against the artery will relieve the onset of attacks.

Tension headaches. In the tension headache group occipital myalgia is the most prominent and this is the result in most instances of a myositis or a fibrositis of one or more of the neck muscles. Usually nervous tension with hypertonicity of the neck muscles produces this type of pain. The pain in this case is usually dull and comes on during periods of stress or worry. On occasion a cervical arthritis may be a factor in producing this type of headache. Dentists are prone to develop this disease because of the constant bending of their head and tension at the dental chair, thus producing a spasm within the neck muscles. Treatment of this condition is best afforded by the use of vitamin B therapy; more specifically, injections of nicotinic acid, along with physical therapy such as diathermy, deep massage, or heat to the affected neck muscles.

Histamine cephalgia. Histamine cephalgia is also known as neurovascular headache or "suicide headache." It is a severe, unilateral type of headache lasting usually less than an hour. It begins and ends suddenly. This headache has a tendency to awaken the patient at night with its severity. It is a constant, excruciatingly painful type of headache involving the neck and face, particularly the temple, nose, and eye, and may extend into the shoulder area. At times it involves even the teeth. Associated with this type of headache is eyewatering, together with stuffiness, watering, and discomfort of the nostril. Usually the attacks of this type of headache can be induced by subcutaneous injection of histamine. The treatment has been attempted by desensitizing the patient with increasing doses of histamine diphosphate, with indifferent success.

Psychogenic headache. The psychogenic headache is a nonorganic and idiopathic phenomenon that is associated with an emotional disturbance such as one of the neuroses. The patient usually describes this type of headache as a sharp, shooting, stabbing type of ache, which appears as pain in the head. He may describe it as very intense, or terrible, or excruciating, etc. The amount of time that the headache may last cannot be specified. It seems to be increased by problematical situations such as the necessity of making a decision, or situations involving great mental strain that induces a certain amount of excitement. Some persons seem to become afflicted during their participation in competitive sports, or sometimes just the excitement of being in a crowd will bring on the headache. This headache is at first responsive to almost any type of treatment. The patient responds not only to medicinal therapy, but also to suggestion; however, as long as the underlying psychoneurosis exists, no treatment is successful. The best treatment is directed at removing the underlying cause of the neurosis.

Psychalgia. Many other types of headache exists with which the dentist could familiarize himself, and the works of Wolff[10] or Pollock[7] are recommended. Aside from the psychogenic type of headache a psychogenic facial neuralgia is occasionally seen, which, again, is an idiopathic, nonspecific, nonorganic type of ailment that does produce pain in the face. This type of facial pain simulates the major and minor neuralgias as well as the headaches, and it is not affected by the position of the patient or by any trigger point, that is, one can touch the patient's face in any location of the peripheral nerve branches and no pain will be specifically elicited in that area. The location of the pain, although severe, may shift. No location specificity is found at all. The pain may be unilateral or bilateral. The duration is often persistent and constant. The patient is always aware that he has some pain, and it occasionally gets worse, like the psychogenic headache, under duress, stress, or tension. Almost all medications in this instance would give a temporary measure of relief, but none will give permanent relief, and usually an equal relief will be obtained by the use of placebos.

The patient who presents a psychogenic neuralgia usually is a type of individual who might be termed nervous and does present other symptoms of a neurosis or a psychogenic disturbance. The dentist should not be quick to label anything that resembles a neuralgia as psychogenic until he has exhausted all the techniques that will stop an ordinary neuralgia, such as the use of local blocks, which will initiate relief in even the major neuralgias for at least a period, and has failed to relieve the pain with the use of inhalation analgesics, high vitamin B therapy, or a Tolseram-Dilantin injection. In other words, after all measures are exhausted, and the pain still persists and presents a nonspecific picture, then perhaps the practitioner is warranted in labeling it a psychogenic type of pain, particularly if all measures, including suggestion, are of some help, but that nothing gives relief for as long as, say, 3 hours.

I think the dentist must be on guard, particularly with the psychogenic facial neuralgias, because often these patients seem to be eager for some surgical intervention, and although they derive temporary benefit from it, they are the first to condemn the dentist if permanency is not the result. The proper treatment for this type of patient is referral to a psychiatrist, who in turn will use either psychotherapy based upon psychoanalysis or one of the convulsive therapies such as electroconvulsive therapy; the patient will necessarily be treated in toto instead of just a local ramification of his persistent illness.

Differential diagnosis

The dentist would do well to categorically place these various types of pain in his mind, because, by knowing the various types, he can take a more critical attitude toward the symptom of pain, and thus prevent misguided therapy. After a pain is definitely established to be in the realm of neuralgia, neuritis, referred pain, central pain, or psychalgia, as a working hypothesis, he can then proceed to differentiate between the more specific entities that might be a cause of each. For instance, it may be ascertained that a neuralgia is present, but which of the neuralgias is it? Or, although it may be ascertained that it is a neuritis, perhaps by the very act of referred pain a neuritis may take on the characteristics of neuralgia. Hence, it behooves one to make a further evaluation based upon additional differentiating factors. Among these, consider the effective position, location, duration, and actual type of locale and, finally, through differentiating techniques, categorically divide these types into a more readily discernible diagnostic form.

Once again, as in dealing with typical dental pain, a few simple questions concerning the characteristics of the pain relating to its onset, intensity, and duration as well as locality often serve to point in the direction of a correct diagnosis. And if a graphic form of classification is kept in mind, the various causes of facial pain may more easily be discerned and, hence, a more differential diagnosis rendered. Space does not permit a running of the gamut in this regard, but the student will, through his experience, be able to formulate in his own mind a more complete differentiating chart. The accompanying chart is only a suggested form. Unless this equation can be satisfied, a definite diagnosis of neuralgia

Table 26-2. Differential diagnosis of pain

Syndrome	Effect of position	Type	Location	Duration	Differentiating techniques
Diseases of temporomandibular joint	Supine or recumbent position increases pain	More often unilateral; may be bilateral, however	In or about joints; may refer to temporal and cervical region	Constant; increases upon opening or closing mouth	0.5 ml. procaine solution injected in temporomandibular joint usually gives relief; hydrocortisone in joint gives relief; temporary splinting gives relief along with heat therapy
Trigeminal neuralgia or tic douloureux	None	Unilateral	Follows distribution of fifth nerve and contiguous sensory areas	Paroxysmal, stabbing, intermittently; 30 seconds to 1 minute duration	Routine mandibular injection with local anesthetic and/or Tolseram plus Dilantin sodium usually relieves; always a definite trigger zone along fifth nerve distribution
Glossopharyngeal neuralgia	None	Unilateral	Fifth nerve and ninth nerve distribution; soft palate, tonsil, and internal ear	Paroxysmal lancinating pain; radiates to ear rather than along fifth nerve, in general	Paint throat with cocaine or lidocaine ointment; trigger zone in tonsillar fossa or base of tongue
Sphenopalatine neuralgia	None	Unilateral	Maxillary division of fifth nerve, more specifically nasal in origin	More or less constant; not paroxysmal; moderately severe	Cocainization of sphenopalatine ganglion through nose affords relief
Auriculotemporal neuralgia	None	Unilateral	Neuralgic pain in temporomandibular joint	2 to 3 minutes' duration; more throbbing and aching	Inhalation of trichlorethylene relieves pain immediately; usually vitamin B_{12} injections improve
Buccal neuralgia (facial artery)	Lying on affected side often starts pain	Unilateral; may be bilateral	Lips, cheek, tongue, and jaws	Paroxysmal; longer lasting, and instituted by chewing and talking	Pressure against segment of facial artery usually relieves; tying off or severing facial artery relieves
Sinus pain Maxillary	Relieved by recumbent position	Unilateral	Tenderness over affected sinus	Hours or days	Antibiotic therapy and dry heat relieves; may be discerned through transillumination and radiographs
Frontal	Improves in upright position	Bilateral	Headache; hurts to jar, as in walking, bending over, etc.	Hours or days	
Psychogenic facial neuralgias	Nonspecific	May be bilateral or unilateral	Persistent and constant; patient always aware of pain	Nonspecific	Only temporary relief to medication; equal relief always to use of placebos

should not be made. Other of the various causes of facial pain should be sought. Neuralgias are of a very specific nature, based upon diagnostic features. Keep in mind, too, that these symptoms never tend to disappear, even when the attention is drawn in some other direction; whereas, as in many of the pseudoneuralgias, such as the psychalgias, the attention of the patient can often be diverted and a cessation of pain result.

It is necessary to again emphasize the importance of being positive that no involvement of a tooth could be producing a severe neuritis. Always keep in mind that a diagnosis rendered from pain patterns alone can often be misleading and erroneous although the symptoms appear to be clearcut and seemingly self-evident. Until all methods of diagnostic technique are instituted, a precursory conclusion should not be drawn. Never be hasty in drawing conclusions or instituting therapy when dealing with such a subjective symptom as pain. If in doubt, after making an exhaustive examination, it is certainly in order to administer sedatives, soporifics, and hypnotics over a period of 24 to 48 hours and then reevaluate the total picture since often in such a short lapse of time a more definite symptomatology may be present that will allow a more easily attained diagnosis.

It is important to recall that any recurrent, lingering pain that occurs mainly when the teeth are pressed together in mastication and gets "sore" occasionally, but seldom exceeds a chronic phase, may be the result of a split or fractured tooth that has not separated at the site of injury. The posterior teeth are most commonly involved, often in a site of traumatic occlusion such as from a plunging cusp. It is difficult to find these "hair line" fractures, but a sharp explorer inserted into the line of anatomical grooves, pits, or fissures and pressed firmly will sometimes reveal the site when bubbles of saliva emerge. A disclosing solution can be used advantageously to reveal a split tooth since it penetrates the crack.

A further admonishment in the treatment of facial pain is to be quite sure that in every case of facial pain the obligation has been fulfilled of performing a careful study to prevent the condition being misinterpreted as psychosomatic and labeled as such, since in most instances, if a patient complains of facial pain, that pain is very real and based upon some physical entity; it is not just imaginary. After a diagnosis of a facial pain of nonspecific dental origin is rendered, then with good faith and strong conviction the patient can be referred to one specially trained to render appropriate treatment. In these cases it is an absolute necessity that the dentist and the physician give full cooperation, one to the other. In so doing, impetus will be given to the dentist-physician-patient relationship that invokes the confidence and good will which are so vitally necessary.

REFERENCES

1. Ballenger, H. C.: Headaches and neuralgias of the face and head, Otology, rhinology and laryngology, Philadelphia, 1954, Lea & Febiger, p. 83.
2. Coolidge, E. D.: Clinical pathology and treatment of the dental pulp and periodontal tissues, ed. 2, Philadelphia, 1946, Lea & Febiger, p. 38.
3. Comroe, B. I., Collins, L. H., Jr., and Crane, M. P.: Internal medicine in dental practice, ed. 4, Philadelphia, 1954, Lea & Febiger, pp. 221, 223, 225.
4. Chor, Herman: Neurologic aspects of temporomandibular disorders, J. Amer. Dent. Ass. **25:**1033, 1938 (quoted by Schweitzer).
5. Frazier, C. H., Lewy, F. H., and Rowe, S. N.: Origin and mechanism of paroxysmal neuralgic pain and the surgical treatment of central pain, Brain **60:**44, 1937.
6. Merritt, H H., and Sciarra, D.: Tumors of the brain and spinal cord; in Harrison, T. R.: Principles of internal medicine, New York, 1950, McGraw-Hill Book Co., pp. 1658-1661.
7. Pollock, L. J.: Neurology, Ann. Otol. **52:**730, 1943.
8. Prinz, H.: Diseases of the soft structures of the teeth and their treatment, Philadelphia, 1947, Lea & Febiger, p. 84.

9. Schweitzer, J. M.: Oral rehabilitation, St. Louis, 1951, The C. V. Mosby Co., p. 430.
10. Wolff, H. G.: Headache and other head pain, New York, 1948, Oxford University Press, pp. 15-16.
11. Wolf, S., and Wolff, H. G.: Human Gastric functions: an experimental study of a man and his stomach, New York, 1943, Oxford University Press.
12. Ishmael, D. M.: Dental pain, J. Okla. Dent. Ass. **46**:5, 1957.
13. Kruger, G. O., and Reynolds, D. C.: Maxillofacial pain. In McCarthy, F. M., editor: Emergencies in dental practice, Philadelphia, 1967, W. B. Saunders Co., pp. 123-143.

INDEX

A

Abrasion
 definition, 268
 treatment, 269
Abscess
 alveolar, 191
 dissecting, 171
 incision and drainage, 168, 174
 indurated, 167, 171
 localization, 168
 medial mandibular, 172
 in oral cavity, 140
 periapical, 167
  extraction, 168
  pulp canal opening, 168
 periodontal, 173
  treatment, 173
 subperiosteal, 171
Acid-base balance, 208
Actinomycosis, 161
 diagnosis, 161
 etiology, 161
 signs and symptoms, 161
 treatment, 162
Addison's disease, 207
Adenitis, 170
 pericoronal infection, 169
Adenocarcinoma, 530, 548
Adenoma, salivary, 545
Adrenal insufficiency, 207
Agranulocytosis, 133
 secondary to antibiotic therapy, 151, 154
Airway, 15, 394
 obstruction, 16
  treatment, 16
Allergy, 130
Alloplasts; see Implants
Alveolar process, fracture of, 289
Alveolectomy; see Alveoloplasty
Alveoloplasty, 72
 interradicular, 76
 radical, 74
 simple, 73
Alveolus, septic, 128
Ameloblastoma, 518
 maxillary sinus, 242
Anaphylactoid reaction, 130
Anemia, aplastic, secondary to antibiotic therapy, 151, 154

Anesthesia, 49, 58
 general, exodontia under, 124
 precaution with gases, 30
 reaction to, 130
 selection for exodontia, 122
Aneurysm, 200
Ankylosis of temporomandibular joint, 345, 383
Antibiotics
 allergic responses to, 143
 dosage, 143
 general considerations, 139
 historical background, 139
 indiscriminate use, 144
 ointments, 144
 resistance, 144
 routes of administration, 142
 topical, 140, 143, 144
 toxic reactions, 144, 145
 use in acute infections, 187
Antihistamines in allergic manifestations of antibiotic therapy, 155
Antimetabolites, 536
Antrostomy, intranasal, 249
Anxiety, 47
Apertognathia, 438, 501
Aphthae, 163
Apicoectomy, 194
Arch bars, 293, 321, 480
Armamentarium, 45
 for exodontia, 52
 for impactions, 87
Arthritis, 370, 574
 in focal infection, 138
Arthroplasty for ankylosis of temporomandibular joint, 383
Asepsis, 14, 24, 50
 office practice, 27, 56
 principles of, 4
Auriculotemporal neuralgia, 580
Autoclaving, 18

B

Bacillus, fusiform, 132
Bacitracin, 143, 153
Bacteremia, 174
 in oral surgery, 135
 in periodontal infection, 197
 transient, 137

Bacteria
  causing pain, 570, 571, 574
  in hematoma, 17
  normal inhabitants of mouth, 132
Bandages, 34
Battle's sign, 358
Behçet's syndrome, 164
Bell's palsy, 570
Bence Jones bodies, 524
Biopsy, 526, 532
Bite planes in temporomandibular dysfunction, 377
Blastomyces dermatitidis, 162
Bleeding time, Duke method, 3
Blood
  analysis, 2
  culture, 187
  dyscrasia, 167
    surgical intervention in, 133
  loss, 13, 208
  plasma, 206
  protein fractions, 199
  replacement, 13
  typing, 199, 206
    cross matching, 199
    Rh determination, 199
Bone grafts, 252, 418, 427
  alveolar ridge, 433
  artificial (alloplast), 419, 423
  autogenous, 259, 428
  complications, 429
  criteria, 253
  evaluation, 260
  fate of, 418
  healing, 307
  heterogenous, 257
  homogenous, 255, 418
  immobilization following, 431
  indications for homogenous grafts, 418
  pin fixation following, 432
  plates following, 332, 432
  in reconstruction of mandible, 427, 428, 429, 430
  splints following, 431
  storage, 254
  technique for obtaining, 428
  types, 418
    block, 418, 419
    chip, 428
    freeze dried, 254, 255
    iliac, 428
    rib, 428
    tibia, 428
Brain tumors, 56
Branchial arch, 387
Branchial cyst, 546
Bruxism, 575
Buccal neuralgia, 580
Burns
  classification, 268, 281
  intraoral, 286
  local treatment, 286, 287
  in mass casualty care, 283
  shock in, 281

Burns—cont'd
  systemic problems, 281
    therapy in, 282, 283, 284
Burow flap, 113

C

Caldwell technique in ridge extension, 119
Caldwell-Luc operation, 246, 248, 249, 365
  indications, 249
  technique, 249
Callus, 307, 308
Canine impaction, 97
Carcinoma, 167, 531
  maxillary sinus, 244
  squamous cell, 531
    in salivary glands, 548
Cardiovascular disease, 135
  congenital, 135
  rheumatic fever, 135
Cartilage grafts, 257, 259, 416, 418
  homogenous transplant, 257
Case history, 1, 22, 207
Cavernous sinus thrombosis, 186
Cellulitis, 141, 169, 174
  acute, 174
  in lateral pharyngeal space, 183
  pericoronal infection, 169
  resolution, 174
  systemic reaction, 174
  treatment, 174
Cementoma, 517
Central pain, 580
Cephalothin, 152
Cerebrospinal rhinorrhea, 302
Cervical radicular tension syndrome, 569
Cheilorrhaphy, 392
Cheiloschisis, 386
Cheyne-Stokes respiration, 570
Children
  fractured jaws in, 351
  removal of teeth in, 120
Chloramphenicol, 150
  indications, 150
  precautions, 150
  preparation and dosage, 150
Chondroma, 521
Chondrosarcoma, 522
Circumferential wiring, 324, 337
Circumzygomatic wiring, 340
Clark's technique for ridge extension, 116
Clefts
  embryology, 386
  etiology, 389
  feeding, 392
  incomplete, 397
  lip repair, 393
  occurrence, 386
  oral, 386
  palate function, 394
  palate repair, 390
  pharyngeal flap, 402
  prosthetic speech aid appliance, 402
  speech therapy, 404
  submucosal, 399

Clefts—cont'd
  surgical correction, 392
  team approach, 405
  time for operation, 392, 396
Clostridium bifermentans, 159
Clostridium novyi, 159
Clostridium perfringens, 159
Clostridium septicum, 159
Clostridium tetani, 158
Closure, soft tissue, 38
Coagulation time, 3
Cocaine
  sensitivity to, 246
  in sinus surgery, 246
Cold applications, 187
Cold sterilization, 19
Complications of exodontia, 126, 127
Condyle, mandibular fracture of, 345
Condylectomy, 379
  technique, 379, 380
Congenital deformities of jaws; see Developmental deformities of jaws
Contraindications for extraction, 50
Contusion
  definition, 267
  treatment, 269
Convulsions, 570
Cornish wool, 408
Cortex, cerebral, 568, 570
Cortisone
  in allergic manifestations, 156
  in temporomandibular joint dysfunction, 377
Craniomaxillary fixation, 359
Crepitus, 317
Crosshatching of incision, 36
Cryosurgery, 537
Culture, organisms, 176
Cysts
  bone, 228
  branchiogenic, 213, 226
  classification, 212
  congenital, 213, 226
  dentigerous, 221
  dermoid, 214, 226
  developmental, 215
  diagnosis, 223
    x-ray findings, 224
  enucleation, 230
  follicular, 220
  in fractures, 297
  general considerations, 223
  globulomaxillary, 217
  hemorrhagic, 213
  incisive canal, 215
  median, 215
  mucous retention, 217
  nasoalveolar, 215
  nasopalatine, 215
  periapical, 193, 195
    exteriorization of, 196
    obturators in, 196
    technique of removal, 195
    treatment, 196

Cysts—cont'd
  periodontal, 218, 220
  postoperative complications, 234
  primordial, 220
  radiopaque materials in diagnosis, 224
  ranula, 218
  retention, 227, 545
  soft tissue, 226
  surgical technique in removal, 225
  thyroglossal, 213, 226
  traumatic, 213
  use of bone chips in, 231
  use of dressings in, 231
  use of Gelfoam in, 231

D

Defects following cancer surgery, 434
Dehydration, 187, 208
  in fever, 137
Denture sore mouth; see Moniliasis
Dermatitis, secondary to antibiotics, 149, 153
Developmental deformities of jaws, 438
  anterior segmental osteotomy, 490
  apertognathia, 438, 501
    sliding osteotomy to lengthen ramus, 486, 497
    V-shaped ostectomy in body of mandible, 505
  fixation appliances, 480
  growth and orthodontics, 440
  horizontal osteotomy of ramus, 465
    Gigli saw osteotomy, 465
    Moose osteotomy, 465
  micrognathia, 484
    L sliding osteotomy, 488
    microgenia, 500
    step sliding osteotomy in body of mandible, 486
    vertical osteotomy of ramus with bone graft, 493
    vertical L or C osteotomy, 497
  musculature relationship to surgical correction, 460, 478
  oblique subcondylar osteotomy, 463
    Gigli saw condylotomy, 450
    subsigmoid notch condylotomy, 449
  ostectomy in body of mandible, 471
    intraoral ostectomy, 475
  postoperative care, 478
  preoperative planning, 440
  preparation of patient for surgery, 444
  roentgenographic survey, 440, 441
  sagittal osteotomy, 468
  vertical osteotomy in ramus, 452
Diabetes mellitus, surgical intervention in, 133
Diarrhea, secondary to antibiotic therapy, 149, 151, 152
Dicumarol, 199
Diet in fractures, 352
Dihydrostreptomycin; see Streptomycin
Dingman two-stage operation, 472
Dislocations, temporomandibular joint, 381
  treatment, 382
Disposable supplies, 28
Dorrance "push-back" operation, 400

Drains
  iodoform, 5
  Penrose, 5
  rubber dam, 5
  surgical, 5
Draping, 27
  for exodontia, 58, 86
Dressings, 10, 34
  pressure, 110
Dry heat sterilization, 19
Dry socket, 128, 140, 574
Duct, parotid, 539
Dysplasia, fibrous, 213

E

Ears, bleeding from, 301
Ecchymosis, 17
Electrolyte balance, 43, 207
  abnormal, in fever, 137
Electrosurgery, 110, 119
Elevator principles, 82
Embryology, oral clefts, 386
Emergencies in dental office, 129
Emphysema, 173
Enamel pearls, 517
Endaural incision, 40
Endocarditis, bacterial, 135
Environment in oral clefts, 390
Epulis
  fibrous, 525
  fissuratum, 110, 202
Erich operation, 471
Erythema multiforme, 163
  differentiate from periodontitis, 197
Erythromycin, 148
  preparation and dosage, 148
Esophagus, tooth displaced in, 131
Essig splint, 293
Ewing's tumor, 523
Examination of patient, 49
Exodontia
  complicated, 72
  forceps extraction, 58
  in hospital, 125
  impacted teeth, 85
  introduction, 46
  special considerations, 120
  under general anesthesia, 124
Exolevers, 54
Exostosis, 520
Exteroceptor, 568
Eye, lesion, 572, 574

F

Face development, 387
Facial nerve, 569, 570
Facial tic, 571
Fascia, 177
Fascial planes, 176
Fever, 137
  clinical symptoms, 137
  physiological changes, 137
Fibrin foam, 205

Fibroma, 525
  neurogenic, 531
  ossifying, 213
Fibro-osteoma, 521
Fibrosarcoma, 521, 531
Fibrous dysplasia, 521
  in fractures, 297
First aid in fractures, 303
Flaps
  Abbe, 413
  advancement or rotation, 409, 410
  distant, 409, 415
  Estlander, 413
  pedicle, 411, 415
  surgical, 5, 76
  transposition, 410
  tube, 416
  V-Y, 410, 411
  Z-plasty, 411
Fluctuance, 175, 176
Fluid balance, 43, 187, 207, 209
  categories of patients, 208
    fluid needs in aged, 209
    fluid needs in youth, 209
  methods of administration, 209
Forceps, 53
  extraction, 59
Foreign body
  localization, 198
  removal, 198
  in wounds, 280
Fractures
  arch bars, 321
  automobile cause of, 296
  bone healing in, 307
  causes, 296, 309
  children, 351
  circumferential wiring, 324, 337
  classification, 297, 356
  comminuted, 298
  complications, 354
  compound, 297
  diet, 352
  elastic traction, 320
  examination for, 298
  favorable, 316
  feeding problems, 353
  first aid, 303
  fixation, 318
  frequency of various types, 298
  frontozygomatic wiring, 362
  functional reconstruction of bone, 309
  greenstick, 297
  history in, 298
  horizontal maxillary, 356, 359
  Ivy loop wiring, 320
  mandible, 309, 333
    angle, 334
    bone plates, 332
    causes, 309
    in children, 351
    circumzygomatic wiring, 340
    complications, 354
    condyle, 345

Fractures—cont'd
　mandible—cont'd
　　coronoid process, 344
　　displacement, 311
　　edentulous, 337
　　examination for, 299
　　favorable fracture, 316
　　location, 311
　　malunion, 355
　　multiple fractures, 341
　　muscle pull, 311
　　nonunion, 333, 355
　　open reduction, 329
　　pernasal wiring, 339
　　piriform fossa wiring, 339
　　signs and symptoms, 317
　　symphysis, 335
　　time for repair, 354
　　treatment, uncomplicated, 333
　　unfavorable fracture, 316
　maxilla
　　causes, 356
　　cerebrospinal rhinorrhea, 302
　　classification, 356
　　complications, 364
　　examination for, 298
　　horizontal, 356
　　　treatment, 359
　　neurological signs in, 302
　　pyramidal, 356
　　　treatment, 361
　　transverse, 358
　　　treatment, 362
　multiple-loop wiring, 318
　nasal, 362
　neurological signs in, 302
　plaster head cap, 360
　predisposing factors, 296
　pyramidal maxillary, 356, 361
　radiographic examination, 302
　reduction
　　closed, 304
　　open, 305, 307, 329, 335
　　　advantages, 305
　　　disadvantages, 305
　Risdon wire, 321
　signs and symptoms, 317
　simple, 397
　skeletal pin fixation, 327, 334
　splints, 323
　temporary fixation, 304
　Thoma bone clamp, 328
　time for repair, 354
　tooth in line of, 333
　transverse, 358, 362
　treatment, 304
　　methods, 318
　unfavorable, 316
　zygoma, 364
　　Caldwell-Luc operation, 365
　　complications, 367
　　diagnosis, 300, 365
　　Gillies operation, 366
　　treatment, 365

Frenum, labial, 113
Frenum, lingual, 113
Frontonasal suture line, 302
Frontozygomatic wiring, 362

G

Ganglioneuroma, 537
Gangrene, gas, 158, 159
　diagnosis, 159
　treatment, 159
Gas sterilization, 19
Gelfoam, 205
Genioplasty, 500
Gentian violet, 159
Giant cell tumor
　central, 525
　peripheral, 527
Gigli saw osteotomy, 450
Gillies operation, 366
Gingivitis, necrotic, 133
Glands
　minor salivary, 541
　parotid, 539
　　anatomy, 539, 541
　　removal, 565
　salivary
　　atrophy, 545
　　tumors, 545
　sublingual, 541
　　anatomy, 541
　submandibular, 539
　　anatomy 539
　　removal, 561, 564
Glossitis
　secondary to antibiotic therapy, 149
　in syphilis, 159
Glossopharyngeal nerve, 569
　neuralgia, 569, 576, 580
Grafts, 252
　alveolar ridge, 433
　artificial (alloplast), 419, 423
　bone, 252, 418; see also Bone grafts
　cartilage, 257, 259, 416, 418
　metal, 420, 423
　resins, 421
　skin, 110, 408
　　free graft, 408
　　full-thickness, 408
　　split-thickness, 408
Granuloma, 191
Gunshot wounds, 298

H

Hand, left, in exodontia, 59
Haversian systems, 307
Head injury, 304
Headache, 570, 577
　tension, 578
Heart disease; see Cardiovascular disease
Heat applications, 187
Hemangioma, 528
　capillary, 528
　cavernous, 528
Hematocrit, 2

Hematoma, 17
Hemorrhage, 16, 200
  amount of blood loss, 208
  capillary, 205
  control measures, 16, 205, 206
    bone, 17, 205
    cautery, 17, 203
    ligation, 17, 200
    phytonadiones, 18
    pressure pack, 17, 203
    secondary, 18, 127, 204
    soft tissue, 200
  general care of patient, 204
  isolation of bleeding site, 204
  postoperative, 204
  types, 200
Hemostasis in wound closure, 272
Hepatitis, 21, 27
Heredity in oral clefts, 389
Herpangina, 164
Herpetic stomatitis, 163
Heterophil agglutination test, 554
Hinds operation, 464
Histamine cephalgia, 578
Histamines in inflammation, 136
Histiocytosis X, 213
Histoplasmosis, 162
Hospital environment control, 22
Hospital, removal of teeth in, 125
Hullihen, L. P., 438
Hydrocortisone, 207
Hypertrophy of labial sulcus, 110
  technique for excision, 110, 111

I

Immune response, 253
Impacted teeth, 85
  classification, 88
  removal
    mandibular distoangular, 93
      horizontal, 91
      mesioangular, 89
      vertical, 92
    maxillary canine, 97
      distoangular, 96
      mesioangular, 95
      vertical, 95
    supernumerary, 99
Implants
  cartilage, 416
  metal, 423
  in surgical defects, 423
  synthetic resins, 425
Incision
  crosshatching, 36
  and drainage, 168, 172, 174, 176
  mucosa, 33
  skin, 32, 33, 36
Indications for extraction, 50
Infection
  acute, 166, 169
    antibiotics, 187
    blood culture, 187
    cold applications, 187

Infection—cont'd
  acute—cont'd
    dehydration, 187
    fluid balance, 187
    heat applications, 187
    patient management in, 187
  allergies, 166
  blood dyscrasias, 167
  cancers, 167
  cellulitis, 174
  chemical poisoning, 166
  chronic, 191
  cranial extension, 174
  fascial planes, 176
  focal, 137
  in oral cavity, 132
  periapical, 191
    apicoectomy, 194
    incision and drainage, 194
    root canal filling, 194
    treatment, 193
  pericoronal, 169
  periodontal, 197
  physical condition in, 15
  physiology of, 136
  stomatitis, 166
  systemic manifestations, 137, 166
Infectious mononucleosis, 554
Inflammation
  physiology, 136
  signs and symptoms, 136
  types, 136
Infratemporal fossa, 184
  drainage, 185
Infratemporal space, loss of tooth in, 127
Injuries, soft tissue, 266
Instruction, postoperative, 210
Instruments for exodontia, 52
Intravenous fluids, 13, 207
Iritis in focal infection, 138
Irradiation therapy, 533
Ivy loop wiring, 320

K

Kanamycin, 152
Kazanjian technique, ridge extension, 115
Kidney disease, surgical intervention, 134
Kirschner wire, 306
Knot ties
  instrument, 10
  one-hand, 9
  two-hand, 8

L

Laboratory tests, 50
Laceration
  definition, 268
  treatment, 270
Langer's lines, 32, 33
Larynx, edema, 183, 185
Lateral pharyngeal space, 182
  cellulitis, 183
  drainage, 183
  edema, larynx, 183
  septicemia, 183

Leukemia, surgical intervention, 133
Leukoplakia, 531
Levarterenol bitartrate, 207
Ligatures, 10
  technique for placing, 11
Lincomycin, 151
Lip defects
  closure of, 413
  shave, 409
Lipoma, 529
Listerism, 14
Liver diseases, 134
Localization
  broken needle, 196
  foreign body, 197
Lockjaw; see Tetanus
Ludwig's angina, 185
  drainage, 186
  induration, 185
Lymphangioma, 529

M

Malnutrition, 134
Mandible
  bone grafting, indications, 427
  fractures; see Fractures, mandible
  reconstruction, 423
    bone, 418
    implants, 423
Marsupialization, 228, 229, 233
Masticator space, 178
  drainage, 179
Maxilla
  fractures; see Fractures, maxilla
  repair after loss of, 416
Maxillary sinus
  accidental openings, 244
    closure of, 245
  acute sinusitis, 242
  ameloblastoma, 244
  anatomy, 237
  Caldwell-Luc operation, 249
  carcinoma, 244
  chronic sinusitis, 242
  cyst, 241, 244
  development, 237
  disease, 239
  empyema, 244
  function, 238
  mucosa, 237
  pathology, 242
  relation of teeth to, 238
  subacute sinusitis, 242
  tooth in, 239, 241
  toothache associated with, 239
  treatment, 244
Meckel's ganglion, 576
Meningitis, 302
Metabolic disturbances, 15, 208
Microgenia, 500
Micrognathia, 438, 440, 484
Migraine headache, 577
Monilia albicans; see Moniliasis

Moniliasis
  diagnosis, 161
  etiology, 161
  oral, 160
  secondary to antibiotic therapy, 149, 151
  treatment, 161
Monsel's solution, 205
Moose operation, 466
Morphine in head injury, 304
Mucocele, 217, 218, 542
Multiple-loop wiring, 318
Muscle
  pull in fracture, 311
  relation to osteotomy, 478
Myeloma, multiple, 524
Mylohyoid ridges, sharp, 102
Myoma, 529
Myxoma, 521

N

Nausea, secondary to antibiotic therapy, 149, 151
Needle aspiration, 176
Needles, 10
  broken, location, 196
  removal, 196
Neomycin, 143, 153
Neoplasms, oral, surgical treatment, 535
Nerve growth, 570
Nerves, motor, 569
Neuralgia, 571, 575, 578, 580
Neurilemoma, 547
Neurinoma, 531
Neuritis, 571, 572, 575
Neurofibroma, 570
Neurological survey, 568, 569, 579
Neurotic patients, 48
Neutropenia secondary to antibiotic therapy, 151
Nevus, pigmented, 529
Nikolsky's sign in pemphigus, 164
Nitrogen, nonprotein, increase in fever, 137
Norepinephrine, 207
Novobiocin
  indications, 151
  precautions, 151
  preparation and dosage, 151
Number of teeth to be extracted, 70
Nystatin, 161

O

Obturator following maxillary resection, 416
Obwegeser
  sagittal osteotomy, 468
  submucous vestibuloplasty, 117
Odontalgia, 572, 573, 574
Odontoma, 517
Office
  aseptic routine in, 27
  for exodontia, 52
Oliguria, 137
Open bite, 438
Operating room, 13, 24
  decorum, 24
  draping, 26, 27
  equipment, 13

Operating room—cont'd
  scrub technique, 24
Operative technique, 35
  submandibular approach, 35
    closure, 38
      deeper soft tissue dissection, 37
    incision, 36
  temporomandibular joint, 39
Optic neuritis in focal infection, 138
Oral surgery, definition, 1
Order of extraction, 70
Oroantral fistula, closure of, 285
  antrostomy, intranasal, 249
  Berger's method, 248
  cartilage in, 248
  causes of failure, 249
  gold disk, 249
  palatal flap, 247
Ostectomy, mandible, 471
Osteitis fibrosa cystica, 213
Osteitis, local, 128
Osteochondroma, 522
Osteoma, 520
Osteomyelitis, 180, 187, 574
  culture, pus, 189
  incision and drainage, 189
  of maxilla, 189
  radiographic diagnosis in, 188
  sequestrum, 190
  staphylococcus, 189
  syphilitic, 160
  treatment, 189
    saucerization, 190
Osteoradionecrosis, 535
Osteotomy
  anterior segmental, 490
  condylar neck, 449
  horizontal, 465
  maxillary
    anterior, 510
    posterior, 512
  sagittal, 468
  step sliding, 488
  subcondylar (oblique), 463
  vertical, 452, 493
  vertical L or C sliding, 497
Otalgia, 371, 574, 631
Oxygen, precautions, 30

P

Paget's disease, 521
Pain, 167, 170, 568, 571
  abscess, periapical, 167
  differential diagnosis, 579
  idiopathic, 571
  pericoronal infections, 169
  referred, 571, 574
Palate
  development, 386
  vessels of, 201
Palatorrhaphy, 394
Palatoschisis, 386
Papanicolaou smears
  in carcinoma, 533

Papanicolaou smears—cont'd
  in salivary tumors, 554
Papillary cystadenoma lymphomatosum, 546
Papilloma, 525
Paralysis, 569
Parapharyngeal space, 182
Paresthesia, 571
  following sinus operation, 250
Parotid duct
  severed, 287
  space, 183
    drainage, 184
Partsch operation, 220, 228, 232
Pathways for eruption of pus, 192
Pels-Macht test in pemphigus, 164
Pemphigus, 164
Penicillin, 142, 146
  intramuscular, 146
  oral, 147
  precautions, 147
  preparations and dosage, 146
  topical, 147
Penicillinase, 156
Pericoronal infections, 169
  cellulitis, 169
Pericoronitis, 85
Periodontal abscess, 573
  infection, 197
  in focal infection, 137
Periostitis, syphilitic, 160
Pharyngeal flap operation, 402
Pin fixation, 307, 326
Piriform fossa wiring, 339
Placebo, 46
Plasma volume expanders, 206
Plaster head cap, 360
Plummer-Vinson syndrome, 531
Polymyxin, 144, 153
Position of patient for exodontia, 58
Postoperative care, 42, 59, 210
Preoperative routine, 23, 48
Preparation of patient, 85
  for exodontia, 58
  history, 22
  preoperative, 22, 23
    orders, 23
    routine, 23
  sedation, 22
Prognathism, 438, 447
Proprioceptor, 568
Proteus vulgaris, 151, 355
Prothrombin time, 3, 199
Psychalgia, 571, 578, 580
Psychogenic headache, 578
Psychology, 46
Pterygopalatine fossa, 184
  drainage, 185
Pulp
  dental, 191
  stones, 572
Pulpitis, 572, 573
Pus, 136, 174
  laudable, 14, 28

R

Radiographic examination
  "double" fracture, 303
  in fractures, 302
  of salivary glands, 552
  temporomandibular view, 302, 373
Radium, 533
Radon seeds, 534
Ranula, 218, 227
Reaction to anesthesia, 130
Reconstruction of commissure of mouth, 411, 412
Referred pain, 571, 574
Reimplantation, tooth, 263
Reiter operation, 450
Renal complications in sulfonamide therapy, 154
Resolution of infection, 174
Rheumatic fever, antibiotic prophylaxis, 135
Ridge extension techniques, 111-119
  flabby, 108
  sharp, in denture construction, 101
Risdon wire, 321
Robinson operation, 350, 463
Root canal therapy, 138, 194
Root, fractured
  recovery
    antrum, 127
    infratemporal space, 127
    mandibular canal, 127
  removal, 76
    closed procedure, 78
    elevator principles in, 82
    open procedure, 80
    residual, 81
  resection in focal infection, 138

S

Sabouraud's medium, 161, 162
Sagittal osteotomy (Obwegeser), 468
Saliva, bactericidal effect, 132, 133
Salivary glands, 539
Sarcoma
  osteoblastic, 523
  osteolytic, 523
  telangiectatic, 523
Saucerization in osteomyelitis, 190
Schwannoma, 547
Sclerosing solutions in temporomandibular joint therapy, 379
Scrub technique, 24
Second set response, 254
Sensation, loss of, 569
Sensitivity of microorganisms, 141
  tests, 142
Sensory nerves, 571
Septicemia, 137
  in lateral pharyngeal space, 183
Sequestrum in osteomyelitis, 189
Shock, 206
  in fractures, 303
  treatment, 206
    blood plasma, 206
    plasma volume expanders, 206
    transfusion, 206
    vasoconstrictor drugs, 207

Shock—cont'd
  types, 206
Sialadenitis
  acute, 542
  chronic, 543
Sialoangiectasis, 545
Sialogram, 552
  interpretation, 555-560
  technique, 552
Sialolithiasis, 544
  management, 544
  symptoms, 544
Sialolithotomy, 560
  parotid duct, 563
  submaxillary duct, 561
Sinus
  maxillary, 237
  pain, 572, 573, 580
  paranasal
    diagram, 240
    function, 238
Sinusitis, 239
Skeletal pin fixation, 307, 326, 334
Sluder's syndrome, 576
Smith operation, 449
Speech, 386, 394, 404
  aid prosthesis, 402
Sphenopalatine neuralgia, 576, 580
Spinal accessory nerve, 571
Splinting tooth injuries, 293
Splints, 105
  acrylic
    in fractures, 323
    in torus removal, 105
  cast cap silver, 323
Staphylococcus albus, 132
Staphylococcus aureus, 132, 151
Staphylococcus cavernous sinus thrombosis, 186
Staphylorrhaphy, 398
Stents in skin grafting, 408
Sterilization, 18
  autoclaving, 18
  boiling water, 18
  cold, 19
  dry heat, 19
  gas, 19
  paper wraps, 18
  principles, 18, 56
  radiation, 20
Stevens-Johnson syndrome, 164
Stomatitis
  aphthous, 163
  secondary to antibiotic therapy, 149
Streptococcus, 132, 134
  alpha, 132, 151
  beta, 132
  Ludwig's angina, 185
  nonhemolytic, 132
Streptomycin 150
  precautions, 150
Subcondylar osteotomy, 463
Sublingual space, 181
Submandibular approach, 35
Submandibular space, 181

Submaxillary space, 181
Submental space, 181
Sulfonamides, 154
  precautions, 155
Supernumerary impaction, 99
Supports, tissue, 109
Surgical flap, 76
Suture materials, 5, 34
Suture techniques, 6-7, 15, 33, 35
  continuous locked, 6
    mattress, 6
  Halstead mattress, 6
  interrupted mattress, 6
    skin, 6
  over-and-over, 6
  subcuticular, 7
Suturing in soft tissue wounds, 272
Swallowing, 386
Syphilis, 158, 159
  chancre, 160
  gumma, 160
  mucous patches, 160
  oral lesions, 160
  osteomyelitis, 160
  periostitis, 160

T

Tantalum mesh, 34
Tattoo, traumatic, 270
Teeth
  avulsion, 290
  luxation, 290
  split, 581
  transplantations of, 261
  traumatic injuries to, 289
    classification, 290
    clinical evaluation, 289
    postoperative care, 294
    splinting, 293
    treatment, 292
Temporal arteritis, 578
Temporal pouches, 180
  drainage, 181
Temporomandibular joint
  anatomy, 369
  ankylosis, 383
  articular disk, 369
  blood supply, 370
  capsule, 370
  condyloid process, 369
  dislocation, 381
  dysfunction
    injection therapy, 377
    symptoms, 371
    treatment, conservative, 374
  innervation, 370
  ligaments, 370
  pain, 574, 580
    clinical findings in, 371
    etiology, 370
    roentgenographic findings in, 373
  radiograph, 302
  surgical approach, 39, 379
  synovial membrane, 370

Tension headache, 578
Tetanus, 158
  antitoxin, 159, 304
  diagnosis, 159
  prophylaxis, 159, 276
  signs and symptoms, 159
  toxoid, 159
Tetracyclines, 148
Thalamus, 568, 571
Thoma bone clamp, 328
Thoma operation, 475
Throat, sore, 170
Thrush; *see* Moniliasis
Tic douloureux, 576
Tics, 571
Tissue damage, 14
Tongue
  diminished taste, 576
  pain in, 576
Toothache, symptom of sinus infection, 239
Torus mandibularis, 103
Torus palatinus, 106
Trachea, tooth displaced in, 131
Tracheostomy, 303
  technique, 12
Transfusion, 206
Transplantation
  bone, 252
  tooth, 261
Trauma
  alveolar process, 289
  teeth, 289
Trauner technique in ridge extension, 118
Trigeminal nerve, 570, 574
  neuralgia, 576, 580
Trigger zone, 575
Trismus, 170, 172
  medial mandibular postoperative abscess, 172
  pericoronal infection, 169
  in tetanus, 159
Tuberculosis, 27, 158
  oral, 160
  ulcers in, 160
Tuberosity, enlarged, 107
Tumors, 517
  in fractures, 297
  mixed, 529, 546
  mucoepidermoid, 548
  odontogenic, 517
  oral, 517
  osteogenic, 520
  in pregnancy, 528
Tyrothricin, 143, 154

U

Ulcers, herpetic, 162
Urinalysis, 2
Urticaria, secondary to antibiotics, 151

V

Vaccination in recurrent herpes, 163
Vertical osteotomy, 452, 493
Vestibuloplasty, 117, 408
  submucous, 117

Vincent's spirillum, 132
Vision, disturbance, 364, 367, 570
Vitamin K, 18
Vitamins
   as adjunctive therapy, 155
   avitaminosis secondary to antibiotic therapy, 155
Vomer, development, 387
Vomer flap, operation, 397
Vomiting, 570
Von Langenbeck operation, 396
V-Y flaps, 111, 113

W

Wardill "push-back" operation, 399
Warthin's tumor, 546
Wound cleansing, 271
   closure
      delayed primary, 274
      drains, 275
      dressings, 275
      failures in primary closure, 276

Wound cleansing—cont'd
   closure—cont'd
      prevention of infection, 275
      primary, 270, 271
   healing, 15
      metabolic disease in, 15
      nutritional state in, 15
Wounds
   avulsive, 268
   general considerations, 268
   gunshot, 268
      treatment, 277
   intraoral, 284
   penetrating, 268
      treatment, 276
   perforating, 268
      treatment, 277

Z

Z-plasty, 411
   for enlarged frenum, 111
Zygoma, fractures; *see* Fractures, zygoma